D1597645

Tumors of
the Pancreas

*AFIP Atlas
of
Tumor Pathology*

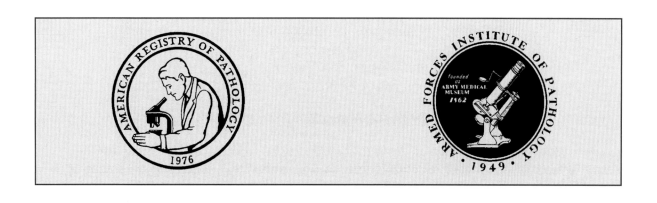

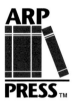

ARP

PRESS™

Editorial Director: Kelley S. Hahn
Production Editor: Dian S. Thomas
Editorial/Scanning Assistant: Mirlinda Q. Caton
Copyeditor: Audrey Kahn

Available from the American Registry of Pathology
Armed Forces Institute of Pathology
Washington, DC 20306-6000
www.afip.org
ISBN 1-933477-02-4
978-1-933477-02-2

AFIP ATLAS OF TUMOR PATHOLOGY

Fourth Series
Fascicle 6

TUMORS OF
THE PANCREAS

by

Ralph H. Hruban, MD
Professor of Pathology and Oncology
The Sol Goldman Pancreatic Cancer Research Center
The Johns Hopkins Medical Institutions
Baltimore, Maryland

Martha Bishop Pitman, MD
Associate Professor of Pathology, Harvard Medical School
Director, Fine Needle Aspiration Biopsy Service
Department of Pathology
Massachusetts General Hospital
Boston, Massachusetts

David S. Klimstra, MD
Attending Pathologist, Chief of Surgical Pathology
Memorial Sloan-Kettering Cancer Center
Professor of Pathology and Laboratory Medicine
Joan and Sanford I. Weill Medical College of Cornell University
New York, New York

Published by the
American Registry of Pathology
Washington, DC
in collaboration with the
Armed Forces Institute of Pathology
Washington, DC
2007

AFIP ATLAS OF TUMOR PATHOLOGY

EDITOR
Steven G. Silverberg, MD
Department of Pathology
University of Maryland School of Medicine
Baltimore, Maryland

ASSOCIATE EDITOR
Leslie H. Sobin, MD
Armed Forces Institute of Pathology
Washington, DC

EDITORIAL ADVISORY BOARD

Manuscript Reviewed by:
Jorge Albores-Saavedra, MD
David A. Owen, MB, BCh, FRCPC, FRCPath

EDITORS' NOTE

The Atlas of Tumor Pathology has a long and distinguished history. It was first conceived at a Cancer Research Meeting held in St. Louis in September 1947 as an attempt to standardize the nomenclature of neoplastic diseases. The first series was sponsored by the National Academy of Sciences-National Research Council. The organization of this Sisyphean effort was entrusted to the Subcommittee on Oncology of the Committee on Pathology, and Dr. Arthur Purdy Stout was the first editor-in-chief. Many of the illustrations were provided by the Medical Illustration Service of the Armed Forces Institute of Pathology (AFIP), the type was set by the Government Printing Office, and the final printing was done at the Armed Forces Institute of Pathology (hence the colloquial appellation "AFIP Fascicles"). The American Registry of Pathology (ARP) purchased the Fascicles from the Government Printing Office and sold them virtually at cost. Over a period of 20 years, approximately 15,000 copies each of nearly 40 Fascicles were produced. The worldwide impact of these publications over the years has largely surpassed the original goal. They quickly became among the most influential publications on tumor pathology, primarily because of their overall high quality but also because their low cost made them easily accessible the world over to pathologists and other students of oncology.

Upon completion of the first series, the National Academy of Sciences-National Research Council handed further pursuit of the project over to the newly created Universities Associated for Research and Education in Pathology (UAREP). A second series was started, generously supported by grants from the AFIP, the National Cancer Institute, and the American Cancer Society. Dr. Harlan I. Firminger became the editor-in-chief and was succeeded by Dr. William H. Hartmann. The second series' Fascicles were produced as bound volumes instead of loose leaflets. They featured a more comprehensive coverage of the subjects, to the extent that the Fascicles could no longer be regarded as "atlases" but rather as monographs describing and illustrating in detail the tumors and tumor-like conditions of the various organs and systems.

Once the second series was completed, with a success that matched that of the first, ARP, UAREP, and AFIP decided to embark on a third series. Dr. Juan Rosai was appointed as editor-in-chief, and Dr. Leslie H. Sobin became associate editor. A distinguished Editorial Advisory Board was also convened, and these outstanding pathologists and educators played a major role in the success of this series, the first publication of which appeared in 1991 and the last (number 32) in 2003.

The same organizational framework will apply to the current fourth series, but with UAREP no longer in existence, ARP will play the major role. New features will include a hardbound cover, illustrations almost exclusively in color, and an accompanying electronic version of each Fascicle. There will also be increased emphasis (wherever appropriate) on the cytopathologic (intraoperative, exfoliative, and/or fine needle aspiration) and molecular features that are important in diagnosis and prognosis. What will not change from the three previous series, however, is the goal of providing the practicing pathologist with thorough, concise, and up-to-date information on the nomenclature and classification; epidemiologic, clinical, and pathogenetic features; and, most importantly, guidance in the diagnosis of the tumors and tumor-like lesions of all major organ systems and body sites.

As in the third series, a continuous attempt will be made to correlate, whenever possible, the nomenclature used in the Fascicles with that proposed by the World Health Organization's Classification of Tumors, as well as to ensure a consistency of style throughout. Close cooperation between the various authors and their respective liaisons from the Editorial Board will continue to be emphasized in order to minimize unnecessary repetition and discrepancies in the text and illustrations.

Particular thanks are due to the members of the Editorial Advisory Board, the reviewers (at least two for each Fascicle), the editorial and production staff, and—first and foremost—the individual Fascicle authors for their ongoing efforts to ensure that this series is a worthy successor to the previous three.

Steven G. Silverberg, MD
Leslie H. Sobin, MD

INTRODUCTION

In 1959, Virginia Kneeland Frantz, MD, wrote the first series Fascicle on tumors of the pancreas. This Fascicle provided a central resource for the diagnosis and classification of neoplasms of the pancreas, as well as the first description of the solid-pseudopapillary neoplasm (2). The first series Fascicle stood as the gold standard for 25 years, until the publication of the second series Fascicle in 1984. Written by Drs. Antonio L. Cubilla and Patrick J. Fitzgerald, the second series Fascicle focused on tumors of the exocrine pancreas (1). This Fascicle was comprehensive and reflected a dramatically improved understanding of the subclassification of serous and mucinous cystic neoplasms of the pancreas (1). This Fascicle stood for 13 years until the third edition, authored by Drs. Enrico Solcia, Carlo Capella, and Günter Klöppel, was published in 1997 (4). The third series Fascicle added an extensive discussion of endocrine tumors, and clarified the importance of separating intraductal papillary mucinous neoplasms and mucinous cystic neoplasms. Here in the fourth series Fascicle on tumors of the pancreas, we cannot improve upon the lucid writing, insight, and thoughtful descriptions of the first three Fascicles. Instead, in our own voice we present our current understanding of the classification and diagnosis of tumors of the exocrine and endocrine pancreas.

This fourth series Fascicle on tumors of the pancreas now has all color illustrations (with the exception of the electron micrographs), and it includes expanded discussions of the cytology and molecular biology of tumors of the pancreas. These expanded sections are integrated into the descriptions of each entity, allowing us to highlight the importance of tumor morphology in guiding molecular analyses, as illustrated in the section on medullary carcinomas. We have also consciously de-emphasized other sections, such as electron microscopy, to reflect the changes that have occurred in the practice of pathology.

The terminology employed here is very similar to the terminology used in the third series Fascicle, and is compatible with that used by the World Health Organization (3). The few changes we have made in terminology reflect our improved understanding of the nature of several entities. For example, the term *solid-pseudopapillary tumor* has been changed to *solid-pseudopapillary neoplasm*, and *pancreatic endocrine tumor* has been replaced with *pancreatic endocrine neoplasm*. Prior attempts to classify well-differentiated pancreatic endocrine neoplasms into benign and malignant groups have been abandoned in preference for a prognostic grading system. In addition, in order to eliminate the incorrect implication that noninvasive mucinous cystic neoplasms (MCNs) and noninvasive intraductal papillary mucinous neoplasms (IPMNs) with moderate atypia have the potential to metastasize, we have replaced the terms *borderline MCN* and *borderline IPMN* with the terms *noninvasive MCN with moderate dysplasia* and *noninvasive IPMN with moderate dysplasia*. Finally, we have expanded the discussion of intraductal neoplasms to include the recently recognized *intraductal tubular adenoma* and *intraductal tubular carcinoma*.

We have also added a chapter outlining a rational and useful approach to the diagnosis of tumors of the pancreas. This chapter is meant to be "user friendly" and very practical.

The ever-increasing numbers of operations performed on the pancreas, coupled with almost daily improvements in our understanding of the molecular biology of pancreatic neoplasia, are rapidly changing the practice of pancreatic pathology. Almost certainly some of the material presented here will become outdated before the next edition of the Fascicle on tumors of the pancreas is published. While such a constantly changing field presents a challenge in writing a text, it is also what makes the study of pancreas pathology exciting.

References

1. Cubilla AL, Fitzgerald PJ. Tumors of the exocrine pancreas. Atlas of tumor pathology, 2nd Series, Fascicle 19. Washington, DC: Armed Forces Institute of Pathology; 1984.
2. Frantz VK. Tumors of the pancreas. Atlas of tumor pathology, 1st Series, Fascicles 27 & 28. Washington, DC: Armed Forces Institute of Pathology; 1959.
3. Hamilton SR, Aaltonen LA, eds. Pathology and genetics of tumours of the digestive system. World Health Organization classification of tumours. Lyon: IARC Press; 2000.
4. Solcia E, Capella C, Klöppel G. Tumors of the pancreas. Atlas of tumor pathology, 3rd Series, Fascicle 20. Washington, DC: Armed Forces Institute of Pathology; 1997.

Ralph H. Hruban, MD
Martha Bishop Pitman, MD
David S. Klimstra, MD

ACKNOWLEDGEMENTS

We are deeply appreciative of the many coworkers and friends who have made the publication of this Fascicle possible. Since this Fascicle is fundamentally based on the study of resected material, we are first indebted to the pancreas surgeons at each of our institutions. In particular, we would like to thank Drs. John Cameron, Charles Yeo, Keith Lillemoe, Steven Leach, Kurtis Campbell, Richard Schulick, Michael Choti, and Mark Talamini at Johns Hopkins; Drs. Andrew Warshaw, Carlos Fernandez-del Castillo, Sarah Thayer, David Rattner, and David Berger at the Massachusetts General Hospital; and Drs. Leslie Blumgart, Murray Brennan, Daniel Coit, Kevin Conlon, Ronald DeMatteo, Yuman Fong, David Jaques, William Jarnagin, and Alan Turnbull at Memorial Sloan-Kettering Cancer Center. Because of their hard work and dedication to excellence, pancreatic surgery is now safe and effective. We would also like to thank Drs. William Brugge and Brenna Bounds for procuring the endoscopic ultrasound–guided fine needle aspiration material for the cytology portion of this Fascicle.

The gross pictures are the product of years of careful gross photography. Many of these photographs were taken by our residents, and by Dante Trusty and Gary March at Johns Hopkins, Steve Conley and Michelle Forrestall at the Massachusetts General Hospital, and Kin Kong and Allyne Manzo Memorial Sloan-Kettering Cancer Center. We are indebted to them, and congratulate them for their excellent work.

We thank Dr. Stanley Siegelman for the numerous radiographic images he provided for this Fascicle, and Dr. Kenji Yamoa for providing the pictures of peroral pancreatoscopy, Dr. Johji Imura for hepatoid carcinoma, and Drs. Giuseppe Zamboni and Polly Lam for acinar cell cystadenoma and paraampullary duodenal wall cyst. We would also like to thank the numerous pathologists who have sent us cases in consultation over the years. These cases are the most challenging and therefore usually the most enlightening.

Two artists deserve our special thanks. We thank Jennifer Parsons Brumbaugh for the gift of her beautiful and informative medical illustrations, and Norman Barker for the countless hours he spent creating many of the photomicrographs, and for his keen photographic eye which enhanced all of the figures in this Fascicle.

We are indebted to our colleagues who took time to read, criticize, and improve the drafts of this manuscript. These include Drs. Frederic Askin, Pedram Argani, Noriyoshi Fukushima, Steven Leach, Anirban Maitra, Elizabeth Montgomery, G. Johan A. Offerhaus, Michael Stanley, Mariko Suchi, and Günter Klöppel.

We are particularly grateful to Sandra Markowitz, Joanne Schiavo, and Jennifer Nobrega for their excellent assistance with the researching, typing, and editing of this Fascicle. We would especially like to acknowledge the administrative assistance of Sandra Markowitz—her patience, organizational skills, and thoughtfulness continue to amaze us.

The authors would like to recognize Drs. Jorge Albores-Saavedra and David A. Owen for their constructive reviews of this Fascicle. We sincerely appreciate their time and effort, and the many suggestions they provided.

This work is built on the shoulders of our predecessors: the authors of the previous editions of this Fascicle and the many pathologists and investigators who contributed to our current knowledge of pancreas pathology.

Dr. Hruban would like to give special thanks to the remarkable families that have supported the pancreatic cancer research team at Johns Hopkins. While space does not allow us to recognize them all, we give special thanks to the family of Sol and Lillian Goldman. The establishment of the Sol Goldman Pancreatic Cancer Research Center at Johns Hopkins is a beacon of hope for patients with pancreatic cancer. We also thank the friends and families of Michael Rolfe, Joseph Monastra, George Rubis, Druel Parker, and Cas Zgonina. Without their support and the support of families like theirs over the years the scientific accomplishments of the past decade would not have been possible.

Finally, and most importantly, we would like to thank our families for their patience, understanding, and support as we have worked on this Fascicle.

Ralph H. Hruban, MD
Martha Bishop Pitman, MD
David S. Klimstra, MD

DEDICATIONS

To my wife Claire and our three wonderful children—Zoe, Emily, and Carolyn.

Ralph H. Hruban, MD

To my husband Peter, and our children Sarah, Katherine, and Benjamin, for their support.

Martha Bishop Pitman, MD

To my wife Sibel, without whose support and encouragement this work would not have been possible.

David S. Klimstra, MD

Permission to use copyrighted illustrations has been granted by:

American Society of Clinical Oncology
　　Journal of Clinical Oncology, 2002;20:2638. For figure 12-31.

Elsevier Saunders
　　Journal of Gastrointestinal Surgery, 2000;4:574. For figures 7-58 and 7-59.
　　Pathologic Basis of Disease, Seventh Edition, 2005. For figure 6-11.

Kanehara & Co.
　　Classification of Pancreatic Carcinoma, 2003. For tables 1-1 and 3-8.

Lippincott Williams & Wilkins
　　American Journal of Surgical Pathology, 2002;26:700. For figure 9-1.
　　American Journal of Surgical Pathology, 1999;23:1324. For figure 5-33.
　　American Journal of Surgical Pathology, 1995;19:1374. For figure 10-1.
　　Annals of Surgery, 2004;239:793. For figure 6-38.
　　Histology for Pathologists, Second Edition, 1997. For figure 1-18.

Springer-Verlag
　　Surgical Pathology Dissection, 2002. For figures 16-1 and 16-2.

CONTENTS

1 THE NORMAL PANCREAS

EMBRYOLOGY

The embryonic pancreas first appears in the 5th week of gestation as dorsal and ventral evaginations of foregut endoderm (21). As suggested by Edlund (12), there are three components of the complex events required for normal pancreatic development. First, foregut endoderm becomes patterned to form dorsal and ventral pancreatic buds; second, cells undergo lineage commitment to either endocrine or exocrine cell fates; and third, pancreatic morphogenesis occurs by way of extensive growth and branching. While recent studies suggest that distinct signaling pathways may control these events, tissue specification, lineage commitment, and growth are highly interdependent and are characterized by considerable spatial and temporal overlap.

Several transcription factors are now known to be required for pancreas specification. Prior to and during budding, the organ primordium expresses the homeodomain protein *pancreatic and duodenal homeobox gene 1* (*Pdx1*) (also known as *insulin promoter factor 1* [*IPF1*]) (12); all three differentiated pancreatic cell types, islet cells, acinar cells, and pancreatic duct cells, are derived from Pdx1-positive progenitors. Deletion of the *Pdx1* gene allows successful specification of pancreatic mesenchyme and initial pancreatic bud formation, but results in severely aborted morphogenesis and failure to generate differentiated islet, acinar, and ductal cell types (2). The early embryonic ductal epithelium expresses Pdx1 uniformly, but later, Pdx1 expression is primarily restricted to the islets of Langerhans, with only low levels detectable in some acinar cells. Under certain conditions, Pdx1 expression again becomes detectable in individual pancreatic ductal epithelial cells, suggesting the persistence of multipotential stem cells within mature pancreatic epithelium (40).

Additional transcriptional factors involved in pancreatic morphogenesis include, but are by no means limited to, Sox17, HLXB9, and PTF1, which appear to be required in early specification. There are also a variety of endocrine lineage–restricted transcription factors such as Ngn3, NeuroD/Beta2, Nkx2.2, and Nkx6.1 (14,28,32,37).

In contrast to the relative abundance of information regarding the transcription factors required for islet development, a paucity of information exists regarding similar factors required for exocrine differentiation. The p48 component of the heterotrimeric PTF1 transcription factor complex is required for normal exocrine differentiation (23). Although initially presumed to be an "exocrine-specific" transcription factor, Pdx1 is now believed to play a far more expansive role in pancreatic specification (28).

In addition to intrinsic transcription factors, the pancreas is also responsive to cell fate determining signals from developmental patterning pathways, such as the Notch and Hedgehog signaling pathways. For example, Notch signals are required for epithelial branching and normal exocrine lineage commitment (29). Notch signaling appears to maintain the undifferentiated state of the putative pool of pancreatic stem cells. These stem cells mediate cellular turnover and repair, and may expand in the face of neoplastic transformation. Indeed, widespread upregulation of Notch transcripts is common in ductal adenocarcinoma of the pancreas as well its precursor lesions, reinforcing the commonality of signaling pathways involved in development and cancer genesis (26).

The Hedgehog gene was first discovered in studies of Drosophila (33). In mammals, three Hedgehog genes are essential for embryogenesis: Sonic Hedgehog (*Shh*), Indian Hedgehog (*Ihh*), and Desert Hedgehog (*Dhh*). *Ihh* and *Dhh* are detected during development as well as in mature pancreatic tissue, consistent with the hypothesis that the hedgehog pathway is active during certain specific phases of pancreas formation (15). In midgestational embryos, the Shh ligand is expressed in nearly all epithelial cells lining the alimentary canal, and its function is critical for proper foregut and gastrointestinal

1

development. In contrast, Shh is excluded from the developing pancreas, but remains expressed in the surrounding gastric and duodenal epithelium. Notochord-derived inhibitory signaling via activin and fibroblast growth factor 2 (FGF2) represses Shh and permits appropriate transcriptional activation of pancreatic gene expression (16). Thus, Shh expression establishes a sharp molecular boundary, which allows for the proper patterning of the duodenal and pancreatic epithelium. If Shh expression in areas adjacent to pancreatic tissue is responsible for restricting pancreas growth, loss of Shh should increase pancreatic mass. Indeed, chemical inhibition of the Shh signaling pathway in experimental models leads to ectopic formation of pancreas buds and an increase in endocrine cell number. Conversely, overexpression of Shh within the developing pancreas of transgenic Pdx1-Shh mice leads to attenuation of the pancreatic phenotype and induction of an intestinal differentiation program (4). The latter phenomenon acquires great significance in the context of human pancreatic neoplasia, where the early precursor lesions of pancreatic adenocarcinoma demonstrate similar histopathologic features as observed in the Pdx1-Shh mice, and also harbor a transcriptional profile that is more akin to foregut epithelium than to native pancreatic ducts (46).

During the development of the pancreas, evaginations (buds) of cuboidal epithelium from the foregut grow to produce a complex branching epithelial tree (25). The larger dorsal pancreatic bud appears first, caudal to the stomach, and grows rapidly in the dorsal mesentery. The smaller ventral pancreatic bud arises from the base of the hepatic diverticulum attached to the entry of the bile duct into the duodenum, and grows between the layers of the ventral mesentery. Initially, the ventral bud is composed of two parts, right and left, but the left bud atrophies early and the right bud, adjacent to the primitive bile duct, persists (fig. 1-1, top).

Around the 7th week of gestation, following rotation of the primitive intestine and its derivatives to the right, a move that gives the duodenum its C shape, the two pancreatic primordia fuse to form a single organ. The dorsal bud gives rise to the tail, body, and the cephalad portion of the pancreatic head; the ventral bud forms the caudal half of the pancreatic head and the unci-

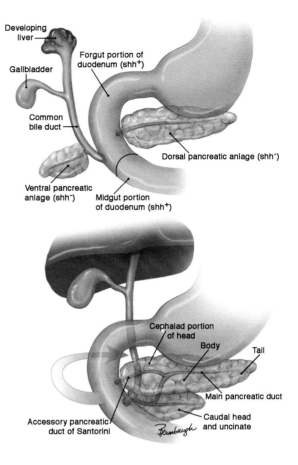

Figure 1-1

ANATOMY OF THE DEVELOPING PANCREAS

Top: The dorsal pancreatic bud appears first as a bud caudal to the stomach. The smaller ventral pancreatic bud arises from the base of the hepatic diverticulum. Neither bud expresses the Sonic Hedgehog (*shh*) gene whereas the adjacent foregut does.

Bottom: Rotation of the duodenum to the right carries the ventral bud to a position posterior to the dorsal bud. The two primitive buds then fuse to form the pancreas. The dorsal bud gives rise to the cephalad portion of the head, as well as the body and tail, whereas the ventral bud gives rise to the caudal portion of the head and the uncinate process. The main pancreatic duct (duct of Wirsung) is formed by the union of the distal portion of the dorsal pancreatic duct and the ventral pancreatic duct. The proximal portion of the dorsal pancreatic duct forms the accessory duct of Santorini. (Artwork by Jennifer Parsons Brumbaugh.)

nate process (fig. 1-1, bottom). The main pancreatic duct (duct of Wirsung) is formed by the union of the distal part of the dorsal pancreatic duct and the smaller ventral pancreatic duct during the 7th week of gestation. As a result, the main duct empties into the major duodenal papilla (the ampulla of Vater). The proximal part

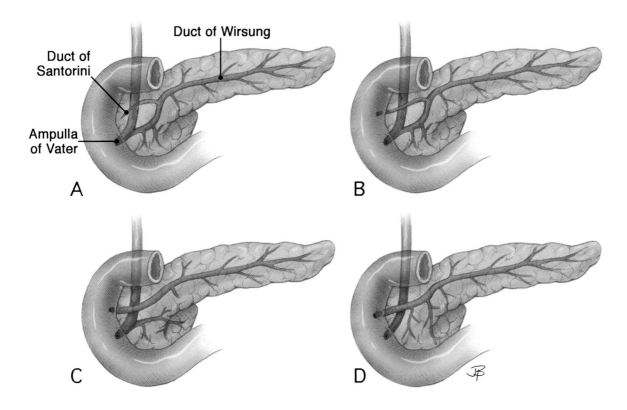

Duct of Wirsung

Duct of
Santorini

Ampulla
of Vater

A

B

C

D

Figure 1-2

ANATOMIC VARIATIONS IN THE PANCREATIC AND COMMON BILE DUCT SYSTEM

A: The proximal portion of the dorsal pancreatic duct regresses completely.

B: The proximal portion of the dorsal pancreatic duct remains patent as the accessory duct of Santorini and drains into the minor papilla.

C: The entire dorsal pancreatic duct drains into the minor papilla and the smaller ventral pancreatic duct joins the common bile duct at the major papilla (pancreas divisum).

D: The ventral pancreatic duct fuses with the dorsal pancreatic duct and drains the gland through the minor papilla leaving the common bile duct to drain into the major papilla. (Artwork by Jennifer Parsons Brumbaugh.)

of the dorsal pancreatic duct may persist as the accessory duct of Santorini. When present, the accessory duct of Santorini drains into the minor papilla located 2 cm cephalad to the ampulla of Vater or it may become a tributary to the duct of Wirsung (fig. 1-1, bottom).

GROSS ANATOMY

The mature pancreas is a uniformly lobulated organ, 14 to 20 cm in length and weighing, on average, 100 g in the adult, with the pancreata of men slightly heavier than those of women. The newborn pancreas weighs only 5 g and the pancreata of the elderly weigh less than those of younger adults.

The four anatomic areas of the pancreas are the head, which comprises the bulk of the pancreas; the neck; the body; and the tail. The main pancreatic duct (of Wirsung) averages 3 mm in diameter (range, 1.8 to 9.0 mm), curves inferiorly at the head, and drains the majority of the gland into the duodenum via the major papilla (ampulla of Vater). Here the diameter of the duct increases to about 4.5 mm. Main ducts greater than 10 mm are considered pathologically dilated.

There are a number of variations in the anatomy of the pancreatic ductal system and in the relationship of the pancreatic ductal system to the common bile duct (fig. 1-2). The usual arrangement is for the main pancreatic duct to drain the bulk of the gland into the duodenum at the major papilla along with the common bile duct (fig. 1-2A). Another arrangement is for the accessory duct of Santorini to be patent and

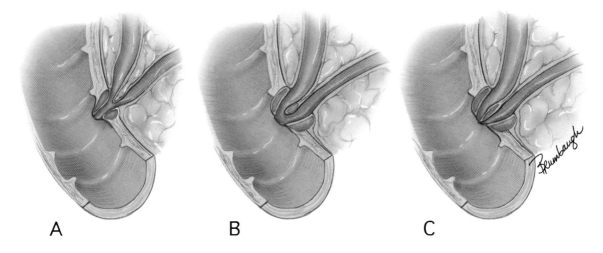

Figure 1-3

ANATOMIC VARIATIONS IN THE UNION OF THE COMMON BILE DUCT
AND THE MAIN PANCREATIC DUCT AT THE MAJOR PAPILLA

A: Early fusion with a long common channel of 3 mm or more.
B: Late fusion with a short common channel of 2 mm or less.
C: No fusion, with separation of the ducts by a septum. (Artwork by Jennifer Parsons Brumbaugh.)

drain through the minor duodenal papilla while maintaining communication with the main pancreatic duct of Wirsung (fig. 1-2B). In a minority of cases, the main pancreatic duct drains through the minor papilla, while the common bile duct, joined only by the small pancreatic duct from the ventral bud, drains through the ampulla (see pancreatic divisum later) (fig. 1-2C). In rare instances, the main duct drains through the minor papilla leaving the common bile duct to drain via the major papilla alone (fig. 1-2D).

The joining of the main pancreatic and common bile ducts at the ampulla of Vater provides a large patent channel for the drainage of pancreatic secretions. The anatomy of the junction of the bile duct and the main pancreatic duct varies. There may be a short common channel, a channel with an interposed septum between the ducts, or two independent channels with separate openings into the duodenum (fig. 1-3). The more typical common channel is called the hepatopancreatic ampulla and is surrounded by a poorly defined smooth muscle sphincter, the sphincter of Oddi.

Anatomic Relationships

The pancreas is situated deep in the retroperitoneum and is enveloped by peritoneum on its anterior surface and connective tissue on its posterior surface. The organ is intimately associated with many different anatomic structures, more so than probably any other organ in the body (fig. 1-4) (39). Surgical access to the pancreas is further complicated because the pancreas lies behind the stomach and transverse colon.

The pancreatic head is the thickest part of the gland, and it is cradled in the C-shaped second part of the duodenum. The head of the pancreas is the portion of the pancreas to the right of the left border of the superior mesenteric-portal vein confluence. The uncinate process extends inferiorly and posteriorly from the head of the gland to pass behind the neck of the pancreas and the superior mesenteric vessels. These vessels frequently produce a sulcus, or indentation, in the uncinate process, giving the uncinate an overall hook shape. Indeed, the term "uncinate" is derived from the Latin word "uncus" meaning hook. The right lateral border of the uncinate process is firmly attached to the third and fourth parts of the duodenum. The common bile duct lies on the posterior-superior surface of the head of the pancreas or is embedded within the gland.

The neck of the pancreas is the short constricted area that rests anterior to the mesenteric

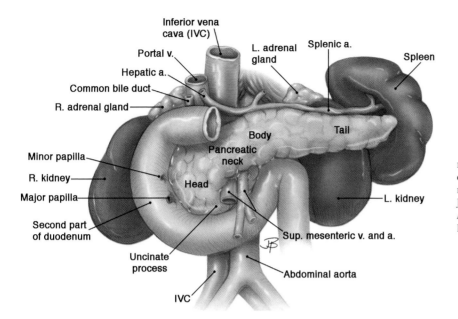

Figure 1-4

ANATOMIC RELATIONSHIP OF THE DEVELOPED PANCREAS WITH SURROUNDING ORGANS AND STRUCTURES

The pancreas has a complex relationship to numerous adjacent structures (a = artery; l = left; r = right; v = vein). (Artwork by Jennifer Parsons Brumbaugh. Adapted from fig. 1-6 from Fascicle 20, Third Series.)

vessels. These vessels may form a groove in the posterior aspect of the neck of the gland, as they do on the anterior surface of the uncinate process; these indentations can be used to orient the resected specimen. The anterior surface of the neck is covered by peritoneum and lies adjacent to the gastric pylorus. The neck is the point at which the gland is surgically transected in pancreatoduodenectomy (Whipple) resections for neoplasms of the pancreatic head.

The body of the pancreas extends from the neck lateral to the left border of the aorta. The body of the pancreas is anterior to the aorta and the L2 vertebra; has contact with the left adrenal gland, left kidney, and left renal vessels; and is covered anteriorly by the posterior peritoneum of the lesser sac. The antrum of the stomach rests on top of the pancreatic body, obscuring it from view.

The tail of the pancreas is the tapered, flat portion of the pancreas to the left of the body (left border of the aorta). The tail has a rounded terminal end that is closely related to the hilum of the spleen. The tail is relatively mobile within the splenorenal ligament, along with the splenic vessels.

Approximately 50 percent of pancreatic tails rest within the central hilum of the spleen, 42 percent inferiorly in the hilum, and 8 percent in the upper hilum (22,24,38).

The Vascular Supply

The arterial blood supply to the pancreas is derived primarily from branches of the celiac trunk and the superior mesenteric artery, and is divided into two main regions: the pancreatic head and the body/tail (fig. 1-5). The arterial supply has many anastomoses between different vessels and numerous anatomic variations.

The pancreatic head is supplied by the anterior and posterior pancreaticoduodenal arteries, which form arcades in the pancreaticoduodenal sulcus. The anterior or prepancreatic arcade is formed by the anterior superior pancreaticoduodenal artery, a branch of the gastroduodenal artery, and the anterior inferior pancreaticoduodenal artery, a branch of the superior mesenteric artery. The posterior arcade is formed by the posterior superior pancreaticoduodenal artery, a branch of the gastroduodenal artery, and the posterior inferior pancreaticoduodenal artery, a branch of the superior mesenteric artery. The inferior vessels tend to be more variable in their origin whereas the superior vessels are more constant. Venous drainage is by the pancreaticoduodenal veins, tributaries of the splenic and superior mesenteric branches of the portal vein (18).

The body and tail of the pancreas are supplied by the dorsal, inferior, transverse, and great pancreatic arteries, and are drained by the inferior and left pancreatic veins. The dorsal

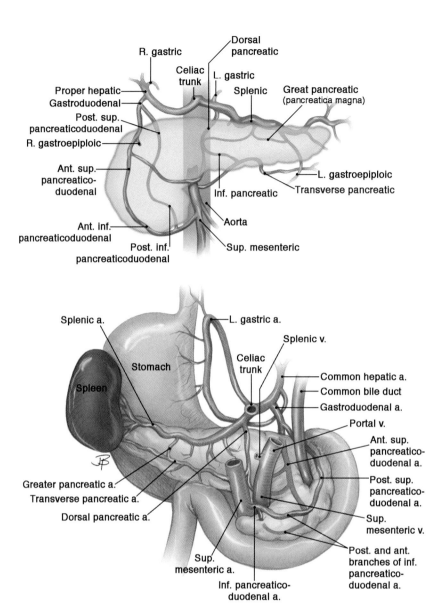

Figure 1-5

THE ARTERIAL BLOOD SUPPLY OF THE PANCREAS

The arterial supply to the pancreas is derived primarily from branches of the celiac trunk and superior mesenteric artery. The head of the pancreas is supplied by the pancreatico-duodenal arteries, which form anterior and posterior arcades around the head. The body and tail are supplied by the dorsal, inferior, and caudate pancreatic arteries (ant = anterior; a = artery; inf = inferior; l = left; post = posterior; r = right; sup = superior; v = vein). (Artwork by Jennifer Parsons Brumbaugh.)

pancreatic artery, also know as the superior pancreatic artery, may arise from either the first 2 cm of the splenic artery, the hepatic artery, the celiac trunk, or the superior mesenteric artery. The right branch of the dorsal pancreatic artery extends across the pancreatic head and supplies the neck of the pancreas, joining the anterior pancreatic arcade. The left branch, known as the inferior pancreatic artery, runs along the inferior border of the body of the pancreas and is often embedded in the posterior aspect of the gland. These major vessels lie posterior to the main pancreatic duct, allowing safe surgical access to the duct anteriorly (18).

Within the pancreas, a large branch of the splenic artery, known as the great pancreatic artery or pancreatica magna, provides left and right branches that course parallel to the main pancreatic duct. The right branch anastomosis with the inferior or dorsal pancreatic artery, and the left branch with the caudal pancreatic artery. Branches of these various pancreatic arteries supply the interlobular arteries and one intralobular artery supplies each lobule. The interlobular arteries run in the periphery of the epithelial lobules. As a result, the ducts at the center of the epithelial lobules are usually separate from the muscular vessels in the pancreas, a feature that can be used to differentiate infiltrating ductal adenocarcinoma, a process that will violate this pattern, and chronic pancreatitis, a process that will retain this architectural pattern (18).

Short arterioles supply blood to the islets. Hormone-rich blood flow from endocrine to exocrine cells is ensured by centrifugal flow. Venous drainage is by small veins that accompany the arteries and drain into splenic and superior mesenteric branches of the portal vein, similar to the venous drainage of the pancreatic head.

The Lymphatic System

The lymphatic system of the pancreas is of critical importance to its homeostasis; however, it is not a system used as a significant pathway for secretory products of the exocrine or endocrine cells. Rather, it is primarily a system to drain substances and excess fluid from the interstitium of the gland.

The majority of lymphatic vessels lie in the interlobular septa of the pancreas. Intralobular and interlobular lymphatic vessels are similarly and strikingly thin walled, with relatively large lumens. Intralobular lymphatics are sparse and are equally distributed in the head, body, and tail of the gland. Intralobular lymphatics are not essential, as excess fluid can track along the intralobular and interlobular connective tissue to the more abundant interlobular lymphatics. The interlobular lymphatics may travel with or independent of blood vessels (35).

Approximately 55 percent of interlobular lymphatic vessels are closely related to the accompanying artery and vein, 25 percent are separated from other structures by a significant amount of connective tissue, and 20 percent are closely related to acinar cells. Only 2 percent border the ductal system (31). Although some lymphatics may be seen on tissue sections to be closely apposed to acini and islets, this finding has no apparent functional significance.

The interlobular lymphatic vessels drain toward the surface of the pancreas and enter a surface network, sometimes referred to as collecting vessels, to converge toward the lymph nodes. The larger lymphatics are generally found beside the larger blood vessels and are similarly named or defined according to their position on the pancreas.

There are two major systems of lymph nodes that drain the pancreas: one rings the pancreas and the other is related to the anterior aspect and sides of the aorta from the level of the celiac trunk to the origin of the superior mesenteric artery. This second set of lymph nodes receives lymph either directly from the pancreas or indirectly from the first level of nodes that surround the pancreas. Although understanding where to look for lymph nodes is helpful, particularly in the gross dissection of a resection specimen, there is no known clinical significance to specifically designating the nodal groups, as only overall nodal status (N0 versus N1) plays a role in the TNM staging system.

Three main systems for classifying lymph node groups have been defined: one is descriptive by location (8,13), one a numerical system (30), and one a combination of the two (9). The descriptive classification of the lymph node groups is illustrated in figure 1-6. The first major group of lymph nodes rings the pancreas (fig. 1-6, top). Starting at the pancreatic tail and moving counterclockwise, this group includes the splenic and gastrosplenic nodes, which are associated with the hilum of the spleen and drain the pancreatic tail and left side of the body of the pancreas; the suprapancreatic nodes scattered along the superior surface of the pancreas; and the gastroduodenal and hepatic nodes, which drain the anterior and posterior aspects of the superior head of the pancreas. A number of lymph nodes rest in the groove between the head of the pancreas and the second part of the duodenum. These are labeled based on the corresponding arteries and veins: anterior and posterior superior pancreaticoduodenal, and anterior and posterior inferior pancreaticoduodenal nodes. Completing this ring of lymph nodes around the pancreas are the infrapancreatic nodes that run along the inferior border of the pancreas, and the mesenteric nodes that lie between the layers of the mesocolon close to its attachment along the anterior surface of the pancreas.

The second major group of lymph nodes includes those related to the aorta and its branches (fig. 1-6, bottom). They are divided into three main groups relative to their relationship with the aorta: the preaortic nodes, which lie anterior to the aorta; the lateral aortic nodes, which lie to the left of the aorta; and the interaorticocaval

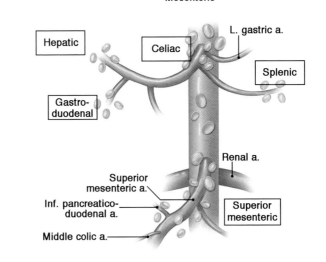

Figure 1-6

LYMPH NODES DRAINING THE PANCREAS AS CLASSIFIED BY THE DESCRIPTIVE NODAL SYSTEM

Top: The first level of lymph drainage is by the nodes that ring the pancreas.

Bottom: The second major group of nodes are named with respect to their relationship to the aorta and its branches (a = artery; ant = anterior; inf = inferior; l = left; post = posterior). (Artwork by Jennifer Parsons Brumbaugh.)

Table 1-1

JAPANESE CLASSIFICATION OF LYMPH NODES ACCORDING TO GROUPS[a,b]

	Head	Body and Tail
Group 1 lymph nodes	13a,13b,17a,17b	8a,8p,10,11p,11d,18
Group 2 lymph nodes	6,8a,8p,12a,12b,12p,14p,14d	7,9,14p,14d,15
Group 3 lymph nodes	1,2,3,4,5,7,9,10,11p,11d,15, 16a2,16b1,18	5,6,12a,12b,12p,13a,13b,17a, 17b, 16a2,16b1

[a]Table 3 from Japan Pancreas Society. Classification of pancreatic carcinoma. Tokyo: Kanehara & Co., Ltd; 2003:9.
[b]See figure 1-7.

nodes, which lie between the aorta and the inferior vena cava. The preaortic nodes can be subdivided into an upper group, the celiac nodes that surround the celiac trunk, and a lower group, the superior mesenteric nodes that surround the origin of this vessel.

In the numbering system, primarily used in Japan (fig. 1-7), the lymph nodes are divided into three groups for dissection (Table 1-1) and numbered 1 to 18. In this system, group 1 nodes consist of those usually removed during resection of the head or body/tail of the pancreas

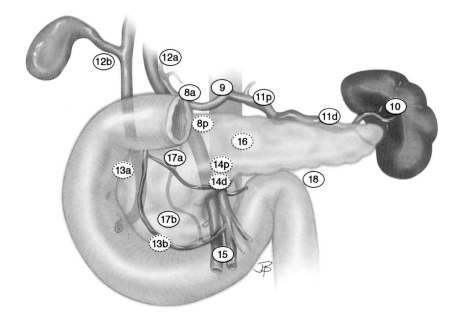

Figure 1-8

PARENCHYMAL ARCHITECTURE OF THE PANCREAS

Low-power magnification of the pancreas illustrates the lobular architecture of the dominating acinar epithelium and the relatively scant interlobular connective tissue.

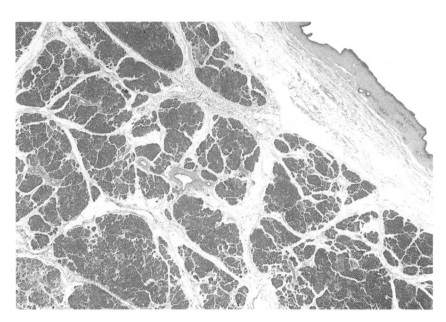

whereas groups 2 and 3 are organized based on lymph flow, rate of involvement by metastatic tumor, and outcome.

Innervation of the Pancreas

The pancreas is innervated by the vagus and thoracic splanchnic nerves that pass through the diaphragm. These nerves contain both parasympathetic and sympathetic nerve fibers and travel with the corresponding vasculature along the celiac and superior mesenteric plexuses (27).

The vagus nerve fibers contribute to the regulation and control of exocrine and endocrine secretory activity as well as capillary blood flow. The sympathetic nerve fibers affect the arteries and veins of the pancreas through the celiac ganglia.

HISTOLOGY, CYTOLOGY, AND FUNCTION

The pancreas is composed of exocrine (acini and ducts) and endocrine (islets of Langerhans) tissue arranged in 1- to 10-mm lobules separated by connective tissue septa (fig. 1-8).

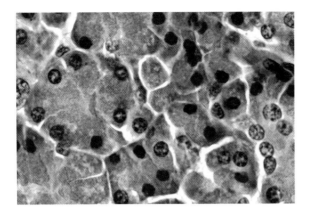

Figure 1-9

ACINAR EPITHELIAL CELLS

High-power magnification of acinar epithelial cells on routine histology highlights the staining differences between the perinuclear basophilic cytoplasm and the granular apical eosinophilic cytoplasm.

The Exocrine Pancreas

Eighty-five percent of the pancreas is exocrine tissue, the vast majority of which is acinar epithelium. Acinar cells are arranged in small rounded groups, tubular structures, and anastomosing loops that bud from the terminal ends and sides of ductules (3). Acinar cells are polarized and polygonal. The nuclei are round and basally located. The perinuclear cytoplasm is basophilic or amphophilic due to the high concentration of rough endoplasmic reticulum, while the more abundant granular apical cytoplasm stains brightly eosinophilic (fig. 1-9) (22).

Ultrastructural analysis shows that the granularity of the apical cytoplasm is due to zymogen granules. These are round, variably sized (range, 250 to 1000 nm) electron-dense granules that are surrounded by a limiting membrane (fig. 1-10). Each granule contains proenzyme forms of the various digestive enzymes, including trypsinogen 1, 2, and 3; chymotrypsinogen A and B; procarboxypeptidase B1 and B2; proelastase 1 and 2; kallikreinogen; prophospholipase A; lipase; and amylase. The apical cytoplasmic border is lined by microvilli, and each acinus is surrounded by a basement membrane without basal or myoepithelial cells. The absence of basal and myoepithelial cells contrasts with the acini of the salivary glands (22,24).

Histochemical stains highlight the zymogen granules, which stain with the periodic acid–

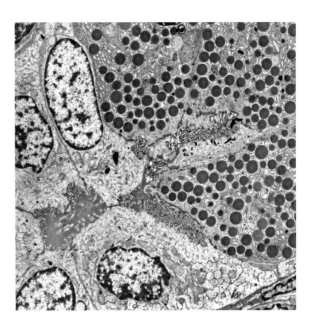

Figure 1-10

ACINAR EPITHELIAL CELLS

This electron micrograph of acinar cells (right) shows microvilli of the luminal edge and round, electron-dense zymogen granules. The acinar cells are juxtaposed to the centroacinar cells (left), also with luminal microvilli but no zymogen granules.

Schiff (PAS) stain and are resistant to diastase digestion. Butyrate esterase also stains the granules in acinar cells, but stains for mucin (Alcian blue at pH 2.5 and high iron diamine) are negative.

The exocrine enzymes produced by the acinar cells can be demonstrated using immunohistochemical labeling with antibodies to trypsin, chymotrypsin, lipase, amylase, and elastase. Antibodies to low molecular weight cytokeratin, CAM5.2, also label acinar cells, as do antibodies to cytokeratins (CKs) 8 and 18. Acinar cells generally do not label with antibodies to cytokeratin AE1/AE3, or with antibodies to CK7 and CK20. The cells also do not label with antibodies to the glycoprotein markers DUPAN-2 and carbohydrate antigen (CA) 19-9 (Table 1-2).

The appearance of acinar cells in cytologic preparations is similar to that seen histologically. In non-neoplastic processes, except in late-stage chronic pancreatitis, acinar cells dominate aspiration smears. The cells appear predominantly as cohesive, small, grape-like clusters with scattered single cells and occasional stripped nuclei (fig. 1-11). The round, regular nuclei are usually central, with uniform chromatin and variably prominent, often quite conspicuous nucleoli. The cells are polygonal and have abundant granular cytoplasm that stains blue-green with the standard Papanicolaou stain (fig. 1-12, left) and purple with a Romanowsky stain (fig. 1-12, right). The cytoplasmic granules may be visible depending on the specific stain. The Romanowsky stain also highlights scattered small vacuoles in the cytoplasm (7,17).

Acinar cells produce the proenzymes used in the digestion of food. These proenzymes are released through exocytosis, a process in which the membranes of the zymogen granule and cell surface fuse, allowing for release of the proenzymes into the acinar lumen where they are transported by the ductal system to the duodenum. In the duodenum, the inactive proenzyme trypsinogen is converted to the active enzyme trypsin by duodenal enteropeptidase (enterokinase). Active trypsin, in turn, catalyzes the cleavage of the other pancreatic proenzymes to their active forms.

The ductal system of the pancreas functions as a conduit for the transport of acinar cell secretions. The epithelial cells lining the ductal system secrete water, chloride, and bicarbonate, which buffer the acidity of the pancreatic juices, thus stabilizing the proenzymes. The ductal system begins with the centroacinar cells. These cells connect the acini to the intercalated ducts, the smallest ducts, and are recognized histologically by their clearly defined,

Table 1-2
IMMUNOREACTIVITY OF NORMAL ADULT PANCREATIC ACINAR, DUCTAL, AND ENDOCRINE CELLS

Antibody	Acinar	Ductal	Endocrine
CAM5.2	+	+	-
AE1	-	+	-
CK7[a]	-	+	-
CK8	+	+	-
CK18	+	+	-
CK19	-	+	-
CK20	-	-	-
Monoclonal CEA	-	-	-
CA19-9	-	+	-
DUPAN-2	-	+	-
Trypsin	+	-	-
Chymotrypsin	+	-	-
Lipase	+	-	-
Elastase	+	-	-
Amylase	+	-	-
Chromogranin	-	-	+
Synaptophysin	-	-	+
Neuron-specific enolase	-	-	+
Specific hormones (insulin, glucagon, somatostatin, PP, VIP)	-	-	+
Progesterone receptor	-	-	+
CD99	-	-	+
Pdx1	-	-	+

[a]CK = cytokeratin; CEA = carcinoembryonic antigen; CA = carbohydrate antigen; VIP = vasoactive intestinal polypeptide; PP = pancreatic polypeptide.

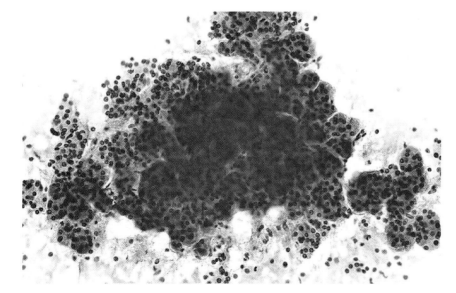

Figure 1-11

ACINAR EPITHELIAL CELLS

Aspirate smear of benign acinar cells demonstrating a relatively cohesive, grape-like clustering architecture. Cells are in sheets with stroma and as single rosettes, with some single cells and stripped epithelial nuclei (direct smear; Papanicolaou stain).

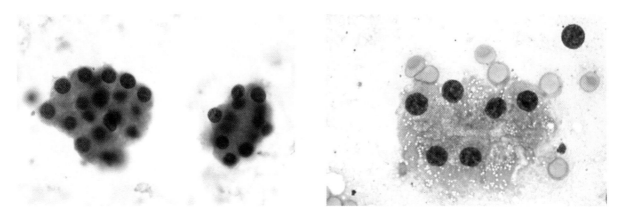

Figure 1-12

ACINAR EPITHELIAL CELLS

Individual acinar cells are polygonal, with round central nuclei, prominent nucleoli, and abundant granular cytoplasm.

Left: Fixation in ethanol and staining with the Papanicolaou stain highlight the nuclear features and may or may not demonstrate cytoplasmic granularity.

Right: Air-dried, Romanowsky-stained smears show the abundant cytoplasm with granular to finely vacuolated basophilic cytoplasm (direct smears).

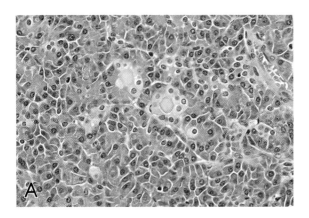

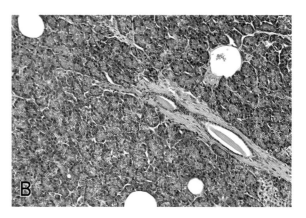

Figure 1-13

DUCTAL EPITHELIAL CELLS

A: Centroacinar cells are recognized by their pale cytoplasm relative to acinar cells and other ductal cells and signify the connection between the acinus and the duct.

B: Intercalated ducts are lined by cuboidal cells and connect the centroacinar cells to the intralobular ducts.

C: Intralobular ducts are lined by nonmucinous cuboidal to columnar cells. They lead to the interlobular ducts, which are also lined by nonmucinous cuboidal to columnar epithelial cells and acquire increasing amounts of periductal collagen.

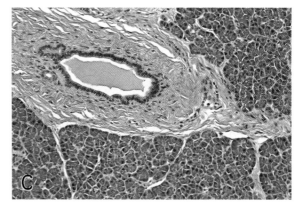

pale cytoplasm and round to oval nuclei (fig. 1-13A). Intercalated ducts fuse to form intralobular ducts; these are lined by nonmucinous, cuboidal epithelial cells that have central, round to oval nuclei and inconspicuous nucleoli (fig. 1-13B). Intralobular ducts drain into interlobular ducts (fig. 1-13C), which are surrounded by collagen once they leave the lobules; this collagen layer becomes increasingly thick as the ducts approach the main ducts of Wirsung and Santorini. Interlobular and main ducts are lined by a low columnar epithelium with round to oval, basally oriented nuclei and small, inconspicuous nucleoli. The cytoplasm of these cells is relatively dense without vacuolization, and as the ducts enlarge en route to the main duct, the cells contain increasing amounts of mucigen granules. Intracytoplasmic mucin is typically not seen with routine hematoxylin and eosin (H&E) stains but can be detected with special histochemical stains for mucin such as PAS, PAS with diastase digestion, and Alcian blue at pH 2.5. Mucinous cytoplasm in ductal cells visible with routine histology is a pathologic change (see Pancreatic Intraepithelial Neoplasia, chapter 7) (22,24).

Ductal cells are strongly labeled by antibodies to high (AE1/AE3) and low (CAM5.2) molecular weight cytokeratins and CK7 and CK19. Normal ductal cells are not labeled with antibodies to CK20 or with monoclonal antibodies to carcinoembryonic antigen. Labeling for exocrine enzymes and endocrine markers is also negative in the ductal cells, although scattered endocrine cells are found by immunolabeling within the epithelium of the larger ducts. Antibodies against CA19-9, DUPAN-2, cystic fibrosis transmembrane conductance regulator (CFTR), and N-terminal gastrin-releasing peptide (N-GRP) also label ductal cells (Table 1-2) (22).

The ultrastructural features of the epithelial cells at various points in the ductal system are similar except for the increasing presence of apical cytoplasmic mucigen granules in epithelial cells in the larger ducts compared to those lining the smaller ducts and the centroacinar cells. As reflected on histology, however, mucin granules are few in most ductal cells. Ductal cells contain significantly less rough endoplasmic reticulum and ribosomes than do acinar cells, but they do contain identifiable rough endoplasmic reticulum, mitochondria, and a Golgi complex, components that reflect their secretory capacity. Short microvilli may also be present on the cell surface, similar to acinar cells (fig. 1-14) (22,24).

The cytologic appearance of normal ductal epithelium is similar to that of ductal epithelium from most other organs. Large, flat, cohesive sheets of uniform, evenly spaced epithelial

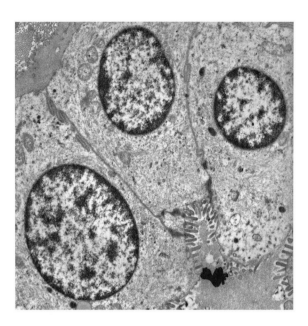

Figure 1-14

DUCTAL EPITHELIAL CELLS

Ultrastructurally, ductal cells contain significantly less rough endoplasmic reticulum and ribosomes than do acinar cells, but they do contain identifiable rough endoplasmic reticulum, mitochondria, and a Golgi complex, components that reflect their secretory capacity. Short microvilli may also be present on the cell surface, similar to acinar cells. Mucigen granules are few.

cells impart the typical "honeycombed" appearance characteristic of ductal epithelium (fig. 1-15A). The cytoplasm of these cells is best seen when the epithelium is present in strips yielding a "picket fence" arrangement, or in sheets with a luminal edge. Ductal cells have uniformly sized, round to oval nuclei, even chromatin, and generally small inconspicuous nucleoli. The relatively abundant, dense, nongranular and nonvacuolated cytoplasm stains aqua-blue with the Papanicolaou stain (fig. 1-15B) and more indigo-blue to purple with a Romanowsky stain (fig. 1-15C) (7,17).

The Endocrine Pancreas

Ninety percent of the endocrine cells in the pancreas reside in collections called the islets of Langerhans. The remainder are extrainsular endocrine cells scattered among the acini and larger ducts. The volume of islet cells in the pancreas is small compared to that of acinar and ductal cells, constituting only 1 to 2 percent of the adult gland. Although the volume of endocrine

Figure 1-15

DUCTAL EPITHELIAL CELLS

On direct smears most ductal epithelial cells are represented by flat, monolayered, honeycombed sheets of nonmucinous glandular cells with evenly spaced, uniformly round nuclei (A; Papanicolaou stain). Ductal cells typically have round to oval nuclei with smooth nuclear envelopes, evenly distributed finely granular chromatin, and nonmucinous cytoplasm that has an aqua blue color with the Papanicolaou stain (B) and a nonvacuolated purple color with an air-dried Romanowsky stain (C).

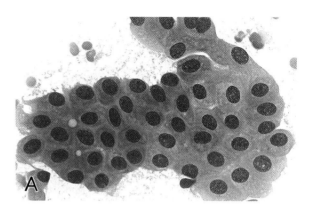

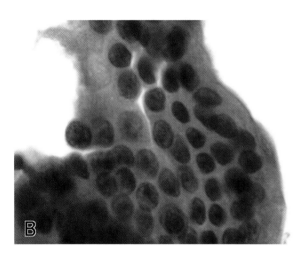

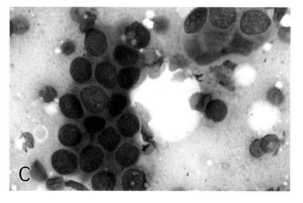

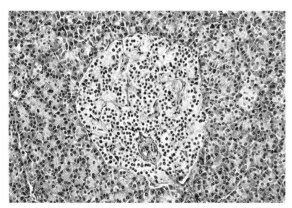

Figure 1-16

COMPACT ISLET OF LANGERHANS

Compact islets are predominantly located in the pancreatic body and tail. They are sharply demarcated from the surrounding acinar epithelium.

cells in the pancreas increases in utero, after birth it declines with age, decreasing from 15 percent in the neonate (less than 2 weeks old) to 5 to 10 percent in infants 6 months old, to 1 to 2 percent in adults. The islets are distributed throughout the pancreas but are more plenti-

ful in the body and tail. The apparent volume of islet cells varies with the presence and extent of exocrine atrophy (22,24).

Individual islets vary in size, shape, and composition of endocrine cells. The majority (about 90 percent), found in the body and tail, are small, generally round, and compact, and range from 50 to 280 µm. These islets are composed of intertwining trabeculae of endocrine cells and capillaries that appear sharply demarcated from the surrounding acini (fig. 1-16). Islets found in the posteroinferior head, the portion of the pancreas that arises from the ventral pancreatic bud, are formed from diffuse and less compact aggregates of endocrine cells (diffuse islets) and can attain sizes up to 450 µm. These islets tend to be composed of cords of cells with more hyperchromatic and irregular nuclei and more basophilic cytoplasm, and the cells can interdigitate among the acinar cells, features that appear infiltrative and, as such, may be mistaken for a neoplastic process (fig. 1-17).

Each islet cell produces a single peptide. The four major peptides are: insulin secreted by beta (β) cells, glucagon secreted by alpha (α) cells,

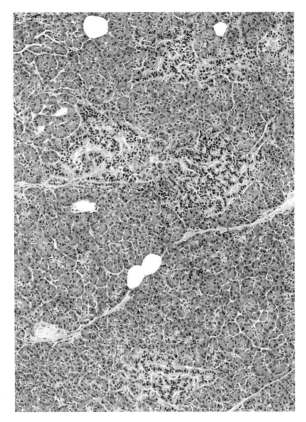

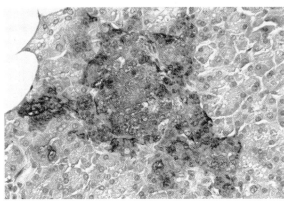

Figure 1-17

DIFFUSE ISLET OF LANGERHANS

Diffuse islets from the posteroinferior head are less clearly defined from the adjacent acinar epithelium than are compact islets. This interdigitation of islet cells and acinar cells can be confused with an infiltrative process (top, hematoxylin and eosin [H&E]; bottom, immunolabeling for chromogranin).

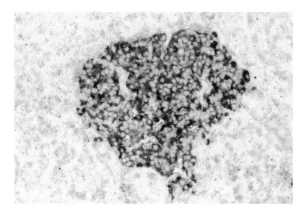

Figure 1-18

COMPACT ISLET

The four types of peptide-producing endocrine cells in a typical islet are the centrally located predominate insulin-producing islet cells (green), the peripherally located glucagon-producing alpha cells (red), and the sporadically placed somatostatin-producing delta cells (blue), and polypeptide-producing cells (immunoperoxidase triple stain). (Fig. 36 from Klimstra DS. Pancreas. In: Sternberg SS, ed. Histology for pathologists, 2nd ed. Philadelphia: Lippincott-Raven; 1997:629.)

somatostatin secreted by delta (δ) cells, and pancreatic polypeptide secreted by pancreatic polypeptide (PP) cells. Gastrin and vasoactive intestinal polypeptide may be expressed in some pancreatic endocrine neoplasms, but these peptides are not found in normal islet cells. The topographic distribution of endocrine cells appears to be functional and not random. The compact islets are largely composed of insulin-secreting β cells (60 to 80 percent) that tend to be centrally located; α (15 to 20 percent), δ (5 to 10 percent), and PP cells (less than 2 percent) are generally peripherally located (fig. 1-18). The diffuse islets are composed primarily of PP cells (70 to 80 percent), with a smaller percentage of β (20 to 30 percent), δ (5 to 10 percent) and α cells (less than 2 percent). The relative proportion of these various endocrine cells changes with age. The proportion of β cells increases from 50 percent in the neonate to 70 percent in the adult whereas the δ cell population decreases from 30 percent in the neonate to 10 percent in the adult (22,24).

In cytologic preparations individual islet cells appear uniform and polygonal, with round nuclei, coarsely clumped chromatin, small inconspicuous nucleoli, and pale amphophilic cytoplasm. These cells are rarely, if ever, appreciated in the aspirate of a nonendocrine neoplasm (7,17).

Histochemical stains can highlight endocrine cells, although somewhat nonspecifically. These include aldehyde fuchsin, a stain for

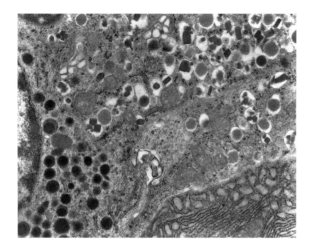

Figure 1-19

ENDOCRINE CELLS

Secretory granules on electron microscopy are distinctive for each cell type. The granules of insulin-producing beta cells are polymorphous, with crystalline cores and a wide halo beneath the limiting membrane (upper right). Glucagon-secreting alpha cell granules are round, with an eccentric dense core and a thin halo beneath the limiting plate (lower left).

insulin-secreting β cells; the Grimelius silver stain, a marker for glucagon-secreting α cells; and the Hellerstrom-Hellman silver stain, a stain that recognizes somatostatin-secreting δ cells. Immunohistochemical markers of islet cells include chromogranin, synaptophysin, neuron-specific enolase, CD56, CD99, and Pdx1, while antibodies for labeling specific endocrine peptides are used to determine the type of individual endocrine cells. Islet cell nuclei are labeled by progesterone receptors using immunohistochemistry. Anticytokeratin antibodies usually do not label islet cells (Table 1-2) (22).

Ultrastructural analysis shows that islet cells are connected by tight and gap junctions with scattered desmosomes. Cytoplasmic organelles reflect a secretory function with rough endoplasmic reticulum (RER), ribosomes, a Golgi complex, and mitochondria. Compared to acinar cells with long parallel arrays of RER, the RER of islet cells has short cisternae. Multivesicular lipid inclusions that resemble ceroid may also be found in β cells (22,24).

The hormone produced by the secretory granule is reflected in its ultrastructural appearance. Insulin-secreting β cells contain 200- to 300-nm membrane-bound dense core granules (fig. 1-19). The granules are characteristically surrounded by a wide halo beneath the limiting membrane that on highest magnification can be seen to contain a finely granular to paracrystalline array. The granules vary in size and shape, most commonly appearing rectangular, square, hexagonal, or polygonal. Glucagon-secreting α cells contain slightly larger granules (250 to 400 nm) with an eccentrically situated, round inner dense core surrounded by a less electron-dense zone that separates the dense core from the limiting membrane (fig. 1-19). Somatostatin-secreting δ cells contain the smallest granules (170 to 220 nm), which tend to be more uniformly electron dense. The granules of the PP cells differ in the portion of the pancreas derived from the dorsal and ventral buds. Granules in the PP cells of the ventrally derived pancreas are more heterogenous in shape and density (180 to 220 nm), whereas those in the PP cells of the dorsally derived pancreas are smaller (120 to 150 nm) and more uniform (22,24).

MINOR ARCHITECTURAL VARIATIONS

Variations in the architecture of the exocrine and endocrine cells within the pancreas, although usually minor, may appear exaggerated and mimic a neoplastic process. This creates a diagnostic pitfall, especially in the setting of a true neoplasm. These variations of normal histology are usually a result of aging, a response to injury, or a physiologic change.

Acinar Cell Nodule

Acinar cell nodules are circumscribed aggregates of acinar cells that stand out from the surrounding acini due to tinctorial differences of the cells (fig. 1-20). Two types have been described (45). The eosinophilic type is much more common and is so named because the loss of basal basophilia produces relative cytoplasmic pallor in the acinar cells. In the less common basophilic type, the acinar cells exhibit greater basophilia due to an increased nuclear to cytoplasmic ratio combined with a loss of zymogen granules in the apical cytoplasm. Both types are more common in adults but may be seen in children, and have been described in up to 20 percent of pancreata examined at autopsy (41). Acinar cell nodules can be confused

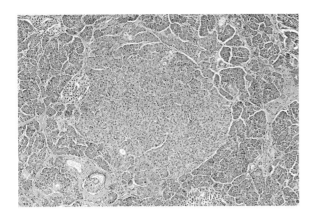

Figure 1-20

EOSINOPHILIC ACINAR CELL NODULE

Acinar cell nodules are enlarged aggregates of benign acinar cells that are distinguished from the surrounding acinar cells by the tinctorial staining qualities of the cytoplasm.

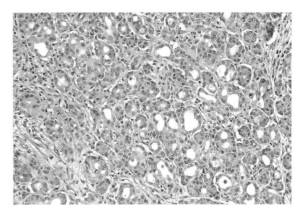

Figure 1-21

ACINAR ECTASIA

Ectatic acini have dilated, patulous lumens that may involve a single acinus or many, as illustrated here. The flattened acinar epithelial cells may resemble a ductule.

with islets of Langerhans as they are similar in size to compact islets. *Focal acinar transformation* and *eosinophilic degeneration* are other terms that have been used to describe these nodules. Dysplasia has also been used in some reports of acinar cell nodules, likely due to the not infrequent presence of nuclear atypia; however, these lesions have no proven preneoplastic significance in humans (35).

Acinar Ectasia

Acinar ectasia is a common finding at autopsy and has been associated with uremia, intestinal obstruction, ulcerative colitis, sepsis, and malignancy. The association with advanced uremia is common, and the term *uremic exocrine pancreatopathy* has been proposed (1). The etiology is poorly understood, but may be secondary to obstruction of pancreatic secretions, neural stimulation of the pancreas causing thick secretions, malnutrition, and dehydration (5).

Dilatation of acini in acinar ectasia may involve a single acinus or an entire lobule, and the acini may or may not contain luminal secretions. The ectasia causes flattening of the acinar cells and an apparent loss of apical zymogen granules, causing the dilated acinus to resemble a ductule (fig. 1-21). Centroacinar cells may proliferate as well. Diffuse ectasia in a small biopsy can cause confusion with well-differentiated adenocarcinoma, particularly on a frozen section specimen. Surgical pathologists must be

aware of this benign process and should carefully look for cytoplasmic granularity in at least some cells to avoid this diagnostic pitfall.

Metaplasia of Ductal Epithelium

Metaplastic changes of the ductal epithelial cells are common and varied. They include mucinous, squamous, acinar, oncocytic, and goblet cell metaplasia.

Mucinous metaplasia, also referred to as *mucinous* or *mucous cell hypertrophy*, is the most commonly encountered metaplastic change (reported in up to 90 percent of pancreata), especially in the pancreatic head (34). It is now recognized that many ducts with mucinous change are not, in fact, metaplastic, but instead are early neoplasms, called *pancreatic intraepithelial neoplasia* (see chapter 7).

Squamous metaplasia, also referred to as *multilayered metaplasia*, due to the typical lack of keratinization (34), is found in up to 45 percent of pancreata and can occur anywhere in the ductal system. It is common in the intercalated ducts where proliferation of the relatively immature-appearing squamous cells may fill and occlude the duct and even extend into the acinus (fig. 1-22A). In the larger ducts, the metaplastic cells may undermine the glandular epithelium while retaining the glandular cells on the luminal edge, and are occasionally keratinized (fig. 1-22B). The most common associations are with chronic pancreatitis and

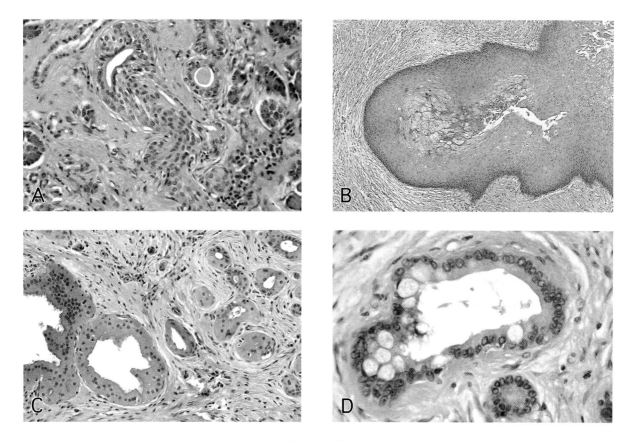

Figure 1-22

DUCTAL METAPLASIA

A: Squamous metaplasia of the intercalated duct extends into the acinus.
B: Squamous metaplasia of an interlobular duct with keratinization.
C: Ductal cells with oncocytic metaplasia.
D: Ductal cells with goblet cell metaplasia.

intraductal calculi. There is no recognized preneoplastic significance.

Acinar metaplasia of ductal epithelium is rare but can occasionally be seen in the smaller ducts. The cells recapitulate the morphology of normal acinar cells, acquiring a granular, eosinophilic cytoplasmic quality.

Oncocytic metaplasia is common in centroacinar cells and may also be seen in the smaller ducts of the lobule. Oncocytic metaplasia reflects an abundance of cytoplasmic mitochondria; thus, the cytoplasm appears finely granular and eosinophilic (fig. 1-22C). This metaplastic change is associated with chronic inflammation, but has been described in pancreata without any other abnormality.

Goblet cell metaplasia can occasionally be seen in the ductal epithelium, usually as isolated cells, and most commonly in the largest ducts, typically near the ampulla of Vater (fig. 1-22D).

CONGENITAL AND DEVELOPMENTAL ANOMALIES

Agenesis and Hypoplasia

Agenesis of the pancreas may be complete or partial, both of which are extremely rare. Complete pancreatic agenesis has been associated with gallbladder agenesis and diaphragmatic hernia, as well as severe growth retardation. Early recognition and treatment with replacement hormones and enzymes in the neonatal period is imperative for survival. Most patients with partial pancreatic agenesis survive, but they usually develop diabetes mellitus, depending on the amount of residual pancreatic tissue.

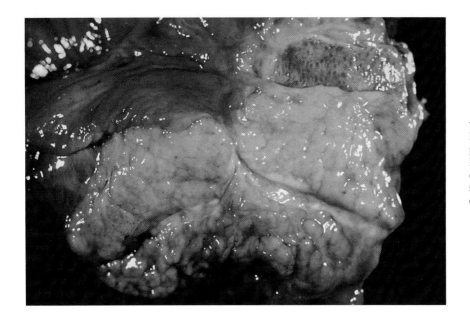

Figure 1-23

PANCREAS DIVISUM

Failure of the dorsal and ventral pancreatic buds to fuse leads to a functionally divided pancreas, as seen here with the larger bile duct (top right) draining into the duodenum separately from the pancreatic ducts (center).

Homozygous deletion of a single nucleotide within codon 63 of the human *IPF1* gene was recently identified in a Caucasian girl born with complete pancreatic agenesis; each parent was a heterozygote for the deletion (44). *IPF1* is critical in the development of the pancreas in mice and its targeted deletion leads to pancreatic agenesis.

More common than pancreatic agenesis is *pancreatic hypoplasia*, also referred to as *congenital short pancreas* and occasionally, *partial pancreatic agenesis* (19). This condition may be part of a congenital syndrome or present as an isolated anomaly. The pancreas appears short and stubby but otherwise retains the normal-appearing lobular architecture. Pancreatic hypoplasia is typically not associated with hypofunction.

Pancreas Divisum

Pancreas divisum is a congenital condition first recognized in the 1700s but initially well described by anatomist Joseph Hyrtl in the late 1800s (42). Pancreas divisum is a functionally divided pancreas caused by the failure of the dorsal and ventral pancreatic duct systems to fuse. It occurs in 5 to 10 percent of the population (43). There are three types: type 1, or classic divisum, refers to total failure of duct fusion causing most of the pancreatic secretions to exit via the duct of Santorini through the smaller minor papilla, with the duct of the small ventral pancreas draining through the major papilla together with the common bile duct; type 2 is a variant with domi-

nant dorsal drainage in which the ventral duct regresses, leaving the duct of Santorini and minor papilla as the only means of egress for exocrine secretions, while the major papilla only drains the bile duct; and type 3 is incomplete divisum where a small communicating branch of the ventral duct remains (see fig. 1-2) (42). The parenchyma of the dorsal and ventral lobes usually fuses in pancreas divisum, so the external appearance of the gland may be normal.

Pancreas divisum is associated with chronic pancreatitis. Patients with pancreas divisum and pancreatitis tend to be younger, more often female, less likely to drink alcohol, and more likely to have a clinical pattern of recurrent pancreatitis compared to patients with pancreatitis and normal ductal anatomy (6,36). The anomaly is also found in 12 to 26 percent of patients with idiopathic pancreatitis (10). The diminutive size of the minor papilla leads to a relative obstruction to proper flow of pancreatic secretions, which in turn is believed to produce chronic pancreatitis, which seems to be limited to the dorsal pancreas in most patients. This relatively common anomaly can be demonstrated on endoscopic retrograde cholangiopancreatography (ERCP); in resected specimens it can be demonstrated using a probe to trace the path of the main pancreatic duct toward the duodenum (fig. 1-23). Surgical or endoscopic sphincterotomy is beneficial in decompressing the minor papilla in some patients (36).

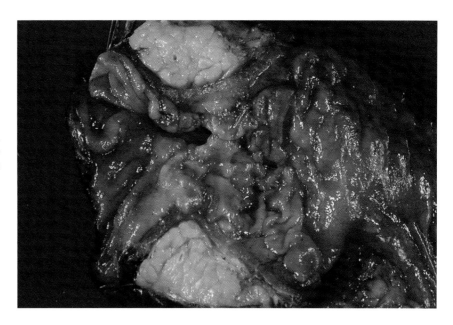

Figure 1-24

ANNULAR PANCREAS

The pancreas completely encircles the duodenum, focally narrowing the lumen of the bowel.

Annular Pancreas

Annular pancreas, also referred to as *pancreas ring*, is an extremely rare anatomic anomaly in which there is partial or complete encircling of the second part of the duodenum by pancreatic tissue (fig. 1-24). Although several theories exist to explain this phenomenon, one likely explanation is the failure of the left portion of the ventral embryonic bud to regress, causing it to encircle the duodenum during the normal rotation of the duodenum. Other explanations include adherence and stretching of the right ventral bud during this rotation, hypertrophy of normally placed pancreatic tissue, and fusion of the normal pancreas with pancreatic rests (20).

Annular pancreas can cause duodenal obstruction and is treated with bypass surgery in which the encircled portion of the duodenum with the pancreatic tissue is removed en block.

Congenital Lipomatosis

Congenital lipomatosis of the pancreas occurs in Shwachman-Diamond syndrome, an extremely rare autosomal recessive syndrome that affects the pancreas, bone marrow, and skeleton (11). The most common manifestations are malabsorption and steatorrhea due to pancreatic insufficiency, low neutrophil count, and short stature. Although neutropenia is the most common hematologic abnormality, all cells of the bone marrow may be affected, leading to anemia and clotting disorders. Thirty percent of children with this syndrome develop leukemia or aplastic anemia.

REFERENCES

1. Abu-Alfa A, Ivanovich P, Mujais SK. Uremic exocrine pancreopathy. Nephron 1988;48:94-100.
2. Ahlgren U, Jonsson J, Edlund H. The morphogenesis of the pancreatic mesenchyme is uncoupled from that of the pancreatic epithelium in IPF1/PDX1-deficient mice. Development 1996;122:1409-16.
3. Akao S, Bockman DE, Lechene de la Porte P, Sarles H. Three-dimensional pattern of ductulo-acinar associations in normal and pathological human pancreas. Gastroenterology 1986;90:661-8.
4. Apelqvist A, Ahlgren U, Edlund H. Sonic hedgehog directs specialised mesoderm differentiation in the intestine and pancreas. Curr Biol 1997;7:801-4.
5. Baggenstoss AH. The pancreas in uremia: a histopathologic study. Am J Pathol 1948;24:1003-11.

6. Bernard JP, Sahel J, Giovannini M, Sarles H. Pancreas divisum is a probable cause of acute pancreatitis: a report of 137 cases. Pancreas 1990;5:248-54.

7. Centeno BA, Pitman MB. Fine needle aspiration biopsy of the pancreas. Boston: Butterworth-Heinemann; 1999.

8. Cubilla AL, Fortner J, Fitzgerald PJ. Lymph node involvement in carcinoma of the head of the pancreas area. Cancer 1978;41:880-7.

9. Deki H, Sato T. An anatomic study of the peripancreatic lymphatics. Surg Radiol Anat 1988;10:121-35.

10. Dhar A, Goenka MK, Kochhar R, Nagi B, Bhasin DK, Singh K. Pancrease divisum: five years' experience in a teaching hospital. Indian J Gastroenterol 1996;15:7-9.

11. Durie PR. Inherited and congenital disorders of the exocrine pancreas. Gastroenterologist 1996;4:169-87.

12. Edlund H. Pancreas: how to get there from the gut? Curr Opin Cell Biol 1999;11:663-8.

13. Evans BP, Ochsner A. The gross anatomy of the lymphatics of the human pancreas. Surg 1954;36:177-91.

14. Gradwohl G, Dierich A, LeMeur M, Guillemot F. Neurogenin3 is required for the development of the four endocrine cell lineages of the pancreas. Proc Natl Acad Sci U S A 2000;97:1607-11.

15. Hebrok M. Hedgehog signaling in pancreas development. Mech Dev 2003;120:45-57.

16. Hebrok M, Kim SK, Melton DA. Notochord repression of endodermal Sonic hedgehog permits pancreas development. Genes Dev 1998;12:1705-13.

17. Hruban RH, Argani P, Ali SZ. The pancreas and extrahepatic biliary system. In: Silverberg SG, DeLellis RL, Frable VA, LiVolsi VA, Wick M, eds. Silverberg's principles and practice of surgical pathology and cytopathology, Vol 2, 4th ed. Philadelphia: Churchill Livingstone; 2005.

18. Ibukuro K. Vascular anatomy of the pancreas and clinical applications. Int J Gastrointest Cancer 2001;30:87-104.

19. Jaffe R. The pancreas. In: Stocker JT, Dehner LP, eds. Pediatric pathology. Philadelphia: JB Lippincott; 1992:791-823.

20. Kiernan PD, ReMine SG, Kiernan PC, ReMine WH. Annular pancreas. Mayo Clinic experience from 1957 to 1976 with review of the literature. Arch Surg 1980;115:46-50.

21. Kim SK, Hebrok M. Intercellular signals regulating pancreas development and function. Genes Dev 2001;15:111-27.

22. Klimstra DS. Pancreas. In: Sternberg SS, ed. Histology for pathologists. Philadelphia: Lippincott-Raven; 1997:613-47.

23. Krapp A, Knofler M, Ledermann B, et al. The bHLH protein PTF1-p48 is essential for the formation of the exocrine and the correct spatial organization of the endocrine pancreas. Genes Dev 1998;12:3752-63.

24. Lack EE. Pathology of the pancreas, gallbladder, extrahepatic biliary tract, and ampullary region. New York: Oxford University Press, Inc.; 2003.

25. Leach SO, Lin JV. Pancreatic development. In: Von Hoff D, Evans D, Hruban R, eds. Pancreatic cancer. Boston: Jones & Bartlett; 2005:71-83.

26. Miyamoto Y, Maitra A, Ghosh B, et al. Notch mediates TGF alpha-induced changes in epithelial differentiation during pancreatic tumorigenesis. Cancer Cell 2003;3:565-76.

27. Moore KL, Agur AM. Essential clinical anatomy. Baltimore: Lippincott Williams & Wilkins; 2002:151-68.

28. Murtaugh LC, Melton DA. Genes, signals, and lineages in pancreas development. Annu Rev Cell Dev Biol 2003;19:71-89.

29. Murtaugh LC, Stanger BZ, Kwan KM, Melton DA. Notch signaling controls multiple steps of pancreatic differentiation. Proc Natl Acad Sci U S A 2003;100:14920-5.

30. Nagakawa T, Kobayashi H, Ueno K, et al. The pattern of lymph node involvement in carcinoma of the head of the pancreas. A histologic study of the surgical findings in patients undergoing extensive nodal dissections. Int J Pancreatol 1993;13:15-22.

31. Navas V, O'Morchoe PJ, O'Morchoe CC. Lymphatic system of the rat pancreas. Lymphology 1995;28:4-20.

32. Naya FJ, Huang HP, Qiu Y, et al. Diabetes, defective pancreatic morphogenesis, and abnormal enteroendocrine differentiation in BETA2/neuroD-deficient mice. Genes Dev 1997;11:2323-34.

33. Nusslein-Volhard C, Wieschaus E. Mutations affecting segment number and polarity in Drosophila. Nature 1980;287:795-801.

34. Oertel JE. The pancreas. Nonneoplastic alterations. Am J Surg Pathol 1989;13(suppl 1):50-65.

35. O'Morchoe CC. Lymphatic system of the pancreas. Microsc Res Tech 1997;37:456-77.

36. Quest L, Lombard M. Pancreas divisum: opinio divisa. Gut 2000;47:317-9.

37. Schwitzgebel VM, Scheel DW, Conners JR, et al. Expression of neurogenin3 reveals an islet cell precursor population in the pancreas. Development 2000;127:3533-42.

38. Skandalakis LJ, Rowe JS, Gray SW, Skandalakis JE. Surgical embryology and anatomy of the pancreas. Surg Clin North Am 1993;73:661-97.

39. Solcia E, Capella C, Klöppel G. Tumors of the endocrine pancreas. Atlas of Tumor Pathology, 3rd Series, Fascicle 20. Washington, D.C.: Armed Forces Institute of Pathology; 1997:145-96.
40. Song SY, Gannon M, Washington MK, et al. Expansion of Pdx1-expressing pancreatic epithelium and islet neogenesis in transgenic mice overexpressing transforming growth factor alpha. Gastroenterology 1999;117:1416-26.
41. Stamm BH. Incidence and diagnostic significance of minor pathologic changes in the adult pancreas at autopsy: a systematic study of 112 autopies in patients without known pancreatic disease. Hum Pathol 1984;15:677-83.
42. Stern CD. A historical perspective on the discovery of the accessory duct of the pancreas, the ampulla 'of Vater' and pancreas divisum. Gut 1986;27:203-12.
43. Stimec B, Bulajic M, Korneti V, Milosavljevic T, Krstic R, Ugljesic M. Ductal morphometry of ventral pancreas in pancreas divisum. Comparison between clinical and anatomical results. Ital J Gastroenterol 1996;28:76-80.
44. Stoffers DA, Zinkin NT, Stanojevic V, Clarke WL, Habener JF. Pancreatic agenesis attributable to a single nucleotide deletion in the human IPF1 gene coding sequence. Nat Genet 1997;15:106-10.
45. Tanaka T, Mori H, Williams GM. Atypical and neoplastic acinar cell lesions of the pancreas in an autopsy study of Japanese patients. Cancer 1988;61:2278-85.
46. Thayer SP, diMagliano MP, Heiser PW, et al. Hedgehog is an early and late mediator of pancreatic cancer tumorigenesis. Nature 2003;425:851-6.

2 CLASSIFICATION OF PANCREATIC TUMORS

The scheme we have adopted to classify neoplasms of the pancreas is based on the classification systems presented in the third edition of this Fascicle and in the 2000 World Health Organization (WHO) "blue book" publication (5,7). In addition, as noted in the Introduction to this Fascicle, we have added to the foundation built by these classification systems using recent improvements in our understanding of the biology and clinical behavior of selected entities. As our knowledge grows we fully anticipate that new entities will be described, and that new facets of previously described entities will be uncovered. As such, we expect that the classification system presented here will require change over time.

The classification system presented is based on direction of differentiation. It is fundamentally a histologic classification based on light microscopic examination of hematoxylin and eosin–stained sections, with recognition of the value of immunohistochemical labeling and, in rare cases, electron microscopy.

The recently recognized category of intraductal tubular neoplasms represents one of the major additions to the classification system. Intraductal tubular neoplasms are grossly cystic epithelial neoplasms that grow within the pancreatic ducts and are composed of back-to-back tubular glands without significant formation of papillae. Those with minimal cytologic atypia, composed of glands resembling pyloric glands, are designated *intraductal tubular neoplasm with low-grade dysplasia* (1,2,4,6,10). Intraductal tubular neoplasms with marked cytoarchitectural atypia, increased mitoses, and necrosis are designated as *intraductal tubular neoplasm with high-grade dysplasia* (8,9).

The classification of mucin-producing neoplasms also has been modified. In the past, noninvasive mucinous cystic neoplasms with moderate dysplasia and noninvasive intraductal papillary mucinous neoplasms with moderate atypia were classified as "borderline" neoplasms, suggesting uncertain malignant potential. It is now clear that completely resected and thoroughly sampled noninvasive mucinous cystic neoplasms follow an entirely benign course (11,12). The term "borderline" has therefore been replaced by "with moderate dysplasia."

The concept of malignancy in pancreatic endocrine neoplasms has also been readdressed. Prior classification systems separated well-differentiated pancreatic endocrine neoplasms into benign, borderline, and malignant categories based on size, mitotic activity, and stage. Recent studies, however, have demonstrated that those pancreatic endocrine neoplasms that fall into the benign and borderline categories may recur or metastasize (3). Thus, the entire group of well-differentiated pancreatic endocrine neoplasms is now classified together, with an emphasis on identification of prognostic groups.

It is our hope that the classification system presented will clarify clinical diagnoses and facilitate comparative studies on pancreatic neoplasia.

I. Epithelial Neoplasms
  A. Exocrine Neoplasms
    1. Serous neoplasms
      a. Microcystic serous cystadenoma
      b. Macrocystic serous cystadenoma
      c. Solid serous adenoma
      d. von Hippel-Landau (VHL)-associated serous cystic neoplasm
      e. Serous cystadenocarcinoma
    2. Mucinous cystic neoplasms
      a. Mucinous cystic neoplasm with low-grade dysplasia
      b. Mucinous cystic neoplasm with moderate dysplasia
      c. Mucinous cystic neoplasm with high-grade dysplasia (carcinoma in situ)
      d. Mucinous cystic neoplasm with an associated invasive carcinoma

3. Intraductal neoplasms
   a. Intraductal papillary mucinous neoplasms
      1) Intraductal papillary mucinnous neoplasm with low-grade dysplasia
      2) Intraductal papillary mucinnous neoplasm with moderate dysplasia
      3) Intraductal papillary mucinnous neoplasm with high-grade dysplasia (carcinoma in situ)
      4) Intraductal papillary mucinnous neoplasm with an associated invasive carcinoma
   b. Intraductal oncocytic papillary neoplasm
   c. Intraductal tubular neoplasms
      1) Intraductal tubular neoplasm with low-grade dysplasia
      2) Intraductal tubular neoplasm with high-grade dysplasia (carcinoma in situ)
      3) Intraductal tubular neoplasm with an associated invasive carcinoma
4. Pancreatic intraepithelial neoplasia (PanIN)
   a. PanIN-1A and PanIN-1B
   b. PanIN-2
   c. PanIN-3
5. Invasive ductal adenocarcinoma
   a. Tubular adenocarcinoma
   b. Adenosquamous carcinoma
   c. Colloid (mucinous noncystic) adenocarcinoma
   d. Hepatoid carcinoma
   e. Medullary carcinoma
   f. Signet ring cell carcinoma
   g. Undifferentiated carcinoma
      1) anaplastic
      2) sarcomatoid
      3) carcinosarcoma
   h. Undifferentiated carcinoma with osteoclast-like giant cells
6. Acinar cell neoplasms
   a. Acinar cell cystadenoma
   b. Acinar cell carcinoma
   c. Acinar cell cystadenocarcinoma

B. Endocrine Neoplasms
   1. Microadenoma (<0.5cm)
   2. Well-differentiated pancreatic endocrine neoplasm
   3. Poorly differentiated endocrine carcinoma
      a. Small cell carcinoma
      b. Large cell endocrine carcinoma
C. Epithelial Neoplasms with Multiple Directions of Differentiation
   1. Mixed acinar-endocrine carcinoma
   2. Mixed acinar-ductal carcinoma
   3. Mixed ductal-endocrine carcinoma
   4. Mixed acinar-endocrine-ductal carcinoma
   5. Pancreatoblastoma
D. Epithelial Neoplasms of Uncertain Direction of Differentiation
   1. Solid-pseudopapillary neoplasm
E. Miscellaneous
   1. Teratoma
   2. Lymphoepithelial cyst
   3. Epidermoid cyst in intrapancreatic heterotopic spleen

II. **Nonepithelial Neoplasms**
   A. Adenomatoid Tumor
   B. Desmoplastic Small Round Cell Tumor
   C. Extragastrointestinal Stromal Tumor
   D. Fibromatosis (Desmoid)
   E. Granular Cell Tumor
   F. Hemangioma/Hemangioendothelioma
   G. Inflammatory Myofibroblastic Tumor
   H. Leiomyoma
   I. Lipoma/Angiolipoma
   J. Lymphangioma
   K. Lymphoma
   L. Malignant Fibrous Histiocytoma
   M. Paraganglioma
   N. PEComa
   O. Primitive Neuroectodermal Tumor (PNET)
   P. Sarcoma (Leiomyosarcoma, Synovial Sarcoma, Osteosarcoma, Angiosarcoma, etc.)
   Q. Schwannoma
   R. Solitary Fibrous Tumor
   S. Other
III. **Secondary Neoplasms (Metastases to the Pancreas)**

IV. Non-Neoplastic Tumors of the Exocrine Pancreas
A. Chronic Pancreatitis
B. Congenital Cyst
C. Duodenal Diverticulum
D. Ectopic Adrenocortical Nodules
E. Endometriotic Cyst
F. Foregut Cyst
G. Hamartoma
H. Heterotopic Pancreas
I. Heterotopic Spleen
J. Lipomatous Pseudohypertrophy
K. Lymphoplasmacytic Sclerosing Pancreatitis (Autoimmune Pancreatitis)
L. Malakoplakia
M. Nodular Lymphoid Hyperplasia
N. Paraampullary Duodenal Wall Cyst (Groove Pancreatitis)
O. Pseudocyst
P. Reactive Fibroinflammatory Pseudotumor
Q. Retention Cyst
R. Sarcoidosis

V. Non-Neoplastic Tumors of the Endocrine Pancreas
A. Islet Aggregation
B. Islet Hyperplasia
C. Nesidioblastosis

REFERENCES

1. Albores-Saavedra J, Sheahan K, O'Riain C, Shukla D. Intraductal tubular adenoma, pyloric type, of the pancreas: additional observations on a new type of pancreatic neoplasm. Am J Surg Pathol 2004;28:233-8.
2. Bakotic BW, Robinson MJ, Sturm PD, Hruban RH, Offerhaus GJ, Albores-Saavedra J. Pyloric gland adenoma of the main pancreatic duct. Am J Surg Pathol 1999;23:227-31.
3. Hochwald SN, Zee S, Conlon KC, et al. Prognostic factors in pancreatic endocrine neoplasms: an analysis of 136 cases with a proposal for low-grade and intermediate-grade groups. J Clin Oncol 2002;20:2633-42.
4. Kato N, Akiyama S, Motoyama T. Pyloric gland-type tubular adenoma superimposed on intraductal papillary mucinous tumor of the pancreas. Pyloric gland adenoma of the pancreas. Virchows Arch 2002;440:205-8.
5. Klöppel G, Hruban RH, Longnecker DS, Adler G, Kern SE, Partanen TJ. Ductal adenocarcinoma of the pancreas. In: Hamilton SR, Aaltonen LA, eds. World Health Organization classification of tumours. Pathology and genetics of tumours of the digestive system. Lyon: IARCPress; 2000: 221-30.
6. Nakayama Y, Inoue H, Hamada Y, et al. Intraductal tubular adenoma of the pancreas, pyloric gland type: a clinicopathologic and immunohistochemical study of 6 cases. Am J Surg Pathol 2005;29:607-16.
7. Solcia E, Capella C, Klöppel G. Tumors of the pancreas. Atlas of Tumor Pathology, 3rd Series, Fascicle 20. Washington, DC: Armed Forces Institute of Pathology; 1997.
8. Tajiri T, Tate G, Inagaki T, et al. Intraductal tubular neoplasms of the pancreas: histogenesis and differentiation. Pancreas 2005;30:115-21.
9. Tajiri T, Tate G, Kunimura T, et al. Histologic and immunohistochemical comparison of intraductal tubular carcinoma, intraductal papillary-mucinous carcinoma, and ductal adenocarcinoma of the pancreas. Pancreas 2004;29: 116-22.
10. Terris B, Dubois S, Buisine MP, et al. Mucin gene expression in intraductal papillary-mucinous pancreatic tumours and related lesions. J Pathol 2002;197:632-7.
11. Wilentz RE, Albores-Saavedra J, Hruban RH. Mucinous cystic neoplasms of the pancreas. Semin Diagn Pathol 2000;17:31-42.
12. Wilentz RE, Albores-Saavedra J, Zahurak M, et al. Pathologic examination accurately predicts prognosis in mucinous cystic neoplasms of the pancreas. Am J Surg Pathol 1999;23:1320-7.

3 STAGING

The staging of carcinomas of the pancreas was revised slightly in the sixth edition of the American Joint Committee on Cancer (AJCC) Cancer Staging Handbook, and the staging schemes of the AJCC and the International Union Against Cancer (IUAC)/Union Internationale Contre le Cancer (UICC) are now uniform (1,4). The staging of carcinoma of the pancreas is based on size and extent of the primary neoplasm (T), the presence or absence of regional lymph node metastases (N), and the presence or absence of metastatic disease (M) (Table 3-1) (1). The TNM staging system is used for carcinomas of the exocrine pancreas. Pure endocrine neoplasms are not included; however, mixed acinar-endocrine and mixed ductal-endocrine carcinomas can be staged using the TNM system (Table 3-2). The neoplasm should be histologically or cytologically confirmed before staging. Clinical staging can be based on physical examination, imaging, cytologic analysis of the neoplasm and surrounding nodes or liver, and/or surgical exploration. Staging based on pathologic findings from surgically resected specimens follows the same TNM categories and should include the prefix "p" (i.e., pT, pN, and pM).

ANATOMIC SUBSITES

The pancreas is divided into three anatomic subsites for staging purposes (Table 3-3) (1). Carcinomas of the head of the pancreas arise to the right of the left border of the superior mesenteric-portal vein confluence. The uncinate process and neck of the pancreas are considered to be part of the head of the pancreas. Carcinomas of the body of the pancreas arise between the left border of the superior mesenteric-portal vein confluence and the left border of the aorta. Carcinomas of the tail of the pancreas arise between the left border of the aorta and the hilum of the spleen. A more detailed description of the anatomic subsites of

---

Table 3-1

TNM CLINICAL CLASSIFICATION

T – Primary Tumor
- TX Primary tumor cannot be assessed
- T0 No evidence of primary tumor
- Tis Carcinoma in situ (high-grade dysplasia)
- T1 Tumor limited to pancreas, 2 cm or less in greatest dimension
- T2 Tumor limited to pancreas, more than 2 cm in greatest dimension
- T3 Tumor extends beyond pancreas, but without involvement of celiac axis or superior mesenteric artery
- T4 Tumor involves celiac axis or superior mesenteric artery (unresectable carcinoma)

N – Regional Lymph Nodes
- NX Regional lymph nodes cannot be assessed
- N0 No regional lymph node metastasis
- N1 Regional lymph node metastasis

M – Distant Metastasis
- MX Distant metastasis cannot be assessed
- M0 No distant metastasis
- M1 Distant metastasis

Table 3-2

NEOPLASMS INCLUDED IN THE TNM STAGING SYSTEM

Acinar cell carcinoma and its variants

Epithelial neoplasms with multiple directions of differentiation (such as mixed acinar-endocrine carcinomas)

In situ carcinoma (pancreatic intraepithelial neoplasia-3)

Intraductal papillary mucinous neoplasms (high-grade dysplasia and invasive)

Intraductal tubular neoplasms (high-grade dysplasia and invasive)

Invasive ductal adenocarcinoma and its variants (adenosquamous, ductal-endocrine carcinoma, hepatoid, medullary, mucinous noncystic, signet ring cell, undifferentiated with osteoclast-like giant cells)

Mucinous cystic neoplasms (high-grade dysplasia and invasive)

Pancreatoblastoma

Serous cystadenocarcinoma

Solid-pseudopapillary neoplasm

Table 3-3

ANATOMIC SUBSITES

Head of the pancreas	Tumors of the head of the pancreas are those arising to the right of the left border of the superior mesenteric vein. The uncinate process is considered as part of the head.
Body of pancreas	Tumors of the body are those arising between the left border of the superior mesenteric vein and left border of the aorta.
Tail of pancreas	Tumors of the tail are those arising between the left border of the aorta and the hilum of the spleen.

Table 3-4

REGIONAL LYMPH NODES

The regional lymph nodes are the peripancreatic nodes, which are subdivided as follows:

Superior	Superior to head and body
Inferior	Inferior to head and body
Anterior	Anterior pancreaticoduodenal, pyloric (for tumors of head only), and some proximal mesenteric
Posterior	Posterior pancreaticoduodenal, common bile duct, and some proximal mesenteric
Splenic	Hilum of spleen and tail of pancreas (for tumors of body and tail only)
Celiac	Surrounding the celiac trunk (for tumors of head only)

the pancreas is given in the section on the normal pancreas (see chapter 1).

The pathologic assignment of subsite can be difficult in surgically resected specimens because the anatomic landmarks that are needed to identify subsite are not present. In these cases, correlation with clinical/radiologic information is used. There are no anatomic barriers separating the subsites within the pancreas. It is therefore not uncommon for carcinomas of the pancreas to involve more than one subsite. In these instances, all of the subsites involved should be documented.

Regional lymph nodes refer to the peripancreatic lymph nodes ordinarily included in a lymphadenectomy specimen and can be subdivided into the superior, inferior, anterior, posterior, splenic, and celiac groups (Table 3-4) (1). Superior group lymph nodes are superior to the head and body of the gland, inferior are inferior to the head and body, and the anterior include the anterior pancreaticoduodenal, the pyloric (for carcinomas of the head only), and the proximal mesenteric nodes. The posterior lymph nodes include the posterior pancreaticoduodenal, the common bile duct, and the proximal mesenteric lymph nodes. The splenic

group includes those at the hilum of the spleen and tail of the pancreas (for carcinomas of the body and tail only), and the celiac group only includes carcinomas of the head of the gland. A more detailed description of the lymph node groups of the pancreas is given in the section on the normal pancreas (see chapter 1).

T CLASSIFICATION

The T designation is based on the primary neoplasm and reflects the important distinction between potentially resectable (T1, T2, and T3) and locally advanced unresectable (T4) disease (1). The T classification system is given in Table 3-1.

TX is the designation given when the primary tumor cannot be assessed, and T0 the designation for no evidence of primary tumor. The Tis designation should be given to pancreatic intraepithelial neoplasia-3, to noninvasive mucinous cystic neoplasms with high-grade dysplasia (carcinoma in situ), and to noninvasive intraductal papillary mucinous neoplasms with high-grade dysplasia (carcinoma in situ).

The greatest diameter of the neoplasm should be recorded as tumor size. The size is generally measured grossly. For carcinomas with abundant desmoplastic stroma (such as infiltrating ductal adenocarcinoma), however, it may be exceedingly difficult grossly to distinguish carcinoma from adjacent areas of chronic pancreatitis. In such cases, the final size should be determined after validation of the extent of the carcinoma based on the microscopic appearance. When an in situ and an invasive component are both present, each component should be measured separately. Only the size of the invasive component should be used to stage invasive carcinomas.

Most carcinomas of the head of the pancreas involve the common bile duct as it courses through the pancreas. The involvement of the intrapancreatic portion of the bile duct does not signify extension beyond the pancreas in the T classification of carcinomas of the pancreas. Involvement of the bile duct should be designated T3 only when the carcinoma extends beyond the pancreas to involve the extrapancreatic biliary tree. The designation T4 is generally reserved for unresectable neoplasms.

N CLASSIFICATION

The N classification is shown in Table 3-1 (1). Involvement of regional lymph nodes, either by metastatic seeding or by direct extension, should be designated N1, as should metastases of any size (even micrometastases). Histopathologic examination of regional lymphadenectomy specimens should ideally include 10 or more lymph nodes. An optional expansion of the N classification includes the separation of metastases to a single regional lymph node (N1a) from metastases to multiple regional lymph nodes (N1b) (1,4).

M CLASSIFICATION

The M classification is shown in Table 3-1 (1). The distant metastasis categories M1 and pM1 may be further subdivided into: pulmonary (PUL), osseous (OSS), hepatic (HEP), brain (BRA), lymph nodes (LYM), bone marrow (MAR), pleura (PLE), peritoneum (PER), adrenal gland (ADR), skin (SKI), and other (OTH). Seeding of the peritoneum, including positive peritoneal cytology, should be designated as M1.

EXTENT OF RESECTION

The presence or absence of residual carcinoma after surgical resection is a very important prognosticator and, although not part of

Table 3-5

R CLASSIFICATION

The absence or presence of residual tumor after surgical resection (designated by the symbol R) is not part of the TNM staging system, but it is clinically important.

RX	Presence of residual tumor cannot be assessed
R0	No residual microscopic or macroscopic tumor
R1	Microscopic residual tumor
R2	Macroscopic residual tumor

the TNM staging system, can be designated by the symbol R (Table 3-5) (1). RX designates that the presence of residual tumor cannot be assessed; R0, complete resection with no residual microscopic or macroscopic tumor; R1, grossly negative but microscopically positive margins of resection; and R2, grossly and microscopically positive margins. The major margins in pancreatoduodenectomy specimens are the bile duct, pancreatic neck, uncinate process, soft tissue, and proximal and distal duodenal margins (see chapter 16). Carcinoma frequently extends to involve the retroperitoneal resection margin, and care should be taken to evaluate this margin in resection specimens.

PREFIXES APPLIED TO THE TNM CLASSIFICATION

Four prefixes can be applied to the TNM classification to designate the basis on which the patient's stage was evaluated (1). *Clinical classification* is based on the clinical assessment of the patient prior to the first definitive treatment, and it includes information gleaned from physical examination, imaging, endoscopy, biopsy, and surgical exploration (1). It is designated with the prefix "c" as cTNM or simply TNM. The *pathologic classification* is designated with the prefix "p" (pTNM) and is based on evidence acquired before treatment, supplemented by additional information acquired during pathologic examination (1). *Retreatment classification*, designated with the lowercase prefix "r" (rTNM), is applied when further treatment is planned for a carcinoma that has recurred after a disease-free interval (1). The prefix "a" (aTNM) is used to designate the *autopsy classification* of a carcinoma based on the postmortem examination of a patient whose cancer was not evident prior to death (1).

Table 3-6
STAGE GROUPING

Stage 0	Tis	N0	M0
Stage IA	T1	N0	M0
Stage IB	T2	N0	M0
Stage IIA	T3	N0	M0
Stage IIB	T1, T2, T3	N1	M0
Stage III	T4	Any N	M0
Stage IV	Any T	Any N	M1

Table 3-7
HISTOPATHOLOGIC GRADING

Neoplasms should be graded based on the most poorly differentiated significant component present.

G – Histopathologic Grading

GX   Grade of differentiation cannot be assessed

G1   Well differentiated

G2   Moderately differentiated

G3   Poorly differentiated

G4   Undifferentiated

Table 3-8
JAPANESE STAGING SYSTEM[a]

	M0			M1
	N0	N1	N2	N3
Tis	0	–	–	–
T1	I	II	III	IVb
T2	II	III	III	IVb
T3	III	III	IVa	IVb
T4	IVa	IVa	IVb	IVb

[a]Table 4 from Japanese Pancreas Society. Classification of pancreatic carcinoma, 2nd English ed. Tokyo: Kanehara & Co., Ltd; 2003:12.

STAGING

The T, N, and M classification can be combined, as shown in Table 3-6, to determine stage (1). Localized resectable disease is classified as stage I or II, locally advanced as stage III, and metastatic disease as stage IV. Clinical staging can usually be accomplished with a careful physical examination, high-quality computerized tomography (CT) images, and endoscopic ultrasound with fine needle aspiration cytology. Surgically resected carcinomas can also be staged pathologically.

HISTOPATHOLOGIC GRADING

Histopathologic grading of pancreatic cancer follows that of other gastrointestinal tract carcinomas (Table 3-7) (1). Multiple histopathologic grades may be observed within a single neoplasm. In these instances, the carcinoma should be graded based on the most poorly differentiated significant component present.

COMPARISON TO THE JAPANESE STAGING SYSTEM

Although there have historically been considerable differences in the way carcinomas of the exocrine pancreas have been classified and staged in Japan and in Western nations, the Second English Edition of the Classification of Pancreatic Carcinoma by the Japan Pancreas Society and the AJCC/IUAC classification are now significantly more compatible (1,3).

The Tis, T1, and T2 designations in the Japanese classification system are the same as the Tis, T1, and T2 designations given in Table 3-1. In the Japanese system, T3 designates a tumor that has extended into the bile duct, duodenum, or peripancreatic tissue (3). Involvement of the intrapancreatic bile duct would therefore be designated T3. The T4 designation in the Japanese system is given to tumors that have extended into large vessels, into the extrapancreatic nerve plexus, or into other organs including the kidney, adrenal gland, stomach, large intestine, spleen, omentum, mesocolon, inferior vena cava, and renal vein (3).

The N designation in the Japanese classification system is divided into additional categories (N1, N2, and N3) based on the lymph node groups involved. The M designations are the same in the two systems.

The overall Japanese staging system is presented in Table 3-8 (3). Although more complex, several studies have shown that the Japanese staging system may be a better predictor of outcome than the AJCC classification system (2).

REFERENCES

1. American Joint Committee on Cancer. Greene FL, Page DL, Fleming ID, et al., eds. AJCC cancer staging handbook, 6th ed. New York: Springer-Verlag; 2002.
2. Isaji S, Kawarada Y, Uemoto S. Classification of pancreatic cancer: comparison of Japanese and UICC classifications. Pancreas 2004;28:231-4.
3. Japanese Pancreas Society. Classification of pancreatic carcinoma, 2nd English ed. Tokyo: Kanehara & Co., Ltd.; 2003.
4. Klöppel G, Hruban RH, Longnecker DS, Adler G, Kern SE, Partanen TJ. Ductal adenocarcinoma of the pancreas. In: Hamilton SR, Aaltonen LA, eds. World Health Organization classification of tumours. Pathology and genetics of tumours of the digestive system. Lyon: IARCPress; 2000: 221-30.

4 SEROUS CYSTIC NEOPLASMS

Serous cystic neoplasms were first reported more than 100 years ago, and a serous cystic neoplasm from the 19th century is still on display in the Viennese collection of pathologic specimens (the "Collectio Rokitansky") (29,62). For decades, however, serous and mucinous cystic neoplasms of the pancreas were lumped together under the designations "cystadenoma" and "cystadenocarcinoma." This was unfortunate because, as we will discuss, almost all serous cystic neoplasms are benign, while mucinous cystic neoplasms have a significant malignant potential. The importance of distinguishing between these two entities has been recognized for half a century (6), but it was not until 1978 that Compagno and Oertel (13), and Hodgkinson (27) and others clearly defined and separated serous cystic neoplasms from mucinous cystic neoplasms.

The vast majority of serous cystic neoplasms are entirely benign; however, a handful of case reports have documented the rare potential for these neoplasms to invade the spleen and stomach, and to involve lymph nodes and liver (1,8, 17,21,33,53,74,75,77). While some have argued that these cases may represent multifocal disease, the existence of rare serous cystadenocarcinomas is now generally accepted.

MICROCYSTIC SEROUS CYSTADENOMA

Definition. *Microcystic serous cystadenoma* is a benign epithelial neoplasm composed of uniform cuboidal, glycogen-rich cells that form numerous small cysts containing serous fluid (9,32,66). Unless otherwise specified, *serous cystadenoma* is synonymous with microcystic serous cystadenoma. Other synonyms include *glycogen-rich cystadenoma* and *microcystic adenoma*.

General Features. Microcystic serous cystadenomas are uncommon. They account for only 1 to 2 percent of all neoplasms of the exocrine pancreas, and for 10 percent of surgically resected cystic lesions of the pancreas (38,66). In most surgical series, the number of micro-

cystic serous cystic neoplasms is about equal to the number of noninvasive mucinous cystic neoplasms (42). Microcystic serous cystadenomas occur more commonly in women (female to male ratio, 7 to 3) and the mean age at diagnosis in most reported series is about 65 years (range, 18 to 91 years) (3,5,13,27,42,63,73). It is reasonable to expect that the mean age at diagnosis will drop as greater numbers of these neoplasms are discovered in asymptomatic patients who undergo whole body "virtual physical" computerized tomography (CT) scanning.

Serous cystadenomas are associated with the von Hippel-Lindau (VHL) syndrome (11,23,28, 47,49,50,72). Pye-Smith (57) documented pancreatic involvement in patients with VHL in 1884, and cystadenomas of the pancreas were present in 8 of the 15 patients in Lindau's original report (45). The VHL syndrome is an autosomal dominant disorder characterized by clear cell neoplasms including hemangioblastomas of the central nervous system (CNS) and retina, renal neoplasms and cysts, clear cell endocrine pancreatic neoplasms, clear cell papillary cystadenomas of the epididymis, clear cell carcinoid tumors of the biliary tree, endolymphatic sac tumors, and pheochromocytomas (22,23,26,64). The gene responsible for the development of VHL syndrome is on chromosome 3p25, and it encodes for a protein that promotes the degradation of hypoxia-inducible factor (HIF) (41). Inactivation of the *VHL* gene increases HIF levels and thereby promotes the formation of blood vessels through the increased production of factors such as vascular endothelial growth factor (VEGF).

Pancreatic involvement is seen in 50 to 80 percent of patients with the VHL syndrome (11, 23,28,47,49,50,72). The cystic pancreatic lesions usually do not cause symptoms and in most cases do not require treatment. Nonetheless, these pancreatic lesions are important to recognize because they can develop before the CNS lesions and, therefore, can be the first clue to

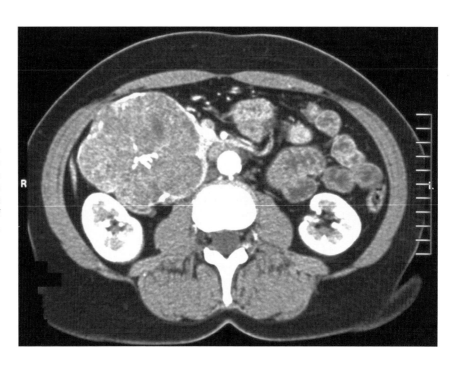

Figure 4-1

MICROCYSTIC SEROUS CYSTADENOMA

As seen on computerized tomography (CT), this well-demarcated, cystic, low attenuation mass in the head of the pancreas has delicate septa and coarse central calcification. (Courtesy of Dr. S. S. Siegelman, Baltimore, MD.)

the diagnosis of VHL syndrome (11,23,28,47, 49,50,72). Patients with VHL syndrome can develop a range of pancreatic lesions including diffuse cystic replacement of the gland, serous cystadenomas, endocrine neoplasms, and the combined well-differentiated endocrine neoplasm-serous cystadenoma (11,23,28,47,49,50,72). The cysts are often multifocal, and the presence of multiple pancreatic cysts should suggest the diagnosis of VHL syndrome (11,23,28,47,49,50,72). Many of these pancreatic cysts have the appearance of macrocystic serous cystadenoma and many express inhibin (11,23,28,47,49,50,72).

A single case of Evans' syndrome, a syndrome characterized by autoimmune hemolytic anemia combined with idiopathic thrombocytic purpura, has been reported in a patient with a serous cystadenoma (15). In this patient the clinical syndrome resolved after the adenoma was resected.

No significant racial associations have been reported. There does not appear to be an association between cigarette smoking and serous cystic neoplasms.

Clinical Features. Most microcystic serous cystadenomas present as large abdominal masses (3,5,13,14,27,42,63,73). Some grow so large that they can be palpated on physical examination. The most common symptoms include abdominal pain, early satiety, weight loss, dyspepsia,

and nausea and vomiting. Less common are obstructive jaundice, acute pancreatitis, and gastrointestinal bleeding. Some patients with the VHL syndrome develop diabetes mellitus from diffuse involvement of the gland. Up to one third of patients with microcystic serous cystadenomas are asymptomatic and the neoplasm is discovered incidentally during abdominal surgery or imaging for an unrelated indication (42).

The radiographic manifestations of microcystic serous cystadenoma can be quite characteristic (5,20,31,42,56). CT shows a well-defined mass with microlacunae separated by delicate septa (fig. 4-1) (31,56). The center of the lesion often has a stellate scar, and 10 to 30 percent of these scars show a "sunburst" pattern of calcification (fig. 4-1). Magnetic resonance imaging (MRI) can also demonstrate the cystic nature of these neoplasms. They tend to have low intensity on T1-weighted images and high intensity on T2-weighted images (59). Endoscopic ultrasound (EUS) reveals an echogenic mass with numerous (usually more than six) small (usually less than 2 cm) cysts that produce a characteristic "soap bubble" pattern (31,56,69). Endoscopic retrograde cholangiopancreatography (ERCP) usually, but not always, demonstrates extrinsic compression or "draping" of the pancreatic duct, and the absence of any communications between the

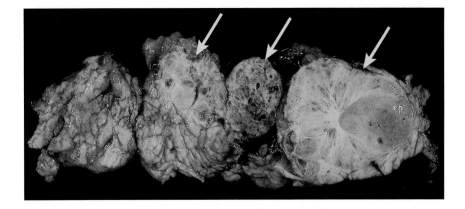

neoplastic cysts and the main pancreatic duct (20, 73). Communication between the cysts and the pancreatic duct can, however, be demonstrated in rare cases (19,24,59). Most microcystic serous cystadenomas are hypervascular on angiography (31,73). Despite the often typical radiographic appearance of most cases, misdiagnosis based on preoperative imaging is still as high as 25 to 50 percent (5,56).

Serum cancer markers, including carcinoembryonic antigen (CEA), carbohydrate antigen (CA) 19-9, and CA125 are almost never elevated in patients with serous cystadenomas (4,42). Analysis of aspirated cyst fluid for pancreatic enzymes and CEA may be helpful in preoperatively distinguishing serous cysts from other cystic lesions in the pancreas (43). The cyst fluid from serous and mucinous cystic neoplasms has both pancreatic and salivary isoenzymes, while pseudocysts contain only pancreatic isoenzymes. The cyst fluid from serous cystadenomas and pseudocysts consistently has low CEA levels (less than 100 ng/ml), while mucinous cysts generally have CEA levels above 100 ng/ml (55,68).

Gross Findings. Microcystic serous cystadenomas involve the head and body/tail of the gland at about the same frequency (3,5,13,14, 27,42,63,73). The majority are solitary; however, multifocal disease has been reported and is especially common in patients with the VHL syndrome (fig. 4-2) (11,23,28,47,49,50,72).

Most microcystic serous cystadenomas have an almost diagnostic gross appearance. They tend to be large (mean, 6 cm; range, microscopic to 30 cm), well-demarcated, somewhat bosselated masses (3,5,13,27,42,63,73). They are composed of innumerable small (usually less than 2

mm up to 1 cm), thin-walled cysts, imparting a sponge-like or honeycomb appearance on cross section (figs. 4-3-4-5). The cysts are filled with clear, watery, straw-colored (serous) fluid and are separated by thin fibrovascular septa. The center of the neoplasms may contain a stellate scar that is often calcified (fig. 4-4). Toward the periphery of the neoplasm the cysts tend to be larger, sometimes measuring centimeters in size. As noted earlier, the cysts do not usually communicate with the pancreatic duct system (fig. 4-3). The pancreatic parenchyma adjacent to the neoplasm often shows obstructive changes from the mass lesion, including chronic pancreatitis and fatty replacement. Rarely, particularly if they have been previously biopsied, some microcystic serous cystadenomas have an infarcted center with subtotal macrocystic degeneration, resembling a pseudocyst.

Rare serous cystadenomas are composed of only a few large (greater than 1.0 cm) cysts or even a single large cyst (see macrocystic variant), and exceptional cases have a solid (noncystic) gross appearance (see solid variant) (54).

Microscopic Findings. The cysts of serous cystadenomas are lined by a single layer of uniform, clear cuboidal cells (fig. 4-6) (3,5,13,14,27, 42,63,73). These cells usually form flat sheets and only rarely form microscopic papillae that project into the cysts (fig. 4-7) (3,5,13,27,42,58,63,73). The neoplastic cells have clear cytoplasm because they contain abundant intracytoplasmic glycogen. In rare cases, the cytoplasm of the neoplastic cells has an eosinophilic, almost oncocytic, appearance (fig. 4-8) (2). Some locules may be lined by a flattened epithelial layer, with cells resembling simple squamous epithelium and lacking significant clear cytoplasm,

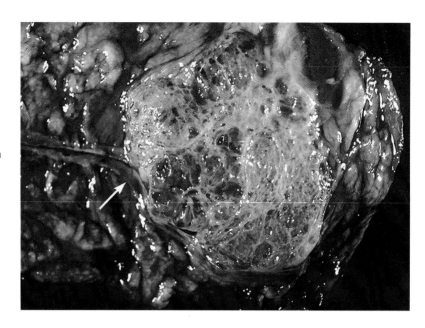

Figure 4-3

**MICROCYSTIC
SEROUS CYSTADENOMA**

The cysts do not communicate with
the main pancreatic duct (arrow).

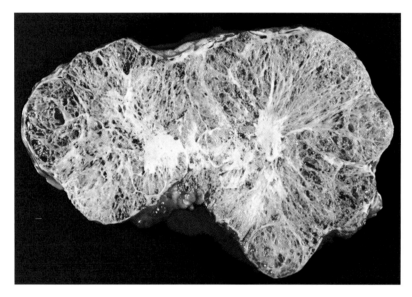

Figure 4-4

**MICROCYSTIC
SEROUS CYSTADENOMA**

The neoplasm is well-demarcated,
composed of innumerable small cysts,
and has a large central stellate scar. This
example measured 27 cm.

but the more typical clear cells can generally be
found elsewhere in the lesion without difficulty.
The nuclei are small and round, and have uniform hyperchromatic chromatin and inconspicuous nucleoli. Atypia and mitoses are usually absent, although nuclear enlargement without pleomorphism may be seen. The central
stellate scar and the stroma separating the cysts
are composed mostly of acellular collagenous
connective tissue, but the stroma may contain
entrapped islets of Langerhans and acini. As
noted earlier, some microcystic serous cystadenomas, particularly those that have been pre-

viously biopsied, have an infarcted center. In
these cases, a rim of surviving neoplastic cells
can usually be appreciated at the outer edge of
the lesion, outside the fibroinflammatory
pseudocapsule that lines the cystic space (fig.
4-9). A rare case with amyloid deposition in the
stroma has been reported (70).

The pancreatic parenchyma adjacent to serous cystadenomas is often atrophic, particularly if the pancreatic duct has been obstructed.
It is also common for the smaller adjacent pancreatic ducts to harbor foci of low-grade pancreatic intraepithelial neoplasia (PanIN) (67a).

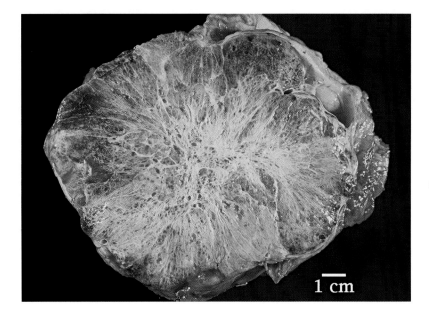

Figure 4-5

**MICROCYSTIC
SEROUS CYSTADENOMA**

The cysts are so small that it is
difficult to distinguish individual cysts.

Figure 4-6

**MICROCYSTIC SEROUS
CYSTADENOMA**

The cysts contain proteinaceous fluid and are lined by
cuboidal epithelium with clear
cytoplasm.

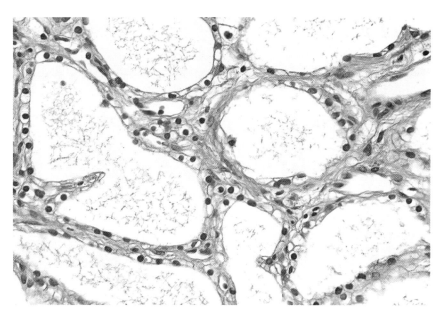

Special stains highlight the abundant
intraepithelial glycogen and absence of stain-
able mucin. The periodic acid–Schiff (PAS) stain
is strongly positive and is sensitive to diastase
digestion (fig. 4-10) (3,5,13,27,42,63,73). Stains
for mucin, including mucicarmine and Alcian
blue, are negative, as are histochemical stains
for neuroendocrine differentiation, including
the Grimelius stain (3,5,13,27,42,63,73).

Histologic Types. Four variants of serous
cystadenoma have been described.

Macrocystic Serous Cystadenoma. This variant
is also known as *oligocystic serous cystadenoma*
and *serous oligocystic and ill-demarcated adenoma*
(12,16,35,38,44,60,67). As these names imply,
this variant of serous cystadenoma is characterized by cysts that are larger, less well defined,
and fewer in number than those of the typical
microcystic serous cystadenoma (fig. 4-11). The
cysts in macrocystic serous cystadenoma measure centimeters, not millimeters, and there can
be as few as one locule (so called unilocular

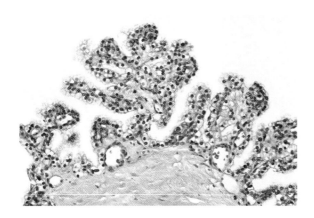

Figure 4-7

MICROCYSTIC SEROUS CYSTADENOMA

The neoplastic epithelium forms micropapillae.

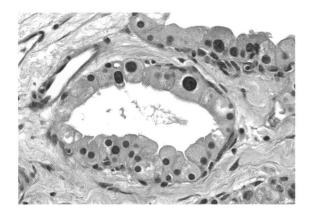

Figure 4-8

MICROCYSTIC SEROUS CYSTADENOMA

Focal oncocytic differentiation and cells with granular pink cytoplasm.

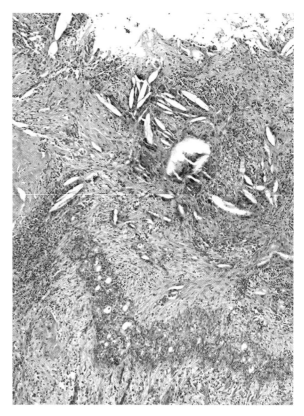

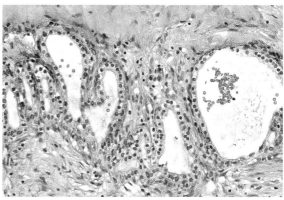

Figure 4-9

MICROCYSTIC SEROUS CYSTADENOMA

Significant degenerative changes are seen at the center of the neoplasm (top) following fine needle aspiration, but a rim of viable neoplastic epithelium remains (bottom).

variant). Because they tend to form larger cysts, macrocystic serous cystadenomas can radiographically and grossly mimic mucinous cystic neoplasms and intraductal papillary mucinous neoplasm of the branch duct type (36,44,67). Macrocystic serous cystadenomas do not have a central stellate scar, and they tend to be poorly circumscribed, often extending into and entrapping adjacent pancreatic parenchyma between the cysts. They involve the head of the gland more than the standard microcystic serous cystadenomas (12). The epithelial cells of this lesion are identical to those in microcystic serous cystadenomas. The cysts are lined by a single layer of uniform clear

cuboidal cells (figs. 4-12, 4-13). The cells contain abundant intracytoplasmic glycogen, and immunohistochemically label for epithelial membrane antigen (EMA), and for cytokeratins (CKs) 7, 8, 18, and 19 (16,60). Macrocystic serous cystadenomas, like their standard microcystic counterparts, are benign.

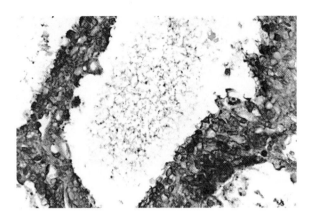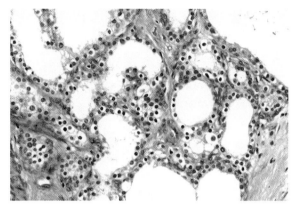

Figure 4-10

MICROCYSTIC SEROUS CYSTADENOMA

Periodic acid–Schiff (PAS) staining without (left) and with (right) diastase digestion highlights the abundant glycogen.

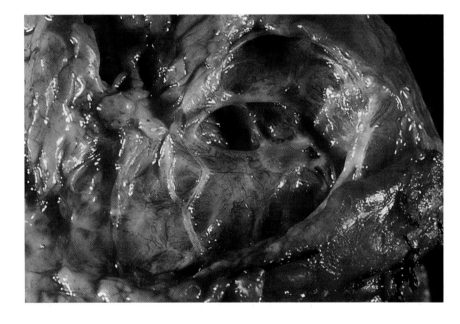

Figure 4-11

**MACROCYSTIC
SEROUS CYSTADENOMA**

The cysts are larger than 1 cm.

Solid Serous Adenoma. This is a grossly solid neoplasm (fig. 4-14) composed of cells morphologically similar to those of microcystic serous cystadenomas (54). In solid serous adenomas, clear to pale polygonal to cuboidal cells form nests, sheets, and trabeculae (figs. 4-15, 4-16) (54). The cells also form small acini, but macroscopic cyst formation is not seen. The nuclear features are identical to those of other serous neoplasms. They are strongly PAS positive and sensitive to diastase digestion (fig. 4-17).

Combined Well-Differentiated Endocrine Neoplasm/Serous Cystadenoma. This variant usually occurs in patients with VHL syndrome (65). As the name suggests, these neoplasms have two components: well-differentiated pancreatic endocrine neoplasm and a serous cystadenoma (fig. 4-18) (65). The two components can be adjacent to each other, or intimately admixed (fig. 4-19). Immunohistochemical labeling highlights the two components of this neoplasm: the well-differentiated endocrine component strongly and diffusely expresses chromogranin, while the serous component does not. It is not clear whether these rare cases represent true mixed neoplasms with both exocrine and endocrine differentiation, or whether they may simply be coincidental "collision" tumors arising

Figure 4-12

MACROCYSTIC SEROUS CYSTADENOMA

A single, large (over 1 cm) cyst is present in the upper left corner.

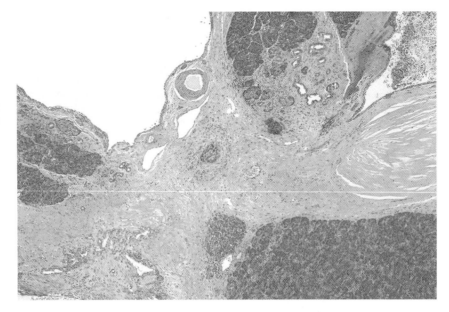

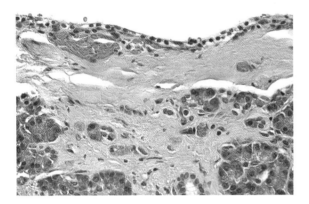

Figure 4-13

MACROCYSTIC SEROUS CYSTADENOMA

Although fewer and larger than in the microcystic variant, the cysts are lined by the same cuboidal cells with clear cytoplasm.

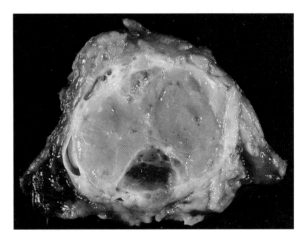

Figure 4-14

SOLID SEROUS ADENOMA

Only a few small cysts are seen.

in VHL patients who are predisposed to both serous cystadenomas and endocrine neoplasms.

VHL-Associated Cystic Neoplasms. It has been suggested that the serous cystic neoplasms seen in patients with VHL syndrome should be separately designated (11,23,28,38,39,47,49,50,72). Serous cystic neoplasms occur at a younger age (mean, 42 years) in patients with VHL syndrome, and, as discussed earlier, they tend to be multifocal and may even diffusely involve the entire gland (38). They often have a macrocystic appearance. The epithelial cells of VHL-associated cystic neoplasms are identical to those in non-VHL-associated serous cystadenomas. A single layer of uniform clear cuboidal cells lines the cysts. The cells contain abundant intracytoplasmic glycogen, and immunohistochemically label for EMA, inhibin, and CK7, CK8, CK18, and CK19. These neoplasms appear to be identical to some of the "congenital pancreatic cysts" of VHL patients.

Immunohistochemical Findings. Serous cystadenomas strongly express cytokeratin. They label with pancytokeratin markers (AE1/

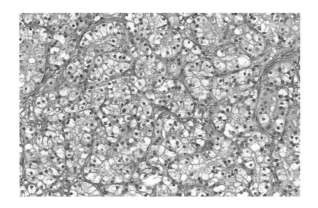

Figure 4-15

SOLID SEROUS ADENOMA

The cells form small acini, but cyst formation is not seen.

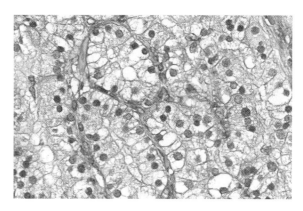

Figure 4-16

SOLID SEROUS ADENOMA

The nuclei are small, round, and uniform.

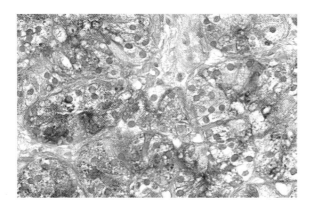

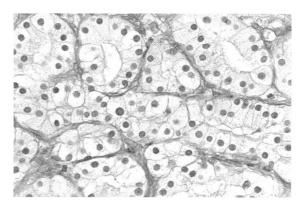

Figure 4-17

SOLID SEROUS ADENOMA

Positivity for PAS without (left) and with (right) diastase digestion confirms the abundant intracytoplasmic glycogen.

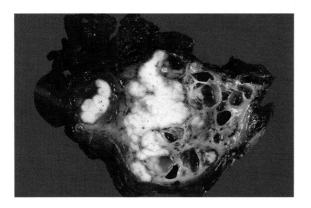

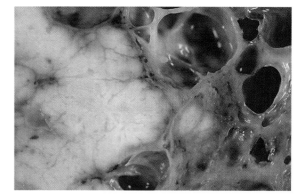

Figure 4-18

COMBINED WELL-DIFFERENTIATED ENDOCRINE NEOPLASM/SEROUS CYSTADENOMA

Gross cross-section (left) and close-up (right) views demonstrate both a cystic component (right) and solid endocrine component (left). (Courtesy of Dr. Noriyoshi Fukushima, Tokyo, Japan.)

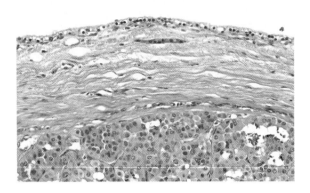

Figure 4-19

COMBINED WELL-DIFFERENTIATED
ENDOCRINE NEOPLASM/SEROUS CYSTADENOMA

The serous epithelium is cuboidal (top), while the endocrine component forms nests (bottom).

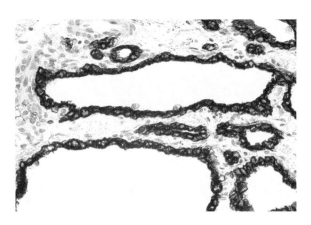

Figure 4-20

MICROCYSTIC SEROUS CYSTADENOMA

Immunolabeling using a pancytokeratin decorates the neoplastic cells.

AE3), as well as with CAM5.2 and antibodies to CK7, CK8, CK18, and CK19 (fig. 4-20) (3,14,16, 39,63). In most cases, the neoplastic cells also express alpha-inhibin and MUC6 (39). A third of the cases express EMA (39). Neuron-specific enolase is not a useful marker as reports on the percentage of serous cystadenomas immunolabeling for this marker have varied from no labeling to 100 percent. Immunolabeling for CEA is usually negative, as is immunolabeling for MUC2, MUC5, chromogranin, synaptophysin, insulin, glucagon, somatostatin, vasoactive intestinal polypeptide (VIP), CD31, factor VIII, HMB-45, S-100 protein, vimentin, and CK20 (39). A few widely scattered endocrine cells, however, are commonly detected within serous cystadenomas by immunolabeling for chromogranin or synaptophysin. The Ki-67 labeling index is usually very low, and immunolabeling for the protein product of the *TP53* gene, p53, is usually negative (normal) (18,30, 48). Immunolabeling for the beta-catenin gene product demonstrates a normal membranous pattern of labeling (37). The stroma contains scattered myofibroblasts that express actin, but, in contrast to mucinous cystic neoplasms, the stromal cells do not express alpha-inhibin, calretinin, and estrogen and progesterone receptors (39,76).

The immunolabeling patterns of the histologic subtypes of serous cystadenoma are similar, with the exception of the combined well-differentiated endocrine neoplasm/serous cys-

tadenoma, which expresses markers of endocrine differentiation, including chromogranin, in the well-differentiated endocrine component (10,16,34,60).

Ultrastructural Findings. As one would expect from the light microscopic appearance of these neoplasms, ultrastructural examination reveals a single layer of cuboidal cells with centrally located round nuclei (fig. 4-21) (3,7,13, 63). These cells sit on a well-formed basement membrane, have short blunt microvilli, and show evidence of epithelial differentiation including well-formed desmosomes and tight junctions. Most organelles are sparse, and instead the neoplastic cells are filled with abundant intracytoplasmic glycogen (3,7,13,63). These ultrastructural findings suggest centroacinar ductal differentiation. The subtypes of serous cystadenomas have a similar ultrastructural appearance (35,60).

A single case in which prominent myoepithelial cells were associated with the neoplastic epithelial cells has been reported (52).

Cytologic Findings. The fluid aspirated from serous cystadenomas is generally clear and thin, not mucoid, but it may be bloody. Smears are characteristically paucicellular and even acellular. Smears may be considered inadequate for interpretation due to insufficient cellularity. Hemosiderin-laden macrophages are often present and may be the only cells in the aspirate. Aspirated epithelial cells form small clusters and flat sheets

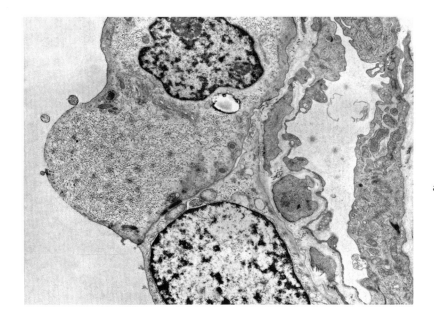

Figure 4-21

MICROCYSTIC SEROUS CYSTADENOMA

Ultrastructural image shows abundant intracellular glycogen.

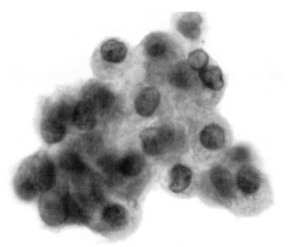

Figure 4-22

MICROCYSTIC SEROUS CYSTADENOMA

Aspirate smears are typically scant, with a nonmucinous background and few, often widely scattered small clusters of cuboidal cells. The cuboidal cells have bland nuclei and nonmucinous cytoplasm (direct smear; Papanicolaou stain).

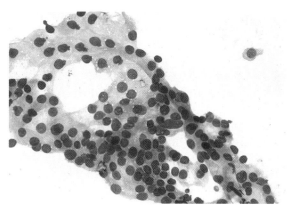

Figure 4-23

MICROCYSTIC SEROUS CYSTADENOMA

The cuboidal cells of the neoplasm appear larger on air-dried smears but maintain their polygonal shape, with a central nucleus and nonmucinous cytoplasm (direct smear; Romanowsky stain).

consisting of uniform cuboidal cells, with round central to slightly eccentric nuclei and scant but visible cytoplasm. The cytoplasm is homogenous to finely vacuolated on Papanicolaou (fig. 4-22) and Romanowsky (fig. 4-23) stains. The nuclei have smooth nuclear membranes, an even chromatin pattern, and inconspicuous to no nucleoli (fig. 4-24) (25,40,46,51). Even a few such groups in a scantily cellular smear can be diagnostic in the appropriate clinical setting. The absence of bloody, inflammatory debris, as would be expected in a pseudocyst, and the absence of background mucin and mucinous glandular epithelium, as would be expected in a mucinous cystic neoplasm or intraductal papillary mucinous neoplasm, are helpful negative cytologic findings. Care must be taken not to interpret gastrointestinal epithelium commonly obtained during endoscopically guided biopsies as originating from the cyst.

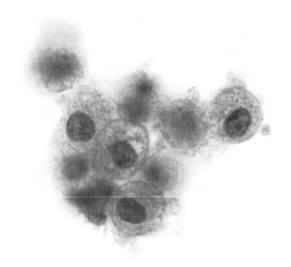

Figure 4-24

MICROCYSTIC SEROUS CYSTADENOMA

The individual cells are bland and obviously benign appearing, with homogeneous chromatin and absent or inconspicuous nucleoli. The cytoplasm may be finely vacuolated but mucin vacuoles are absent (direct smear; Papanicolaou stain).

Molecular and Other Special Techniques. As mentioned earlier, serous cystadenomas are associated with the VHL syndrome (11,23,28,47, 49,50,72). From Knudson's hypothesis it should not be surprising that biallelic inactivation of the *VHL* gene has been reported both in serous cystadenomas that arise in patients with VHL (syndromic adenomas) and in patients without VHL (nonsyndromic or sporadic adenomas) (37,47). Mohr et al. (47) reported deletion of the wild-type *VHL* allele in a series of pancreatic cystic lesions that arose in three patients with the VHL syndrome, and loss of heterozygosity on chromosome 3p25 has been reported in 40 to 70 percent of sporadic serous cystadenomas (37, 48,72). Frequent (50 percent) loss of heterozygosity has also been reported on chromosome 10q (48). By contrast, activating point mutations in the *KRAS* oncogene and inactivation of the *TP53* tumor suppressor gene have not been reported in serous cystadenomas, and these neoplasms exhibit a normal membranous pattern of labeling for the beta-catenin gene product (18,30,37,48,60).

Almost all serous cystadenomas are microsatellite stable and have a remarkably low mean fractional allelic loss of only 0.08 (48). It fol-lows that most are diploid and have a low S-phase by flow cytometry (18). Occasional aneuploid serous cystic neoplasms have been reported, but this finding appears to have no prognostic significance (71).

Differential Diagnosis. Given the characteristic gross and microscopic appearance of serous cystadenomas, diagnosing a resected specimen is usually relatively straightforward. Establishing the correct preoperative diagnosis of a cystic lesion in the pancreas is important for clinical management, and a broad differential diagnosis should be kept in mind.

Mucinous cystic neoplasms, because of their significantly greater malignant potential, are probably the most important neoplasms to consider in the differential diagnosis. In particular, macrocystic serous cystadenomas, because they are composed of larger cysts, can grossly mimic mucinous cystic neoplasms. While both serous and mucinous cystic neoplasms are cystic, the cysts in mucinous cystic neoplasms tend to be larger, thicker walled, and filled with thick tenacious fluid, not the clear watery fluid of serous cystadenomas. Microcystic serous cystadenomas often have a central stellate scar; however, this helpful feature is not always present and is usually not present in the macrocystic serous variant. At the microscopic level, mucinous cystic neoplasms are lined by tall columnar cells containing abundant mucin, while the lining of serous cystadenomas is cuboidal and glycogen-rich. Mucicarmine and other stains for mucin will stain mucinous cystic neoplasms but not serous cystadenomas. Both neoplasms express cytokeratin, but only the mucinous cystic neoplasms are CEA positive. In cases in which the epithelium is extensively denuded, the presence of ovarian-type stroma establishes the diagnosis of a mucinous cystic neoplasm.

Lymphangioma should also be considered in the differential diagnosis. Both lymphangiomas and serous cystadenomas can be cystic and both can contain serous fluid. Although some locules of serous cystadenomas have cells with minimal cytoplasm, the cells lining the cysts in lymphangiomas are uniformly flat, without a population of cuboidal clear cells, and lymphangiomas characteristically contain lymphoid aggregates in the cyst walls. When needed, immunohistochemical labeling can be used to distinguish between the two entities. Lymphangiomas label for CD31 and factor VIII–related antigen, while serous cystadenomas express cytokeratin.

Macrocystic serous cystadenomas need to be distinguished from ductal retention cysts. Retention cysts are non-neoplastic, unilocular cysts lined by normal ductal epithelium, and they may be multiple. Since not all locules of serous cystadenomas have an obvious clear cell lining, careful examination of multiple sections may be necessary to differentiate these lesions.

Most serous cystadenomas are clearly lined by epithelium, but in some cases there is extensive central macrocystic degeneration, resulting in a pseudocyst-like lining (see fig. 4-9). Recognition that there remain in the wall of the cyst strands of tubular glands lined by characteristic clear cells will help avoid the misdiagnosis as a pseudocyst.

Solid serous adenomas need to be distinguished from well-differentiated pancreatic endocrine neoplasms and from metastatic renal cell carcinoma, especially in patients with the VHL syndrome. Neuroendocrine markers, including chromogranin A and synaptophysin, are positive in well-differentiated pancreatic endocrine neoplasms, and metastatic renal cell carcinoma usually demonstrates significant pleomorphism, more frequent mitoses, more prominent nucleoli, and immunolabeling for vimentin, renal cell carcinoma marker (RCCma), and CD10.

Finally, although they are extremely rare, PEComas of the pancreas (primary extrapulmonary sugar tumors) should also be considered in the differential diagnosis (78). PEComas can have clear cytoplasm, but are cytokeratin negative and HMB-45 positive.

Treatment. Because the malignant potential of serous cystadenomas is so low, the treatment is largely dictated by the patient's symptoms (5,61). Surgical resection is the treatment of choice for large, symptomatic tumors, while smaller asymptomatic serous lesions are often followed clinically. In most instances, patients who are followed clinically do not require surgery. Le Borgne et al. (42) reported 26 patients with unresected serous cystadenomas who were followed for a mean of 38 months, and none required surgery. In some cases, however, the neoplasm may grow gradually (median growth rate about 0.6 cm/year) (70a) and eventually

require surgical intervention. The clinical diagnosis of cystic neoplasms is imperfect, and most of the other cystic neoplasms of the pancreas have a significant malignant potential. It is imperative that the diagnosis is well established before observing a patient with a cystic neoplasm in the pancreas.

Prognosis. The prognosis for patients with serous cystadenomas of the pancreas is excellent (3,5,13,27,42,63,73). Compagno and Oertel (13), in their landmark study, followed 34 patients for a mean of 6½ years. Only four patients died from their disease. The causes of death included gastrointestinal bleeding from erosion of the neoplasm into the duodenum, malabsorption, and obstruction of the biliary tree. An equal number of patients died from complications of their surgery. Complete surgical resection almost always leads to a cure; less than 2 percent of serous cystadenomas recur (8,42,53,75,77). There are no known gross and morphologic features, other than the clinical behavior of the neoplasms, that can be used to distinguish serous cystadenoma from serous cystadenocarcinoma.

SEROUS CYSTADENOCARCINOMA

Definition. *Serous cystadenocarcinoma* is a malignant epithelial neoplasm composed of uniform cuboidal, glycogen-rich cells that usually form numerous small cysts containing serous fluid (9,32,66). Malignancy is defined by the presence of metastases to extrapancreatic organs or tissues.

General Features. Although extremely rare, serous cystic neoplasms of the pancreas involving lymph nodes and the liver have been reported and form the basis for the designation serous cystadenocarcinoma (1,21,53,74,75,77). Most patients are slightly older (range, 56 to 72 years) than patients with serous cystadenoma, and males and females are equally represented in reported cases.

Vascular and perineural invasion, and invasion into the duodenum or stomach, although signs of potentially aggressive behavior, are not sufficient to diagnose malignancy.

Clinical Features. In addition to the clinical presentation described for serous cystadenomas, these patients are more likely to present with gastrointestinal bleeding, jaundice, or a very large abdominal mass.

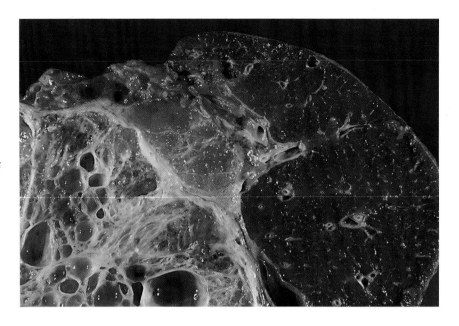

Figure 4-25

SEROUS CYSTADENOCARCINOMA

Invasion into the splenic hilum.

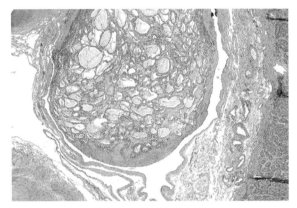

Figure 4-26

SEROUS CYSTADENOCARCINOMA

Invasion into the stomach (right).

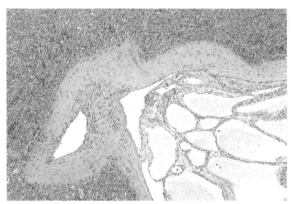

Figure 4-27

SEROUS CYSTADENOCARCINOMA

Invasion into the spleen.

Gross Findings. Serous cystadenocarcinomas tend to be large and frequently invade adjacent organs, including the duodenum, stomach, and spleen (figs. 4-25–4-27). Metastases are by definition present. Common sites of metastasis include the lymph nodes, the peritoneum, and the liver.

Microscopic Findings. Most reported cases of serous cystadenocarcinoma are remarkably bland and histologically identical to serous cystadenomas. Mitoses are not numerous, and only mild cytologic atypia is seen. Perineural and vascular invasion may be identified, and when

present in a serous cystic neoplasm, should suggest the possibility of aggressive behavior.

The diagnosis of malignancy in a serous cystic neoplasm should be established only when there are unequivocal metastases to extrapancreatic organs or tissues.

Immunohistochemical Findings. The immunolabeling profile of serous cystadenocarcinomas is identical to that of serous cystadenomas.

Ultrastructural Findings. The ultrastructural features of serous cystadenocarcinomas are identical to those of serous cystadenomas.

Cytologic Findings. The cytologic features of this tumor have not been well described. Given the histologic similarity between benign and malignant serous tumors, the cytologic features would also be expected to be the same.

Molecular and Other Special Techniques. No genetic alterations have been identified that can distinguish serous cystadenomas from serous cystadenocarcinomas.

Differential Diagnosis. The major neoplasm to consider in the differential diagnosis of serous cystadenocarcinoma is its benign counterpart, serous cystadenoma. The behavior of the neoplasm is the only way to make this distinction. Only those serous cystic neoplasms that metastasize to extrapancreatic organs or tissues should be considered malignant.

Treatment and Prognosis. These are slow-growing, indolent neoplasms and the vast majority of patients do not die of their disease (1,21, 53,74,75,77). Surgical resection of symptomatic disease may be helpful. Staging follows the staging of carcinomas of the exocrine pancreas. Locally aggressive serous cystic neoplasms are technically not classified as serous cystadenocarcinoma. Nonetheless, patients with locally aggressive tumors probably should be monitored clinically for disease recurrence following surgical resection.

REFERENCES

1. Abe H, Kubota K, Mori M, et al. Serous cystadenoma of the pancreas with invasive growth: benign or malignant? Am J Gastroenterol 1998;93:1963-6.

2. Albores-Saavedra J, Gould EW, Angeles-Angeles A, Henson DE. Cystic tumors of the pancreas. Pathol Annu 1990;25:19-50.

3. Alpert LC, Truong LD, Bossart MI, Spjut HJ. Microcystic adenoma (serous cystadenoma) of the pancreas. A study of 14 cases with immunohistochemical and electron-microscopic correlation. Am J Surg Pathol 1988;12:251-63.

4. Bassi C, Salvia R, Gumbs AA, Butturini G, Falconi M, Pederzoli P. The value of standard serum tumor markers in differentiating mucinous from serous cystic tumors of the pancreas: CEA, Ca 19-9, Ca 125, Ca 15-3. Langenbecks Arch Surg 2002;387:281-5.

5. Bassi C, Salvia R, Molinari E, Biasutti C, Falconi M, Pederzoli P. Management of 100 consecutive cases of pancreatic serous cystadenoma: wait for symptoms and see at imaging or vice versa? World J Surg 2003;27:319-23.

6. Becker WF, Welsh RA, Pratt HS. Cystadenoma and cystadenocarcinoma of the pancreas. Ann Surg 1965;161:845-63.

7. Bogomoletz WV, Adnet JJ, Widgren S, Stavrou M, McLaughlin JE. Cystadenoma of the pancreas: a histological, histochemical and ultrastructural study of seven cases. Histopathology 1980;4:309-20.

8. Brenin DR, Talamonti MS, Yang EY, et al. Cystic neoplasms of the pancreas. A clinicopathologic study, including DNA flow cytometry. Arch Surg 1995;130:1048-54.

9. Capella C, Solcia E, Klöppel G, Hruban RH. Serous cystic neoplasms of the pancreas. In: Hamilton SR, Aaltonen LA, eds. World Health Organization classification of tumours. Pathology and genetics of tumours of the digestive system. Lyon: IARC Press; 2000:231-3.

10. Chatelain D, Hammel P, O'Toole D, et al. Macrocystic form of serous pancreatic cystadenoma. Am J Gastroenterol 2002;97:2566-71.

11. Cheng TY, Su CH, Shyr YM, Lui WY. Management of pancreatic lesions in von Hippel-Lindau disease. World J Surg 1997;21:307-12.

12. Cohen-Scali F, Vilgrain V, Brancatelli G, et al. Discrimination of unilocular macrocystic serous cystadenoma from pancreatic pseudocyst and mucinous cystadenoma with CT: initial observations. Radiology 2003;228:727-33.

13. Compagno J, Oertel JE. Microcystic adenomas of the pancreas (glycogen-rich cystadenomas): a clinicopathologic study of 34 cases. Am J Clin Pathol 1978;69:289-98.

14. Compton CC. Serous cystic tumors of the pancreas. Semin Diagn Pathol 2000;17:43-55.

15. Doll DC, List AF, Yarbro JW. Evans' syndrome associated with microcystic adenoma of the pancreas. Cancer 1987;59:1366-8.

16. Egawa N, Maillet B, Schroder S, Mukai K, Klöppel G. Serous oligocystic and ill-demarcated adenoma of the pancreas: a variant of serous cystic adenoma. Virchows Arch 1994;424:13-7.

17. Eriguchi N, Aoyagi S, Nakayama T, et al. Serous cystadenocarcinoma of the pancreas with liver metastases. J Hepatobiliary Pancreat Surg 1998;5:467-70.

18. Flejou JF, Boulange B, Bernades P, Belghiti J, Henin D. p53 protein expression and DNA ploidy in cystic tumors of the pancreas. Pancreas 1996;13:247-52.

19. Furukawa H, Takayasu K, Mukai K, et al. Serous cystadenoma of the pancreas communicating with a pancreatic duct. Int J Pancreatol 1996;19:141-4.

20. Gazelle GS, Mueller PR, Raafat N, Halpern EF, Cardenosa G, Warshaw AL. Cystic neoplasms of the pancreas: evaluation with endoscopic retrograde pancreatography. Radiology 1993;188:633-6.

21. George DH, Murphy F, Michalski R, Ulmer BG. Serous cystadenocarcinoma of the pancreas: a new entity? Am J Surg Pathol 1989;13:61-6.

22. Gilcrease MZ, Schmidt L, Zbar B, Truong L, Rutledge M, Wheeler TM. Somatic von Hippel-Lindau mutation in clear cell papillary cystadenoma of the epididymis. Hum Pathol 1995;26:1341-6.

23. Hammel PR, Vilgrain V, Terris B, et al. Pancreatic involvement in von Hippel-Lindau disease. The Groupe Francophone d'Etude de la Maladie de von Hippel-Lindau. Gastroenterology 2000;119:1087-95.

24. Hashimoto M, Watanabe G, Miura Y, Matsuda M, Takeuchi K, Mori M. Macrocystic type of serous cystadenoma with a communication between the cyst and pancreatic duct. J Gastroenterol Hepatol 2001;16:836-8.

25. Hittmair A, Pernthaler H, Totsch M, Schmid KW. Preoperative fine needle aspiration cytology of a microcystic adenoma of the pancreas. Acta Cytol 1991;35:546-8.

26. Hoang MP, Hruban RH, Albores-Saavedra J. Clear cell endocrine pancreatic tumor mimicking renal cell carcinoma: a distinctive neoplasm of von Hippel-Lindau disease. Am J Surg Pathol 2001;25:602-9.

27. Hodgkinson DJ, ReMine WH, Weiland LH. Pancreatic cystadenoma. A clinicopathologic study of 45 cases. Arch Surg 1978;113:512-9.

28. Hough DM, Stephens DH, Johnson CD, Binkovitz LA. Pancreatic lesions in von Hippel-Lindau disease: prevalence, clinical significance, and CT findings. AJR Am J Roentgenol 1994;162:1091-4.

29. Howard JM, Hess W. History of the pancreas: mysteries of a hidden organ. New York: Kluwer Academic/Plenum Publishers; 2002.

30. Ishikawa T, Nakao A, Nomoto S, et al. Immunohistochemical and molecular biological studies of serous cystadenoma of the pancreas. Pancreas 1998;16:40-4.

31. Itai Y, Ohhashi K, Furui S, et al. Microcystic adenoma of the pancreas: spectrum of computed tomographic findings. J Comput Assist Tomogr 1988;12:797-803.

32. Japanese Pancreas Society. Classification of pancreatic carcinoma, 2nd English ed. Tokyo: Kanehara & Co., Ltd.; 2003.

33. Kamei K, Funabiki T, Ochiai M, Amano H, Kasahara M, Sakamoto T. Multifocal pancreatic serous cystadenoma with atypical cells and focal perineural invasion. Int J Pancreatol 1991; 10:161-72.

34. Keel SB, Zukerberg L, Graeme-Cook F, Compton CC. A pancreatic endocrine tumor arising within a serous cystadenoma of the pancreas. Am J Surg Pathol 1996;20:471-5.

35. Khadaroo R, Knetman N, Joy S, Nguyen GK. Macrocystic serous adenoma of the pancreas. Pathol Res Pract 2002;198:485-8.

36. Khurana B, Mortele KJ, Glickman J, Silverman SG, Ros PR. Macrocystic serous adenoma of the pancreas: radiologic-pathologic correlation. AJR Am J Roentgenol 2003;181:119-23.

37. Kim SG, Wu TT, Lee JH, et al. Comparison of epigenetic and genetic alterations in mucinous cystic neoplasm and serous microcystic adenoma of pancreas. Mod Pathol 2003;16:1086-94.

38. Klöppel G, Kosmahl M. Cystic lesions and neoplasms of the pancreas. The features are becoming clearer. Pancreatology 2001;1:648-55.

39. Kosmahl M, Wagner J, Peters K, Sipos B, Klöppel G. Serous cystic neoplasms of the pancreas: an immunohistochemical analysis revealing alpha-inhibin, neuron-specific enolase and MUC6 as new markers. Am J Surg Pathol 2004;28:339-46.

40. Lal A, Bourtsos EP, DeFrias DV, Nemcek AA, Nayar R. Microcystic adenoma of the pancreas: clinical, radiologic, and cytologic features. Cancer 2004;102:288-94.

41. Latif F, Tory K, Gnarra J, et al. Identification of the von Hippel-Lindau disease tumor suppressor gene. Science 1993;260:1317-20.

42. Le Borgne J, de Calan L, Partensky C. Cystadenomas and cystadenocarcinomas of the pancreas: a multiinstitutional retrospective study of 398 cases. French Surgical Association. Ann Surg 1999;230:152-61.

43. Lewandrowski K, Lee J, Southern J, Centeno BA, Warshaw A. Cyst fluid analysis in the differential diagnosis of pancreatic cysts: a new approach to the preoperative assessment of pancreatic cystic lesions. AJR Am J Roentgenol 1995;164:815-9.

44. Lewandrowski KB, Warshaw A, Compton C. Macrocystic serous cystadenoma of the pancreas: a morphologic variant differing from microcystic adenoma. Hum Pathol 1992;23: 871-5.

45. Lindau A. Studien über Kleinhirncysten. Bau, Pathogenese und Beziehungen zur Angiomatosis Retinae. Acta Pathol Microbiol Scand 1926; 3(Suppl 1):1-128.

46. Logrono R, Vyas SH, Molina CP, Waxman I. Microcystic adenoma of the pancreas: cytologic appearance on percutaneous and endoscopic ultrasound-guided fine-needle aspiration: report of a case. Diagn Cytopathol 1999;20:298-301.

47. Mohr VH, Vortmeyer AO, Zhuang Z, et al. Histopathology and molecular genetics of multiple cysts and microcystic (serous) adenomas of the pancreas in von Hippel-Lindau patients. Am J Pathol 2000;157:1615-21.

48. Moore PS, Zamboni G, Brighenti A, et al. Molecular characterization of pancreatic serous microcystic adenomas: evidence for a tumor suppressor gene on chromosome 10q. Am J Pathol 2001;158:317-21.

49. Mukhopadhyay B, Sahdev A, Monson JP, Besser GM, Reznek RH, Chew SL. Pancreatic lesions in von Hippel-Lindau disease. Clin Endocrinol (Oxf) 2002;57:603-8.

50. Neumann HP, Dinkel E, Brambs H, et al. Pancreatic lesions in the von Hippel-Lindau syndrome. Gastroenterology 1991;101:465-71.

51. Nguyen GK, Vogelsang PJ. Microcystic adenoma of the pancreas. A report of two cases with fine needle aspiration cytology and differential diagnosis. Acta Cytol 1993;37:908-12.

52. Nyongo A, Huntrakoon M. Microcystic adenoma of the pancreas with myoepithelial cells. A hitherto undescribed morphologic feature. Am J Clin Pathol 1985;84:114-20.

53. Okada T, Nonami T, Miwa T, et al. [Hepatic metastasis of serous cystadenocarcinoma resected 4 years after operation—a case report.] Nippon Shokakibyo Gakkai Zasshi 1991;88: 2719-23. [Japanese.]

54. Perez-Ordonez B, Naseem A, Lieberman PH, Klimstra DS. Solid serous adenoma of the pancreas. The solid variant of serous cystadenoma? Am J Surg Pathol 1996;20:1401-5.

55. Pinto MM, Meriano FV. Diagnosis of cystic pancreatic lesions by cytologic examination and carcinoembryonic antigen and amylase assays of cyst contents. Acta Cytol 1991;35:456-63.

56. Procacci C, Graziani R, Bicego E, et al. Serous cystadenoma of the pancreas: report of 30 cases with emphasis on the imaging findings. J Comput Assist Tomogr 1997;21:373-82.

57. Pye-Smith PH. Cyst of the cerebellum with numerous small cysts in the pancreas and the kidneys. Trans R Pathol Soc 1884;36:17-21.

58. Rampy BA, Waxman I, Xiao SY, Logrono R. Serous cystadenoma of the pancreas with papillary features: a diagnostic pitfall on fine-needle aspiration biopsy. Arch Pathol Lab Med 2001;125:1591-4.

59. Samel S, Horst F, Becker H, et al. Serous adenoma of the pancreas with multiple microcysts communicating with the pancreatic duct. HPB Surg 1998;11:43-9.

60. Santos LD, Chow C, Henderson CJ, et al. Serous oligocystic adenoma of the pancreas: a clinicopathological and immunohistochemical study of three cases with ultrastructural findings. Pathology 2002;34:148-56.

61. Sarr MG, Murr M, Smyrk TC, et al. Primary cystic neoplasms of the pancreas. Neoplastic disorders of emerging importance—current state-of-the-art and unanswered questions. J Gastrointest Surg 2003;7:417-28.

62. Sedivy R, Patzak B. Pancreatic diseases past and present: a historical examination of exhibition specimens from the Collectio Rokitansky in Vienna. Virchows Arch 2002;441:12-8.

63. Shorten SD, Hart WR, Petras RE. Microcystic adenomas (serous cystadenomas) of pancreas. A clinicopathologic investigation of eight cases with immunohistochemical and ultrastructural studies. Am J Surg Pathol 1986;10:365-72.

64. Sinkre PA, Murakata L, Rabin L, Hoang MP, Albores-Saavedra J. Clear cell carcinoid tumor of the gallbladder: another distinctive manifestation of von Hippel-Lindau disease. Am J Surg Pathol 2001;25:1334-9.

65. Slukvin II, Hafez GR, Niederhuber JE, Warner TF. Combined serous microcystic adenoma and well-differentiated endocrine pancreatic neoplasm: a case report and review of the literature. Arch Pathol Lab Med 2003;127:1369-72.

66. Solcia E, Capella C, Klöppel G. Tumors of the pancreas. Atlas of Tumor Pathology, 3rd Series, Fascicle 20. Washington, DC: Armed Forces Institute of Pathology; 1997.

67. Sperti C, Pasquali C, Perasole A, Liessi G, Pedrazzoli S. Macrocystic serous cystadenoma of the pancreas: clinicopathologic features in seven cases. Int J Pancreatol 2000;28:1-7.

67a. Stelow EB, Adams RB, Moskaluk CA. The prevalence of pancreatic intraepithelial neoplasia in pancreata with uncommon types of primary neoplasms. Am J Surg Pathol 2006;30:36-41.

68. Tatsuta M, Iishi H, Ichii M, et al. Values of carcinoembryonic antigen, elastase 1, and carbohydrate antigen determinant in aspirated pancreatic cystic fluid in the diagnosis of cysts of the pancreas. Cancer 1986;57:1836-9.

69. Torresan F, Casadei R, Solmi L, Marrano D, Gandolfi L. The role of ultrasound in the differential diagnosis of serous and mucinous cystic tumours of the pancreas. Eur J Gastroenterol Hepatol 1997;9:169-72.

70. Tripodi SA, Civitelli S, Schurfeld K, Cintorino M. Microcystic adenoma of the pancreas (glycogen-rich cystadenoma) with stromal amyloid deposits. Histopathology 2000;37:147-9.

70a. Tseng JF, Warshaw AL, Sahani DV, Lauwers GY, Rattner DW, Fernandez-del Castillo C. Serous cystadenoma of the pancreas: tumor growth rates and recommendations for treatment. Ann Surg 2005;242:413-9.

71. Unger PD, Danque PO, Fuchs A, Kaneko M. DNA flow cytometric evaluation of serous and mucinous cystic neoplasms of the pancreas. Arch Pathol Lab Med 1991;115:563-5.

72. Vortmeyer AO, Lubensky IA, Fogt F, Linehan WM, Khettry U, Zhuang Z. Allelic deletion and mutation of the von Hippel-Lindau (VHL) tumor suppressor gene in pancreatic microcystic adenomas. Am J Pathol 1997;151:951-6.

73. Warshaw AL, Compton CC, Lewandrowski KB, Cardenosa G, Mueller PR. Cystic tumors of the pancreas. New clinical, radiologic, and pathologic observations in 67 patients. Ann Surg 1990;212:432-45.

74. Widmaier U, Mattfeldt T, Siech M, Beger HG. Serous cystadenocarcinoma of the pancreas. Int J Pancreatol 1996;20:135-9.

75. Wu CM, Fishman EK, Hruban RH, Schlott WD, Cameron JL. Serous cystic neoplasm involving the pancreas and liver: an unusual clinical entity. Abdom Imaging 1999;24:75-7.

76. Yasuhara Y, Sakaida N, Uemura Y, Senzaki H, Shikata N, Tsubura A. Serous microcystic adenoma (glycogen-rich cystadenoma) of the pancreas: study of 11 cases showing clinicopathological and immunohistochemical correlations. Pathol Int 2002;52:307-12.

77. Yoshimi N, Sugie S, Tanaka T, et al. A rare case of serous cystadenocarcinoma of the pancreas. Cancer 1992;69:2449-53.

78. Zamboni G, Pea M, Martignoni G, et al. Clear cell "sugar" tumor of the pancreas. A novel member of the family of lesions characterized by the presence of perivascular epithelioid cells. Am J Surg Pathol 1996;20:722-30.

5 MUCINOUS CYSTIC NEOPLASMS

DEFINITION

The *mucinous cystic neoplasm* is a neoplasm composed of mucin-producing epithelial cells associated with an ovarian-type of stroma (35,76, 94). The neoplastic epithelial cells form one or more cysts that contain mucoid fluid and, in virtually all cases, these cysts do not communicate with the larger pancreatic ducts. Noninvasive mucinous neoplasms can be categorized into *mucinous cystic neoplasm with low-grade dysplasia, mucinous cystic neoplasm with moderate dysplasia,* and *mucinous cystic neoplasm with high-grade dysplasia (carcinoma in situ)* based on the degree of architectural and cytologic atypia of the epithelial cells (76,94). *Mucinous cystic neoplasms with an associated invasive carcinoma* are also known as *invasive mucinous cystadenocarcinomas.*

GENERAL FEATURES

Mucinous cystic neoplasms were first described more than a century ago (30), but the importance of distinguishing between serous cystic neoplasms, which have an extremely low malignant potential, and mucinous cystic neoplasms, which have a significant malignant potential, was not recognized until the 1970s (15). Within the group of mucin-producing neoplasms of the pancreas, intraductal papillary mucinous neoplasms and mucinous cystic neoplasms were lumped together until the 1980s, when Ohhashi et al. (58) emphasized the unique features of those mucin-producing neoplasms that involve the larger pancreatic ducts. It is now well accepted that intraductal papillary mucinous neoplasms are clinically, pathologically, and biologically distinct from mucinous cystic neoplasms (21,74). Many neoplasms reported as "mucinous cystic neoplasms" before the mid 1980s were, in fact, probably intraductal papillary mucinous neoplasms, and neoplasms reported as "cystadenomas" before 1978 could have been either mucinous or serous cystic neoplasms.

Mucinous cystic neoplasms are relatively uncommon. They accounted for 5.7 percent of all primary pancreatic tumors seen in consultation at the Armed Forces Institute of Pathology (AFIP) (82) and for 6 percent of all pancreatic cystic lesions reviewed by G. Klöppel (44). Similarly, in a series reported from Germany by Ridder et al. (67), 5.5 percent of all resectable carcinomas of the exocrine pancreas were mucinous cystadenocarcinomas.

Using current diagnostic criteria, all of the patients in some reported series of mucinous cystic neoplasms have been female, however, well-documented cases have been reported in men, and a female to male ratio of 20 to 1 is probably reasonable (1,15,23,48,70,82,84,90, 95). The mean age at diagnosis is between 40 and 50 years, with a range of 14 to 95 years (1,15,23, 48,70,82,84,90,95). In most series, patients with mucinous cystic neoplasms and an associated invasive carcinoma are on average 5 to 10 years older than the patients with noninvasive mucinous cystic neoplasms (48,70,84, 95). This age difference has been used to support the hypothesis that some noninvasive mucinous cystic neoplasms progress to invasive carcinoma over time.

Mucinous cystic neoplasms do not show a racial predominance, they are not associated with cigarette smoking, and they have not been associated with any genetic syndromes. A single case of a patient with the Zollinger-Ellison syndrome and an associated mucinous cystadenocarcinoma has been reported, as has a patient with simultaneous mucinous cystic neoplasms of the pancreas and ovary (25,52).

CLINICAL FEATURES

The clinical symptoms depend on the size of the mucinous neoplasm. Most patients with large neoplasms present with vague abdominal symptoms related to compression of adjacent organs and tissues. These symptoms include epigastric pain and a sense of abdominal fullness (15,18, 48,70,82,95). Less commonly, patients develop nonspecific gastrointestinal symptoms such as nausea and vomiting, diarrhea, anorexia, and

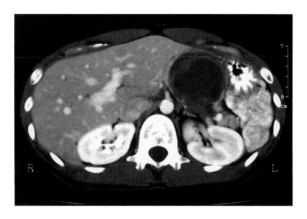

Figure 5-1

MUCINOUS CYSTIC NEOPLASM
WITH LOW-GRADE DYSPLASIA

Cystic low attenuation computerized tomography (CT)
scan of a lesion in the tail of the pancreas with a soft tissue
component. (Courtesy of Dr. S. S. Siegelman, Baltimore, MD.)

weight loss (15,18,48,70,82,95). Only a few
patients present with jaundice, usually due to
an associated invasive carcinoma involving the
head of the gland. Symptoms may be present
years before a diagnosis is established (82,84).

Twenty to 30 percent of mucinous cystic neoplasms, especially those under 3 cm, are discovered incidentally during abdominal imaging for
an unrelated indication (18,82,95). With the
increased use of abdominal imaging it is reasonable to expect that the proportion of detectable mucinous cystic neoplasms that are small
and asymptomatic will increase over time. Very
large mucinous cystic neoplasms can sometimes
be palpated in the left upper quadrant on physical examination.

Twenty percent of mucinous cystic neoplasms have a rim of peripheral calcification
that can be detected on plain radiographs (20,
48,82). Plain radiographs may also reveal the
displacement of the stomach, duodenum, and
colon by the neoplastic mass. Computerized
tomography (CT) scans usually demonstrate a
well-demarcated, thick-walled multilocular cystic mass (fig. 5-1) (16,20,48). The cysts are usually large (1 to 3 cm) and, as expected from the
plain films, peripheral calcification is sometimes
seen within the capsule of the neoplasm. The
attenuation of the cysts vary depending on their
content. Some cysts contain mucin, some con-

tain watery fluid, and others contain hemorrhagic fluid. As a result, the attenuation of individual cysts within a mucinous cystic neoplasm varies (20,48). Mural nodules and papillary excrescences into the cysts are more common in mucinous cystic neoplasms with an associated invasive carcinoma (64). Ultrasound
demonstrates the cystic nature of these neoplasms and has the advantage that it can be used
to facilitate biopsy of the lesion and sampling
of the cyst contents (9,12,16,20).

Most mucinous cystic neoplasms appear
hypovascular on angiography and the cysts
themselves obviously are avascular (20,48). The
pancreatic duct is usually displaced or com-
pressed on endoscopic retrograde cholangiopancreatography (ERCP) and in the vast majority of cases, the larger pancreatic ducts do not
communicate with the cysts. This latter feature
is very helpful in distinguishing mucinous cystic neoplasms from intraductal papillary mucinous neoplasms, which arise in the larger ducts.
Magnetic resonance cholangiopancreatography
(MRCP) is used to image mucinous cystic neoplasms and is less invasive than ERCP. MRCP
has the advantage that it can visualize the pancreatic ducts as well as lesions outside of the
ductal system. Unfortunately, as is true for most
cystic neoplasms of the pancreas, preoperative
imaging diagnoses are often incorrect (27).

Serum carbohydrate antigen (CA) 19-9 levels are elevated in some (20 percent) patients
with mucinous cystadenomas, and in most (70
percent) patients with mucinous cystadenocarcinomas (8,48,79). The cyst fluid often has a
normal amylase level and elevated levels of
carcinoembryonic antigen (CEA), CA19-9, and
CA72-4 (48,79). The levels of these glycoproteins tend to be higher in mucinous cystic neoplasms with an associated invasive carcinoma
than in noninvasive neoplasms (48).

PATHOLOGIC FEATURES

Gross Findings

The majority (90 percent) of mucinous cystic neoplasms arise in the body or tail of the
pancreas, and only a minority (10 percent) involve the head of the gland (1,15,23,48,70,
82,90). Mucinous cystic neoplasms with an associated invasive carcinoma involve the head

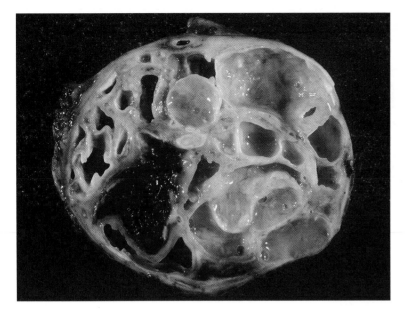

Figure 5-2

MUCINOUS CYSTIC NEOPLASM WITH LOW-GRADE DYSPLASIA

The cysts are separated by thick fibrous septa. Some cysts contain mucin, others blood.

of the gland slightly more often than do noninvasive neoplasms (70,81). Rare examples of mucinous cystic neoplasms arising in ectopic pancreatic tissues have been reported (14).

Mucinous cystic neoplasms are usually solitary and quite large (2 to 36 cm; mean, 7 to 10 cm), and those with an associated invasive carcinoma are even larger (81,84,91,95). Mucinous cystic neoplasms often have a thick pseudocapsule, and the outer surface is usually smooth and well-demarcated.

On cut section, the neoplasm is usually multilocular (figs. 5-2–5-5), but is occasionally unilocular, a feature that can mimic a pseudocyst (fig. 5-6). The individual locules are typically between 1 and 3 cm, but locules as small as a few millimeters and as large as 23 cm have been reported. The locules have thick walls and are typically filled with thick tenacious mucoid material, although some may contain watery fluid, hemorrhagic fluid, or even necrotic debris (fig. 5-2). The lining of the cysts or locules can be smooth, particularly in mucinous cystic neoplasms with low-grade dysplasia, or there can be intracystic papillary excrescences (projections) and even solid mural nodules, features that suggest the diagnosis of high-grade dysplasia or an associated invasive carcinoma (fig. 5-4). Focal calcifications are sometimes present in the periphery of the neoplasms. When there is associated extensive hemorrhage or necrosis, the normal

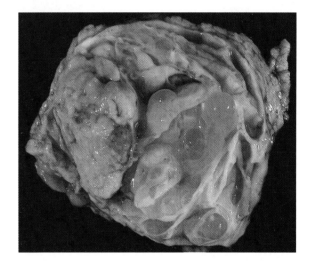

Figure 5-3

MUCINOUS CYSTIC NEOPLASM WITH CARCINOMA IN SITU

A solid mural nodule is seen on the left.

smooth epithelial lining of the cyst may be replaced by a brown, shaggy, friable lining reminiscent of a pseudocyst.

The locules of mucinous cystic neoplasms usually do not communicate with the pancreatic ducts (fig. 5-7). For the rare mucinous cystic neoplasm reported to communicate with the pancreatic ducts (7,48), the communication is

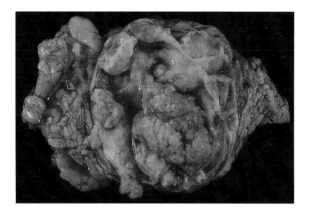

Figure 5-4

MUCINOUS CYSTIC NEOPLASM
WITH FOCAL INVASIVE CARCINOMA

More solid areas are seen in addition to cysts with thick linings.

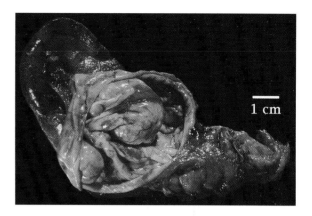

Figure 5-6

MUCINOUS CYSTIC NEOPLASM
WITH LOW-GRADE DYSPLASIA

Tumor in the tail of the pancreas with adjacent spleen. A single cyst with a smooth lining predominates.

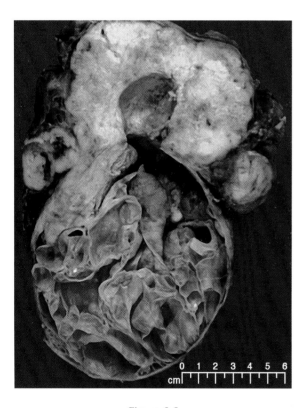

Figure 5-5

MUCINOUS CYSTIC NEOPLASM WITH
INVASIVE SPINDLE CELL CARCINOMA

A large solid mural nodule is associated with the large cystic neoplasm. (Fig. 4-28 from Fascicle 20, Third Series.)

usually due to erosion of the expanding neoplasm into the duct, rather than true intraductal origin.

Extensive involvement of the duct system should suggest the diagnosis of an intraductal papillary mucinous neoplasm. Some mucinous cystic neoplasms obstruct the pancreatic duct; the pancreatic parenchyma upstream from this obstruction is atrophic and the pancreatic duct dilated.

Mucinous cystic neoplasms with an associated invasive carcinoma may infiltrate into adjacent organs, including the stomach, duodenum, colon, bile duct, and spleen.

Microscopic Findings

Mucinous cystic neoplasms are usually surrounded by a thick band of heavily collagenized tissue, which separates the cysts from the nonneoplastic pancreas (fig. 5-8). The cysts are lined by tall, columnar, mucin-producing epithelium (fig. 5-9) (76,94). These columnar cells have basal nuclei and abundant intracytoplasmic apical mucin, and form flat sheets or papillae (fig. 5-10) (2). Gastric foveolar differentiation may be seen and in some cases goblet cells are scattered among the columnar cells.

The epithelium is often focally denuded (fig. 5-11) (especially if it has been vigorously rubbed by an eager resident during specimen grossing!) and several histologic sections may be needed to demonstrate an epithelial lining (48,82,84). The epithelium can be quite bland, with uniform, small, basally located nuclei (fig. 5-9), or can show significant architectural and cytologic atypia (i.e., dysplasia) with cribriforming,

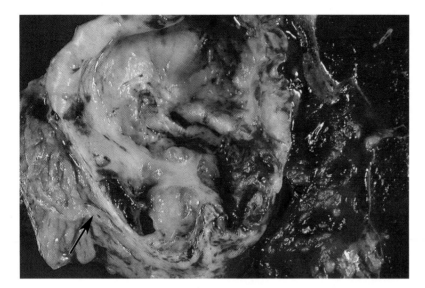

Figure 5-7

MUCINOUS CYSTIC NEOPLASM

The pancreatic duct (arrow) does not communicate with the locules of the neoplasm.

Figure 5-8

MUCINOUS CYSTIC NEOPLASM WITH LOW-GRADE DYSPLASIA

The cysts are lined by tall columnar epithelial cells with prominent underlying ovarian-type stroma. The thick fibrous capsule separates the neoplasm from the adjacent pancreas on the right.

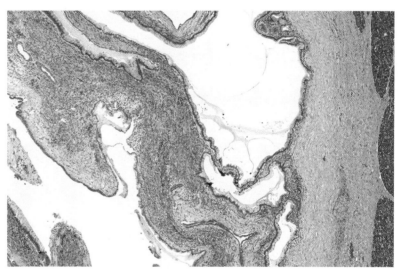

crowding of the cells, an increased nuclear to cytoplasm ratio, loss of nuclear polarity, mitoses, and nuclear pleomorphism (figs. 5-12, 5-13) (1). Dysplasia can be multifocal, and, most remarkably, in a single neoplasm there is often an abrupt, at times striking, transition from completely bland epithelium to epithelium with significant dysplasia (figs. 5-12–5-14) (1).

The cysts, as expected from their gross appearance, usually do not communicate microscopically with the pancreatic ducts. In the rare case in which a microscopic connection can be demonstrated between a cyst and a pancreatic duct, the neoplastic epithelium, in contrast to intraductal papillary mucinous neoplasms, does not spread extensively into the duct system (fig.

5-15). It is common, however, for the adjacent pancreatic ducts to exhibit foci of pancreatic intraepithelial neoplasia (PanIN), with the epithelium closely resembling the lining of the mucinous cystic neoplasm (4,79a). Such foci of PanIN are regarded as independent lesions rather than intraductal extensions of the mucinous cystic neoplasm.

The septa of the cysts, at least focally, contain a distinctive ovarian-type stroma (figs. 5-9, 5-14, 5-15) (15,26b,95). This stroma is composed of densely packed spindle cells with sparse cytoplasm and uniform, elongated wavy nuclei. Mitoses are rare to absent. Intermingled clusters of plump, eosinophilic epithelioid cells resemble leutinized cells (fig. 5-16) (29,34,95). This stroma

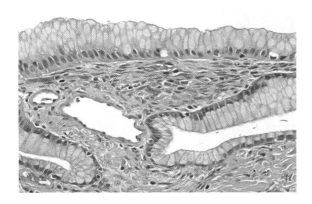

Figure 5-9

MUCINOUS CYSTIC NEOPLASM
WITH LOW-GRADE DYSPLASIA

The cysts are lined by flat, columnar, mucin-producing epithelium without atypia.

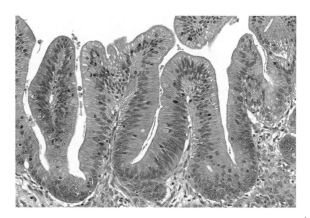

Figure 5-10

MUCINOUS CYSTIC NEOPLASM
WITH MODERATE DYSPLASIA

The epithelium has a papillary architecture.

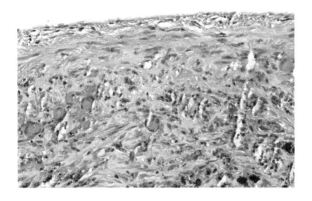

Figure 5-11

MUCINOUS CYSTIC NEOPLASM

The epithelium is denuded and the stroma contains hemosiderin-laden macrophages, mimicking a pseudocyst.

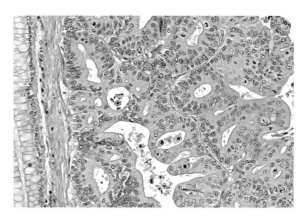

Figure 5-12

MUCINOUS CYSTIC NEOPLASM
WITH HIGH-GRADE DYSPLASIA

Cribriform architecture with significant nuclear atypia. Adjacent epithelium (far left) from the same neoplasm has only mild dysplasia.

is so distinctive that it is almost diagnostic in cases in which the epithelium is denuded, and it is seen in mucinous cystic neoplasms in both women and men. A similar stroma can be seen in mucinous cystic neoplasms of the hepatobiliary tree (hepatobiliary cystadenomas), ovary, and retroperitoneum. The stroma is partially hyalinized in some cases, and some foci have the appearance of corpora albicantia (fig. 5-17). It is not unusual for the stroma to contain noninvasive microcystic buds of neoplastic epithelium from the larger cysts (fig. 5-18). The stroma may also contain entrapped nor-

mal pancreatic tissue including islets of Langerhans, ducts, and acini. Although larger mucinous cystic neoplasms generally are surrounded by a fibrotic pseudocapsule, in some instances, the ovarian-type stroma is abundant and extends into the adjacent pancreatic parenchyma, well away from the mucinous epithelial component of the neoplasm. In areas where the epithelial lining is denuded, elements of the ovarian-type stroma may be admixed with hemorrhage, inflammation, and fibrosis, resembling the wall of a pseudocyst (see fig. 5-11).

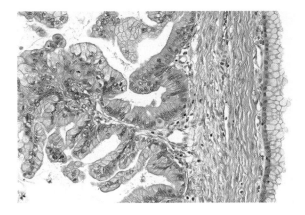

Figure 5-13

**MUCINOUS CYSTIC NEOPLASM
WITH CARCINOMA IN SITU**

Complex papillary architecture with significant nuclear atypia. Adjacent epithelium (far right) from the same neoplasm has only mild atypia.

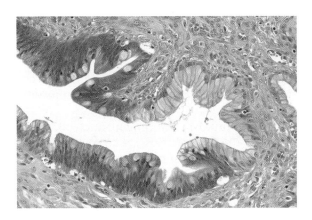

Figure 5-14

**MUCINOUS CYSTIC NEOPLASM
WITH MODERATE DYSPLASIA**

There is an abrupt transition from epithelium with only minimal atypia to epithelium with moderate atypia.

Noninvasive mucinous neoplasms are categorized into *mucinous cystic neoplasm with low-grade dysplasia, mucinous cystic neoplasms with moderate dysplasia,* and *mucinous cystic neoplasms with high-grade dysplasia (carcinoma in situ)* based on the degree of architectural and cytologic atypia of the epithelial cells (94). The neoplasm is classified based on the highest degree of atypia identified, not the average. This categorization follows the classification of mucinous cystic neoplasms of the ovary.

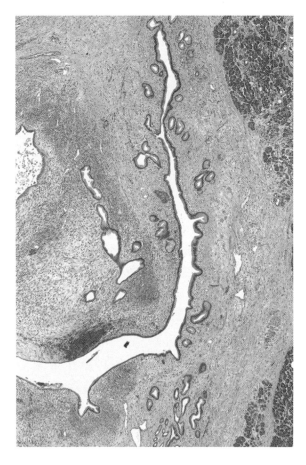

Figure 5-15

**MUCINOUS CYSTIC NEOPLASM
INVOLVING A PANCREATIC DUCT**

Although distinctly unusual, there is clear communication between the lumen of a pancreatic duct (top center) and the lumen of a cyst associated with ovarian-type stroma (lower left).

Mucinous cystic neoplasms with low-grade dysplasia have only minimal to mild architectural and cytologic atypia (see fig. 5-9). The cells are cuboidal to columnar and form a single cell layer. They are well oriented; contain small, uniform, basally oriented nuclei; do not have mitoses; and, if papillae are present, the papillae contain fibrovascular cores. Mucinous cystic neoplasms with mild dysplasia were referred to as "mucinous cystadenomas" in the previous edition of this Fascicle. We have changed the nomenclature here slightly to keep the nomenclature of all of the noninvasive mucinous neoplasms consistent.

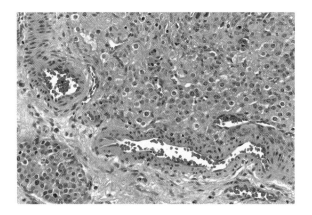

Figure 5-16

MUCINOUS CYSTIC NEOPLASM

The stroma in the cyst wall shows prominent luteinization.

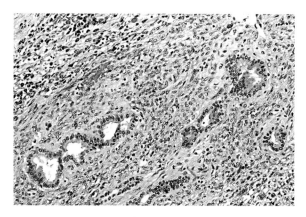

Figure 5-18

MUCINOUS CYSTIC NEOPLASM

Entrapped benign epithelium mimics an invasive cancer.

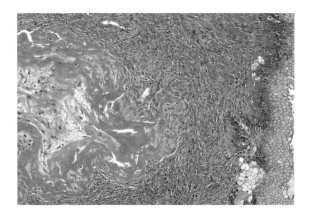

Figure 5-17

MUCINOUS CYSTIC NEOPLASM

Area of fibrosis resembling corpora albicantia.

The epithelial cells of *mucinous cystic neoplasms with moderate dysplasia* show mild to moderate architectural and cytologic atypia (fig. 5-14). The cells may form gross or microscopic papillae, the epithelium may be several cells thick, and the cells may be crowded. The nuclear to cytoplasmic ratio is increased and the nuclei vary slightly in size and shape; nucleoli may be present, as can occasional mitoses. There may be a slight loss of polarity. Mucinous cystic neoplasms with moderate dysplasia were referred to as "borderline tumors" and "mucinous cystic tumors of borderline malignant potential" in the previous edition of this Fascicle. We prefer the term mucinous cystic neoplasms with mod-

erate dysplasia as it more precisely conveys the histologic findings characteristic of these lesions, and because it does not imply that these lesions have the capacity to metastasize.

Significant nuclear and cytologic atypia is seen in *mucinous cystic neoplasms with high-grade dysplasia (carcinoma in situ)* (figs. 5-12, 5-13). The cells are crowded, and the nuclei show a significantly increased nuclear to cytoplasmic ratio, significant pleomorphism, prominent nucleoli, mitoses, and, importantly, loss of nuclear polarity. Architecturally, cribriforming and papillae without fibrovascular cores are evident.

Approximately one third of all mucinous cystic neoplasms are associated with invasive carcinoma (23,70). These neoplasms are classified as *mucinous cystic neoplasm with an associated invasive carcinoma* or *invasive mucinous cystadenocarcinoma*. The invasive carcinomas are usually of tubular (conventional ductal)-type adenocarcinomas (fig. 5-19) (50). Undifferentiated carcinomas with osteoclast-like giant cells, adenosquamous carcinomas, colloid carcinomas, rhabdoid carcinomas, and even choriocarcinomas have also been reported (13,45,93,95). As is discussed later, mucinous cystic neoplasms are also associated with invasive high-grade spindle cell neoplasms ("sarcomatoid carcinomas"). The diagnosis of an invasive carcinoma should only be made when there is clear-cut invasion into the stroma. This invasion is often associated with a desmoplastic reaction, and a stromal desmoplastic reaction can be used to distinguish true invasion from noninvasive

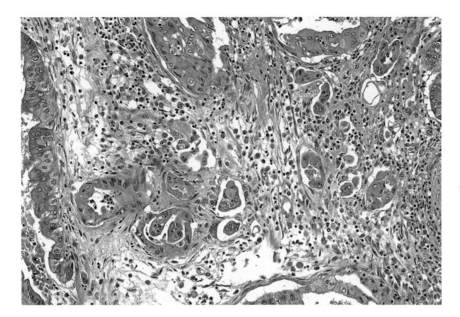

Figure 5-19

INVASIVE ADENOCARCINOMA ARISING IN A MUCINOUS CYSTIC NEOPLASM

Carcinoma has invaded the septum.

microcystic buds of neoplastic epithelium coming off the larger cysts.

The invasive and in situ carcinoma components of mucinous cystic neoplasms can be very focal (48). In two cases in the original report from the AFIP on mucinous cystic neoplasms, 47 and 66 blocks of tissue, respectively, were examined before the presence of carcinoma could be demonstrated (15). Indeed, the focality of carcinomas and the frequent abrupt transition from completely bland epithelium to epithelium with significant dysplasia (see figs. 5-12–5-14), dictate that mucinous cystic neoplasms have to be entirely resected and entirely submitted for histologic examination before a carcinoma can be excluded (89,90). A benign diagnosis cannot be established on biopsy alone, nor can it be established in an inadequately examined specimen (90). This being said, completely sampling a large mucinous cystic neoplasm for histologic examination can be a daunting task. Grossly nodular and papillary areas should be sampled first, as these are the areas most likely to harbor an invasive carcinoma. If an invasive carcinoma is not identified in this initial sampling, then the entire neoplasm should be submitted for histologic examination.

Mucicarmine and periodic acid–Schiff (PAS) stains confirm the presence of substantial quantities of intracellular and extracellular mucin (69). These are predominantly sulfated acid mucins with some neutral mucins; two thirds of the neoplasms are Alcian blue (pH 2.5) positive. In most cases, Grimelius/Churukin-Schenk (argyrophilic) and Fontana-Masson (argentaffin) stains reveal scattered endocrine cells at the base of the epithelium. These endocrine cells are often more numerous in mucinous cystic neoplasms with moderate and high-grade dysplasia (3,69).

Histologic Types of Invasive Carcinoma

Several distinct histologic types of invasive carcinoma may arise in mucinous cystic neoplasms (26). The most common type (other than conventional tubular-type ductal adenocarcinoma) is undifferentiated carcinoma with osteoclast-like giant cells (53,62,88,95). These neoplasms have infiltrating atypical mononuclear cells and large osteoclast-like giant cells with multiple uniform nuclei (55,62,88). The infiltrating mononuclear cells variably express cytokeratin and epithelial membrane antigen (EMA), while the osteoclast-like giant cells express common leukocyte antigen (CD45) as well as markers of macrophage differentiation including CD68 and KP1 (55). Recent molecular analyses have shown that the infiltrating atypical mononuclear cells harbor the same genetic alterations as do the neoplastic mucinous epithelial cells, helping to establish that the mononuclear cells and neoplastic epithelial cells have the same clonal origin (88). By contrast, the osteoclast-like giant cells appear to be non-neoplastic.

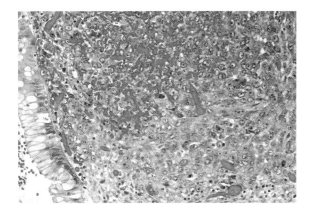

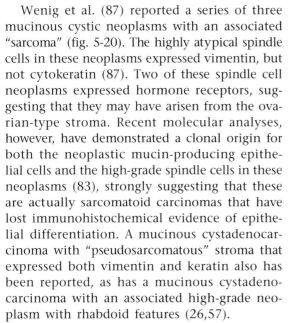

Figure 5-20

**MUCINOUS CYSTIC NEOPLASM
WITH SARCOMATOID STROMA**

Mucinous epithelium (left) and a high-grade invasive spindle cell neoplasm (right).

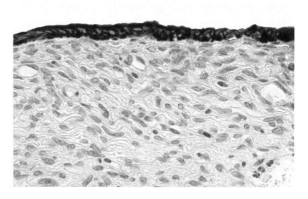

Figure 5-21

**MUCINOUS CYSTIC NEOPLASM
WITH LOW-GRADE DYSPLASIA**

Neoplastic epithelium is strongly labeled with an antibody to cytokeratin.

Wenig et al. (87) reported a series of three mucinous cystic neoplasms with an associated "sarcoma" (fig. 5-20). The highly atypical spindle cells in these neoplasms expressed vimentin, but not cytokeratin (87). Two of these spindle cell neoplasms expressed hormone receptors, suggesting that they may have arisen from the ovarian-type stroma. Recent molecular analyses, however, have demonstrated a clonal origin for both the neoplastic mucin-producing epithelial cells and the high-grade spindle cells in these neoplasms (83), strongly suggesting that these are actually sarcomatoid carcinomas that have lost immunohistochemical evidence of epithelial differentiation. A mucinous cystadenocarcinoma with "pseudosarcomatous" stroma that expressed both vimentin and keratin also has been reported, as has a mucinous cystadenocarcinoma with an associated high-grade neoplasm with rhabdoid features (26,57).

These variants are important to recognize because they appear to have a very poor prognosis.

Frozen Section

Several features of mucinous cystic neoplasms should be kept in mind when evaluating frozen sections from cystic neoplasms of the pancreas. First, the patient's gender and the location of the neoplasm can both suggest the diagnosis. Mucinous cystic neoplasms (and solid-pseudopapillary neoplasms) should be at the top of the differential diagnosis for cystic

neoplasms in the tail of the pancreas in middle-aged women. Second, although cyst contents are often ignored, they can be essential in establishing a diagnosis. Tenacious mucoid material should suggest either a mucinous cystic neoplasm or an intraductal papillary mucinous neoplasm. Third, the relationship of the cysts to the larger pancreatic ducts can be used to distinguish mucinous cystic neoplasms from intraductal papillary mucinous neoplasms. In contrast to intraductal papillary mucinous neoplasms, the cysts of mucinous cystic neoplasms do not involve the pancreatic ducts. Fourth, as mentioned earlier, the mucin-producing epithelium of mucinous cystic neoplasms is often focally, and occasionally extensively, denuded (fig. 5-11). In these instances, the underlying ovarian stroma can be a strong clue to the diagnosis and should prompt the search for intact mucinous epithelium.

Immunohistochemical Findings

Immunohistochemical labeling confirms epithelial differentiation and characterizes the mucin produced. The epithelial cells label with antibodies to pancytokeratin; cytokeratins (CKs) 7, 8, 18 and 19; CAM5.2; and CEA (fig. 5-21) (59,82). Labeling for DUPAN-2 and for CA19-9 is also positive (82,95). The neoplastic epithelial cells also label with markers of gastric-type mucin (MUC5AC), and scattered intraepithelial goblet-like cells express MUC2 (50). Only rare

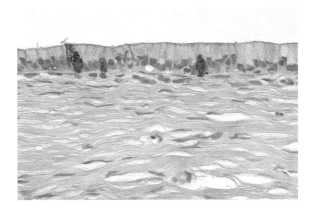

Figure 5-22

MUCINOUS CYSTIC NEOPLASM
WITH LOW-GRADE DYSPLASIA

Rare cells within the epithelium label for chromogranin.

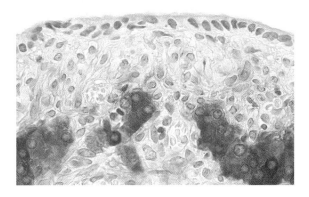

Figure 5-23

MUCINOUS CYSTIC NEOPLASM
WITH LOW-GRADE DYSPLASIA

Some ovarian-type stromal cells, particularly those with a luteinized morphology, label with an antibody to inhibin.

cases express MUC6; MUC1 expression is seen primarily in cases with an invasive component (50). Mucinous cystic neoplasms only rarely express CDX2 and CK20, and therefore do not demonstrate the sort of intestinal differentiation common in intraductal papillary mucinous neoplasms (39).

Immunohistochemical labeling for endocrine markers reveals scattered endocrine cells within the epithelium of most cases (fig. 5-22) (1,50,82,95). These endocrine cells usually express serotonin and chromogranin, and a minority express somatostatin, pancreatic polypeptide, and gastrin (3). The expression of gastrin may explain the case of Zollinger-Ellison syndrome reported in association with a mucinous cystic neoplasm of the pancreas (52). Labeling for insulin and glucagon is usually negative.

The ovarian-type stromal cells label with antibodies to vimentin, smooth muscle actin, muscle-specific actin, desmin (focally), calretinin, tyrosine hydroxylase, alpha-inhibin (in two thirds of the cases) (fig. 5-23), Melan-A, CD99, and bcl2 (22,34,40,66); this immunophenotype is strikingly similar to that of normal ovarian stroma (40). Estrogen receptors are expressed by the stromal cells in 25 percent of mucinous cystic neoplasms and progesterone receptors in 50 to 75 percent (fig. 5-24) (82,95). The leutinized cells label with antibodies to tyrosine hydroxylase, alpha-inhibin, Melan-A, and calretinin, markers that also label normal

hilar cells in the ovary (95). Labeling for S-100 protein and CD34 is usually negative (22).

Ultrastructural Findings

Ultrastructurally, mucinous cystic neoplasms are mucin-producing epithelial neoplasms (fig. 5-25, left). The columnar epithelial cells are attached to each other by junctional complexes, they contain abundant apical mucin vacuoles, and they have short and long microvilli on their apical surfaces (1). Filamentous glycocalyx material is often associated with the microvilli.

Two types of stromal cells have been reported (1). Spindle-shaped cells with fibroblastic differentiation have abundant rough endoplasmic reticulum and surrounding collagen (fig. 5-25, right). Other stromal cells appear relatively undifferentiated and have nuclei with deep indentations of the nuclear envelope.

Cytologic Findings

Cytologic samples of mucinous cystic neoplasm are most often obtained by fine needle aspiration biopsy via either a percutaneous route or, increasingly, by endoscopic ultrasound-guided biopsy. ERCP with brush cytology and pancreatic duct aspiration are not useful techniques given the lack of continuity of this neoplasm with the pancreatic ductal system.

Mucinous cystic neoplasms demonstrate significant variability in mucin content and degree of cytologic atypia of the cyst lining, and, as

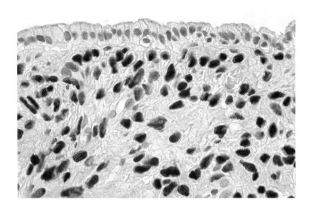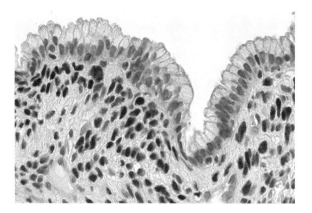

Figure 5-24

MUCINOUS CYSTIC NEOPLASM WITH LOW-GRADE DYSPLASIA

Some of the ovarian-type stromal cells label with antibodies to progesterone receptor (left) and with antibodies to estrogen receptor (right).

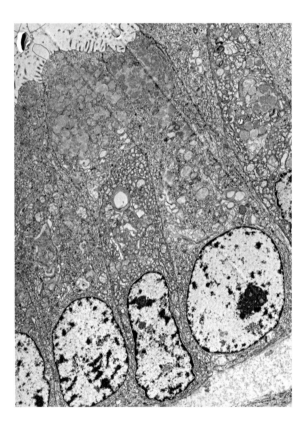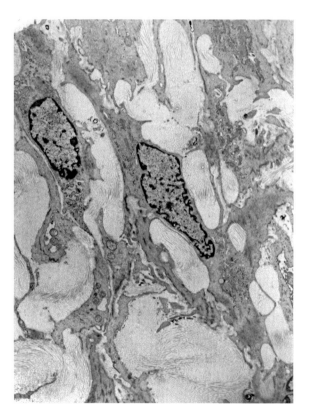

Figure 5-25

MUCINOUS CYSTIC NEOPLASM WITH LOW-GRADE DYSPLASIA

Electron microscopy of the epithelium (left) and stroma (right).

such, the cyst aspirates may not accurately reflect the true nature of the cyst. A specific diagnosis of mucinous cystic neoplasm, therefore, is

less common with a fine needle aspiration biopsy than a more general diagnosis of *mucin-producing cystic neoplasm*, a term that encompasses both intraductal papillary mucinous neoplasm and mucinous cystic neoplasm. This is primarily due to the hypocellularity of the mucinous contents aspirated and/or a lack of architectural specificity of the glandular epithelium, i.e., the absence of papillary fragments that would help to define an intraductal papillary mucinous neoplasm. Additionally, cytologic samples tend to underestimate the degree of atypia present in the neoplasm, e.g., low-grade, moderate, and high-grade dysplasia (47,48,54,65). Finally, the characteristic ovarian-type cellular stroma is usually not represented on fine needle aspiration biopsies.

The introduction of gastrointestinal contamination in the form of both extracellular mucin and glandular epithelium by the endoscopic ultrasound-guided technique adds to the diagnostic difficulty in some cases (see Differential Diagnosis) (17,47,54,80). It is almost impossible to site an accurate range of sensitivity and specificity for the cytologic diagnosis of mucinous cystic neoplasm owing to the rather recent subclassification of pancreatic cysts that separates mucinous from serous cysts in general and mucinous cystic neoplasm from intraductal papillary mucinous neoplasm in particular. The method of sampling, and the experience of the aspirator and the cytopathologist impact on the sensitivity and specificity. The overall accuracy of endoscopic ultrasound-guided pancreatic fine needle aspiration biopsy is lower for cystic than for solid neoplasms in general, and is higher if a cytopathologist is present during the procedure (10,17, 36,43,51,65,73).

Integration of the clinical and radiologic features of the cyst being aspirated aids the cytopathologist in arriving at an accurate diagnosis. The presence of a neoplastic mucinous cyst is often first suspected at the time of aspiration owing to the difficulty in both aspirating cyst fluid into and expressing fluid from the needle. The high viscosity of the cyst fluid is reflected on the slide as thick,"colloid-like" mucin that frequently covers most of the slide (fig. 5-26). Mucin contamination from the gastrointestinal tract will not be colloid-like. Entrapped degenerated cells and histiocytes within the mucin, a feature of mucin from a cyst, also help to distinguish contaminating mucin from the mucin of mucinous cystic neoplasms (46,47,54,80). Not all mucinous cystic neoplasms have such

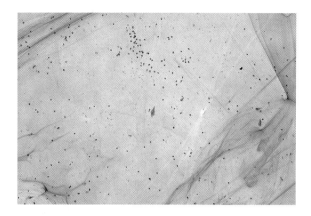

Figure 5-26

MUCINOUS CYSTIC NEOPLASM

Thick "colloid-like" mucin, often with entrapped cellular debris and histiocytes, as seen here, defines the cyst as a mucin-producing cystic neoplasm and distinguishes the mucin from gastrointestinal mucin (direct smear; Papanicolaou stain).

tenacious cyst contents, however, and as noted previously, the contents may appear clear and thin, and even bloody, mimicking the contents of a pseudocyst. Extracellular mucin can appear as focally thick clumps, thin wisps, or focal or diffuse thin background mucin that may be difficult to visualize without stains (46,47,54). Mucin can also appear inspissated (fig. 5-27). An aliquot of the cyst fluid, if sufficient in quantity, can be used to prepare cytospin slides for mucicarmine or Alcian blue pH 2.5 staining. In our experience, stains for mucin aid in the identification of background mucin and intracytoplasmic mucin in cases where these features are difficult to appreciate on routinely prepared slides. The absence of mucin by these special stains, however, does not exclude the diagnosis of a mucin-producing cystic neoplasm.

Mucinous epithelial cells, as noted above, are not necessary for a general diagnosis of a mucin-producing cystic neoplasm and the presence of nonpapillary mucinous glandular epithelium, expected for mucinous cystic neoplasm, does not exclude the diagnosis of intraductal papillary mucinous neoplasm (47,54,80). In addition, the increased cellularity and hyperchromasia of the cyst lining cells in moderate dysplasia and higher-grade neoplasms can mimic papillary lesions, leading to a misdiagnosis of intraductal papillary mucinous neoplasm (fig. 5-27). As such, the radiologic and clinical features of the

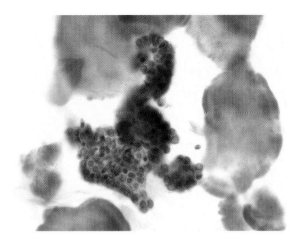

Figure 5-27

**MUCINOUS CYSTIC NEOPLASM
WITH MODERATE DYSPLASIA**

Cellular epithelial clusters of dysplastic cells can mimic papillary clusters of an intraductal papillary mucinous neoplasm. The mucin is condensed and inspissated (ThinPrep®; Papanicolaou stain).

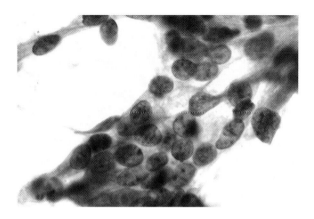

Figure 5-28

**MUCINOUS CYSTIC NEOPLASM
WITH MODERATE DYSPLASIA**

The epithelial cells are in crowded groups and have a high nuclear to cytoplasmic ratio (cytospin; Papanicolaou stain).

neoplasm are necessary for a specific diagnosis of mucinous cystic neoplasm.

Mucinous cystic neoplasms with low-grade dysplasia have single cells, small clusters of cells, and flat sheets of bland glandular epithelial cells that typically demonstrate cytoplasmic mucin on routine light microscopy. The nuclei are basally located, round and regular, with even chromatin and inconspicuous to occasionally prominent nucleoli. Scant cellularity is common in most cases, and only foamy histocytes may be present, with or without background mucin.

The glandular epithelium aspirated from mucinous cystic neoplasms with moderate or high-grade dysplasia demonstrates nuclear crowding, loss of polarity, nuclear elongation or rounding, hyperchromasia, and an increased nuclear to cytoplasmic ratio (fig. 5-28). Cells in small clusters or singly, with or without cytoplasmic mucin, are also consistent with a higher-grade neoplasm. The finding of crowded groups of cells with open chromatin, irregular nuclear membranes and nucleoli, significant background inflammation, and necrosis supports the interpretation of at least high-grade dysplasia (carcinoma in situ), however, invasive carcinomas may also demonstrate markedly atypical cells with visible mucinous cytoplasm

(fig. 5-29). Invasion can only be determined by the aspiration of a mural nodule, since the cytologic features distinguishing high-grade dysplasia from invasive carcinoma have not been established (28,54,71,72,80). Given the atypia present in these cyst-lining epithelial cells, gastric- or duodenal-contaminating epithelium does not usually pose a diagnostic pitfall in higher-grade mucinous cystic neoplasms.

Chemical analysis of the cyst fluid can aid in the diagnosis and subclassification of pancreatic cysts. CEA levels above 200 ng/mL have been found to distinguish nonmucinous from mucinous cysts; very high levels of CEA correlate with malignancy (49,60,61). Amylase levels are not typically elevated in mucinous cystic neoplasms due to their lack of connectivity with the pancreatic duct.

Molecular and Other Special Techniques

Molecular analyses of mucinous cystic neoplasms have revealed mutations in several cancer-associated genes and, in general, have revealed an accumulation of genetic alterations in the progression from mucinous cystic neoplasms with low-grade dysplasia to mucinous cystic neoplasms with an associated invasive carcinoma (6,19). Activating point mutations in codon 12 of the *KRAS* gene appear early and increase in frequency proportional to the degree of dysplasia, while mutations in the *TP53* tumor suppressor gene appear to occur relatively

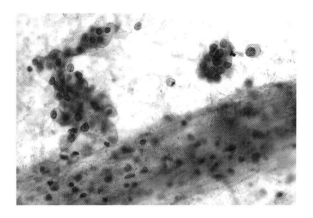

Figure 5-29

MUCINOUS CYSTIC NEOPLASM

This cystic neoplasm with an invasive carcinoma produced abundant extracellular mucin on aspiration. The malignant cells contain visible mucinous cytoplasmic vacuoles (direct smear; Papanicolaou stain).

late in in situ and invasive mucinous cystadenocarcinomas (6,19,37,41,50,95). Inactivation of the *SMAD4/DPC4* tumor suppressor gene also appears to be a late event as almost all noninvasive mucinous cystic neoplasms show intact labeling with antibodies to the *SMAD4/DPC4* gene product, Dpc4, while approximately half of the associated invasive carcinomas show loss of Dpc4 expression (32,50). The stromal cells almost always show intact Dpc4 labeling, even in cases in which the invasive carcinoma shows loss of Dpc4 expression (32). This latter finding further suggests that the ovarian-type stroma is non-neoplastic (32).

These molecular alterations are paralleled by ploidy studies (11,19,77,82). Most noninvasive mucinous cystic neoplasms are diploid, while some of those with an associated invasive carcinoma are aneuploid (11). In some series, patients with diploid invasive mucinous cystadenocarcinomas have a significantly better survival rate than do patients with aneuploid invasive mucinous cystadenocarcinomas (11).

The clonality of the epithelium in mucinous cystic neoplasms has been established by the analysis of the inactivation of the X-linked phosphoglycerate kinase gene (92).

Less than 15 percent of mucinous cystic neoplasms show aberrant methylation of the *p16/CDKN2A* and *p14* genes (41), and, in contrast to serous cystadenomas, only a minority show

loss of heterozygosity at the *VHL* gene locus on chromosome 3p25 (41). Global analyses of gene expression in mucinous cystic neoplasms have revealed the overexpression of a number of proteins by the neoplastic epithelium, including S-100 protein, cathepsin E, prostate stem cell antigen, highly expressed in cancer, STK6/STK15, and pepsinogen (24). In these same studies, the stromal cells were shown to overexpress proteins implicated in estrogen-mediated growth such as steroidogenic acute regulatory protein (STAR) and estrogen receptor 1 (ESR1) (24).

DIFFERENTIAL DIAGNOSIS

Most mucinous cystic neoplasms are clearly cystic and the differential diagnosis therefore includes the other cystic lesions of the pancreas (Table 5-1). The correct diagnosis is usually easy to establish, especially if one considers the patient's gender, the location of the neoplasm within the gland (head versus body/tail), the nature of the cyst contents, the relationship of the cysts to the larger pancreatic ducts, the type of epithelial lining (if any), and the character of the stroma.

Pseudocysts are the most important lesions to consider in the differential diagnosis because the treatment and outcome for this lesion compared to mucinous cystic neoplasm is so different (68,84,86). The drainage of a mucinous cystic neoplasm misdiagnosed as a pseudocyst can lead to a missed opportunity for a cure and can therefore have devastating consequences for the patient (86). Pseudocysts and mucinous cystic neoplasms can both produce thick-walled large cysts; however, the two entities are distinguished by the clinical, gross, and microscopic findings (68). Pseudocysts are more common in men than in women, and patients typically have a history of pancreatitis and elevated serum amylase levels. By contrast, mucinous cystic neoplasms are much more common in women, most of the patients do not develop pancreatitis, and serum amylase levels are usually normal. Most pseudocysts are unilocular and actually extrapancreatic, while most mucinous cystic neoplasms are multilocular and involve the parenchyma of the body/tail of the gland. Pseudocysts contain necrotic/hemorrhagic debris with high levels of amylase, while the cysts of mucinous cystic neoplasms usually contain

Table 5-1

COMPARISON OF COMMON CYSTIC NEOPLASMS

	Mucinous Cystic Neoplasm	IPMN[a]	Serous Cystic Neoplasm
Age	40–50 years	60s	60–70
Gender	Female>>Male	Male>Female	Female>Male
Head vs. body/tail	Usually body/tail	Usually head	Body/tail=head
Connectivity to large ducts	Usually not	Always	Usually not
Cyst contents	Mucoid	Mucoid	Serous
Mucin oozing from ampulla	No	Often	No
Stroma	Ovarian-type	Collagen	Collagen
Multifocal disease	Very rare	20–30%	Very Rare

[a]IPMN = intraductal papillary mucinous neoplasm.

tenacious mucoid material with an amylase level equal to or lower than the patient's serum amylase level. Caution should be exercised in establishing a diagnosis of a pseudocyst on the cyst contents alone, as some of the locules in a mucinous cystic neoplasm can contain hemorrhagic fluid and even necrotic material. Microscopically, pseudocysts lack an epithelial lining, while columnar mucin-containing epithelial cells line mucinous cystic neoplasms. Finally, even when the epithelium of a mucinous cystic neoplasm is partially denuded, the presence of ovarian-type stroma can help separate mucinous cystic neoplasms from pseudocysts (see fig. 5-11). Fine needle aspiration biopsies of mucinous cystic neoplasms that do not produce identifiable mucin or epithelial cells can be mistaken for a pseudocyst. Cyst fluid analysis and both clinical and radiologic correlation become especially important in these cases.

The distinction between a mucinous cystic neoplasm and an intraductal papillary neoplasm (IPMN) will impact on the interpretation of margins, the likelihood of multifocal disease, patient prognosis, and the types of associated infiltrating carcinomas (21,74). IPMNs occur more often in men than woman, and tend to involve the head of the gland more frequently than the body/tail (23,74). The reverse is true for mucinous cystic neoplasms (74). IPMNs, by definition, involve the pancreatic ductal system, while the cysts in the vast majority of mucinous cystic neoplasms do not communicate with the larger pancreatic ducts (74). Microscopically, the cysts of both neoplasms are lined by columnar

mucinous epithelium, but only mucinous cystic neoplasms have the dense ovarian-type of stroma. Also, they usually lack the uniform, regular, intestinal-type papillae that closely resemble villous adenomas of the large bowel and are commonly found in IPMNs (39).

It is important to distinguish between mucinous and serous cystic neoplasms because almost all serous cystadenomas are benign, while mucinous cystic neoplasms have a significant malignant potential. Smaller cysts, a central stellate scar, and cuboidal epithelial lining all support the diagnosis of serous cystadenoma. Macrocystic serous cystadenomas, because they are composed of only a few larger cysts, can mimic mucinous cystic neoplasms when they arise in the pancreatic tail (26a). The cyst contents, the epithelial lining, and the stroma can help distinguish between these two entities. Macrocystic serous cystadenomas contain watery serous fluid; the cysts are lined by optically clear, cuboidal, glycogen-rich cells; and the stroma between the cysts is composed of loose connective tissue. By contrast, the cysts of mucinous cystic neoplasms contain thick tenacious mucoid material, are lined by columnar mucin-producing cells, and the stroma, as discussed before, is dense and has the appearance of ovarian-type stroma. Special stains and immunohistochemical labeling can help in difficult cases. Oligocystic serous cystadenomas are sensitive to diastase digested PAS stains and a mucicarmine stain is negative. Mucinous cystic neoplasms are diastase resistant and mucicarmine positive. Serous cystic neoplasms immunohistochemically label with

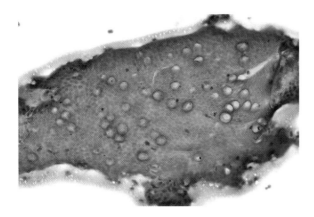

Figure 5-30

NORMAL DUODENUM

Sheets of contaminating duodenal epithelium are recognized by the uniformly distributed nuclei in flat monolayered sheets, and scattered goblet cells that stand out as round clear spaces on this air-dried smear (direct smear; Romanowsky stain).

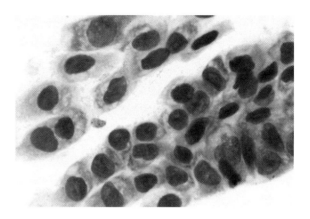

Figure 5-31

NORMAL STOMACH

Gastric epithelial cells tend to present more often as smaller groups and single cells than duodenal epithelium and cause more diagnostic difficulty with mucinous cystic neoplasm. Compared to the cells in a mucinous cystic neoplasm, the single gastric epithelial cells here have denser, less vacuolated cytoplasm (direct smear of gastric mucosa; Romanowsky stain).

antibodies to cytokeratin and EMA, but, in contrast to mucinous cystic neoplasms, not CEA. The aspirate smears of most serous cystic neoplasms produce thin, clear, nonviscous fluid and scant epithelium. The epithelial cells are bland cuboidal cells with nonmucinous cytoplasm in contrast to the columnar cells with basal nuclei and mucinous cytoplasm of mucinous cystic neoplasms with low-grade dysplasia. Higher-grade mucinous cystic neoplasms display atypia well beyond that of serous cystadenoma.

Both solid-pseudopapillary neoplasms and mucinous cystic neoplasms occur much more commonly in women than they do in men. Both of these entities should, therefore, be near the top of the differential diagnosis for cystic neoplasms in women. Fortunately, it is relatively easy to distinguish between these two entities. The spaces in solid-pseudopapillary neoplasms are not true cysts; instead, they are areas of necrosis and hemorrhage associated with a drop-out of poorly cohesive neoplastic cells. By contrast, the cysts in mucinous cystic neoplasms are true cysts and are filled with thick tenacious mucoid material. Microscopically, solid-pseudopapillary neoplasms are composed of relatively uniform cells with granular eosinophilic cytoplasm and uniform oval nuclei. Mucinous cystic neoplasms are lined by a well-oriented layer

of mucin containing columnar epithelial cells. Although it is almost never needed, immunohistochemical labeling can distinguish between these two entities. Mucinous cystic neoplasms have a normal membranous pattern of labeling with antibodies to beta-catenin, and they express CEA and MUC5AC, while solid-pseudopapillary neoplasms express CD10, vimentin, CD56, and alpha-1-antitrypsin, and have an abnormal nuclear accumulation of beta-catenin.

A particular challenge in the interpretation of fine needle aspiration biopsies is the distinction of mucinous cystic neoplasms from gastrointestinal epithelium, especially gastric epithelium. Duodenal epithelium is recognized by the presence of large, uniform, flat sheets of glandular epithelium with a brush-bordered luminal edge, studded with goblet cells containing clear cytoplasm (fig. 5-30) (47,56). Gastric epithelium more often presents as small groups and, occasionally, as single columnar glandular epithelial cells that can be easily confused with the epithelium of mucinous cystic neoplasms (fig. 5-31), especially foveolar cells with caps of apical mucin filling the upper portion of the cytoplasm (see fig. 6-36) (56).

A variety of other cystic neoplasms arise in the pancreas and they need to be distinguished from mucinous cystic neoplasms. These include

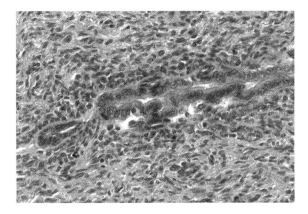

Figure 5-32

NORMAL FETAL PANCREAS

The stroma in the fetal pancreas is morphologically similar to that of mucinous cystic neoplasms.

cystic well-differentiated pancreatic endocrine neoplasms and acinar cell cystadenocarcinoma. Histologically, these neoplasms are easily distinguished from each other. Cytologically, the small, often individual cells of a mucinous cystic neoplasm with moderate dysplasia or carcinoma are similar to the cells of a cystic well-differentiated pancreatic endocrine neoplasm. The most helpful distinguishing features are those of the nucleus. In cystic pancreatic endocrine neoplasms, the nuclei are round with relatively smooth nuclear membranes and have chromatin that is coarse and stippled in the typical "salt and pepper" endocrine pattern. The cells are often arranged individually and have a plasmacytoid configuration. By contrast, the nuclei of mucinous cystic neoplasms with significant dysplasia have a more irregular nuclear membrane with hyperchromatic or hypochromatic chromatin. The presence of even focal intracytoplasmic mucin vacuoles supports a diagnosis of mucinous cystic neoplasm over cystic pancreatic endocrine neoplasm.

PATHOGENESIS

Neoplasms virtually identical to mucinous cystic neoplasms of the pancreas can arise in the ovaries, the hepatobiliary tree (where they are designated hepatobiliary cystadenomas), and the retroperitoneum (5,33,34). The origin of neoplasms with ovarian-type stroma outside of the ovary has been the subject of much speculation, and currently several theories predominate for the development of mucinous cystic neoplasms in the pancreas. First, it has been noted that embryologically the left primordial gonad comes in close proximity to the dorsal pancreatic anlage during the 4th and 5th weeks of development (95). This raises the possibility that cells from the primitive ovary may be incorporated into the embryonic pancreas, and that these ectopic ovarian cells give rise to mucinous cystic neoplasms (34,95). Since, as noted in the chapter on the normal pancreas, the dorsal pancreatic anlage gives rise to the body and tail of the pancreas, this hypothesis would explain both the preponderance of mucinous cystic neoplasms in women, and the tendency for mucinous cystic neoplasms to occur in the body and tail of the gland. Alternatively, it has been suggested that the neoplastic epithelial cells of mucinous cystic neoplasms induce ovarian stromal differentiation in cells that normally reside in the pancreas. The histologic similarity of the stromal cells of mucinous cystic neoplasms to the periductal mesenchyme of the fetal pancreas (fig. 5-32) suggests the possibility that expression of hormone receptors in the periductal stromal cells may cause stromal cells to acquire sensitivity to estrogen and progesterone after menarche, with subsequent stromal proliferation and the induction of neoplasia in the associated ductal epithelium. Direct evidence for any of these theories has yet to be found, however (40).

SPREAD AND METASTASES

Mucinous cystic neoplasms with an associated invasive carcinoma infiltrate into the pancreatic parenchyma and frequently into the peripancreatic connective tissues. Perineural and angiolymphatic invasion are common. Larger mucinous cystic neoplasms with an associated invasive carcinoma can infiltrate into adjacent organs, including the bile duct, stomach, spleen, and transverse colon. Lymph node metastases are identified in about 25 percent of patients with mucinous cystic neoplasms with an associated invasive carcinoma, and the liver is usually the first organ involved by distant metastases. Metastases consist only of the invasive epithelial component.

A number of lines of evidence now make it clear that noninvasive mucinous cystic neoplasms can, over time, progress to mucinous cystic neoplasm with an associated invasive carcinoma (invasive mucinous cystadenocarcinomas) (31,48,63). This evidence includes: 1) the progressive accumulation of genetic alterations in the *KRAS, TP53* and *SMAD4/DPC4* genes associated with progression from mucinous cystic neoplasm with low-grade dysplasia to mucinous cystic neoplasm with an associated invasive carcinoma (19,32,37,50); 2) case reports in which patients with incompletely resected mucinous cystic neoplasms with low-grade dysplasia subsequently developed an invasive adenocarcinoma (31,63); and 3) the younger age at diagnosis and smaller size of most mucinous cystic neoplasms with low-grade dysplasia compared to most mucinous cystic neoplasms with an associated invasive carcinoma (19,48,91).

STAGING

Staging of both mucinous cystic neoplasms with an in situ carcinoma and mucinous cystic neoplasms with an associated invasive carcinoma follows that for carcinomas of the exocrine pancreas (see chapter 3).

TREATMENT

The potential for noninvasive mucinous cystic neoplasms to progress to invasive cancers significantly impacts on the optimal treatment regimen. If clinically possible, all mucinous cystic neoplasms should be completely surgically resected (48). Mucinous cystic neoplasms should never be drained internally into a viscus, nor should they be partially resected. If noninvasive mucinous cystic neoplasms are incompletely resected, they may progress to an invasive cancer, and an opportunity for cure will be lost (86). Fortunately, with improvements in diagnosis and surgical care, the resectability rate for mucinous cystic neoplasms has improved over the last two decades (38).

Recently, partial/segmental pancreatic resection with preservation of the spleen has been introduced as a treatment option for noninvasive mucinous cystic neoplasms, lessening the risk of diabetes mellitus and subsequent infection (42,78,85). Adjuvant therapy should be considered if an invasive carcinoma is present,

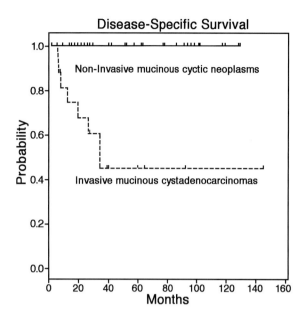

Figure 5-33

**DISEASE-SPECIFIC SURVIVAL
AFTER SURGICAL RESECTION**

The presence or absence of an associated invasive carcinoma is the best predictor of survival following surgical resection of a mucinous cystic neoplasm. (Fig. 5 from Wilentz RE, Albores-Saavedra J, Zahurak M, et al. Pathologic examination accurately predicts prognosis in mucinous cystic neoplasms of the pancreas. Am J Surg Pathol 1999; 23:1324.)

even in cases in which negative surgical margins are attained (70).

PROGNOSIS

The presence of an associated invasive carcinoma, the extent (depth) of invasion, and resectability are the best predictors of outcome (48, 90,95). Although some studies erroneously concluded that it was possible for metastatic carcinoma to develop from primary mucinous cystic neoplasms lacking an invasive component (13,79), most such neoplasms were probably under sampled, and some were not completely resected. Thus, it is likely that undetected foci of invasive carcinoma were present in the primary neoplasms. Based on studies of thoroughly sampled mucinous cystic neoplasms, it is clear that almost all noninvasive neoplasms are cured if they are completely resected (fig. 5-33) (48, 70,75,81,90,95). By contrast, the 2-year survival rate for patients with a mucinous cystic neoplasm with an associated invasive carcinoma is about

67 percent and the 5-year survival rate about 50 percent (48,70,75,81). Because of the significantly worse prognosis associated with the presence of an invasive carcinoma, it is not appropriate to lump invasive and noninvasive mucinous cystic neoplasms together (89).

If an invasive cancer is present, the extent of the invasive component is a predictor of patient outcome. Patients with an invasive carcinoma that is confined to the tumor stroma and capsule do significantly better than do patients with invasive carcinomas that have extended beyond the tumor capsule and into adjacent tissues (95). The extent and size of both the noninvasive and invasive components should therefore be documented. For example, a pathology report could read "Invasive moderately differentiated adenocarcinoma (2 cm) arising in association with a 5-cm mucinous cystic neoplasm with carcinoma in situ. The invasive carcinoma infiltrates into splenic parenchyma."

The 2-year survival rate for patients with unresectable mucinous cystic neoplasms with an associated invasive carcinoma is only 10 to 20 percent. Other reported adverse prognostic factors include tumor aneuploidy, patient age over 50 years, and lymph node and distant metastases (77). Importantly, even though mucinous cystic neoplasms with an associated invasive carcinoma are fully malignant neoplasms, the survival rate for patients with invasive mucinous cystic neoplasms is still significantly better than that associated with conventional infiltrating ductal adenocarcinoma (89).

As discussed earlier, infiltrating carcinomas have been documented to arise from incompletely resected noninvasive mucinous cystic neoplasms. In contrast to intraductal papillary mucinous neoplasms, however, multifocal disease is not a significant concern for these patients.

REFERENCES

1. Albores-Saavedra J, Angeles-Angeles A, Nadji M, Henson DE, Alvarez L. Mucinous cystadenocarcinoma of the pancreas. Morphologic and immunocytochemical observations. Am J Surg Pathol 1987;11:11-20.
2. Albores-Saavedra J, Gould EW, Angeles-Angeles A, Henson DE. Cystic tumors of the pancreas. Pathol Annu 1990;25:19-50.
3. Albores-Saavedra J, Nadji M, Henson DE, Angeles-Angeles A. Entero-endocrine cell differentiation in carcinomas of the gallbladder and mucinous cystadenocarcinomas of the pancreas. Pathol Res Pract 1988;183:169-75.
4. Andea AA, Cheng J, Lauwers GY, Klimstra DS, Adsay NV. Pancreatic intraepithelial neoplasia (PanIN) in pancreata involved by mucinous cystic neoplasms. Mod Pathol 2002;15:282A.
5. Balat O, Aydin A, Sirikci A, Kutlar I, Aksoy F. Huge primary mucinous cystadenoma of the retroperitoneum mimicking a left ovarian tumor. Eur J Gynaecol Oncol 2001;22:454-5.
6. Bartsch D, Bastian D, Barth P, et al. K-ras oncogene mutations indicate malignancy in cystic tumors of the pancreas. Ann Surg 1998;228:79-86.
7. Baruch Y, Levy Y, Goldsher D, Munichor M, Eidelman S. Massive haematemesis—presenting symptoms of cystadenocarcinoma of the pancreas. Postgrad Med J 1989;65:42-4.
8. Bassi C, Salvia R, Gumbs AA, Butturini G, Falconi M, Pederzoli P. The value of standard serum tumor markers in differentiating mucinous from serous cystic tumors of the pancreas: CEA, Ca 19-9, Ca 125, Ca 15-3. Langenbecks Arch Surg 2002;387:281-5.
9. Bastid C, Sahel J, Sastre B, Schurgers P, Sarles H. Mucinous cystadenocarcinoma of the pancreas. Ultrasonographic findings in 5 cases. Acta Radiol 1989;30:45-7.
10. Brandwein SL, Farrell JJ, Centeno BA, Brugge WR. Detection and tumor staging of malignancy in cystic, intraductal, and solid tumors of the pancreas by EUS. Gastrointest Endosc 2001;53:722-7.
11. Brenin DR, Talamonti MS, Yang EY, et al. Cystic neoplasms of the pancreas. A clinicopathologic study, including DNA flow cytometry. Arch Surg 1995;130:1048-54.
12. Brugge WR. Role of endoscopic ultrasound in the diagnosis of cystic lesions of the pancreas. Pancreatology 2001;1:637-40.
13. Campman SC, Fajardo MA, Rippon MB, Kraegel SA, Ruebner BH. Adenosquamous carcinoma arising in a mucinous cystadenoma of the pancreas. J Surg Oncol 1997;64:159-62.

14. Carp NZ, Paul AR, Kowalyshyn MJ, Petersen RO, Hoffman JP. Heterotopic mucinous cystadenoma of the pancreas. Dig Dis Sci 1992;37:1297-301.

15. Compagno J, Oertel JE. Mucinous cystic neoplasms of the pancreas with overt and latent malignancy (cystadenocarcinoma and cystadenoma). A clinicopathologic study of 41 cases. Am J Clin Pathol 1978;69:573-80.

16. de Calan L, Levard H, Hennet H, Fingerhut A. Pancreatic cystadenoma and cystadenocarcinoma: diagnostic value of preoperative morphological investigations. Eur J Surg 1995;161:35-40.

17. Faigel DO, Ginsberg GG, Bentz JS, Gupta PK, Smith DB, Kochman ML. Endoscopic ultrasound-guided real-time fine-needle aspiration biopsy of the pancreas in cancer patients with pancreatic lesions. J Clin Oncol 1997;15:1439-43.

18. Fernandez-del Castillo C, Targarona J, Thayer SP, Rattner DW, Brugge WR, Warshaw AL. Incidental pancreatic cysts: clinicopathologic characteristics and comparison with symptomatic patients. Arch Surg 2003;138:427-3.

19 Flejou JF, Boulange B, Bernades P, Belghiti J, Henin D. p53 protein expression and DNA ploidy in cystic tumors of the pancreas. Pancreas 1996;13:247-52.

20. Friedman AC, Lichtenstein JE, Dachman AH. Cystic neoplasms of the pancreas. Radiological-pathological correlation. Radiology 1983;149:45-50.

21. Fukushima N, Mukai K. Differential diagnosis between intraductal papillary-mucinous tumors and mucinous cystic tumors of the pancreas. Int J Surg Pathol 2000;8:271-8.

22. Fukushima N, Mukai K. 'Ovarian-type' stroma of pancreatic mucinous cystic tumor expresses smooth muscle phenotype. Pathol Int 1997;47:806-8.

23. Fukushima N, Mukai K, Kanai Y, et al. Intraductal papillary tumors and mucinous cystic tumors of the pancreas: clinicopathologic study of 38 cases. Hum Pathol 1997;28:1010-7.

24. Fukushima N, Sato N, Prasad N, Leach SD, Hruban RH, Goggins M. Characterization of gene expression in mucinous cystic neoplasms of the pancreas using oligonucleotide microarrays. Oncogene 2004;23:9042-51.

25. Gagne LJ, Colacchio T, Longnecker DS. Simultaneous mucinous cystadenoma of ovary and mucinous cystadenocarcinoma of pancreas. Int J Pancreatol 2000;28:9-13.

26. Garcia Rego JA, Valbuena Ruvia L, Alvarez Garcia A, Santiago Freijanes MP, Suarez Penaranda JM, Rois Soto JM. Pancreatic mucinous cystadenocarcinoma with pseudosarcomatous mural nodules. A report of a case with immunohistochemical study. Cancer 1991;67:494-8.

26a. Goh BK, Tan YM, Yap WM, et al. Pancreatic serous oligocystic adenomas: clinicopathologic features and a comparison with serous microcystic adenomas and mucinous cystic neoplasm. World Jr Surg 2006;30:1553-9.

26b. Goh BK, Tan YM, Chung YF, Chow PK, Cheow PC, Wong WK, Ooi LL. A review of mucinous cystic neoplasms of the pancreas defined by ovarian-type stroma: clinicopathological features of 344 patients. World J Surg 2006;30:2236-45.

27. Grieshop NA, Wiebke EA, Kratzer SS, Madura JA. Cystic neoplasms of the pancreas. Am Surg 1994;60:509-14.

28. Hara H, Suda K, Oyama T. Cytologic study of noninvasive intraductal papillary-mucinous carcinoma of the pancreas. Acta Cytol 2002;46:519-26.

29. Hara T, Kawashima H, Ishigooka M, et al. Mucinous cystic tumors of the pancreas. Surg Today 2002;32:965-9.

30. Howard JM, Hess W. History of the pancreas: mysteries of a hidden organ. New York: Kluwer Academic/Plenum Publishers; 2002.

31. Hyde GL, Davis JB, McMillin RD, McMillin M. Mucinous cystic neoplasm of the pancreas with latent malignancy. Am Surg 1984;50:225-9.

32. Iacobuzio-Donahue CA, Wilentz RE, Argani P, et al. Dpc4 protein in mucinous cystic neoplasms of the pancreas: frequent loss of expression in invasive carcinomas suggests a role in genetic progression. Am J Surg Pathol 2000;24:1544-8.

33. Ishak KG, Willis GW, Cummins SD, Bullock AA. Biliary cystadenoma and cystadenocarcinoma: report of 14 cases and review of the literature. Cancer 1977;39:322-38.

34. Izumo A, Yamaguchi K, Eguchi T, et al. Mucinous cystic tumor of the pancreas: immunohistochemical assessment of "ovarian-type stroma." Oncol Rep 2003;10:515-25.

35. Japanese Pancreas Society. Classification of pancreatic carcinoma, 2nd English ed. Tokyo: Kanehara & Co., Ltd.; 2003.

36. Jhala NC, Jhala D, Eltoum I, et al. Endoscopic ultrasound-guided fine-needle aspiration biopsy: a powerful tool to obtain samples from small lesions. Cancer 2004;102:239-46.

37. Jimenez RE, Warshaw AL, Z'graggen K, et al. Sequential accumulation of K-ras mutations and p53 overexpression in the progression of pancreatic mucinous cystic neoplasms to malignancy. Ann Surg 1999;230:501-11.

38. Katoh H, Rossi RL, Braasch JW, Munson JL, Shimozawa E, Tanabe T. Cystadenoma and cystadenocarcinoma of the pancreas. Hepatogastroenterology 1989;36:424-30.

39. Khalifeh I, Basturk O, Zamboni G, et al. Villous-intestinal differentiation and progression to colloid carcinoma, characteristic of a major subset of IPMNs, are not features of mucious cystic neoplasms. Mod Pathol 2005;18(Suppl 1):281A.

40. Khalifeh I, Klimstra DS, Qureshi F, et al. The nature and potential role of ovarian-type stroma (OTS) in pancreatic mucinous cystic neoplasms and hepatobiliary cystic neoplasms: a recapitulation of the periductal fetal mesenchyme? Am J Surg Pathol. (In press.)

41. Kim SG, Wu TT, Lee JH, et al. Comparison of epigenetic and genetic alterations in mucinous cystic neoplasm and serous microcystic adenoma of pancreas. Mod Pathol 2003;16:1086-94.

42. Kimura W, Inoue T, Futakawa N, Shinkai H, Han I, Muto T. Spleen-preserving distal pancreatectomy with conservation of the splenic artery and vein. Surgery 1996;120:885-90.

43. Klapman JB, Logrono R, Dye CE, Waxman I. Clinical impact of on-site cytopathology interpretation on endoscopic ultrasound-guided fine needle aspiration. Am J Gastroenterol 2003;98:1289-94.

44. Klöppel G, Kosmahl M. Cystic lesions and neoplasms of the pancreas. The features are becoming clearer. Pancreatology 2001;1:648-55.

45. Lane RB, Sangueza OP. Anaplastic carcinoma occurring in association with a mucinous cystic neoplasm of the pancreas. Arch Pathol Lab Med 1997;121:533-5.

46. Lau SK, Lewandrowski KB, Brugge WR, Warshaw AL, Cenieno BA. Diagnostic significance of mucin in fine needle aspiration samples of pancreatic cysts. Mod Pathol 2000;13:48A.

47. Layfield LJ, Cramer H. Fine-needle aspiration cytology of intraductal papillary-mucinous tumors: a retrospective analysis. Diagn Cytopathol 2005;32:16-20.

48. Le Borgne J, de Calan L, Partensky C. Cystadenomas and cystadenocarcinomas of the pancreas: a multiinstitutional retrospective study of 398 cases. French Surgical Association. Ann Surg 1999;230:152-61.

49. Lewandrowski KB, Southern JF, Pins MR, Compton CC, Warshaw AL. Cyst fluid analysis in the differential diagnosis of pancreatic cysts. A comparison of pseudocysts, serous cystadenomas, mucinous cystic neoplasms, and mucinous cystadenocarcinoma. Ann Surg 1993;217:41-7.

50. Lüttges J, Feyerabend B, Buchelt T, Pacena M, Klöppel G. The mucin profile of noninvasive and invasive mucinous cystic neoplasms of the pancreas. Am J Surg Pathol 2002;26:466-71.

51. Mallery JS, Centeno BA, Hahn PF, Chang Y, Warshaw AL, Brugge WR. Pancreatic tissue sampling guided by EUS, CT/US, and surgery: a comparison of sensitivity and specificity. Gastrointest Endosc 2002;56:218-24.

52. Margolis RM, Jang N. Zollinger-Ellison syndrome associated with pancreatic cystadenocarcinoma. N Engl J Med 1984;311:1380-1.

53. Mentes A, Yuce G. Osteoclast-type giant cell tumor of the pancreas associated with mucinous cystadenoma. Eur J Surg Oncol 1993;19:84-6.

54. Michaels PJ, Brachtel EF, Bounds BC, Brugge WR, Pitman MB. Intraductal papillary mucinous neoplasm of the pancreas: cytologic features predict histologic grade. Cancer 2006;108:174-9.

55. Molberg KH, Heffess CS, Delgado R, Albores-Saavedra J. Undifferentiated carcinoma with osteoclast-like giant cells of the pancreas and periampullary region. Cancer 1998;82:1279-87.

56. Nagle J, Wilbur DC. Cytomorphology of gastric and duodenal epithelium and reactivity to B72.3: a baseline for comparison to pancreatic neoplasms aspirated by EUS-FNAB. Diagn Cytopathol 2005;33:381-6.

57. Nishihara K, Katsumoto F, Kurokawa Y, Toyoshima S, Takeda S, Abe R. Anaplastic carcinoma showing rhabdoid features combined with mucinous cystadenocarcinoma of the pancreas. Arch Pathol Lab Med 1997;121:1104-7.

58. Ohhashi K, Murakami Y, Takekoshi T. Four cases of "mucin producing" cancer of the pancreas on specific findings of the papilla of Vater [abstract]. Prog Diagn Endosc 1982;20:348-51.

59. Ohta T, Nagakawa T, Fukushima W, et al. Immunohistochemical study of carcinoembryonic antigen in mucinous cystic neoplasm of the pancreas. Eur Surg Res 1992;24:37-44.

60. O'Toole D, Palazzo L, Hammel P, et al. Macrocystic pancreatic cystadenoma: the role of EUS and cyst fluid analysis in distinguishing mucinous and serous lesions. Gastrointest Endosc 2004;59:823-9.

61. Pinto MM, Meriano FV. Diagnosis of cystic pancreatic lesions by cytologic examination and carcinoembryonic antigen and amylase assays of cyst contents. Acta Cytol 1991;35:456-63.

62. Posen JA. Giant cell tumor of the pancreas of the osteoclastic type associated with a mucous secreting cystadenocarcinoma. Hum Pathol 1981;12:944-7.

63. Probstein JG, Blumenthal HT. Progressive malignant degeneration of a cystadenoma of the pancreas. Arch Surg 1960;81:683-9.

64. Procacci C, Carbognin G, Accordini S, et al. CT features of malignant mucinous cystic tumors of the pancreas. Eur Radiol 2001;11:1626-30.

65. Recine M, Kaw M, Evans DB, Krishnamurthy S. Fine-needle aspiration cytology of mucinous tumors of the pancreas. Cancer 2004;102:92-9.

66. Ridder GJ, Maschek H, Flemming P, Nashan B, Klempnauer J. Ovarian-like stroma in an invasive mucinous cystadenocarcinoma of the pancreas positive for inhibin. A hint concerning its possible pathogenesis. Virchows Arch 1998;432:451-4.

67. Ridder GJ, Maschek H, Klempnauer J. Favourable prognosis of cystadeno- over adenocarcinoma of the pancreas after curative resection. Eur J Surg Oncol 1996;22:232-6.

68. Sachs JR, Deren JJ, Sohn M, Nusbaum M. Mucinous cystadenoma: pitfalls of differential diagnosis. Am J Gastroenterol 1989;84:811-6.

69. Santini D, Bazzocchi F, Ricci M, Mazzoleni G, Campione O, Marrano D. Mucinous cystic tumour of the pancreas. A histological and histochemical study. Pathol Res Pract 1988;183:767-70.

70. Sarr MG, Carpenter HA, Prabhakar LP, et al. Clinical and pathologic correlation of 84 mucinous cystic neoplasms of the pancreas: can one reliably differentiate benign from malignant (or premalignant) neoplasms? Ann Surg 2000;231:205-12.

71. Shabaik A. Endoscopic ultrasound-guided fine needle aspiration cytology of intraductal papillary mucinous tumor of the pancreas. A case report. Acta Cytol 2003;47:657-62.

72. Shimizu M, Hirokawa M, Manabe T, et al. Cytologic findings in noninvasive intraductal papillary-mucinous carcinoma of the pancreas. A report of two cases. Acta Cytol 1999;43:243-6.

73. Shin HJ, Lahoti S, Sneige N. Endoscopic ultrasound-guided fine-needle aspiration in 179 cases: the M. D. Anderson Cancer Center experience. Cancer 2002;96:174-80.

74. Shyr YM, Su CH, Tsay SH, Lui WY. Mucin producing neoplasms of the pancreas. Intraductal papillary and mucinous cystic neoplasms. Ann Surg 1996;223:141-6.

75. Siech M, Tripp K, Schmidt-Rohlfing B, et al. Cystic tumours of the pancreas: diagnostic accuracy, pathological observations and surgical consequences. Langenbecks Arch Surg 1998;383:56-61.

76. Solcia E, Capella C, Klöppel G. Tumors of the pancreas. Atlas of Tumor Pathology, 3rd Series, Fascicle 20. Washington, DC: Armed Forces Institute of Pathology; 1997.

77. Southern JF, Warshaw AL, Lewandrowski KB. DNA ploidy analysis of mucinous cystic tumors of the pancreas. Correlation of aneuploidy with malignancy and poor prognosis. Cancer 1996;77:58-62.

78. Sperti C, Pasquali C, Ferronato A, Pedrazzoli S. Median pancreatectomy for tumors of the neck and body of the pancreas. J Am Coll Surg 2000;190:711-6.

79. Sperti C, Pasquali C, Guolo P, Polverosi R, Liessi G, Pedrazzoli S. Serum tumor markers and cyst fluid analysis are useful for the diagnosis of pancreatic cystic tumors. Cancer 1996;78:237-43.

79a. Stelow EB, Adams RB, Moskaluk CA. The prevalence of pancreatic intraepithelial neoplasia in pancreata with uncommon types of primary neoplasms. Am J Surg Pathol 2006;30:36-41.

80. Stelow EB, Stanley MW, Bardales RH, et al. Intraductal papillary-mucinous neoplasm of the pancreas. The findings and limitations of cytologic samples obtained by endoscopic ultrasound-guided fine-needle aspiration. Am J Clin Pathol 2003;120:398-404.

81. Sugiyama M, Atomi Y, Kuroda A. Two types of mucin-producing cystic tumors of the pancreas: diagnosis and treatment. Surgery 1997;122:617-25.

82. Thompson LD, Becker RC, Przygodzki RM, Adair CF, Heffess CS. Mucinous cystic neoplasm (mucinous cystadenocarcinoma of low-grade malignant potential) of the pancreas: a clinicopathologic study of the pancreas. Am J Surg Pathol 1999;23:1-16.

83. van den Berg W, Tascilar M, Offerhaus GJ, et al. Pancreatic mucinous cystic neoplasms with sarcomatous stroma: molecular evidence for monoclonal origin with subsequent divergence of the epithelial and sarcomatous components. Mod Pathol 2000;13:86-91.

84. Warshaw AL, Compton CC, Lewandrowski KB, Cardenosa G, Mueller PR. Cystic tumors of the pancreas. New clinical, radiologic, and pathologic observations in 67 patients. Ann Surg 1990;212:432-45.

85. Warshaw AL, Rattner DW, Fernandez-del Castillo C, Z'graggen K. Middle segment pancreatectomy: a novel technique for conserving pancreatic tissue. Arch Surg 1998;133:327-31.

86. Warshaw AL, Rutledge PL. Cystic tumors mistaken for pancreatic pseudocysts. Ann Surg 1987;205:393-8.

87. Wenig BM, Albores-Saavedra J, Buetow PC, Heffess CS. Pancreatic mucinous cystic neoplasm with sarcomatous stroma: a report of three cases. Am J Surg Pathol 1997;21:70-80.

88. Westra WH, Sturm PJ, Drillenburg P, et al. K-ras oncogene mutations in osteoclast-like giant cell tumors of the pancreas and liver: genetic evidence to support origin from the duct epithelium. Am J Surg Pathol 1998;22:1247-54.

89. Wilentz RE, Albores-Saavedra J, Hruban RH. Mucinous cystic neoplasms of the pancreas. Semin Diagn Pathol 2000;17:31-42.

90. Wilentz RE, Albores-Saavedra J, Zahurak M, et al. Pathologic examination accurately predicts prognosis in mucinous cystic neoplasms of the pancreas. Am J Surg Pathol 1999;23:1320-7.

91. Yamaguchi K, Enjoji M. Cystic neoplasms of the pancreas. Gastroenterology 1987;92:1934-43.

92. Yoshizawa K, Nagai H, Sakurai S, et al. Clonality and K-ras mutation analyses of epithelia in intraductal papillary mucinous tumor and mucinous cystic tumor of the pancreas. Virchows Arch 2002;441:437-43.

93. Zamboni G, Castelli P, Pea M, et al. Mucinous cystic tumor of the pancreas recurring after 11 years as cystadenocarcinoma with foci of cho-riocarcinoma and osteoclast-like giant cell tumor. Surg Pathol 1994;5:253-62.

94. Zamboni G, Klöppel G, Hruban RH, Longnecker DS, Adler G. Mucinous cystic neoplasms of the pancreas. In: Hamilton SR, Aaltonen LA, eds. World Health Organization Classification of Tumours. Pathology and genetics of tumours of the digestive system. Lyon: IARCPress; 2000: 234-6.

95. Zamboni G, Scarpa A, Bogina G, et al. Mucinous cystic tumors of the pancreas: clinicopathological features, prognosis, and relationship to other mucinous cystic tumors. Am J Surg Pathol 1999;23:410-22.

6 INTRADUCTAL NEOPLASMS

A number of distinct pancreatic neoplasms have an intraductal growth pattern. Most arise in the native pancreatic ducts, but some typically solid neoplasms, such as pancreatic endocrine neoplasms and acinar cell carcinomas, extend intraductally on rare occasion. Among the primary intraductal neoplasms, intraductal papillary mucinous neoplasms are the most common and best characterized. They have a range of histologic patterns that include different morphologic types of papillae, including intestinal, pancreatobiliary, and gastric foveolar differentiation. A subset of intraductal neoplasms with oncocytic cytology is separately designated as intraductal oncocytic papillary neoplasms. A new category of intraductal tubular neoplasms recently has been recognized in which the neoplastic cells are not arranged in papillary structures but instead are arranged as tightly packed tubular glands forming a polypoid intraluminal mass.

INTRADUCTAL PAPILLARY MUCINOUS NEOPLASM

Intraductal papillary mucinous neoplasm (IPMN) is one of the more exciting pancreatic entities to be characterized in the last few decades. Slow, noninvasive growth provides an opportunity to surgically resect these neoplasms while they are still curable. Even when an associated invasive carcinoma is present, patients with IPMN have a significantly better prognosis than those with invasive ductal adenocarcinoma of the pancreas. It is not surprising that IPMNs have drawn the attention of radiologists, gastroenterologists, pathologists, oncologists, and surgeons. While this interest has helped characterize the neoplasm, it has also led to significant confusion, as each specialty, and sometimes even each investigator, seems to emphasize a different aspect of the neoplasm, often using a different nomenclature. Fortunately, it has now been internationally agreed that mucin-producing pancreatic neoplasms, with prominent intraductal growth and frequent papillary architecture are best united under the single designation, intraductal papillary mucinous neoplasm.

In the previous edition of this Fascicle and in the current World Health Organization (WHO) classification, IPMNs with in situ carcinoma are designated *intraductal papillary mucinous carcinoma* whereas those with an invasive component are simply designated *papillary mucinous carcinoma*, without separate designation of the intraductal and invasive components (67,117). A number of clinical studies have made it clear that the presence of an associated invasive carcinoma and the size of the invasive component are important prognostic factors for patients with an IPMN. The current international classification system for IPMNs therefore clearly separates the noninvasive and invasive components of IPMNs (35). Noninvasive IPMNs are further categorized into three groups based on the degree of cytologic and architectural dysplasia in the lesion: *IPMN with low-grade dysplasia* (or *intraductal papillary mucinous adenoma*), *IPMN with moderate dysplasia*, and *IPMN with high-grade dysplasia* (or *intraductal papillary mucinous carcinoma in situ*). IPMN with low-grade dysplasia replaces the old term IPMN-adenoma to keep the nomenclature of all of the noninvasive mucin-producing cystic neoplasms consistent. IPMN with moderate dysplasia replaces the old term, IPMN-borderline because the term borderline incorrectly implies that noninvasive IPMNs have the ability to metastasize.

Definition. IPMN is a grossly visible, mucin-producing epithelial neoplasm that predominantly grows within the main pancreatic duct or one of its branches; it often, although not always, has a papillary architecture (35,45,67, 117). IPMNs frequently produce copious quantities of mucin, and this mucin usually significantly dilates the pancreatic ducts. In some cases, the mucin can be seen extruding from the ampulla of Vater, a finding virtually diagnostic of IPMN. There are numerous synonyms for this entity, including *intraductal papilloma, diffuse papillomatosis, villous adenoma, diffuse villous carcinoma, intraductal papillary neoplasm, mucinous duct ectasia, duct ectatic mucinous cystadenoma* and *cystadenocarcinoma, intraductal cystadenoma* and *cystadenocarcinoma, mucin-producing tumor, intraductal mucin-producing tumor*, and *mucin-hypersecreting tumor*; however, the use of these terms is discouraged.

General Features. In retrospect, IPMNs were reported by Haben more than 70 years ago, but it wasn't until 1982 that Ohhashi et al. (29,93) clearly emphasized the importance of separating IPMNs from mucinous cystic neoplasms and ductal adenocarcinomas. These investigators reported the clinical findings of four patients with diffuse dilatation of the main pancreatic duct and mucin extruding from a patulous, enlarged ampulla of Vater. IPMNs have been recognized with growing frequency since this seminal report; over 2,000 cases have been reported to date and it is now estimated that IPMNs account for 3 to 5 percent of all pancreatic neoplasms, and 20 percent of all cystic neoplasms of the pancreas (58,125). In an autopsy study, small cystic lesions possibly representing early IPMNs were identified in 24 percent of elderly patients (55). With the growing awareness of this entity, some neoplasms that were previously classified as mucinous cystic neoplasms are now being correctly designated as IPMNs. As a result, the proportion of IPMNs relative to mucinous cystic neoplasms is increasing in most series.

IPMNs occur in men slightly more often than in women, with a male to female ratio in reported cases of 3 to 2 (14,20,24,50,54,56,79,88). The mean age at diagnosis is 63 years, with a range of 25 to 94 years (14,20,24,50,54,79,88). In some series, patients with noninvasive IPMNs are 3 to 5 years younger than patients with an IPMN associated with an invasive cancer (14, 100,115a). Many of the reports on IPMNs come from Japan, although this concentration probably reflects early recognition of the entity by Japanese investigators and not necessarily an increased prevalence of the disease in Asia (54).

Most IPMNs are localized, but they can diffusely involve the entire gland. Gross and microscopic multifocally have been reported in 20 to 30 percent of cases (16,17,39,50,51,75,116, 126,152).

There are no clearly established environmental risk factors for the development of IPMNs, although many patients are cigarette smokers (139). Patients with IPMN have an increased risk of extrapancreatic malignancies, particularly cancers of the colorectum and stomach (18a, 49a,121,144). IPMNs have been reported in patients with the Peutz-Jeghers syndrome; these patients show biallelic inactivation of the Peutz-Jeghers gene (*STK11/LKB1*), helping to establish a causal relationship between the inherited mutation in the *STK11/LKB1* gene and IPMN (119). Similarly, an IPMN has been reported in a patient with familial adenomatous polyposis, and genetic analysis showed loss of the wild-type *APC* allele in the IPMN (71).

Clinical Features. The clinical presentation of patients with an IPMN is usually related to intermittent obstruction of the pancreatic duct by the tenacious mucin produced by the neoplasm. Common presenting symptoms include abdominal pain, back pain, anorexia, weight loss, and recurrent episodes of pancreatitis (8,17, 18,20,23,28,56,88). Some patients, particularly those with longstanding symptoms, develop pancreatic insufficiency resulting in steatorrhea and diabetes mellitus (8,13). A minority (less than 20 percent) of patients develop jaundice, presumably from either tenacious mucin slowing the flow of bile as it courses through the ampulla of Vater, or from the neoplasm itself obstructing the distal common bile duct. Jaundice is more common in patients with an IPMN associated with an invasive cancer than it is in patients with a noninvasive IPMN (56). Remarkably, most patients have symptoms for more than a year (mean, 12 to 37 months in several reported series) before a diagnosis is established (8,13,28, 56). There is even a case report of a patient followed for 27 years with a noninvasive IPMN (112). This finding speaks both to the slow growth of some of these neoplasms and to the nonspecific and indolent nature of the symptoms, which make establishing a clinical diagnosis of an IPMN difficult. Today, a growing number of patients are diagnosed when they are asymptomatic because their neoplasm is discovered incidentally during imaging for another indication.

Computerized tomography (CT) typically reveals a markedly distended main pancreatic duct or numerous cysts that represent dilated

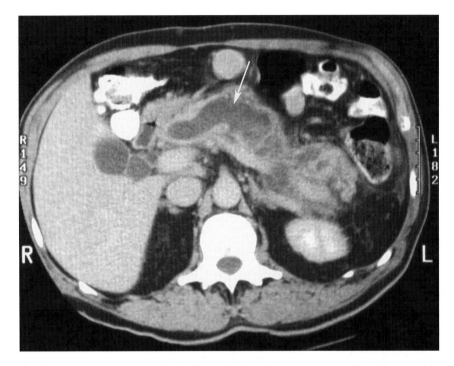

Figure 6-1

INTRADUCTAL PAPILLARY MUCINOUS NEOPLASM

The pancreatic duct (arrow) is massively dilated in this computerized tomography (CT) scan. (Courtesy of Dr. S. S. Siegelman, Baltimore, MD.)

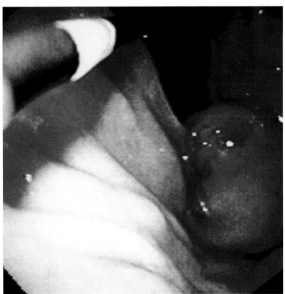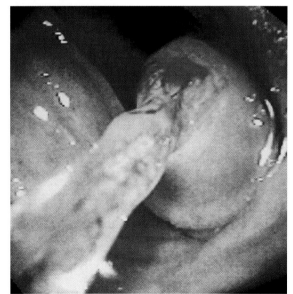

Figure 6-2

INTRADUCTAL PAPILLARY MUCINOUS NEOPLASM

Endoscopic view shows a prominent ampulla of Vater (left) with copious amounts of mucin exuding from it (right).

secondary (branch) ducts (fig. 6-1) (53a,115). In some instances, these dilated branch ducts communicate with the larger pancreatic ducts. Endoscopy classically reveals mucin excretion from a patulous ampulla of Vater (fig. 6-2) (8,146). In patients with pancreas divisum, mucin can flow out of the minor papilla (143). Endoscopic retrograde cholangiopancreatography (ERCP) usually demonstrates a dilated pancreatic duct or ducts in the absence of a stricture, as well as filling

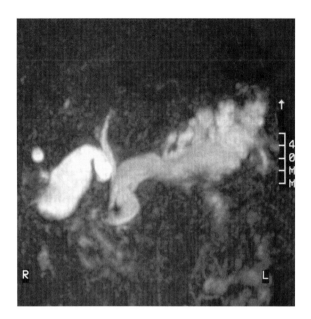

Figure 6-3

INTRADUCTAL PAPILLARY MUCINOUS NEOPLASM

As seen on magnetic resonance cholangiopancreatography (MRCP), there is a markedly dilated pancreatic duct and side branches. (Courtesy of Dr. S. S. Siegelman, Baltimore, MD.)

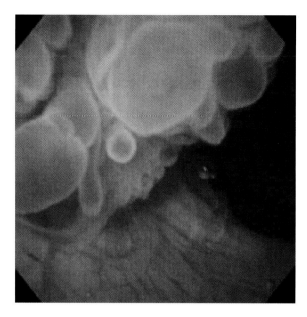

Figure 6-4

INTRADUCTAL PAPILLARY MUCINOUS NEOPLASM

Peroral pancreatoscopy (POPS) shows villous projections within the pancreatic duct. (Courtesy of Dr. K. Yamoa, Nogoya, Japan.)

defects caused by intraluminal mucous plugs or by papillary projections of the neoplasm itself (8,69). Magnetic resonance cholangiopancreatography (MRCP), a T2-weighted technique, demonstrates ductal dilatation and mural nodules significantly better than ERCP, and MRCP is less invasive (fig. 6-3) (60). Gadolinium enhancement on MRI is an indication of increased vascularity and should suggest the possibility of an invasive carcinoma arising in association with an IPMN.

Peroral pancreatoscopy (POPS) can be used to visualize even small intraductal lesions in the pancreas and to guide selective biopsy of these lesions (32,51,145). POPS typically reveals granular or polypoid exophytic lesions in the pancreatic duct (fig. 6-4). This technique has also been used to establish multifocality and diffuse involvement of the pancreatic duct.

Clinical laboratory data are generally nonspecific. Patients with pancreatitis have elevated serum amylase and lipase levels, and there have even been reports of patients developing the Christian-Weber syndrome (asymmetric subcutaneous nodules, fever, polyarthralgias) from the release of lipase and amylase into the circulation (65). Only a minority of patients with IPMNs have elevated carcinoembryonic antigen (CEA) or carbohydrate antigen (CA)19-9 levels, and even when elevated, these serum markers are usually only slightly elevated unless there is an associated large infiltrating tubular (ductal) adenocarcinoma (18).

Unfortunately, current imaging modalities and clinical tests cannot preoperatively distinguish between invasive and noninvasive IPMNs with certainty, although larger neoplasms, mural nodules, and a significantly enlarged main pancreatic duct diameter are seen more commonly in malignant tumors (53a,125a).

Gross Findings. Seventy percent of IPMNs arise in the head of the gland, 20 percent in the body/tail, and 5 to 10 percent diffusely involve the entire gland (8,13,50,56). Discrete cysts may protrude from the surface of the gland, but more frequently, a segment of the pancreas is enlarged. On sectioning, the main pancreatic duct or one of its branches is usually diffusely or segmentally dilated (fig. 6-5). This dilatation can extend into the ampulla and produce the patulous ampulla seen endoscopically. In rare

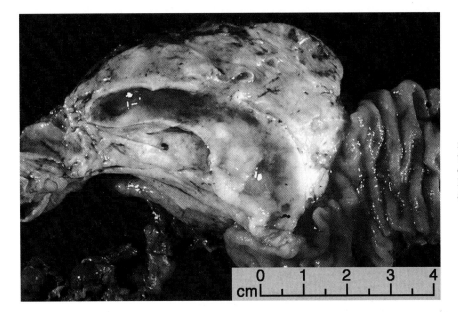

Figure 6-5

INTRADUCTAL PAPILLARY MUCINOUS NEOPLASM

Longitudinal section of the main pancreatic duct as it enters the duodenum. The wall of the duct is fibrotic and the epithelium has a thickened, velvety appearance.

Figure 6-6

INTRADUCTAL PAPILLARY MUCINOUS NEOPLASM

Papillae (arrow) project onto the surface of the duodenum.

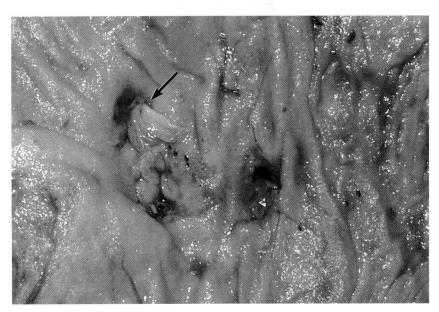

cases, projections of neoplastic papillary epithelium and thick mucin grow out of the ampulla and onto the surface of the duodenum (figs. 6-6, 6-7), or even up into the distal common bile duct. The dilated ducts in most IPMNs contain copious quantities of thick tenacious mucin. Documenting the quality of cyst contents can, therefore, be extremely helpful in establishing the diagnosis. This is particularly true during preoperative fine needle aspiration biopsy when the mucin, which may be acellular, is the only material for diagnosis.

It should be possible to demonstrate a connection between an IPMN and the main pancreatic duct or one of its branches, either grossly or microscopically. The dilated ducts, however, can appear to be true cysts because the relationship between the dilated spaces and the pancreatic ducts can be difficult to discern. This is particularly true when the neoplasm is limited to the secondary ducts. In these cases, a probe inserted into the main pancreatic duct can establish the relationship between the main pancreatic duct and the dilated spaces of the neoplasm.

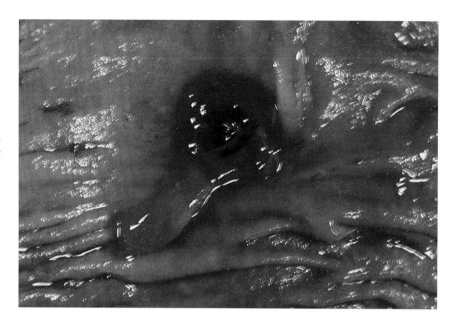

Figure 6-7

INTRADUCTAL PAPILLARY MUCINOUS NEOPLASM

Mucin oozes from the ampulla of Vater onto the surface of the duodenum.

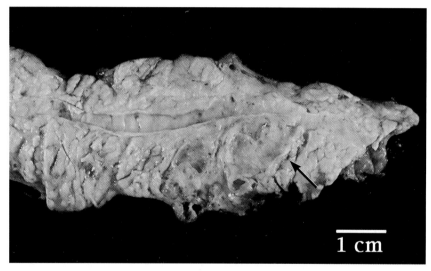

Figure 6-8

BRANCH DUCT-TYPE INTRADUCTAL PAPILLARY MUCINOUS NEOPLASM

The main pancreatic duct is uninvolved by the neoplasm arising in a side branch duct (arrow).

All IPMNs connect to larger pancreatic ducts, however, not all IPMNs arise in the main pancreatic duct. IPMNs are grossly subclassified into those that primarily involve the main pancreatic duct (*main duct type*) (fig. 6-5), those that involve the secondary branches of the main pancreatic duct (*branch duct type*) (fig. 6-8), and those that involve both the main and branch ducts (*combined type*) (10,59,62,83,87,132). This distinction is important because the branch duct type of IPMN tends to arise in younger patients, is more likely to involve the head of the gland, and is less frequently associated with an invasive carcinoma than is the main duct type IPMN (10,41,132). The wide disparity in the reported proportion of branch duct and main duct types of IPMNs, however, suggests that the diagnostic criteria for distinguishing between these two variants need to be defined better.

Normal pancreatic ducts are lined by a thin, almost translucent, flat mucosa (fig. 6-9). By contrast, most IPMNs are grossly papillary and the papillae project into the dilated pancreatic ducts (called a papillary or villous growth pattern) (figs. 6-10, 6-11). Other IPMNs are relatively flat and impart an almost velvety appearance to the involved duct (called ductectatic

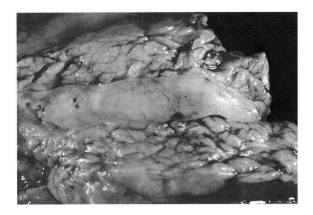

Figure 6-9

NORMAL PANCREATIC DUCT

The duct is thin walled and has flat, almost translucent epithelium.

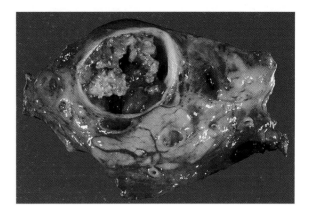

Figure 6-10

INTRADUCTAL PAPILLARY MUCINOUS NEOPLASM

Distended pancreatic duct with papillary projections is seen on cross-section.

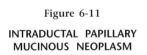

Figure 6-11

INTRADUCTAL PAPILLARY MUCINOUS NEOPLASM

Numerous prominent papillary projections massively distend the pancreatic duct. (Fig. 19-12 from Kumar V, Abbas AK, Fausto N, eds. Pathologic basis of disease, 7th ed. Philadelphia: Elsevier Saunders; 2005:949.)

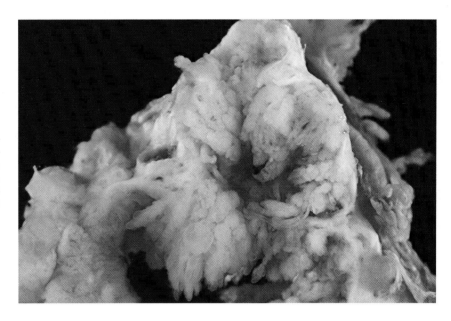

pattern) (fig. 6-12). IPMNs can also form fistulous tracts into the duodenal or gastric lumen.

IPMNs range in size from less than 1 cm to the entire length of the pancreas; most are larger than 1 cm. In some series, malignant IPMNs are reported to be larger than benign IPMNs (about 5 cm versus about 3 cm on average), but size alone cannot be used to make this distinction (88,141).

The adjacent pancreatic parenchyma is usually firm and pale white, reflecting scarring and atrophy from chronic obstruction of the pancreatic duct by thick tenacious mucin. An associated solid or gelatinous nodule should suggest the presence of an invasive component.

Small invasive carcinomas can arise focally in a large IPMN, even in the absence of a grossly defined stromal mass. All IPMNs should, therefore, be carefully examined grossly and extensively, if not completely, sampled for microscopic examination. This being said, completely sampling a large IPMN for histologic examination can be a daunting task. Grossly solid or gelatinous nodules should be sampled first, as these are the areas most likely to harbor an invasive carcinoma. If an invasive carcinoma is not identified in this initial sampling, then the entire neoplasm should be submitted for histologic examination.

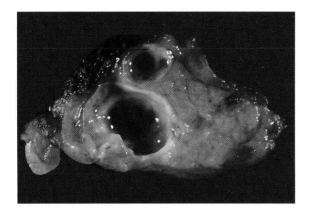

Figure 6-12

INTRADUCTAL PAPILLARY MUCINOUS NEOPLASM

A flat neoplasm has distended the pancreatic duct with thick tenacious mucin.

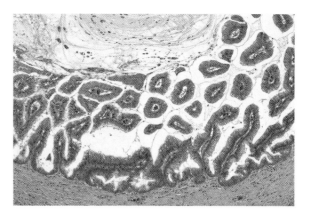

Figure 6-13

INTRADUCTAL PAPILLARY MUCINOUS NEOPLASM

Long finger-like papillae and associated intraluminal mucin are seen.

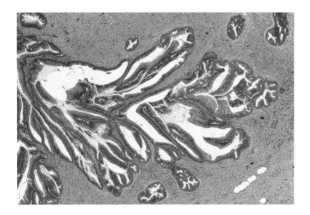

Figure 6-14

INTRADUCTAL PAPILLARY MUCINOUS NEOPLASM

Involvement of the pancreatic duct system can be appreciated as the larger ducts (left) branch into smaller ducts (right).

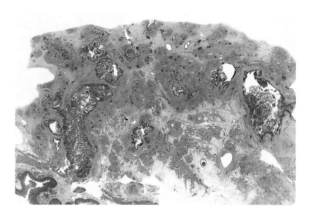

Figure 6-15

INTRADUCTAL PAPILLARY MUCINOUS NEOPLASM

Involvement of the pancreatic ducts in a whole mount section.

Microscopic Findings. Most IPMNs are composed of mucin-secreting columnar epithelial cells with varying degrees of atypia (fig. 6-13). The neoplastic cells conform to the branching of the pancreatic duct system, confirming the intraductal growth of these neoplasms (figs. 6-14–6-16). Most involve the main duct (fig. 6-16), while others involve one of the side branches of the main pancreatic duct (figs. 6-17, 6-18). The spectrum of microscopic findings parallels the spectrum of gross changes seen in IPMNs. Some IPMNs form prominent papillae (figs. 6-13, 6-14), while ectasia of rela-

tively flat ducts predominates in others (fig. 6-18). The size of the papillae ranges from subtle microscopic projections to grossly visible papillae measuring several centimeters in length. The papillae are usually well-developed and have a fibrovascular core (fig. 6-19), but micropapillae also occur.

Most IPMNs involve only a portion of the pancreatic duct. Some diffusely involve the gland. Twenty to 30 percent are multifocal, with morphologically distinct IPMNs separated by an uninvolved segment of pancreatic duct (16,17, 39,75,92).

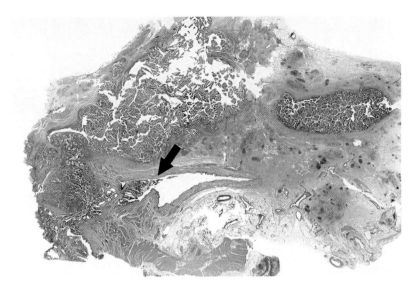

Figure 6-16

INTRADUCTAL PAPILLARY MUCINOUS NEOPLASM

Neoplasm in the main pancreatic duct (top) extends into the ampulla of Vater (left) and focally into the bile duct (arrow) in a whole mount section of the ampulla.

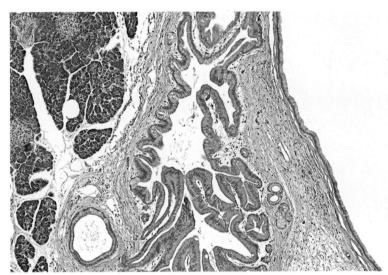

Figure 6-17

BRANCH DUCT-TYPE INTRADUCTAL PAPILLARY MUCINOUS NEOPLASM

The neoplasm involves a branch duct (center), while the main pancreatic duct is not involved (right).

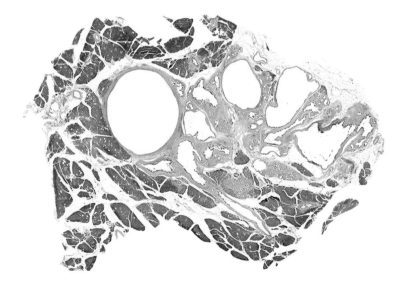

Figure 6-18

BRANCH DUCT-TYPE INTRADUCTAL PAPILLARY MUCINOUS NEOPLASM

The main duct is not involved (center) by a neoplasm involving side branch ducts (right).

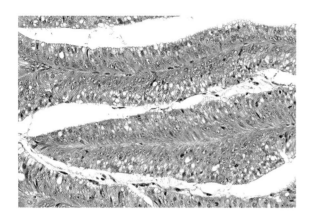

Figure 6-19

INTRADUCTAL PAPILLARY MUCINOUS NEOPLASM

Well-formed papillae project into the pancreatic duct.

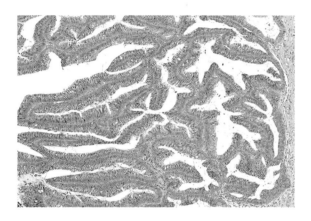

Figure 6-20

INTESTINAL-TYPE INTRADUCTAL PAPILLARY MUCINOUS NEOPLASM

Well-formed papillae are lined by columnar mucin-producing neoplastic cells with cigar-shaped nuclei.

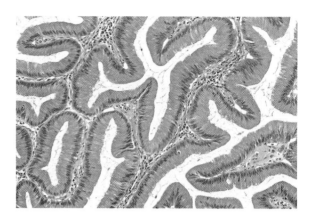

Figure 6-21

GASTRIC FOVEOLAR-TYPE INTRADUCTAL PAPILLARY MUCINOUS NEOPLASM

Columnar epithelium with slightly eosinophilic cytoplasm.

The neoplastic epithelial cells in an IPMN can have a variety of directions of differentiation (26a); however, the biologic and clinical significance of patterns of differentiation remain controversial (26a). Most IPMNs show intestinal differentiation (4,5,17). Intestinal-type papillae are well-formed, long villous projections, lined by columnar mucin-producing neoplastic cells with cigar-shaped nuclei, resembling villous adenomas of the large intestine (figs. 6-13, 6-19, 6-20). Most of the columnar cells contain abundant apical mucin, while others have the appearance of goblet cells.

IPMNs can also have gastric foveolar differentiation (5). The gastric foveolar type of IPMN tends to be histologically low-grade, with slightly eosinophilic cytoplasm, basally oriented nuclei, and abundant apical cytoplasmic mucin (fig. 6-21). Gastric foveolar-type IPMNs are either flat or papillary, in which case they have thick finger-like papillae. Branch duct-type IPMNs often show gastric foveolar differentiation.

The pancreatobiliary type of IPMN is less common and is characterized by the presence of cuboidal neoplastic cells that form more complex papillae with bridging and cribriforming (fig. 6-22) (17). The nuclei are rounder than in the intestinal type and the chromatin pattern is open, often with prominent nucleoli. This type contains less intracellular mucin and tends to be of a higher histologic grade than the intestinal type. Both the intestinal and pancreatobiliary types of IPMN may transition to areas with gastric foveolar morphology; however, it is uncommon to find both intestinal- and pancreatobiliary-type papillae within the same IPMN. Although intestinal- and pancreatobiliary-type papillae have different immunolabeling patterns (see below), the fact that most pancreatobiliary-type IPMNs are high grade has raised questions about whether the morphologic differences between the various papilla types may be simply a reflection of the degree of dysplasia, or whether each type represents a distinct entity.

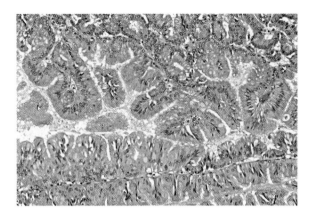

Figure 6-22

**PANCREATOBILIARY-TYPE INTRADUCTAL
PAPILLARY MUCINOUS NEOPLASM**

Cuboidal neoplastic epithelium forms complex papillae.

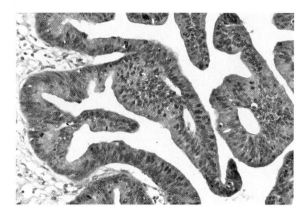

Figure 6-23

**INTRADUCTAL PAPILLARY MUCINOUS NEOPLASM
WITH HIGH-GRADE DYSPLASIA (IN SITU CARCINOMA)**

Significant architectural and nuclear atypia, including
loss of nuclear polarity and pleomorphism, is present.

The non-neoplastic pancreatic parenchyma adjacent to an IPMN frequently shows changes of chronic obstruction, including atrophy, fibrosis, and chronic inflammation. In extreme cases, there is complete atrophy of the surrounding parenchyma, and sections reveal isolated ductal profiles, each filled with papillary neoplasm and separated only by fibrotic stroma. In contrast to mucinous cystic neoplasms, IPMNs lack a distinctive stroma (24).

Noninvasive IPMNs have a spectrum of cytoarchitectural atypia that is classified as low-grade dysplasia, moderate dysplasia, and high-grade dysplasia (carcinoma in situ). *IPMN with low-grade dysplasia* is composed of uniform cells with only a mild degree of epithelial dysplasia (fig. 6-21). The neoplastic cells form a single layer of well-oriented, small and uniform nuclei. Nucleoli and mitoses are not prominent (35,45,67,117). *IPMN with moderate dysplasia* has nuclear stratification and a high nuclear to cytoplasmic ratio that may result in the appearance of nuclei filling the epithelial layer. There is also a slight loss of polarity, nuclear enlargement, and some nuclear pleomorphism (figs. 6-19, 6-20). The papillae retain their fibrovascular cores (35,45,67,117). *IPMN with high-grade dysplasia (carcinoma in situ)*, as the name suggests, has more severe architectural complexity and nuclear atypia. There is a significant loss of polarity, significant nuclear pleomorphism, and architectural atypia with cribriforming and bud-

ding off of clusters of neoplastic cells into the lumen (fig. 6-23). Mitotic figures are often present and can be located towards the luminal surface of the epithelium (35,45,67,117). If there is significant variation in the degree of dysplasia within an IPMN, as is often the case, the neoplasm should be graded based on the highest degree of dysplasia.

Three dimensional mapping of IPMNs has demonstrated that areas of carcinoma in situ arise within zones of lower-grade dysplasia, suggesting a progression from low-grade dysplasia, to high-grade dysplasia, to invasive carcinoma (27). In addition, noninvasive IPMNs often extend microscopically several centimeters beyond the area of gross ductal dilatation and in many instances the neoplastic epithelium also extends into smaller ducts (figs. 6-14, 6-24) (27). As will be discussed in the section on differential diagnosis, it can be very difficult to distinguish between an IPMN extending into a small duct and a separate focus of pancreatic intraepithelial neoplasia.

Approximately 35 percent of IPMNs have an associated invasive adenocarcinoma (14). As noted earlier, invasive carcinoma can be very focal, and a benign diagnosis cannot be established on biopsy alone, nor can it be established in an inadequately examined specimen. In half the cases, the invasive carcinoma has a colloid, or muconodular, pattern of invasion and in half a tubular, or conventional, ductal pattern (6,14).

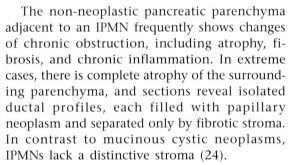

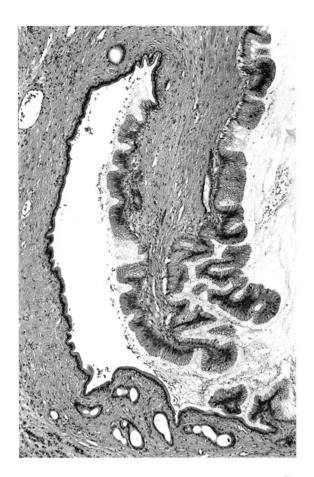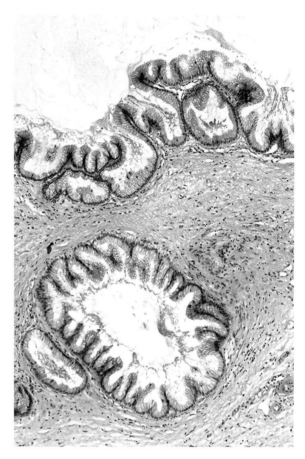

Figure 6-24

INTRADUCTAL PAPILLARY MUCINOUS NEOPLASM

Intraductal papillary mucinous neoplasms (IPMNs) (right in left figure, top in right figure) can extend into smaller ducts (left in left figure and bottom in the right figure) and mimic pancreatic intraepithelial neoplasia.

Figure 6-25

INVASIVE COLLOID CARCINOMA

Neoplastic cells embedded in pools of mucin (bottom) arise in association with an intraductal papillary mucinous neoplasm (top).

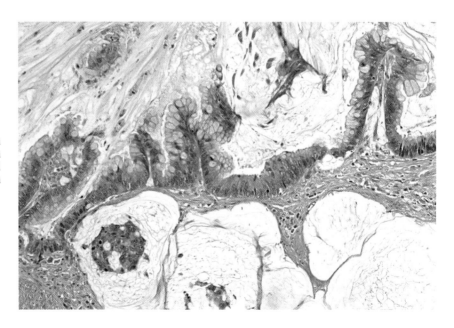

Invasive colloid carcinomas, also known as *mucinous noncystic carcinomas*, form large pools of extracellular mucin containing free-floating neoplastic epithelial cells (fig. 6-25). This form of invasive cancer has to be distinguished from benign spillage of mucin into the stroma. Mucin spillage presumably is a manifestation of duct rupture and results in extraductal stromal pools of acellular mucin that dissect into the substance of the pancreas (fig. 6-26). Often there is a brisk inflammatory response (in contrast to invasive colloid carcinoma). These pools of mucus do not represent invasive carcinoma. In order to diagnose invasive colloid carcinoma, the mucin in the stroma should either contain free-floating neoplastic epithelial cells, or pools of mucin lined by neoplastic epithelial cells should be in a location incompatible with the normal branching ductal system of the pancreas. When carefully examined, almost all invasive colloid carcinomas of the pancreas have been shown to arise in association with an IPMN (107) (see chapter 8, Colloid Carcinomas).

The other pattern of invasive carcinoma associated with IPMN has a conventional or tubular ductal histology (figs. 6-27, 6-28). These infiltrating carcinomas are morphologically identical to infiltrating ductal adenocarcinomas that do not arise in association with an IPMN. The neoplastic cells form small tubules that infiltrate an intensely desmoplastic stroma.

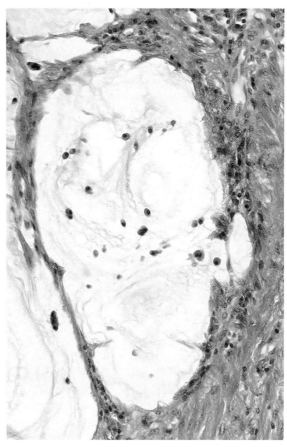

Figure 6-26

ACELLULAR MUCIN EXTRUDED INTO STROMA

In the absence of neoplastic cells this does not represent invasive cancer.

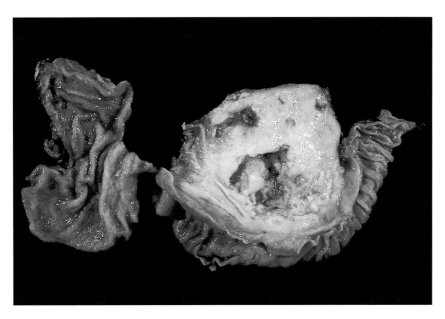

Figure 6-27

INVASIVE ADENOCARCINOMA ARISING IN AN INTRADUCTAL PAPILLARY MUCINOUS NEOPLASM

Dilated pancreatic duct in combination with a firm sclerotic mass in the head of the pancreas.

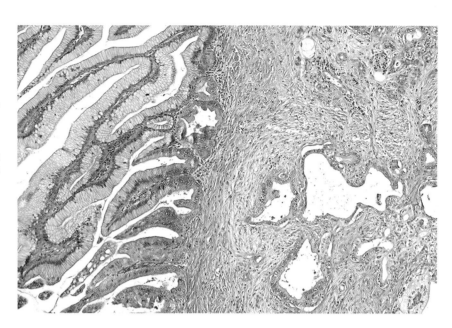

Figure 6-28

INVASIVE ADENOCARCINOMA ARISING IN AN INTRADUCTAL PAPILLARY MUCINOUS NEOPLASM

Infiltrating neoplastic glands (right) arise in association with an intraductal neoplasm (left).

Invasive carcinomas associated with IPMNs can be "microinvasive" (only a small portion of the carcinoma extends beyond the duct) or they can be more extensive (called "invasive" in the Japanese classification system). Size criteria for defining microinvasive carcinoma and the clinical importance of distinguishing between microinvasive and invasive carcinomas have not been established.

Stains demonstrate the abundant quantities of mucin produced by the neoplastic cells. Most IPMNs are strongly periodic acid–Schiff (PAS) positive, and resistant to diastase digestion (94). The neoplastic cells are usually also mucicarmine and Alcian blue positive. Silver stains for endocrine differentiation (Grimelius or Churukian/Schenk) usually reveal scattered argyrophil- and argentaffin-positive cells at the base of the neoplastic epithelium.

Frozen Section. Intraoperative frozen section consultation plays a critical role in ensuring that IPMNs are completely resected (14,15a, 16,28,56,88,96). Results of intraoperative frozen section analysis extend the portion of the pancreas resected in 20 to 40 percent of cases (14,16,28). This reflects the inaccuracy of preoperative imaging as well as the frequent extension of the neoplastic epithelium beyond the grossly dilated portion of the pancreatic duct. Conversely, the main pancreatic duct may remain dilated upstream from the neoplasm, so gross evaluation of the diameter of the pan-

creatic duct at the margin is not sufficient to define the extent of an IPMN.

The interpretation of pancreatic parenchymal margins in patients with IPMNs can be extremely difficult. Margins should be evaluated for the presence of a noninvasive IPMN and for an associated invasive adenocarcinoma. The frozen section evaluation of margins for invasive adenocarcinoma is discussed in chapter 7. Evaluating a margin is treacherous to say the least. Noninvasive IPMNs can be histologically very bland and can mimic reactive epithelial changes, and IPMNs can extend into the smaller ducts and ductules thereby mimicking pancreatic intraepithelial neoplasia (35).

A paucity of mucin and the presence of a significant intraepithelial inflammatory cell infiltrate should suggest the possibility of reactive epithelial changes, particularly when there are numerous polymorphonuclear leukocytes. Reactive changes typically lack the well-formed long papillae of IPMNs, and the nuclei, although enlarged, are usually round with smooth contours and finely dispersed chromatin.

It can be extremely difficult to distinguish between pancreatic intraepithelial neoplasia (PanIN) and an IPMN on frozen section; even on paraffin sections there are ductal lesions that fall in between the defined criteria for these intraductal neoplasms (35). IPMNs tend to be larger (over 1 cm) and the papillae are taller and more complex than those of PanIN

(35). Abundant intracellular and luminal mucin suggests the diagnosis of IPMN. PanINs generally do not display the intestinal features common in IPMNs. When evaluating a pancreatic margin, these features may not be sufficient to determine whether a duct involved by a papillary mucinous epithelial proliferation represents intraductal extension of an IPMN (that has more obvious diagnostic features elsewhere in the pancreas) or a separate focus of PanIN. The finding of PanIN-1 or PanIN-2 at the margin generally does not indicate the need for further resection, but involvement of the margin by IPMN usually suggests that more pancreas should be resected. Comparison of a ductal lesion in a frozen section of the margin with a section of the established IPMN may help in the distinction. In addition, if the IPMN is predominantly in the main duct but the margin is grossly separate from the IPMN and the lesion at the margin is in a small duct, the possibility of a PanIN is more likely.

Some investigators have found that margin involvement by either IPMN or PanIN does not correlate with recurrence of IPMN (17), especially if the intraductal lesion at the margin has less than high-grade dysplasia. Thus, exclusion of invasive carcinoma and high-grade dysplasia (in situ carcinoma) in the margin section may be sufficient information for some surgeons. Other surgeons, however, are reluctant to leave any elements of IPMN behind, and resect additional pancreatic parenchyma until a completely negative margin is obtained.

A dilated main pancreatic duct completely denuded of its epithelium is also problematic. While the temptation is to consider this a negative margin, our experience is that in many instances this represents denuded IPMN. Deeper sections into the block are warranted to determine if adherent epithelium can be identified.

In difficult cases, we find it useful to determine the gross extent of the lesion by examining the entire specimen and defining the gross relationship of the margin in question to the grossly identifiable IPMN. If the IPMN is far from the margin in question, then the lesion is more likely a PanIN. Conversely, a papillary mucinous lesion at a margin is more worrisome if the IPMN is grossly close to the margin. This information, along with the microscopic findings and the patient's clinical status, can all be discussed with the surgeon and a rational decision on whether or not to resect additional pancreatic parenchyma can then be made based on an integration of the gross, microscopic, and clinical findings. For example, if the patient has an associated high-grade infiltrating carcinoma, the margin is grossly far from the IPMN, and a noninvasive lesion with only minimal atypia is present in the pancreatic duct, it may be prudent not to resect additional pancreatic parenchyma as the patient's clinical course will likely be determined by the invasive carcinoma.

Immunohistochemical Findings. IPMNs express markers of epithelial differentiation. Virtually all IPMNs express cytokeratin, and label with pancytokeratin antibodies (AE1/AE3), as well as for CAM5.2, and cytokeratins (CKs) 7, 8, 18 and 19, and variably for CK20 (94,127). Most IPMNs also express carcinoembryonic antigen (CEA) and CA19.9 (79,80,129). Twenty percent of IPMNs label for DUPAN-2 and 25 percent for Adnab-9 (94,129,133).

Most IPMNs produce copious amounts of mucin and a great deal of effort has gone into characterizing this mucin. IPMNs have been immunolabeled for MUC1, MUC2, MUC3, MUC4, MUC5AC, and MUC7 (4,68,84,131). Most IPMNs are strongly MUC2 and MUC5AC positive (fig. 6-29) (68,131,148,149). They show weaker labeling for MUC4 (70 percent), MUC3 (60 percent), and MUC5B (35 percent) (131). Almost all IPMNs are MUC7 negative, and only 15 percent are MUC1 positive (fig. 6-30).

Three patterns of MUC expression have emerged in IPMNs, and these have correlated with the morphologic directions of differentiation discussed earlier (Table 6-1) (26a). More than two thirds of IPMNs are MUC2 and MUC5AC positive, and MUC1 negative (4,68,131). These IPMNs tend to have intestinal-type papillae by light microscopy and they co-express CDX2, a transcriptional factor and determinant of intestinal differentiation (5). When these MUC2-positive/MUC1-negative IPMNs are associated with an invasive cancer, the cancer tends to be a colloid carcinoma, and colloid carcinomas also usually express MUC2 and CDX2 but not MUC1 (4,6,68). A smaller number of IPMNs express MUC5AC, and are MUC1 and MUC2 negative. These show gastric foveolar papillae

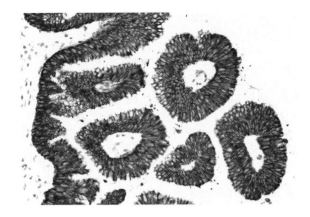

Figure 6-29

INTRADUCTAL PAPILLARY MUCINOUS NEOPLASM

Immunohistochemical labeling for MUC2 in the intestinal-type papillae.

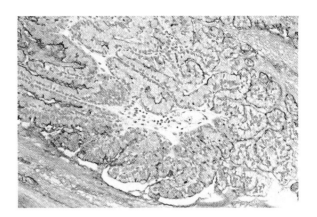

Figure 6-30

INTRADUCTAL PAPILLARY MUCINOUS NEOPLASM

Immunohistochemical labeling for MUC1 in pancreatobiliary-type papillae.

Table 6-1

SUBTYPES OF INTRADUCTAL PAPILLARY NEOPLASMS

Histologic Differentiation	MUC1 Expression	MUC2 Expression	MUC5AC Expression	CDX2 Expression	Type of Associated Invasive Cancer
Intestinal	-	+	+	+	Colloid
Gastric foveolar	-	-	+	-	Rare
Pancreatobiliary	+	-	+	-	Ductal
Oncocytic (IOPN)[a]	+	Focal	Focal	?	Oncocytic

[a]IOPN = intraductal oncocytic papillary neoplasm.

by light microscopy. Finally, IPMNs with pancreatobiliary papillae by light microscopy are usually MUC2 negative, and MUC1 and MUC5AC positive (68). When these IPMNs are associated with an invasive cancer, the cancer is usually a tubular-type ductal adenocarcinoma, and ductal adenocarcinomas are also usually MUC1 positive and MUC2 negative (68).

The patterns of MUC expression have not only helped identify possible subtypes of IPMNs, but they also suggest a dichotomy in the progression from dysplasia to invasive carcinoma in the pancreas (4,68). Noninvasive IPMNs that strongly express MUC2 and are negative for MUC1 may give rise to invasive colloid carcinomas that also strongly express MUC2 and are MUC1 negative. By contrast, PanINs and those noninvasive IPMNs that are MUC1 positive and MUC2 negative may be more likely give rise to invasive conventional tubular-type ductal adenocarcinoma. It is also

possible that some PanINs grow slowly and give rise to IPMNs. This latter possibility may explain why it can be so difficult to distinguish some large PanINs from small IPMNs (67a).

Immunolabeling also reveals scattered (5 percent) chromogranin A-, serotonin-, insulin-, and even gastrin-positive cells at the base of the neoplastic epithelium (128). Cyclooxygenase-2 (Cox-2) is expressed in 60 to 80 percent of IPMNs (89).

IPMNs have a relatively low proliferation rate. Approximately 3 percent of the neoplastic cells in an IPMN with low-grade dysplasia label for Ki-67 and proliferating cell nuclear antigen (PCNA). The percentage of cells that label increases with increasing degrees of dysplasia (78,127).

Ultrastructural Findings. Ultrastructural examination is rarely performed for IPMNs. The neoplastic cells sit on a well-defined basement membrane and are connected by junctional complexes; numerous microvilli are present on the

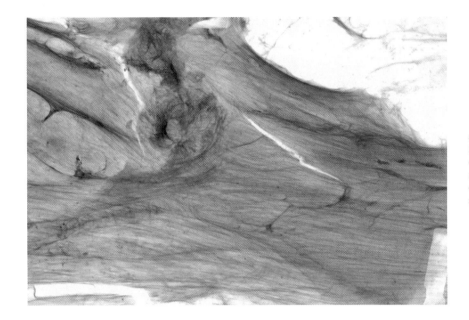

Figure 6-31

INTRADUCTAL PAPILLARY MUCINOUS NEOPLASM

Thick, "colloid-like" mucin aspirated from a pancreatic cyst is diagnostic of a mucin-producing cystic neoplasm but does not distinguish IPMN from mucinous cystic neoplasm (direct smear; Papanicolaou stain).

apical surface (77). The neoplastic cells contain numerous apical mucin granules up to 300 nm in size, well-developed endoplasmic reticulum, abundant Golgi complexes, and numerous mitochondria (77).

Cytologic Findings. Cytologic samples of IPMN are most often obtained by fine needle aspiration biopsy by either a percutaneous route or, more recently and increasingly, by endoscopic ultrasound (EUS)-guided biopsy. ERCP with brush cytology and pancreatic duct aspiration are also used to sample ductal contents for cytologic interpretation (18b,70,134).

Intraductal papillary mucinous neoplasms demonstrate significant variability in the amount of mucin present and the degree of cytologic atypia of the epithelial lining, and, as such, sampling of an IPMN by aspiration may not accurately reflect the true nature of the neoplasm. A specific diagnosis of IPMN, therefore, is less common with fine needle aspiration biopsy than a more general diagnosis of a *mucin-producing cystic neoplasm*, a term that encompasses both IPMN and mucinous cystic neoplasm. Additionally, cytologic samples tend to underestimate the degree of atypia present in the neoplasm, making it difficult to specifically distinguish low-grade dysplasia, moderate dysplasia, and carcinoma (in situ and invasive) (64,74,98). As discussed in greater detail in chapter 5, the introduction of gastrointestinal contamination in the form of both extracellular mucin and

glandular epithelium by the EUS-guided technique adds to the diagnostic difficulty in some cases (12,19,46,57,64,73,74,98,113,118).

The clinical and radiologic features of the lesion being aspirated need to be kept in mind when interpreting aspiration biopsy specimens of mucin-producing cystic neoplasms. This cannot be overemphasized, as the ability to sonographically see a lesion is a feature that can be used to distinguish an IPMN from PanIN. Another important feature is the connectivity of the cyst to the pancreatic duct, the presence of which distinguishes an IPMN from a mucinous cystic neoplasm. A mucin-producing cystic neoplasm (IPMN or mucinous cystic neoplasm) is often first suspected at the time of aspiration owing to the difficulty in both aspirating cyst fluid into and expressing fluid from the needle. Such thick and viscous cyst fluid is reflected on the slide as thick, "colloid-like" mucin that frequently covers most of the slide (fig. 6-31). Mucin contamination from the gastrointestinal tract will not be "colloid-like." The entrapment of degenerated cells and histiocytes within the mucin is a feature of mucin from a cyst and can help distinguish contaminating mucin from mucin aspirated from a cyst (63,64,74,118). Not all mucin-producing cystic neoplasms in general, and IPMNs in particular, will have such tenacious cyst contents. The extracellular mucin can appear as focally thick clumps, thin wisps, and diffuse thin background mucin that may be difficult to visualize

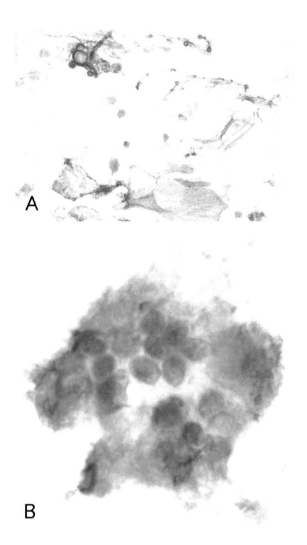

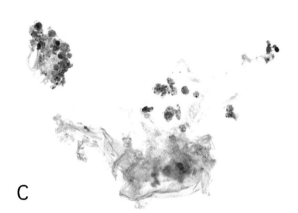

Figure 6-32

INTRADUCTAL PAPILLARY MUCINOUS NEOPLASM

A: Thin background mucin is highlighted by mucicarmine stain on a cytospin preparation of the aspirated cyst fluid. The fluid was not viscous and was not clearly identifiable as mucin on the routinely prepared aspirate (see C).

B: Intracytoplasmic mucin is demonstrated in these benign-appearing epithelial cells from an IPMN with low-grade dysplasia. The background mucin was thin, epithelial cells were sparse, and cytoplasmic mucin is not obvious on the routinely prepared specimen (see C) (cytospin; Alcian blue pH 2.5 stain).

C: Thin wisps of mucin resemble fibrin in this paucicellular aspirate from an IPMN with low-grade dys-plasia. The neoplasm produced thin fluid, and no obvious background or intracytoplasmic mucin in the rare epithelial cells (cytospin; Papanicolaou stain).

without special stains for mucin (63,64,74). An aliquot of the cyst fluid, if sufficient in quantity, can be used to prepare cytospin slides for mucicarmine or Alcian blue pH 2.5 staining to assess for mucin. Although no study has systemically assessed the diagnostic utility of these mucin stains, in our experience, they can aide in the identification of background mucin (fig. 6-32A) and intracytoplasmic mucin (fig. 6-32B) in cases where these features are difficult to appreciate on the routinely prepared specimen (fig. 6-32C). It is important to remember, however, that the absence of mucin by these special stains does not exclude the diagnosis of IPMN.

Mucinous epithelial cells are necessary for a specific cytologic diagnosis of IPMN. The presence of papillary epithelial fragments (fig. 6-33)

supports the diagnosis of IPMN over mucinous cystic neoplasm, but clearly evident papillary fragments may not be identified (64,74,118). More common is the presence of small clusters and flat sheets of glandular epithelial cells that may (fig. 6-34, left), or may not (fig. 6-34, right), demonstrate cytoplasmic mucin on routine light microscopy. Higher-grade IPMNs have less cytoplasmic mucin (74), and therefore the presence of visible intracytoplasmic mucin is not necessary for the diagnosis.

The epithelial lining of IPMN with low-grade dysplasia appears as columnar mucinous glandular cells with basally located nuclei, minimal nuclear atypia, and inconspicuous nucleoli arranged in flat to folded sheets with a honeycombed pattern (fig. 6-35, left), singly (fig. 6-35, right) or in small clusters. Distinction from

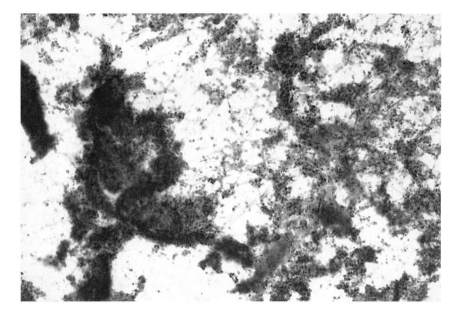

Figure 6-33

INTRADUCTAL PAPILLARY MUCINOUS NEOPLASM

Papillary fragments of glandular epithelium distinguish an IPMN from a mucinous cystic neoplasm. The IPMN here has an associated invasive carcinoma (direct smear; Papanicolaou stain).

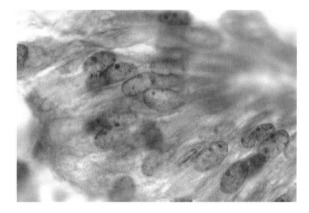 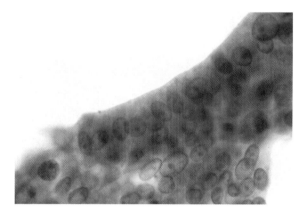

Figure 6-34

INTRADUCTAL PAPILLARY MUCINOUS NEOPLASM

Left: The delicate mucinous cytoplasm is clearly visible (direct smear; Papanicolaou stain).

Right: The epithelial cells in this IPMN with moderate dysplasia demonstrate denser cytoplasm, without visible mucin. The nuclear atypia and crowding distinguish the epithelium of this cyst from duodenal epithelium (direct smear; Papanicolaou stain).

gastrointestinal epithelium is particularly challenging in this setting, especially gastric epithelium. As discussed in chapter 5, duodenal epithelium is generally readily recognized by the presence of large, uniform, flat sheets of glandular epithelial cells often, but not always, studded with goblet cells containing clear cytoplasm and occasionally, with a brush-bordered luminal edge (fig. 6-36A) (64,81). Gastric epithelium, on the other hand, often appears as small groups of glandular epithelial cells that usually do not demonstrate visible intracytoplasmic mucin

(fig. 6-36B), however, an apical cytoplasmic mucin compartment in the upper third of the cytoplasmic compartment can be seen in some foveolar cells (fig. 6-36C).

IPMN with moderate dysplasia and IPMN with high-grade dysplasia (carcinoma in situ) are characterized either by a glandular epithelium with nuclear crowding, loss of polarity, and nuclear elongation and hyperchromasia (fig. 6-37A), or by smaller cells with a high nuclear to cytoplasmic ratio forming small clusters or single cells (fig. 6-37B) (74). The presence of large

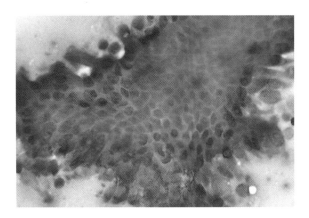 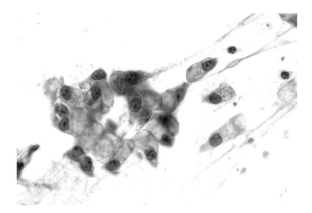

Figure 6-35

INTRADUCTAL PAPILLARY MUCINOUS NEOPLASM

Left: The epithelial lining cells of IPMN with low-grade dysplasia can present as flat, uniform, honeycombed sheets with generally evenly spaced nuclei. Mucin is evident in the cytoplasm of the cells at the edge of the sheet and extracellular mucin surrounds the sheet (direct smear; Romanowsky stain).

Right: This example is composed of small clusters of cells and single columnar cells with round basal nuclei, prominent but uniform nucleoli, and visibly mucinous cytoplasm that fills the cytoplasmic compartment (direct smear; Papanicolaou stain).

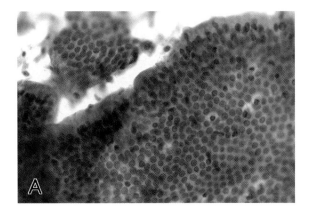 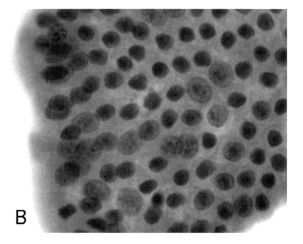

Figure 6-36

GASTROINTESTINAL EPITHELIUM

A: Contaminating duodenal epithelium is most readily recognized when the epithelial cells form large, flat, monolayered sheets in which the clear goblet cells stand out and a luminal edge can be seen (direct smear; Papanicolaou stain).

B: Contaminating gastric epithelial cells typically form smaller sheets than duodenal epithelial cells. A nonmucinous luminal edge is present. Note the uniform and evenly spaced nuclei (direct smear; Papanicolaou stain).

C: Although the cytoplasm of gastric epithelial cells is most often dense and nonmucinous, apical mucin caps may be seen, mimicking IPMN with low-grade dysplasia (direct smear; Papanicolaou stain).

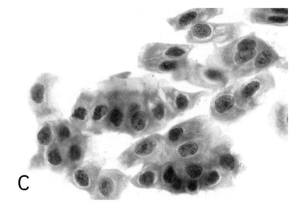

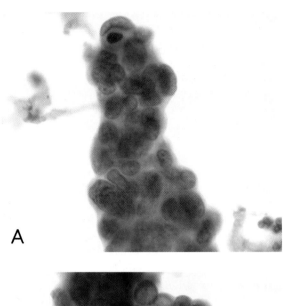

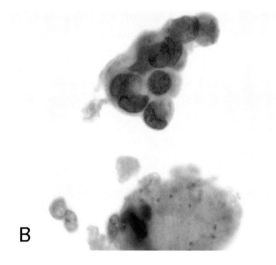

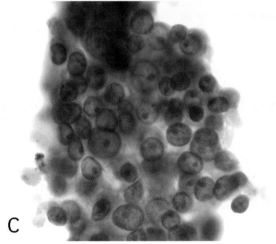

Figure 6-37

INTRADUCTAL PAPILLARY MUCINOUS NEOPLASM

A: The atypical, crowded and hyperchromatic nuclei in this papillary cluster of epithelial cells characterize the cyst as at least dysplastic (direct smear; Papanicolaou stain).

B: Most IPMNs with moderate dysplasia and IPMNs with carcinoma in situ are characterized by atypical cells, either singly or in small clusters, with a high nuclear to cytoplasmic ratio that may not demonstrate visible cytoplasmic mucin (direct smear; Papanicolaou stain).

C: In contrast to IPMNs with moderate dysplasia, IPMNs with carcinoma in situ are characterized by cellular, crowded clusters of enlarged, variably sized cells with parachromatin clearing, irregular nuclear membranes, and prominent nucleoli, similar to the cytologic features of well-differentiated ductal adenocarcinoma (direct smear; Papanicolaou stain).

papillary fragments or crowded groups, with cells having open chromatin, irregular nuclear membranes and nucleoli, significant background inflammation, and necrosis, supports the interpretation of an in situ or invasive carcinoma (fig. 6-37C), whereas only necrosis appears to correlate with the presence of invasion (31,74,109,110,118). Given the atypia present in these higher-grade neoplastic epithelial cells, gastric- or duodenal-contaminating epithelium does not usually pose a diagnostic problem even when smaller fragments have lost their honeycombed appearance.

The presence of a mural nodule and thickened septa is suggestive of an invasive carcinoma. Currently, aspiration of this nodule (as opposed to the cyst contents alone) is necessary to document cytologically an invasive carcinoma, given the overlap in the cytologic features of in situ and invasive carcinomas (12,74,118).

Molecular and Other Special Techniques. Most noninvasive IPMNs are diploid. There is a suggestion that aneuploid IPMNs are more likely to be malignant than are diploid IPMNs (21).

A number of molecular genetic alterations have been reported in IPMNs and most occur at a lower frequency than they do in invasive ductal adenocarcinomas. Activating point mutations in codons 12 or 13 of the *KRAS* oncogene have been reported in 13 to 100 percent (mean, 30 to 40 percent) of IPMNs (33,44,76,85,105, 106,108,122,140,147,150). These mutations have been identified in "early" IPMNs, that is, IPMNs without significant dysplasia, and in most reports the frequency of *KRAS* gene mutations increases with the increasing grade of dysplasia (150,151). Mutant *KRAS* genes from IPMNs are shed into the lumens of the pancreatic ducts and are detected in the pancreatic juice of patients with IPMNs, although the presence of mutant *KRAS* genes in pancreatic juice is not specific for the presence of IPMN (48,61). Some studies have identified more than one *KRAS* gene mutation in a single IPMN, suggesting genetic heterogeneity (44). The phosphotidylinositol-3-kinases (PI3Ks) are regulators of cell growth, transformation, adhesion, survival, apoptosis, and motility. Missense mutations in the phosphoinositide-3-kinase catalytic-alpha (*PIK3CA*) gene have been reported in 11 percent of IPMNs (106a).

Several tumor suppressor genes appear to be targeted for inactivation in IPMNs. Analyses of microdissected IPMNs for loss of heterozygosity (LOH) has revealed frequent losses of chromosome arms 9p, 6q, 17p, and 18q, suggesting that the *p16/CDKN2A* gene on chromosome 9p, the *TP53* gene on 17p, and the *SMAD4/DPC4* gene on 18q may all be targeted for inactivation in IPMNs (22,135). In addition, these LOH analyses provide evidence of clonal progression in IPMNs, as well as LOH patterns suggestive of substantial allelic heterogeneity in several cases (22,136).

The frequency of *TP53* gene mutations reported in IPMNs varies greatly from 0 to 50 percent (11,21,33,42,43,53,56,76,78,85,101,106, 108). In general, mutations in the *TP53* gene appear to occur only in IPMNs with significant dysplasia, suggesting that inactivation of the *TP53* gene is a late event in the development of IPMNs. Similarly, the frequency of *p16/CDKN2A* gene alterations varies greatly between reported series (11,76,85,101). The expression of the p16 protein was reported to be intact in one study of IPMNs (76), while others have reported that *p16/CDKN2A* gene inactivation increases with increasing dysplasia (11,85).

In contrast to invasive ductal adenocarcinomas and PanIN-3 (high grade), the *SMAD4/DPC4* tumor suppressor gene is only rarely inactivated in IPMNs (11,38,76,85). Almost all noninvasive IPMNs, particularly of the intestinal type, express the Dpc4 protein at normal immunohistochemically detectable levels, as do 85 to 95 percent of invasive carcinomas associated with IPMNs (11,38), especially those of the colloid type. By contrast, 30 percent of high-grade PanINs (PanIN-3 lesions) and 55 percent of invasive ductal adenocarcinomas not arising in association with an IPMN show loss of Dpc4 expression (30, 137,138). Loss of Dpc4 expression, therefore, appears to distinguish IPMNs from ductal adenocarcinomas. In IPMNs, the loss of Dpc4 expression is an indirect marker of invasion.

As noted earlier, IPMNs that arise in patients with the Peutz-Jeghers syndrome show biallelic inaction of the Peutz-Jeghers gene (*STK11/LKB1*). About 25 percent of sporadic IPMNs show biallelic somatic inactivation of the *STK11/LKB1* gene (103). Similarly, as noted earlier, an IPMN has been reported in a patient with familial adenomatous polyposis and genetic analysis of this neoplasm showed loss of the wild-type *APC* allele in the IPMN (71). Abnormalities in the wnt-signaling pathway have been reported in sporadic IPMNs (14a).

Clonality of IPMNs has been assessed with differing results. Using methylation-induced polymorphic inactivation of the X-linked phosphoglycerate gene, the incidence of monoclonality has been reported to increase with increasing dysplasia (normal, 27 percent; grade 1 IPMN, 43 percent; grade 2-3 IPMN, 100 percent) (150). By contrast, X-chromosome inactivation of the androgen receptor gene (*HUMARA*) has been reported to show a polyclonal or oligoclonal pattern in 80 percent of IPMNs (44). The differences in these analyses likely reflect the presence of multiple clones in some IPMNs and clonal genetic progression in others.

Microsatellite instability occurs in less than 10 percent of IPMNs. Not surprisingly, most IPMNs show intact expression of the hmlh1 and hmsh2 proteins (85).

Elevated telomerase activity, as measured by the telomeric repeat amplification protocol (TRAP) assay, are detected in pancreatic juice samples taken from patients with malignant IPMNs, but not in juice samples from patients with benign IPMNs (40).

Most (90 percent) IPMNs show aberrant hypermethylation of at least one gene, and the number of hypermethylated loci increases with increasing dysplasia (26,34,104). Aberrant methylation of the *p16/CDKN2A* and *ppENK* genes in IPMNs is associated with loss of expression of these genes (104).

Recent global analyses of gene expression have demonstrated that IPMNs overexpress genes expressed in normal gastric mucosa (*MUC5AC, pepsinogen C, claudin 18,* and *cathepsin E*), as well as some of the same genes found in ductal adenocarcinomas of the pancreas, including *lipocalin 2, mesothelin, claudin 4,* and *S-100A4* (102,130). The most highly upregulated genes in IPMNs in one study included three members of the trefoil factor family (*TFF1, TFF2,* and *TFF3*) (130). *TFF1* and *TFF2* are also expressed in normal gastric epithelium, and *TFF3* in intestinal epithelium.

Differential Diagnosis. IPMNs should be considered in the differential diagnosis of a cystic lesion in the pancreas. Mucinous cystic neoplasms can closely mimic IPMNs. Both neoplasms are cystic and both can produce copious amounts of extracellular mucin. Mucinous cystic neoplasms, however, tend to occur in younger patients (40 to 50 versus 60 to 70 years), they usually arise in the body/tail of the gland rather than the head, they are larger on average (7 versus 3.5 cm), the vast majority arise in women (about 95 percent), they have ovarian-type stroma, and they do not usually communicate with the pancreatic ducts (144). The presence or absence of ovarian-type stroma is the single most useful histologic feature in distinguishing between a mucinous cystic neoplasm and an IPMN (see Table 5-1).

PanINs also have to be distinguished from IPMNs (35). While these two lesions can easily be differentiated at the extremes in lesional size, there clearly is a gray zone and possibly even significant overlap (35,67a). A size cut-off of 0.5 to 1.0 cm is a useful start. Most lesions smaller than 0.5 cm in greatest ductal diameter are PanINs, while those greater than 1.0 cm are usually IPMNs. This size cut-off was chosen not for biologic reasons but because lesions greater than or equal to 1 cm can generally be seen grossly and radiologically (35). Lesions that fall between 0.5 cm and 1.0 cm may be either PanIN or IPMN, and evaluation of their cytoarchitectural features are helpful. As discussed earlier in the section on frozen section evaluation of margins, the papillae in IPMNs are taller and more complex than those of PanIN. The presence of abundant luminal mucin and the expression of MUC2 should suggest the diagnosis of IPMN (35).

Serous cystic neoplasms, with their characteristic gross and microscopic appearance, are readily distinguished from IPMNs in surgical material. Cytologically, the presence of thick, viscous mucin excludes the diagnosis of a serous cyst, but thin or focally thick mucin, which could also be gastrointestinal contamination, does not. The aspirates of most serous cysts produce thin, clear, nonviscous fluid and scant epithelium. The epithelial cells are bland cuboidal cells with scant nonmucinous cytoplasm in contrast to the columnar cells of IPMNs, with basal nuclei and mucinous cytoplasm. Higher-grade IPMNs display atypia well beyond that of serous cystadenoma.

Retention cysts caused by an obstruction of a pancreatic duct can mimic an IPMN, especially those of the branch duct type. Many retention cysts are unilocular and lined by a single layer of normal (nonmucinous) ductal epithelium. Low-grade PanIN, however, may involve a retention cyst (mucinous non-neoplastic cyst, see chapter 15), simulating an IPMN. The vast majority of retention cysts have flat, or at the very most, a low papillary epithelium, and retention cysts do not contain abundant luminal mucin (35). The thin quality of the mucin is important to recognize on fine needle aspiration, since thick, viscous mucinous cyst contents would tend to exclude retention cyst from the differential diagnosis. The epithelial cells of a retention cyst usually have no or only minimal atypia, although when PanIN is also present, there may be mild atypia and mucinous cytoplasm (35). This finding on cytology would preclude the preoperative distinction between an IPMN with low-grade dysplasia and a retention cyst (in the absence of thick, viscous mucin). A stricture or a mass lesion obstructing the pancreatic duct may be identifiable downstream from a retention cyst. By contrast, most IPMNs are papillary and are lined by epithelial cells with some degree of atypia, and most IPMNs have abundant luminal and intracellular mucin. The presence of multiple cysts, reflecting the involvement of a branching duct system, also favors the diagnosis of an IPMN.

Cystic pancreatic endocrine neoplasms (PENs) can mimic an IPMN in cytologic preparations. In the absence of background mucin diagnostic of a mucin-producing cystic neoplasm, the small, often individual cells of an IPMN with moderate dysplasia or carcinoma are similar to the cells of cystic PEN. The most helpful distinguishing features are those of the nucleus. In cystic PENs, the nuclei are round with relatively smooth nuclear membranes and have chromatin that is coarse and stippled in the typical "salt and pepper" endocrine pattern. By contrast, the nuclei of IPMNs with dysplasia or carcinoma have a more irregular nuclear membrane with hyperchromatic (dysplastic, see fig. 6-37B) or hypochromatic (low-grade carcinoma, see fig. 6-37C) chromatin. The presence of even focal intracytoplasmic vacuoles also supports a diagnosis of IPMN over cystic PEN.

As discussed in chapter 5, gastrointestinal mucin or epithelial contamination can be misinterpreted as indicative of a mucin-producing cystic neoplasm of the pancreas in cytologic samples. Close clinical and radiologic correlation is required to avoid this pitfall.

Chemical analysis of the cyst fluid can aid in the diagnosis and subclassification of pancreatic cysts. CEA levels above 200 ng/mL have been found to distinguish nonmucinous from mucinous cysts, with very high levels of CEA correlating with malignancy (66,97). Amylase levels are high in IPMN, due to the connection with the pancreatic duct, but tend to be low in a mucinous cystic neoplasm.

Spread and Metastases. Most IPMNs are noninvasive and do not spread or metastasize. When IPMNs are associated with an invasive carcinoma, the invasive carcinoma can infiltrate into the peritoneum, bile duct, stomach, and duodenum (111).

The lymph nodes are the most common site of metastases for invasive IPMNs. Lymph node metastases are seen in 30 percent of surgically resected IPMNs with an associated invasive carcinoma (14,16). By contrast, lymph node metastases are seen in 75 percent of surgically resected invasive ductal adenocarcinomas not associated with an IPMN. The liver and lung are the most common sites of more distant metastases. A metastasis to the thyroid gland has been reported (36).

Margin status is a relatively poor predictor of local recurrence. Noninvasive IPMNs can recur after surgical resection, even with negative margins (114,116). Conversely, noninvasive IPMNs with positive margins often do not re-cur (17). Sites of recurrence after surgical resection include the remnant pancreas, most likely representing synchronous or metachronous multifocal neoplasia (114,116).

Staging. Staging should follow the staging for carcinomas of the exocrine pancreas (see chapter 3).

Treatment. Surgical resection is the treatment of choice for IPMNs. The surgical resectability rate is much higher than it is for infiltrating ductal adenocarcinomas. Between 80 and 98 percent of IPMNs are surgically resectable. As discussed earlier, the extent of surgery should be guided with the use of intraoperative frozen section consultation. Because even noninvasive IPMNs can recur after partial pancreatectomy, patients with surgically resected noninvasive IPMNs should be carefully followed (39).

In cases with an associated infiltrating carcinoma, the postoperative therapy is usually determined by the type of infiltrating carcinoma (see chapter 7).

Prognosis. Not only are IPMNs more often surgically resectable than infiltrating ductal carcinomas, but the prognosis for patients with an infiltrating carcinoma arising in association with an IPMN is also significantly better than it is for infiltrating ductal adenocarcinomas not arising in association with an IPMN (fig. 6-38) (14,54,72,116). The overall 5-year survival rate reported for all surgically resected patients with an IPMN (noninvasive and invasive lumped together) ranges from 57 to 95 percent, with a mean of 75 percent (16,32,50,54,82,120). Approximately half will still be alive at 10 years (82). These figures are particularly impressive if one remembers that IPMNs tend to occur in the elderly (mean age, 63 years) and some of these patients will die of causes unrelated to their neoplasms.

The presence or absence of an associated invasive carcinoma is critically important in determining patient prognosis (fig. 6-38) (17,54,115a). Patients with surgically resected noninvasive IPMNs have a 90 to 100 percent 5-year survival rate (14,17,56,120), while the 5-year survival rate for patients with an IPMN associated with an invasive carcinoma is 40 percent (14,28,56,109a).

Although patients with surgically resected noninvasive IPMNs do significantly better than do patients with an IPMN associated with an invasive carcinoma, not all of the former are cured.

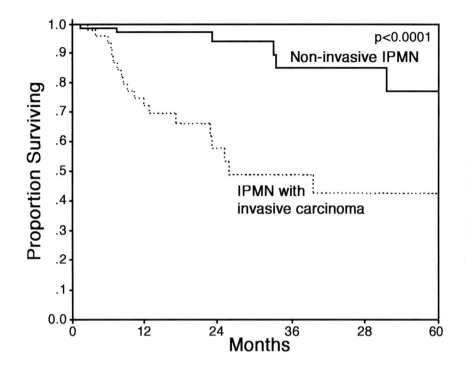

Figure 6-38

**INTRADUCTAL PAPILLARY
MUCINOUS NEOPLASM**

Kaplan-Meier actuarial survival curves compare patients
with surgically resected noninvasive and invasive IPMNs. (Fig.
5 from Sohn TA, Yeo CJ, Cameron JL, et al. Intraductal papillary
mucinous neoplasms of the pancreas: an updated experience.
Ann Surg 2004;239:793.)

Some patients with surgically resected noninvasive IPMNs eventually die of metastatic carcinoma (2,114,116). In some of these cases, inadequate sampling for histology may have re-
sulted in failure to detect an invasive component.
We recommend complete sampling of IPMNs for
histologic examination. As is true for mucinous
cystic neoplasms, grossly nodular and papillary
areas should be sampled first, as these are the areas most likely to harbor an invasive carcinoma.

Some of the recurrences observed in patients
with surgically resected noninvasive IPMNs
appear to be from multifocal disease. Two lines
of evidence support this conclusion. First,
multifocality with morphologically distinct
IPMNs separated by an uninvolved segment of
pancreatic duct has been observed (16,17,39,75,
92). Second, complete resection of the pancreas
eliminates the risk of recurrence. Patients who
undergo total pancreatectomy for a noninvasive
IPMN have close to a 100 percent 5-year disease-free survival rate (14,16,142).

There have been several reports on the long-
term follow-up of patients with an IPMN who
did not have surgery, and many, although not
all, did well (49,112,144a). For example,
Kamisawa et al. (49) reported two patients with
IPMNs who were followed for 7.5 and 10 years

without progression. Tanaka et al. (125a) have
recently proposed guidelines for when to follow and when to resect an IPMN. Nonetheless,
the inability preoperatively to determine with
certainty whether an invasive carcinoma component is present suggests that the decision to
observe a patient with a known IPMN should
not be taken lightly.

The survival rate for patients with IPMNs
with an associated invasive carcinoma depends
on the size of the invasive component
(17,72,120). It is therefore important to document the presence or absence of invasion and
the size of both the noninvasive and the invasive components of an IPMN, just as one would
for ductal neoplasms of the breast. It has also
been suggested that the prognosis for patients
with an IPMN with an associated invasive colloid carcinoma is significantly better than it is
for patients with an associated infiltrating ductal adenocarcinoma (6,17). The 5-year survival
rate for patients with colloid carcinomas are as
high as 60 percent when the criteria for the
diagnosis of colloid carcinoma outlined in
chapter 8 are strictly applied. Pathology reports
should clearly designate the type of any invasive carcinomas associated with an IPMN. A pathology report could read "IPMN-carcinoma in

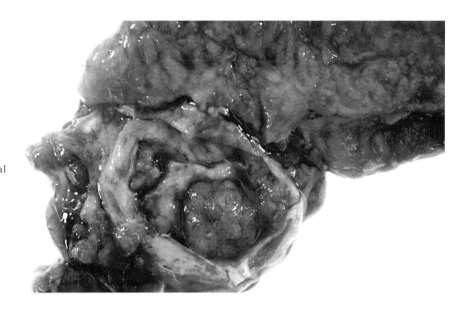

Figure 6-39

**INTRADUCTAL
ONCOCYTIC
PAPILLARY NEOPLASM**

A red-brown intraductal neoplasm.

situ (5 cm) with an associated well-differentiated infiltrating colloid carcinoma (3 cm)."

In most reported series, patients with branch duct type IPMNs have a better prognosis than patients with main duct type (10,17,18,41,59, 99,111,132). This most likely is related to the higher frequency of an associated invasive carcinoma in main duct type IPMNs.

Not surprisingly, patients with lymph node metastases do worse than patients without lymph node metastases (16,17,25,72). Similarly, patients with distant metastases do worse than those without distant metastases.

INTRADUCTAL ONCOCYTIC
PAPILLARY NEOPLASM

Definition. *Intraductal oncocytic papillary neoplasm* (IOPN) is a grossly cystic epithelial neoplasm that grows within the pancreatic ducts and is composed of architecturally complex papillary masses of oxyphilic cells (1,47,91,95).

General Features. This intraductal neoplasm with distinctive cytoarchitectural features, considered a variant of IPMN by some authors, was described by Adsay et al. (1,47,91,95). Most IOPNs display sufficient cytoarchitectural atypia to be considered in situ carcinomas (*intraductal oncocytic papillary neoplasm with carcinoma in situ*), and some are associated with an invasive carcinoma that may also display oncocytic features. IOPNs occur in adults (mean age, 67 years; range, 39 to 78 years) and affect men and women equally (3).

Clinical Features. The clinical features of IOPNs are similar to those of IPMNs. Most patients present with nonspecific symptoms, and jaundice is uncommon.

Gross Findings. Grossly, IOPNs are usually unilocular or multilocular and cystic, and contain soft red-brown luminal papillary masses (fig. 6-39). They measure between 1.6 and 15.0 cm (mean, 6.0 cm). The intraductal location may be difficult to recognize grossly, and most do not involve the main pancreatic ducts (1,90).

Microscopic and Cytologic Findings. Microscopically, IOPNs are architecturally complex, with arborizing papillae, cribriform formations, and solid nests, all growing into the lumens of massively dilated ducts. In the simplest areas, uniform papillae or even flat epithelium may be found, but most IOPNs have papillae with multiple layers of epithelium. The neoplastic epithelial cells of IOPNs have abundant granular eosinophilic cytoplasm (figs. 6-40-6-42) (1).

The oncocytic nature of the cells can also be appreciated in cytologic preparations (fig. 6-43). Both intraepithelial and intracellular lumens are found, many containing mucin, and scattered goblet cells may be identified (1). In the most complex areas, the papillary structures appear fused, resulting in apparently solid sheets of oncocytic cells with an abundant capillary network (fig. 6-41). The stroma at the tips of the papillae may be edematous and myxoid.

Invasive carcinomas are only found in about 25 percent of IOPNs, although the solid areas

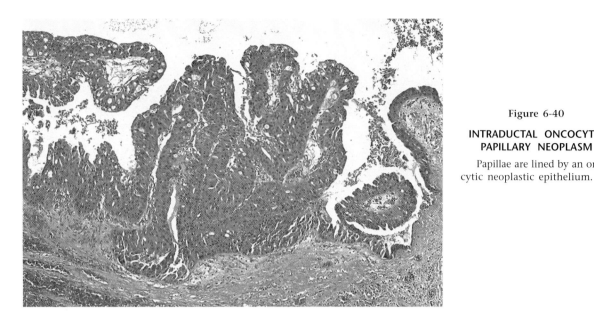

Figure 6-40

INTRADUCTAL ONCOCYTIC PAPILLARY NEOPLASM

Papillae are lined by an oncocytic neoplastic epithelium.

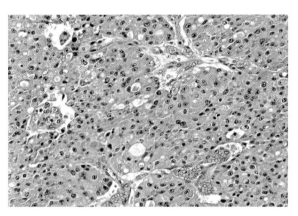

Figure 6-41

INTRADUCTAL ONCOCYTIC PAPILLARY NEOPLASM

Focal solid growth.

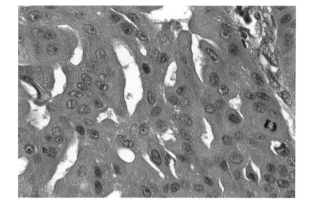

Figure 6-42

INTRADUCTAL ONCOCYTIC PAPILLARY NEOPLASM

Enlarged, somewhat hyperchromatic, nuclei.

may be difficult to recognize as intraductal. Some invasive carcinomas retain the oncocytic cytology, growing as small solid nests of cell and glands infiltrating the periductal stroma (fig. 6-44). Extracellular mucin accumulation may also occur, resembling the pattern of colloid carcinomas. IOPNs with an invasive component should be reported in the same way as IPMNs with an associated invasive carcinoma; i.e., both components should be recognized and the extent of the invasive carcinoma should be specified.

The oncocytic nature of the cells is highlighted by staining with phosphotungstic acid-hematoxylin (PTAH), which results in dense blue cytoplasmic granularity (fig. 6-45) (1). Intracellular and luminal mucin is demonstrated with mucicarmine and PAS stains.

Immunohistochemical Findings. IOPNs label strongly with antibodies against mitochondrial antigens such as 111.3 (1,15). IOPNs usually label for B72.3, however, most label inconsistently for CEA and CA19-9 (1). Immunolabeling for MUC5AC and MUC2 is largely restricted to goblet cells, whereas MUC1 is often more widely expressed (15,68,131). Focal endocrine and acinar differentiation can be

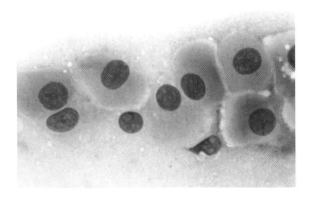

Figure 6-43

INTRADUCTAL PAPILLARY ONCOCYTIC NEOPLASM

The presence of dense, oncocytic cytoplasm is consistent with the rare intraductal oncocytic papillary neoplasm (direct smear; Diff Quik stain).

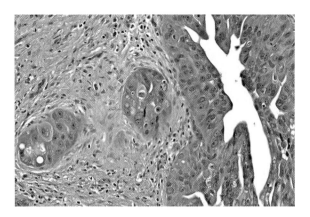

Figure 6-44

INVASIVE CARCINOMA ARISING IN AN INTRADUCTAL ONCOCYTIC PAPILLARY NEOPLASM

Invasive adenocarcinoma with oncocytic features (left) arising in association with an intraductal oncocytic papillary neoplasm (right).

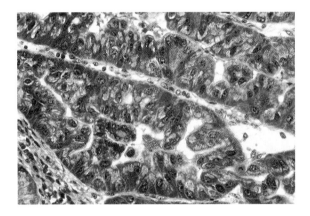

Figure 6-45

INTRADUCTAL ONCOCYTIC PAPILLARY NEOPLASM

Staining with phosphotungstic acid-hematoxylin (PTAH).

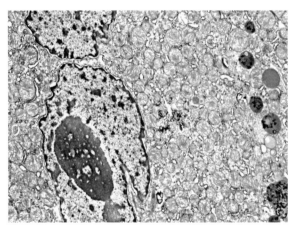

Figure 6-46

INTRADUCTAL ONCOCYTIC PAPILLARY NEOPLASM

Electron microscopy reveals numerous mitochondria.

detected by immunolabeling for chromogranin and trypsin (1). There is consistent immunolabeling with hepatocyte paraffin-1 antibodies; the apparent suggestion of hepatocellular differentiation is not supported by in situ hybridization for albumin, a more specific test for hepatocellular differentiation that is consistently negative (15). Most IOPNs immunolabel for mesothelin, CDX2 is rarely expressed, and claudin 4 is not expressed (15).

Ultrastructural Findings. Electron microscopy has demonstrated numerous mitochondria in the oncocytic cells as well as focal mucin (fig. 6-46) (47).

Molecular and Other Special Techniques. Molecular studies of nine intraductal oncocytic papillary neoplasms failed to identify mutations in the *KRAS* oncogene (15,95), an unusual finding in a pancreatic neoplasm of ductal type. Also, no LOH was found at the loci of the *TP53* and *SMAD4* genes in the only case studied (95), although immunohistochemical evidence of abnormal p53 expression was found in 21 percent of IOPNs (15). Loss of p16 expression is relatively common, but there is no immunohistochemical evidence of abnormalities in Smad4 or beta-catenin (15).

Differential Diagnosis. IOPNs should be distinguished from IPMNs. The complex architecture and eosinophilic cytoplasm allow easy distinction from IPMNs with gastric foveolar- or intestinal-type papillae; there is overlap, however, with IPMNs with pancreatobiliary-type papillae. In fact, there are cases that are transitional between these morphologic patterns. Abundant granular eosinophilic cytoplasm should be a prominent feature in cases designated IOPN.

IOPNs with a predominantly solid growth pattern may be difficult to recognize as intraductal neoplasms. They resemble other solid pancreatic neoplasms such as acinar cell carcinoma, pancreatic endocrine neoplasm, and solid-pseudopapillary neoplasm. Immunohistochemistry is helpful in this distinction; widespread labeling for chromogranin or synaptophysin favors an endocrine neoplasm, labeling for trypsin or chymotrypsin favors acinar cell carcinoma, and labeling for vimentin, CD10, and beta-catenin (nuclear) suggests a solid-pseudopapillary neoplasm. If the intraductal location of the neoplasm is not appreciated, solid IOPNs may be misinterpreted as invasive oncocytic carcinomas; it is possible that some previously reported "oncocytic carcinomas" of the pancreas were IOPNs with a solid growth pattern (37).

Prognosis. Although many of the IOPNs reported to date have been noninvasive, invasive IOPNs do occur, but too few have been reported to determine if their clinical behavior differs significantly from that of conventional IPMNs (1). Metastases have occurred in patients with invasive carcinoma, as has local recurrence following partial pancreatectomy for noninvasive IOPN (3).

INTRADUCTAL TUBULAR NEOPLASM

Definition. *Intraductal tubular neoplasm* is a grossly cystic epithelial neoplasm that grows within the pancreatic ducts and is composed of back-to-back tubular glands without the significant formation of papillae. Most reported cases have minimal cytologic atypia and are composed of glands resembling pyloric glands; they are designated *intraductal tubular neoplasm with low-grade dysplasia* (or *intraductal tubular adenoma, pyloric gland type*) (7,9,52,86,131). More recently, intraductal tubular neoplasms with marked cytoarchitectural atypia, high mitotic rates, and necrosis have been reported, and are best classified as *intraductal tu-

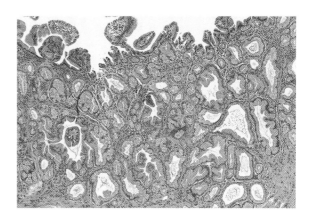

Figure 6-47

INTRADUCTAL TUBULAR ADENOMA
Prominent pyloric gland differentiation.

bular neoplasm with high-grade dysplasia (or *intraductal tubular carcinoma*) (123,124).

Pathologic Findings. Intraductal tubular neoplasms with low-grade dysplasia are grossly and microscopically similar to pyloric gland adenomas of the gallbladder. They can be sessile or pedunculated, and can lead to occlusion and secondary dilatation of the pancreatic duct (7,9,52,86,131).

Microscopically, these lesions are composed of lobules of closely packed tubular glands similar to the pyloric glands of the stomach (fig. 6-47) (7,9,52,86,131). The epithelial cells are columnar, with abundant clear apical mucin and basally oriented nuclei without atypia (7,9,52,86,131). Mucicarmine and PAS stains are positive, and immunohistochemical labeling reveals the expression of CK7 but not CK20 (7,9,52,131). Focal linear immunoreactivity for CEA has been reported along the apical cytoplasm, and these neoplasms tend to have a low proliferation rate (MIB-1 labeling index) (7,9,52,131). Immunolabeling for both MUC1 and MUC2 has been reported to be negative, while labeling for MUC6, MUC5AC, and pepsinogen II is positive in most cases (7,9,52,86,131). A synchronous intraductal papillary mucinous neoplasm can be found in the adjacent pancreas (86).

All reported patients with an intraductal tubular neoplasm with low-grade dysplasia have done well and are free of disease following surgical resection.

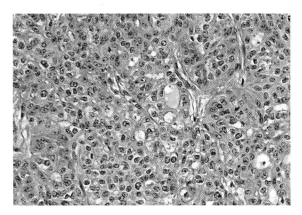

Figure 6-48

INTRADUCTAL TUBULAR CARCINOMA

Marked architectural and cytologic atypia.

In contrast, intraductal tubular neoplasm with high-grade dysplasia displays unequivocal architectural and cytologic evidence of malignancy, with markedly complex cribriform glands and solid areas, variation in nuclear size and shape, pleomorphism, abundant mitoses, and necrosis (fig. 6-48) (123,124). Although the overall pattern within the ducts is hypercellular, focal desmoplastic stroma may be found between the complex glands. In many cases, it is difficult to appreciate the intraductal location of the neoplasm, and on high-power examination, intraductal tubular carcinomas may resemble invasive ductal adenocarcinomas. Transition to normal ductal epithelium shows the intraductal location of the neoplasm. True extraductal stromal invasion occurs, and such neoplasms should be designated as *intraductal tubular neoplasms with an associated invasive carcinoma*. Despite the highly dysplastic appearance of these neoplasms, available clinical follow-up suggests an indolent course in those intraductal tubular carcinomas lacking an invasive component.

REFERENCES

1. Adsay NV, Adair CF, Heffess CS, Klimstra DS. Intraductal oncocytic papillary neoplasms of the pancreas. Am J Surg Pathol 1996;20:980-94.
2. Adsay NV, Conlon KC, Zee SY, Brennan MF, Klimstra DS. Intraductal papillary-mucinous neoplasms of the pancreas (IPMN): an analysis of in situ and invasive carcinomas in 28 patients. Cancer 2002;94:62-77.
3. Adsay NV, Longnecker DS, Klimstra DS. Pancreatic tumors with cystic dilatation of the ducts: intraductal papillary mucinous neoplasms and intraductal oncocytic papillary neoplasms. Semin Diagn Pathol 2000;17:16-30.
4. Adsay NV, Merati K, Andea A, et al. The dichotomy in the preinvasive neoplasia to invasive carcinoma sequence in the pancreas: differential expression of MUC1 and MUC2 supports the existence of two separate pathways of carcinogenesis. Mod Pathol 2002;15:1087-95.
5. Adsay NV, Merati K, Basturk O, et al. Pathologically and biologically distinct types of epithelium in intraductal papillary mucinous neoplasms: delineation of an "intestinal" pathway of carcinogenesis in the pancreas. Am J Surg Pathol 2004;28:839-48.
6. Adsay NV, Pierson C, Sarkar F, et al. Colloid (mucinous noncystic) carcinoma of the pancreas. Am J Surg Pathol 2001;25:26-42.
7. Albores-Saavedra J, Sheahan K, O'Riain C, Shukla D. Intraductal tubular adenoma, pyloric type, of the pancreas: additional observations on a new type of pancreatic neoplasm. Am J Surg Pathol 2004;28:233-8.
8. Azar C, Van de Stadt J, Rickaert F, et al. Intraductal papillary mucinous tumours of the pancreas. Clinical and therapeutic issues in 32 patients. Gut 1996;39:457-64.
9. Bakotic BW, Robinson MJ, Sturm PD, Hruban RH, Offerhaus GJ, Albores-Saavedra J. Pyloric gland adenoma of the main pancreatic duct. Am J Surg Pathol 1999;23:227-31.
10. Bernard P, Scoazec JY, Joubert M, et al. Intraductal papillary-mucinous tumors of the pancreas: predictive criteria of malignancy according to pathological examination of 53 cases. Arch Surg 2002;137:1274-8.
11. Biankin AV, Biankin SA, Kench JG, et al. Aberrant p16(INK4A) and DPC4/Smad4 expression in intraductal papillary mucinous tumours of the pancreas is associated with invasive ductal adenocarcinoma. Gut 2002;50:861-8.
12. Brandwein SL, Farrell JJ, Centeno BA, Brugge WR. Detection and tumor staging of malignancy in cystic, intraductal, and solid tumors of the pancreas by EUS. Gastrointest Endosc 2001;53:722-7.

13. Cellier C, Cuillerier E, Palazzo L, et al. Intraductal papillary and mucinous tumors of the pancreas: accuracy of preoperative computed tomography, endoscopic retrograde pancreatography and endoscopic ultrasonography, and long-term outcome in a large surgical series. Gastrointest Endosc 1998;47:42-9.

14. Chari ST, Yadav D, Smyrk TC, et al. Study of recurrence after surgical resection of intraductal papillary mucinous neoplasm of the pancreas. Gastroenterology 2002;123:1500-7.

14a. Chetty R, Serra S, Salahshor S, et al. Expression of Wnt-signaling pathway proteins in intraductal papillary mucinous neoplasms of the pancreas: a tissue microarray analysis. Hum Pathol 2006;37:212-7.

15. Chung SM, Hruban RH, Iacobuzio-Donahue CA, Adsay NV, Zee SY, Klimstra DS. Analysis of molecular alterations and differentiation pathways in intraductal oncocytic papillary neoplasm of the pancreas. Mod Pathol 2005;18(Suppl 1):277A-8.

15a. Couvelard A, Sauvanet A, Kianmanesh R, et al. Frozen sectioning of the pancreatic cut surface during resection of intraductal papillary mucinous neoplasms of the pancreas is useful and reliable: a prospective evaluation. Ann Surg 2005;242:774-8.

16. Cuillerier E, Cellier C, Palazzo L, et al. Outcome after surgical resection of intraductal papillary and mucinous tumors of the pancreas. Am J Gastroenterol 2000;95:441-5.

17. D'Angelica M, Brennan MF, Suriawinata AA, Klimstra DS, Conlon KC. Intraductal papillary mucinous neoplasms of the pancreas: an analysis of clinicopathologic features and outcome. Ann Surg 2004;239:400-8.

18. Doi R, Fujimoto K, Wada M, Imamura M. Surgical management of intraductal papillary mucinous tumor of the pancreas. Surgery 2002;132:80-5.

18a. Eguchi H, Ishikawa O, Ohigashi H, et al. Patients with pancreatic intraductal papillary mucinous neoplasms are at high risk of colorectal cancer development. Surgery 2006;139:749-54.

18b. Emerson RF, Randolph ML, Cramer HM. Endoscopic ultrasound-guided fine-needle aspiration cytology diagnosis of intraductal papillary mucinous neoplasm of the pancreas is highly predictive of pancreatic neoplasia. Diagn Cytopathol 2006;34:457-62.

19. Faigel DO, Ginsberg GG, Bentz JS, Gupta PK, Smith DB, Kochman ML. Endoscopic ultrasound-guided real-time fine-needle aspiration biopsy of the pancreas in cancer patients with pancreatic lesions. J Clin Oncol 1997;15:1439-43.

20. Falconi M, Salvia R, Bassi C, Zamboni G, Talamini G, Pederzoli P. Clinicopathological features and treatment of intraductal papillary mucinous tumour of the pancreas. Br J Surg 2001;88:376-81.

21. Flejou JF, Boulange B, Bernades P, Belghiti J, Henin D. p53 protein expression and DNA ploidy in cystic tumors of the pancreas. Pancreas 1996;13:247-52.

22. Fujii H, Inagaki M, Kasai S, et al. Genetic progression and heterogeneity in intraductal papillary-mucinous neoplasms of the pancreas. Am J Pathol 1997;151:1447-54.

23. Fukushima N, Mukai K. Pancreatic neoplasms with abundant mucus production: emphasis on intraductal papillary-mucinous tumors and mucinous cystic tumors. Adv Anat Pathol 1999; 6:65-77.

24. Fukushima N, Mukai K, Kanai Y, et al. Intraductal papillary tumors and mucinous cystic tumors of the pancreas: clinicopathologic study of 38 cases. Hum Pathol 1997;28:1010-7.

25. Fukushima N, Mukai K, Sakamoto M, et al. Invasive carcinoma derived from intraductal papillary-mucinous carcinoma of the pancreas: clinicopathologic and immunohistochemical study of eight cases. Virchows Arch 2001;439:6-13.

26. Fukushima N, Sato N, Sahin F, Su GH, Hruban RH, Goggins M. Aberrant methylation of suppressor of cytokine signalling-1 (SOCS-1) gene in pancreatic ductal neoplasms. Br J Cancer 2003;89:338-43.

26a. Furukawa T, Klöppel G, Volkan AN, et al. Classification of types of intraductal papillary-mucinous neoplasm of the pancreas: a consensus study. Virchows Arch 2005;447:794-9.

27. Furukawa T, Takahashi T, Kobari M, Matsuno S. The mucus-hypersecreting tumor of the pancreas. Development and extension visualized by three-dimensional computerized mapping. Cancer 1992;70:1505-13.

28. Gigot JF, Deprez P, Sempoux C, et al. Surgical management of intraductal papillary mucinous tumors of the pancreas: the role of routine frozen section of the surgical margin, intraoperative endoscopic staged biopsies of the Wirsung duct, and pancreaticogastric anastomosis. Arch Surg 2001;136:1256-62.

29. Haban G. Papillomatose und Carcinom des Gangsystems der Bauchspeicheldruse. Virchows [A] Pathol Anat 1936;297:207-20.

30. Hahn SA, Schutte M, Hoque AT, et al. DPC4, a candidate tumor suppressor gene at human chromosome 18q21.1. Science 1996;271:350-3.

31. Hara H, Suda K, Oyama T. Cytologic study of non-invasive intraductal papillary-mucinous carcinoma of the pancreas. Acta Cytol 2002;46: 519-26.

32. Hara T, Yamaguchi T, Ishihara T, et al. Diagnosis and patient management of intraductal papillary-mucinous tumor of the pancreas by using peroral pancreatoscopy and intraductal ultrasonography. Gastroenterology 2002;122:34-43.

33. Hoshi T, Imai M, Ogawa K. Frequent K-ras mutations and absence of p53 mutations in mucin-producing tumors of the pancreas. J Surg Oncol 1994;55:84-91.

34. House MG, Guo M, Iacobuzio-Donahue CA, Herman JG. Molecular progression of promoter methylation in intraductal papillary mucinous neoplasms (IPMN) of the pancreas. Carcinogenesis 2003;24:193-8.

35. Hruban RH, Takaori K, Klimstra DS, et al. An illustrated consensus on the classification of pancreatic intraepithelial neoplasia and intraductal papillary mucinous neoplasms. Am J Surg Pathol 2004;28:977-87.

36. Hsiao PJ, Tsai KB, Lai FJ, Yeh KT, Shin SJ, Tsai JH. Thyroid metastasis from intraductal papillary-mucinous carcinoma of the pancreas. A case report. Acta Cytol 2000;44:1066-72.

37. Huntrakoon M. Oncocytic carcinoma of the pancreas. Cancer 1983;51:332-6.

38. Iacobuzio-Donahue CA, Klimstra DS, Adsay NV, et al. Dpc-4 protein is expressed in virtually all human intraductal papillary mucinous neoplasms of the pancreas: comparison with conventional ductal carcinomas. Am J Pathol 2000;157:755-61.

39. Inagaki M, Maguchi M, Kino S, et al. Mucin-producing tumors of the pancreas: clinicopathological features, surgical treatment, and outcome. J Hepatobiliary Pancreat Surg 1999;6:281-5.

40. Inoue H, Tsuchida A, Kawasaki Y, Fujimoto Y, Yamasaki S, Kajiyama G. Preoperative diagnosis of intraductal papillary-mucinous tumors of the pancreas with attention to telomerase activity. Cancer 2001;91:35-41.

41. Irie H, Yoshimitsu K, Aibe H, et al. Natural history of pancreatic intraductal papillary mucinous tumor of branch duct type: follow-up study by magnetic resonance cholangiopancreatography. J Comput Assist Tomogr 2004;28: 117-22.

42. Islam HK, Fujioka Y, Tomidokoro T, et al. Immunohistochemical analysis of expression of molecular biologic factors in intraductal papillary-mucinous tumors of pancreas—diagnostic and biologic significance. Hepatogastroenterology 1999;46:2599-605.

43. Islam HK, Fujioka Y, Tomidokoro T, et al. Immunohistochemical study of genetic alterations in intraductal and invasive ductal tumors of the pancreas. Hepatogastroenterology 2001;48:879-83.

44. Izawa T, Obara T, Tanno S, Mizukami Y, Yanagawa N, Kohgo Y. Clonality and field cancerization in intraductal papillary-mucinous tumors of the pancreas. Cancer 2001;92:1807-17.

45. Japanese Pancreas Society. Classification of pancreatic carcinoma, 2nd English ed. Tokyo: Kanehara & Co., Ltd.; 2003.

46. Jhala NC, Jhala D, Eltoum I, et al. Endoscopic ultrasound-guided fine-needle aspiration biopsy: a powerful tool to obtain samples from small lesions. Cancer 2004;102:239-46.

47. Jyotheeswaran S, Zotalis G, Penmetsa P, Levea CM, Schoeniger LO, Shah AN. A newly recognized entity: intraductal "oncocytic" papillary neoplasm of the pancreas. Am J Gastroenterol 1998;93:2539-43.

48. Kaino M, Kondoh S, Okita S, et al. Detection of K-ras and p53 gene mutations in pancreatic juice for the diagnosis of intraductal papillary mucinous tumors. Pancreas 1999;18:294-9.

49. Kamisawa T, Fujiwara T, Tu Y, et al. Long-term follow-up of intraductal papillary adenoma of the pancreas. J Gastroenterol 2002;37:868-73.

49a. Kamisawa T, Tu Y, Egawa N, Nakajima H, Tsuruta K, Okamoto A. Malignancies associated with intraductal papillary mucinous neoplasm of the pancreas. World J Gastroenterol 2005;11:5688-90.

50. Kanazumi N, Nakao A, Kaneko T, et al. Surgical treatment of intraductal papillary-mucinous tumors of the pancreas. Hepatogastroenterology 2001;48:967-71.

51. Kaneko T, Nakao A, Nomoto S, et al. Intraoperative pancreatoscopy with the ultrathin pancreatoscope for mucin-producing tumors of the pancreas. Arch Surg 1998;133:263-7.

52. Kato N, Akiyama S, Motoyama T. Pyloric gland-type tubular adenoma superimposed on intraductal papillary mucinous tumor of the pancreas. Pyloric gland adenoma of the pancreas. Virchows Arch 2002;440:205-8.

53. Kawahira H, Kobayashi S, Kaneko K, Asano T, Ochiai T. p53 protein expression in intraductal papillary mucinous tumors (IPMT) of the pancreas as an indicator of tumor malignancy. Hepatogastroenterology 2000;47:973-7.

53a. Kawamoto S, Lawler LP, Horton KM, Eng J, Hruban RH, Fishman EK. MDCT of intraductal papillary mucinous neoplasm of the pancreas: evaluation of features predictive of invasive carcinoma. AJR Am J Roentgenol 2006;186:687-95.

54. Kimura W, Makuuchi M, Kuroda A. Characteristics and treatment of mucin-producing tumor of the pancreas. Hepatogastroenterology 1998; 45:2001-8.

55. Kimura W, Nagai H, Kuroda A, Muto T, Esaki Y. Analysis of small cystic lesions of the pancreas. Int J Pancreatol 1995;186:197-206.

56. Kitagawa Y, Unger TA, Taylor S, Kozarek RA, Traverso LW. Mucus is a predictor of better prognosis and survival in patients with intraductal papillary mucinous tumor of the pancreas. J Gastrointest Surg 2003;7:12-8.

57. Klapman JB, Logrono R, Dye CE, Waxman I. Clinical impact of on-site cytopathology interpretation on endoscopic ultrasound-guided fine needle aspiration. Am J Gastroenterol 2003;98: 1289-94.

58. Klöppel G, Kosmahl M. Cystic lesions and neoplasms of the pancreas. The features are becoming clearer. Pancreatology 2001;1:648-55.

59. Kobari M, Egawa S, Shibuya K, et al. Intraductal papillary mucinous tumors of the pancreas comprise 2 clinical subtypes: differences in clinical characteristics and surgical management. Arch Surg 1999;134:1131-6.

60. Koito K, Namieno T, Ichimura T, et al. Mucin-producing pancreatic tumors: comparison of MR cholangiopancreatography with endoscopic retrograde cholangiopancreatography. Radiology 1998;208:231-7.

61. Kondo H, Sugano K, Fukayama N, et al. Detection of K-ras gene mutations at codon 12 in the pancreatic juice of patients with intraductal papillary mucinous tumors of the pancreas. Cancer 1997;79:900-5.

62. Kuroda A. [A recent progress in clinicopathology of pancreatic tumors.] Tan to Sui. [Biliary Tract & Pancreas] 1988;9:1459-72. Japanese.

63. Lau SK, Lewandrowski KB,Brugge WR, Warshaw AL, Cenieno BA. Diagnostic significance of mucin in fine needle aspiration samples of pancreatic cysts. Mod Pathol 2000;13:48A.

64. Layfield LJ, Cramer H. Fine-needle aspiration cytology of intraductal papillary-mucinous tumors: a retrospective analysis. Diagn Cytopathol 2005;32:16-20.

65. Le Borgne J, Partensky C, Dupas B, Chavaillon A. Weber-Christian syndrome revealing intraductal papillary mucinous tumor of the pancreas. Pancreas 1999;18:322-4.

66. Lewandrowski KB, Southern JF, Pins MR, Compton CC, Warshaw AL. Cyst fluid analysis in the differential diagnosis of pancreatic cysts. A comparison of pseudocysts, serous cystadenomas, mucinous cystic neoplasms, and mucinous cystadenocarcinoma. Ann Surg 1993;217:41-7.

67. Longnecker DS, Adler G, Hruban RH, Klöppel G. Intraductal papillary-mucinous neoplasms of the pancreas. In: Hamilton SR, Aaltonen LA, eds. World Health Organization Classification of Tumours. Pathology and genetics of tumours of the digestive system. Lyon: IARC Press; 2000: 237-40.

67a. Longnecker DS, Adsay NV, Fernandez-del Castillo C, et al. Histopathological diagnosis of pancreatic intraepithelial neoplasia and intraductal papillary-mucinous neoplasms: interobserver agreement. Pancreas 2005;31:344-9.

68. Lüttges J, Zamboni G, Longnecker DS, Klöppel G. The immunohistochemical mucin expression pattern distinguishes different types of intraductal papillary mucinous neoplasms of the pancreas and determines their relationship to mucinous noncystic carcinoma and ductal adenocarcinoma. Am J Surg Pathol 2001;25:942-8.

69. Madura JA, Wiebke EA, Howard TJ, et al. Mucin-hypersecreting intraductal neoplasms of the pancreas: a precursor to cystic pancreatic malignancies. Surgery 1997;122:786-92.

70. Maire F, Couvelard A, Hammel P, et al. Intraductal papillary mucinous tumors of the pancreas: the preoperative value of cytologic and histopathologic diagnosis. Gastrointest Endosc 2003;58:701-6.

71. Maire F, Hammel P, Terris B, et al. Intraductal papillary and mucinous pancreatic tumour: a new extracolonic tumour in familial adenomatous polyposis. Gut 2002;51:446-9.

72. Maire F, Hammel P, Terris B, et al. Prognosis of malignant intraductal papillary mucinous tumours of the pancreas after surgical resection. Comparison with pancreatic ductal adenocarcinoma. Gut 2002;51:717-22.

73. Mallery JS, Centeno BA, Hahn PF, Chang Y, Warshaw AL, Brugge WR. Pancreatic tissue sampling guided by EUS, CT/US, and surgery: a comparison of sensitivity and specificity. Gastrointest Endosc 2002;56:218-24.

74. Michaels PJ, Brachtel EF, Bounds BC, Brugge WB, Pitman MB. Intraductal papillary mucinous neoplasm of the pancreas: cytologic features predict histologic grade. Cancer 2006;108:163-73.

75. Milchgrub S, Campuzano M, Casillas J, Albores-Saavedra J. Intraductal carcinoma of the pancreas. Cancer 1992;69:651-6.

76. Moore PS, Orlandini S, Zamboni G, et al. Pancreatic tumours: molecular pathways implicated in ductal cancer are involved in ampullary but not in exocrine nonductal or endocrine tumorigenesis. Br J Cancer 2001;84:253-62.

77. Morohoshi T, Kanda M, Asanuma K, Klöppel G. Intraductal papillary neoplasms of the pancreas. A clinicopathologic study of six patients. Cancer 1989;64:1329-35.

78. Mukawa K, Kawa S, Aoki Y, Zhai Y, Nikaido T. Reduced expression of p53 and cyclin A in intraductal mucin-hypersecreting neoplasm of the pancreas compared with usual pancreatic ductal adenocarcinoma. Am J Gastroenterol 1999;94:2263-7.

79. Nagai E, Ueki T, Chijiiwa K, Tanaka M, Tsuneyoshi M. Intraductal papillary mucinous neoplasms of the pancreas associated with so-called "mucinous ductal ectasia." Histochemical and immunohistochemical analysis of 29 cases. Am J Surg Pathol 1995;19:576-89.

80. Nagasaka T, Nakashima N. Problems in histological diagnosis of intraductal papillary-mucinous tumor (IPMT). Hepatogastroenterology 2001;48:972-6.

81. Nagle J, Wilbur DC, Pitman MB. Cytomorphology of gastric and duodenal epithelium and reactivity to B72.3: a baseline for comparison to pancreatic neoplasms aspirated by EUS-FNAB. Diagn Cytopathol 2005;33:381-6.

107

82. Nakagohri T, Asano T, Kenmochi T, Urashima T, Ochiai T. Long-term surgical outcome of noninvasive and minimally invasive intraductal papillary mucinous adenocarcinoma of the pancreas. World J Surg 2002;26:1166-9.

83. Nakagohri T, Kenmochi T, Kainuma O, Tokoro Y, Asano T. Intraductal papillary mucinous tumors of the pancreas. Am J Surg 1999;178:344-7.

84. Nakamura A, Horinouchi M, Goto M, et al. New classification of pancreatic intraductal papillary-mucinous tumour by mucin expression: its relationship with potential for malignancy. J Pathol 2002;197:201-10.

85. Nakata B, Yashiro M, Nishioka N, et al. Very low incidence of microsatellite instability in intraductal papillary-mucinous neoplasm of the pancreas. Int J Cancer 2002;102:655-9.

86. Nakayama Y, Inoue H, Hamada Y, et al. Intraductal tubular adenoma of the pancreas, pyloric gland type: a clinicopathologic and immunohistochemical study of 6 cases. Am J Surg Pathol 2005;29:607-16.

87. Nakazawa S, Yamao K, Yamada M, et al. [Study of the classification of mucin-producing cystic tumor of the pancreas.] Nippon Shokakibyo Gakkai Zasshi 1988;85:924-32. [Japanese.]

88. Navarro F, Michel J, Bauret P, et al. Management of intraductal papillary mucinous tumours of the pancreas. Eur J Surg 1999;165:43-8.

89. Niijima M, Yamaguchi T, Ishihara T, et al. Immunohistochemical analysis and in situ hybridization of cyclooxygenase-2 expression in intraductal papillary-mucinous tumors of the pancreas. Cancer 2002;94:1565-73.

90. Nobukawa B, Suda K, Suyama M, Ariyama J, Beppu T, Futagawa S. Intraductal oncocytic papillary carcinoma with invasion arising from the accessory pancreatic duct. Gastrointest Endosc 1999;50:864-6.

91. Noji T, Kondo S, Hirano S, et al. Intraductal oncocytic papillary neoplasm of the pancreas shows strong positivity on FDG-PET. Int J Gastrointest Cancer 2002;32:43-6.

92. Obara T, Saitoh Y, Maguchi H, et al. Multicentric development of pancreatic intraductal carcinoma through atypical papillary hyperplasia. Hum Pathol 1992;23:82-5.

93. Ohhashi K, Murakami Y, Takekoshi T. Four cases of "mucin producing" cancer of the pancreas on specific findings of the papilla of Vater [abstract]. Prog Diagn Endosc 1982;20:348-51.

94. Paal E, Thompson LD, Przygodzki RM, Bratthauer GL, Heffess CS. A clinicopathologic and immunohistochemical study of 22 intraductal papillary mucinous neoplasms of the pancreas, with a review of the literature. Mod Pathol 1999;12:518-28.

95. Patel SA, Adams R, Goldstein M, Moskaluk CA. Genetic analysis of invasive carcinoma arising in intraductal oncocytic papillary neoplasm of the pancreas. Am J Surg Pathol 2002;26:1071-7.

96. Paye F, Sauvanet A, Terris B, et al. Intraductal papillary mucinous tumors of the pancreas: pancreatic resections guided by preoperative morphological assessment and intraoperative frozen section examination. Surgery 2000;127: 536-44.

97. Pinto MM, Meriano FV. Diagnosis of cystic pancreatic lesions by cytologic examination and carcinoembryonic antigen and amylase assays of cyst contents. Acta Cytol 1991;35:456-63.

98. Recine M, Kaw M, Evans DB, Krishnamurthy S. Fine-needle aspiration cytology of mucinous tumors of the pancreas. Cancer 2004;102:92-9.

99. Sai JK, Suyama M, Kubokawa Y, et al. Management of branch duct-type intraductal papillary mucinous tumor of the pancreas based on magnetic resonance imaging. Abdom Imaging 2003;28:694-9.

100. Salvia R, Fernandez-del Castillo C, Bassi C, et al. Main-duct intraductal papillary mucinous neoplasms of the pancreas: clinical predictors of malignancy and long-term survival following resection. Ann Surg 2004;239:678-85.

101. Sasaki S, Yamamoto H, Kaneto H, et al. Differential roles of alterations of p53, p16, and SMAD4 expression in the progression of intraductal papillary-mucinous tumors of the pancreas. Oncol Rep 2003;10:21-5.

102. Sato N, Fukushima N, Maitra A, et al. Gene expression profiling identifies genes associated with invasive intraductal papillary mucinous neoplasms of the pancreas. Am J Pathol 2004; 164:903-14.

103. Sato N, Rosty C, Jansen M, et al. STK11/LKB1 Peutz-Jeghers gene inactivation in intraductal papillary-mucinous neoplasms of the pancreas. Am J Pathol 2001;159:2017-22.

104. Sato N, Ueki T, Fukushima N, et al. Aberrant methylation of CpG islands in intraductal papillary mucinous neoplasms of the pancreas. Gastroenterology 2002;123:365-72.

105. Satoh K, Sawai T, Shimosegawa T, et al. The point mutation of c-Ki-ras at codon 12 in carcinoma of the pancreatic head region and in intraductal mucin-hypersecreting neoplasm of the pancreas. Int J Pancreatol 1993;14:135-43.

106. Satoh K, Shimosegawa T, Moriizumi S, Koizumi M, Toyota T. K-ras mutation and p53 protein accumulation in intraductal mucin-hypersecreting neoplasms of the pancreas. Pancreas 1996;12:362-8.

106a. Schonleben F, Qiu W, Ciau NT, et al. PIK3CA mutations in intraductal papillary mucinous neoplasm/carcinoma of the pancreas. Clin Cancer Res 2006;12:3851-5.

107. Seidel G, Zahurak M, Iacobuzio-Donahue CA, et al. Almost all infiltrating colloid carcinomas of the pancreas and periampullary region arise from in situ papillary neoplasms: a study of 39 cases. Am J Surg Pathol 2002;26:56-63.

108. Sessa F, Solcia E, Capella C, et al. Intraductal papillary-mucinous tumours represent a distinct group of pancreatic neoplasms: an investigation of tumour cell differentiation and K-ras, p53 and c-erbB-2 abnormalities in 26 patients. Virchows Arch 1994;425:357-67.

109. Shabaik A. Endoscopic ultrasound-guided fine needle aspiration cytology of intraductal papillary mucinous tumor of the pancreas. A case report. Acta Cytol 2003;47:657-62.

109a. Shimada K, Sakamoto Y, Sano T, Kosuge T, Hiraoka N. Invasive carcinoma originaging in an intraductal papillary mucinous neoplasm of the pancreas: a clinicopathologic comparison with a common type of invasive ductal carcinoma. Pancreas 2006;32:281-7.

110. Shimizu M, Hirokawa M, Manabe T, et al. Cytologic findings in noninvasive intraductal papillary-mucinous carcinoma of the pancreas. A report of two cases. Acta Cytol 1999;43:243-6.

111. Shimizu M, Manabe T. Mucin-producing pancreatic tumors: historical review of its nosological concept. Zentralbl Pathol 1994;140:211-23.

112. Shimizu Y, Yasui K, Morimoto T, Torii A, Yamao K, Ohhashi K. Case of intraductal papillary mucinous tumor (noninvasive adenocarcinoma) of the pancreas resected 27 years after onset. Int J Pancreatol 1999;26:93-8.

113. Shin HJ, Lahoti S, Sneige N. Endoscopic ultrasound-guided fine-needle aspiration in 179 cases: the M. D. Anderson Cancer Center experience. Cancer 2002;96:174-80.

114. Sho M, Nakajima Y, Kanehiro H, et al. Pattern of recurrence after resection for intraductal papillary mucinous tumors of the pancreas. World J Surg 1998;22:874-8.

115. Silas AM, Morrin MM, Raptopoulos V, Keogan MT. Intraductal papillary mucinous tumors of the pancreas. AJR Am J Roentgenol 2001;176:179-85.

115a. Sohn TA, Yeo CJ, Cameron JL, et al. Intraductal papillary mucinous neoplasms of the pancreas: an updated experience. Ann Surg 2004;239:788-97.

116. Sohn TA, Yeo CJ, Cameron JL, Iacobuzio-Donahue CA, Hruban RH, Lillemoe KD. Intraductal papillary mucinous neoplasms of the pancreas: an increasingly recognized clinicopathologic entity. Ann Surg 2001;234:313-21.

117. Solcia E, Capella C, Klöppel G. Tumors of the pancreas. AFIP Atlas of Tumor Pathology, 3rd Series, Fascicle 20. Washington, DC: American Registry of Pathology; 1997.

118. Stelow EB, Stanley MW, Bardales RH, et al. Intraductal papillary-mucinous neoplasm of the pancreas. The findings and limitations of cytologic samples obtained by endoscopic ultrasound-guided fine-needle aspiration. Am J Clin Pathol 2003;120:398-404.

119. Su GH, Hruban RH, Bova GS, et al. Germline and somatic mutations of the STK11/LKB1 Peutz-Jeghers gene in pancreatic and biliary cancers. Am J Pathol 1999;154:1835-40.

120. Sugiura H, Kondo S, Islam HK, et al. Clinicopathologic features and outcomes of intraductal papillary-mucinous tumors of the pancreas. Hepatogastroenterology 2002;49:263-7.

121. Sugiyama M, Atomi Y. Extrapancreatic neoplasms occur with unusual frequency in patients with intraductal papillary mucinous tumors of the pancreas. Am J Gastroenterol 1999;94:470-3.

122. Tada M, Omata M, Ohto M. Ras gene mutations in intraductal papillary neoplasms of the pancreas. Analysis in five cases. Cancer 1991;67:634-7.

123. Tajiri T, Tate G, Inagaki T, et al. Intraductal tubular neoplasms of the pancreas: histogenesis and differentiation. Pancreas 2005;30:115-21.

124. Tajiri T, Tate G, Kunimura T, et al. Histologic and immunohistochemical comparison of intraductal tubular carcinoma, intraductal papillary-mucinous carcinoma, and ductal adenocarcinoma of the pancreas. Pancreas 2004;29:116-22.

125. Tanaka M. Intraductal papillary mucinous neoplasm of the pancreas: diagnosis and treatment. Pancreas 2004;28:282-8.

125a. Tanaka M, Chari S, Adsay NV, et al. International consensus guidelines for management of intraductal papillary mucinous neoplasms and mucinous cystic neoplasms of the pancreas. Pancreatology 2006;6:17-32.

126. Taouli B, Vilgrain V, Vullierme MP, et al. Intraductal papillary mucinous tumors of the pancreas: helical CT with histopathologic correlation. Radiology 2000;217:757-64.

127. Terada T, Ohta T, Kitamura Y, Ashida K, Matsunaga Y. Cell proliferation activity in intraductal papillary-mucinous neoplasms and invasive ductal adenocarcinomas of the pancreas: an immunohistochemical study. Arch Pathol Lab Med 1998;122:42-6.

128. Terada T, Ohta T, Kitamura Y, Ashida K, Matsunaga Y, Kato M. Endocrine cells in intraductal papillary-mucinous neoplasms of the pancreas. A histochemical and immunohistochemical study. Virchows Arch 1997;431:31-6.

129. Terada T, Ohta T, Nakanuma Y. Expression of oncogene products, anti-oncogene products and oncofetal antigens in intraductal papillary-mucinous neoplasm of the pancreas. Histopathology 1996;29:355-61.

130. Terris B, Blaveri E, Crnogorac-Jurcevic T, et al. Characterization of gene expression profiles in intraductal papillary-mucinous tumors of the pancreas. Am J Pathol 2002;160:1745-54.

131. Terris B, Dubois S, Buisine MP, et al. Mucin gene expression in intraductal papillary-mucinous pancreatic tumours and related lesions. J Pathol 2002;197:632-7.

132. Terris B, Ponsot P, Paye F, et al. Intraductal papillary mucinous tumors of the pancreas confined to secondary ducts show less aggressive pathologic features as compared with those involving the main pancreatic duct. Am J Surg Pathol 2000;24:1372-7.

133. Tobi M, Hatfield J, Adsay NV, et al. Prognostic significance of the labeling of Adnab-9 in pancreatic intraductal papillary mucinous neoplasms. Int J Pancreatol 2001;29:141-50.

134. Uehara H, Nakaizumi A, Iishi H, et al. Cytologic examination of pancreatic juice for differential diagnosis of benign and malignant mucin-producing tumors of the pancreas. Cancer 1994;74:826-33.

135. Wada K. p16 and p53 gene alterations and accumulations in the malignant evolution of intraductal papillary-mucinous tumors of the pancreas. J Hepatobiliary Pancreat Surg 2002;9: 76-85.

136. Wada K, Takada T, Yasuda H, et al. Does "clonal progression" relate to the development of intraductal papillary mucinous tumors of the pancreas? J Gastrointest Surg 2004;8:289-96.

137. Wilentz RE, Iacobuzio-Donahue CA, Argani P, et al. Loss of expression of Dpc4 in pancreatic intraepithelial neoplasia: evidence that DPC4 inactivation occurs late in neoplastic progression. Cancer Res 2000;60:2002-6.

138. Wilentz RE, Su GH, Dai JL, et al. Immunohistochemical labeling for Dpc4 mirrors genetic status in pancreatic adenocarcinomas: a new marker of DPC4 inactivation. Am J Pathol 2000; 156:37-43.

139. Yamada M, Kozuka S, Yamao K, Nakazawa S, Naitoh Y, Tsukamoto Y. Mucin-producing tumor of the pancreas. Cancer 1991;68:159-68.

140. Yamaguchi K, Chijiiwa K, Noshiro H, Torata N, Kinoshita M, Tanaka M. Ki-ras codon 12 point mutation and p53 mutation in pancreatic diseases. Hepatogastroenterology 1999;46: 2575-81.

141. Yamaguchi K, Ogawa Y, Chijiiwa K, Tanaka M. Mucin-hypersecreting tumors of the pancreas: assessing the grade of malignancy preoperatively. Am J Surg 1996;171:427-31.

142. Yamaguchi K, Ohuchida J, Ohtsuka T, Nakano K, Tanaka M. Intraductal papillary-mucinous tumor of the pancreas concomitant with ductal carcinoma of the pancreas. Pancreatology 2002;2:484-90.

143. Yamaguchi K, Tanaka M. Mucin-hypersecreting tumor of the pancreas with mucin extrusion through an enlarged papilla. Am J Gastroenterol 1991;86:835-9.

144. Yamaguchi K, Yokohata K, Noshiro H, Chijiiwa K, Tanaka M. Mucinous cystic neoplasm of the pancreas or intraductal papillary-mucinous tumour of the pancreas. Eur J Surg 2000;166: 141-8.

144a. Yamaguchi T, Baba T, Ishihara T, et al. Long-term follow-up of intraductal papillary mucinous neoplasm of the pancreas with ultrasonography. Clin Gastroenterol Hepatol 2005;3:1136-43.

145. Yamao K, Ohashi K, Nakamura T, et al. Efficacy of peroral pancreatoscopy in the diagnosis of pancreatic diseases. Gastrointest Endosc 2003;57:205-9.

146. Yamao K, Ohashi K, Nakamura T, et al. Evaluation of various imaging methods in the differential diagnosis of intraductal papillary-mucinous tumor (IPMT) of the pancreas. Hepatogastroenterology 2001;48:962-6.

147. Yanagisawa A, Kato Y, Ohtake K, et al. c-Ki-ras point mutations in ductectatic-type mucinous cystic neoplasms of the pancreas. Jpn J Cancer Res 1991;82:1057-60.

148. Yonezawa S, Sueyoshi K, Nomoto M, et al. MUC2 gene expression is found in noninvasive tumors but not in invasive tumors of the pancreas and liver: its close relationship with prognosis of the patients. Hum Pathol 1997;28:344-52.

149. Yonezawa S, Taira M, Osako M, et al. MUC-1 mucin expression in invasive areas of intraductal papillary mucinous tumors of the pancreas. Pathol Int 1998;48:319-22.

150. Yoshizawa K, Nagai H, Sakurai S, et al. Clonality and K-ras mutation analyses of epithelia in intraductal papillary mucinous tumor and mucinous cystic tumor of the pancreas. Virchows Arch 2002;441:437-43.

151. Z'graggen K, Rivera JA, Corris PA, et al. Prevalence of activating K-ras mutations in the evolutionary stages of neoplasia in intraductal papillary mucinous tumors of the pancreas. Ann Surg 1997;226:491-8.

152. Zamora C, Sahel J, Cantu DG, et al. Intraductal papillary or mucinous tumors (IPMT) of the pancreas: report of a case series and review of the literature. Am J Gastroenterol 2001;96: 1441-7.

7 DUCTAL ADENOCARCINOMA

The first description of pancreatic cancer is usually attributed to Giovani Battista Morgagni (1682–1771). In 1769, he aptly described the pain experienced by many patients with cancer of the pancreas, "just as if he were being torn to pieces by dogs" (127). It wasn't until more than a century later, in 1898, that William Stuart Halsted performed the first successful ampullectomy for an ampullary cancer, and the modern surgical era in the treatment of periampullary malignancies began. In 1918, the Italian physician Ottorino Tenani reported the first successful pancreatoduodenectomy, and in the 1930s, Allan Oldfather Whipple (127) popularized the surgery that now bears his name. Today, thousands of pancreatoduodenectomies (Whipple procedures) are performed every year, and our knowledge of the pathology of cancer of the pancreas continues to grow. Despite progress, infiltrating ductal adenocarcinoma, the most common malignancy of the pancreas, remains an almost uniformly fatal disease (59,146).

It is now clear that pancreatic cancer is fundamentally a genetic disease, and that some infiltrating adenocarcinomas of the pancreas arise from histologically well-defined, noninvasive epithelial proliferations called *pancreatic intraepithelial neoplasia*. The identification of the genes targeted in pancreatic cancer has helped to classify variants of pancreatic cancer, and has formed a foundation for new diagnostic tests and novel therapies. The recognition of noninvasive precursors to infiltrating pancreatic carcinomas provides a rational basis for their early detection.

DEFINITION

Infiltrating ductal adenocarcinoma is an invasive malignant epithelial neoplasm with glandular (ductal) differentiation and without a predominant component of any of the other types of carcinoma (145,161a,279). Synonyms include *duct cell adenocarcinoma, tubular-type adenocarcinoma, duct cell carcinoma,* or simply *pancreatic cancer*. The term *mucinous adenocarcinoma* has been used inappropriately to refer to conventional infiltrating ductal adenocarcinomas with intracellular or luminal mucin accumulation. The use of this term is discouraged because it can potentially be confused with the less aggressive colloid (mucinous noncystic) carcinoma. For simplicity, in this chapter we interchangeably use the terms infiltrating ductal adenocarcinoma and pancreatic cancer.

GENERAL FEATURES

Infiltrating ductal adenocarcinoma is by far the most common type of carcinoma of the pancreas. Worldwide, pancreatic cancer causes approximately 213,000 deaths per year, making pancreatic cancer the eighth leading cause of cancer death (246). The age-adjusted incidence rate for pancreatic cancer in the United States is 11/100,000, resulting in 33,730 new cases and 32,300 deaths in 2006 (1,146). In the United States, pancreatic cancer is the fourth leading cause of cancer deaths in men, in women, and overall. The 5-year survival rate for all patients with pancreatic cancer is only 4 percent; as a result, the mortality rate is almost equal to the incidence rate (146). The incidence of pancreatic cancer appears to have risen three-fold from the 1920s to the 1970s, but it has remained relatively stable since the 1970s (6). Much of the increase in the incidence of documented pancreatic cancer is likely a combination of a real increase in the incidence caused by increased cigarette smoking, and an apparent increase due to technological advances in imaging that have improved the identification of tumor origin. Many cancers previously called "abdominal malignancy" or "stomach cancer," are now being correctly classified as pancreatic cancers.

The incidence of pancreatic cancer does not vary dramatically from country to country (6). The incidence appears higher in Western industrialized countries than in undeveloped

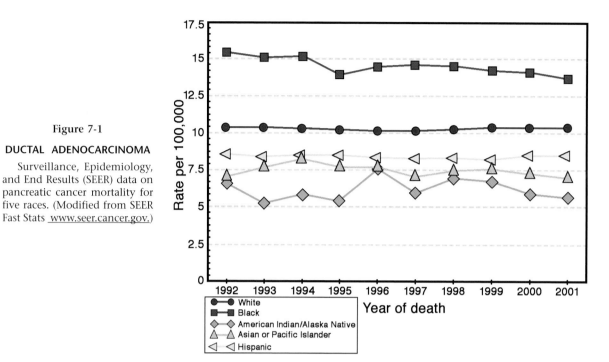

Figure 7-1

DUCTAL ADENOCARCINOMA

Surveillance, Epidemiology, and End Results (SEER) data on pancreatic cancer mortality for five races. (Modified from SEER Fast Stats www.seer.cancer.gov.)

countries, but much of this likely represents underdiagnosis in the latter. Pancreatic cancer is more common in the Maoris in New Zealand, in native Hawaiians, and in African-Americans living in the United States (104). The age-adjusted incidence in whites in the Untied States is 10.8/ 100,000, compared to 15.4/100,000 for African-Americans, 9.3/100,000 for Asian-Americans, 9.85 for Hispanics, and 8.33/100,000 for American Indians/Alaskan Natives (fig. 7-1) (www. seer.cancer.gov). Not only is the incidence in African-Americans 50 percent higher than in whites in the United States, but their cancers tend to present at a higher stage and are less often surgically resectable than are cancers in Caucasians (54,232). The incidence in native African populations is generally low, suggesting that environment or lifestyle may account for the increased incidence in African-Americans. Indeed, much of the increased risk of pancreatic cancer in African-American males in the United States is attributable to established risk factors, including cigarette smoking and long-term diabetes mellitus (276).

Age is a significant risk factor for pancreatic cancer. The peak incidence of the disease is in the 7th to 8th decades of life, and most cases (80 percent) occur between the ages of 60 and 80 years (fig. 7-2) (204). Pancreatic cancer is rare

before 40 years of age, and extremely rare before the age of 20 years (189); patients under 20 years of age commonly have an associated known risk factor, such as Peutz-Jeghers syndrome (189). Pancreatic cancer is more common in men than in women (male to female ratio, 1.30 to 1.0), and this gender predominance is seen across racial groups (fig. 7-2) (1). The incidence of pancreatic cancer has been reported to be higher in Jews than in Catholics and Protestants (229).

Cigarette smoking has been consistently identified as a risk factor for pancreatic cancer (6,54,63,96,129,270). In most studies, cigarette smoking is associated with a doubling of the risk of pancreatic cancer (relative risk = 2), and there appears to be a dose response with a trend toward greater risk with greater lifetime consumption of cigarettes. Fortunately, smoking cessation has been shown to reduce the risk of pancreatic cancer, and the risk of pancreatic cancer drops to that of nonsmokers after 10 years of abstinence (63).

A number of dietary factors are associated with pancreatic cancer (6,76,77,104,128,208). Diets high in meat, pork products, fats, nitrates, and total energy intake increase risk, while diets high in fruits, vegetables, fiber, folate, and vitamin C appear to be protective. Paralleling

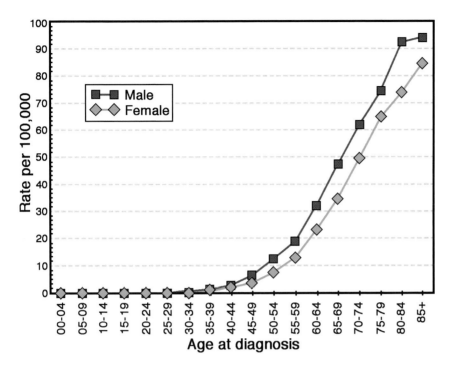

Figure 7-2

DUCTAL ADENOCARCINOMA

SEER data on pancreatic cancer incidence for males and females. (Modified from SEER Fast Stats www.seer.cancer.gov.)

the findings with dietary folate, higher serum folate levels have been suggested to be protective in some studies (283,284). The regular use of aspirin has been associated with a reduced risk of pancreatic cancer in some, but not all, studies (14). Obesity (body mass index 30 kg/m² or greater) and physical inactivity increase risk, as does height in the top quartile (28,54, 207). Regular physical activity appears to decrease risk (207).

Although a well-publicized study suggested a link between coffee consumption and pancreatic cancer, this study had methodological flaws, and subsequent studies have shown no link between coffee (regular or decaffeinated) or alcohol consumption and pancreatic cancer (107).

Case-control studies have suggested an association between certain occupations and the development of pancreatic cancer (6,104). These include workers exposed to coal gas, metal workers, workers in the leather tanning industry, and dry cleaners. Exposure to certain chemicals, including β-naphthylamine, benzidine, solvents, dichlorodiphenyltrichloroethane (DDT), and gasoline may also increase risk.

Several medical conditions increase the risk of pancreatic cancer. Longstanding diabetes mellitus is associated with a two-fold increased risk (46,54,63,75,277). The association of diabetes

mellitus and obesity with pancreatic cancer suggests a role for altered glucose/insulin metabolism in disease development. Chronic pancreatitis, particularly familial chronic pancreatitis (see below) and tropical calcifying chronic pancreatitis, is also associated with pancreatic cancer (43,72,184,185). The association between the more common forms of chronic pancreatitis, such as alcoholic pancreatitis, and pancreatic cancer is less clear. In addition to increasing pancreatic cancer risk, both diabetes mellitus and chronic pancreatitis can be caused by pancreatic cancer. Caution should be exercised, therefore, when interpreting epidemiologic studies causally linking recent onset diabetes or recent chronic pancreatitis with the development of pancreatic cancer.

Several studies have found an increased risk of pancreatic cancer many years after cholecystectomy or partial gastrectomy (237,277). Allergies may reduce risk, and there may even be a trend for decreased risk with increasing number of allergies (123). Tonsillectomy may be protective, as it has been associated with a decreased incidence of pancreatic cancer in several studies (6,104). Radiation to the pancreas, as a consequence of either clinical therapy or nuclear bomb blast, has been weakly associated with the development of pancreatic cancer (6).

Table 7-1

GERMLINE GENETIC ALTERATIONS ASSOCIATED WITH AN INCREASED RISK OF PANCREATIC CANCER

Individual	Gene	Relative Risk	Risk by Age 70
No history	None	1	0.5%
Breast cancer	BRCA2	3.5–10X	5%
	BRCA1	2X	1%
FAMMM[a]	p16 (CDKN2A)	20–34X	10–17%
3 FDR with pc	Unknown	32X	16%
Familial pancreatitis	PRSS1	50–80X	25–40%
Peutz-Jeghers syndrome	STK11/LKB1	132X	30–60%
HNPCC	MLH1, MSH2, others	unknown	<5%
Young age onset pc	FANC-C, FANC-G, others	unknown	unknown
Family X	Palladin	unknown	unknown

[a]FAMMM = familial atypical multiple mole melanoma syndrome; 3 FDR with pc = three or more first-degree relatives with pancreatic cancer; HNPCC= hereditary nonpolyposis colorectal cancer syndrome.

Synchronous and even metachronous pancreatic cancers have been reported, but it is hard to distinguish between an intraglandular metastasis and a synchronous cancer. Metachronous pancreatic cancers are very rare, most likely because of the very high mortality rate of the disease (74,173,202,308). Pancreatic cancers have been reported in patients with a history of an extrapancreatic primary cancer (73,92,228), the most common of which, in men, are lung and prostate cancers. In women, second primaries include lung, head and neck, and bladder cancers. Most of these cancers are associated with cigarette smoking.

A case of pancreatic cancer transmitted in a renal allograft has been reported (93).

FAMILIAL PANCREATIC CANCER

Pancreatic cancer aggregates in some families and the genetic basis for this aggregation is only now being elucidated. For years, anecdotal case reports have documented the familial aggregation of pancreatic cancer and numerous case-control studies have shown that patients with pancreatic cancer are more likely to have a family history of pancreatic cancer than are controls (20,54,76,79,95,118,270,277). Prospective analyses of the incidence of pancreatic cancer confirm the increased risk associated with a family history of the disease (159,302). For persons with three first-degree relatives with pancreatic cancer, this increased risk is 32-fold greater than the

risk in the general population; for individuals with two first-degree relatives with pancreatic cancer, the risk is elevated 6-fold; and for individuals with a single first-degree relative with pancreatic cancer, the risk is elevated 2.3-fold (12,159). While the aggregation of a cancer in some families can have an environmental or genetic basis, segregation analyses have suggested that the clustering of pancreatic cancer in kindreds has a genetic (inherited) basis (158). It is roughly estimated that approximately 10 percent of pancreatic cancers are familial. A number of genetic syndromes have already been identified in which germline mutations in specific genes are associated with an increased risk of pancreatic cancer (Table 7-1).

Germline mutations in the second breast cancer gene (BRCA2) account for about 16 percent of the familial aggregation of pancreatic cancer; those with germline BRCA2 gene mutations have a 3- to 10-fold increased risk of pancreatic cancer (26,41a,102,113,172,177,217,242,307). Some of the increased incidence of pancreatic cancer in the Jewish population may be caused by a "founder" germline BRCA2 gene mutation, the 6174 delT mutation, which is present in about 1 percent of the Ashkenazi Jewish population (242). Importantly, the penetrance of these germline mutations is incomplete, and therefore, many pancreatic cancer patients with germline BRCA2 gene mutations do not have a family history of breast or pancreatic cancer

(102,217). The protein product of the *BRCA2* gene interacts with the protein products of the Fanconi anemia complementation genes (the *FANC* genes), and mutations in the *FANC-C* and *FANC-G* genes have been reported in young patients with pancreatic cancer (53,314). Mutations in genes of the Fanconi anemia pathway are not only important for screening and genetic counseling, but, when present, may also have therapeutic implications (313). Germline mutations in the first breast cancer gene, *BRCA1*, have also been associated with an increased risk of pancreatic cancer (172,177,194,304).

Germline mutations in the *p16/CDKN2A* gene are associated with the familial atypical multiple mole melanoma (FAMMM) syndrome. These individuals develop melanocytic nevi and atypical melanocytic nevi, have an increased risk of melanoma, and a 20- to 34-fold increased risk of pancreatic cancer (21,24,33,64,105,172,193,245, 318). Almost all patients with a germline *p16/CDKN2A* gene mutation and pancreatic cancer have a family or personal history of melanoma.

The Peutz-Jeghers syndrome is characterized by mucocutaneous melanocytic macules and hamartomatous polyps of the gastrointestinal tract, caused by germline mutations in the *STK11/LKB1* gene. Patients with Peutz-Jeghers syndrome have a remarkable 132-fold increased risk of developing pancreatic cancer (97,287). Of interest, intraductal papillary mucinous neoplasms of the pancreas have been reported in a number of these patients (269).

Familial pancreatitis is caused by germline mutations in either the cationic trypsinogen (*PRSS1*) or the serine protease inhibitor, Kazal-type 1 (*SPINK1*) gene. Patients with familial pancreatitis develop multiple severe episodes of pancreatitis starting at a young age, and these patients have a 50- to 80-fold increased risk of pancreatic cancer (184). Twenty-five to 40 percent of these patients will develop pancreatic cancer by the age of 70, and the risk appears to be particularly high among cigarette smokers (184). Because they are often diabetic and lack significant pancreatic exocrine function, prophylactic pancreatectomy may be a reasonable option for selected patients with familial pancreatitis.

Pancreatic cancer has been reported in some kindreds with hereditary nonpolyposis colorectal cancer (HNPCC) (195). HNPCC is caused by germline mutations in one of the DNA mismatch repair genes (e.g., *MLH1*), and about 4 percent of pancreatic cancers show microsatellite instability, the hallmark of an inactivating mutation in a DNA mismatch repair gene (101, 329). As will be discussed in greater detail in chapter 8, pancreatic carcinomas with microsatellite instability frequently have a distinct histologic appearance, indicating that tumor morphology can be used to suggest the possibility of HNPCC in a patient with pancreatic cancer (325,329). The risk of pancreatic cancer has also been reported to be elevated in patients with familial adenomatous polyposis, ataxia-telangiectasia, and the von Hippel-Lindau syndrome, but these risks are less well defined, and patients with these syndromes are at risk for other pancreatic neoplasms as well (98).

Recently, Pogue-Geile et al. (248a) reported that inherited mutations in the *Palladin* gene on chromosome 4q are responsible for the familial aggregation of pancreatic cancer in a large kindred designated "Family X."

These known genetic syndromes collectively account for only a fraction (less than 20 percent) of the familial aggregation of pancreatic cancer. The genetic basis for most cases of familial pancreatic cancer is not known at this time.

CLINICAL FEATURES

Pancreatic cancer, unfortunately, usually presents nonspecifically, and many patients are not correctly diagnosed until many months or even years after they first develop symptoms. The most common symptom associated with carcinoma of the head of the pancreas is epigastric pain that radiates to the back (60,239). Patients with pancreatic cancer also have unexplained weight loss, painless jaundice, light clay-colored stools, dark urine, pruritus, and nausea, and 10 percent develop spontaneously appearing and disappearing thromboses (60). The French physician Armand Trousseau first described the association of pancreatic cancer with migratory thrombophlebitis, now known as the Trousseau's syndrome, in 1861 (127). Ironically, Trousseau diagnosed his own pancreatic cancer when he himself developed migratory thrombophlebitis. Less common presentations of pancreatic cancer include acute pancreatitis, hypoglycemia, hypercalcemia, metastatic carcinoma of unknown

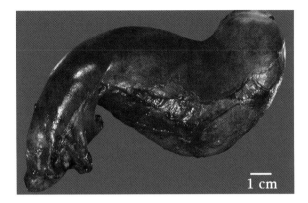

1 cm

Figure 7-3

DUCTAL ADENOCARCINOMA

A massively distended gallbladder in a patient with pancreatic cancer. When palpable on physical exam this is referred to as Courvoisier's sign.

primary, and endocarditis. Up to a third of the patients develop a palpable distended gallbladder (fig. 7-3), called Courvoisier's sign after the Swiss surgeon who lived from 1843–1918 (127).

Patients with carcinoma of the body or tail of the gland often present with unexplained weight loss, abdominal and/or back pain, or distant metastases (60). Periumbilical nodules may be palpated in patients with advanced metastatic disease. This finding is called the Sister Mary Joseph sign after the surgical assistant of Dr. William Mayo who associated palpable periumbilical nodules with the presence of a widely metastatic abdominal malignancy (127).

Diabetes mellitus not only increases the risk of pancreatic cancer, but it also can be a presenting complication of the disease. More than 70 percent of patients with pancreatic cancer have fasting blood glucose levels over 120 mg/dL at presentation. Similarly, chronic pancreatitis can both contribute to the development of pancreatic cancer and it can be a consequence of tissue destruction and duct obstruction from the cancer itself.

Depression is common in pancreatic cancer patients (42,247). Although in some cases, recognition of the dire prognosis of the disease may contribute to the depressive symptoms, studies have suggested that the severity of the depression is often out of proportion to the severity of the disease, when compared to other immediately life-threatening illnesses. Thus, depression is regarded as a bona fide symptom of pan-

creatic cancer, and it may be one of the presenting manifestations (247).

The radiographic diagnosis and staging of pancreatic cancer has improved dramatically in the last decade. Currently, spiral (helical) computerized tomography (CT), magnetic resonance imaging (MRI), endoscopic ultrasound (EUS), and endoscopic retrograde cholangiopancreatography (ERCP) are all used to evaluate pancreatic masses. CT is the most commonly utilized modality to diagnose and stage pancreatic neoplasms. CT technology has improved dramatically, and the new spiral CT scanners have an overall accuracy of over 90 percent (30,205,240,244,312). Pancreatic cancer on CT appears as a hypodense mass that deforms the normal size, contour, and borders of the pancreas (figs. 7-4, 7-5). There is often a central area of decreased attenuation and the periphery of the lesion is usually poorly defined. If the carcinoma involves the head of the gland, the pancreatic tail will show a dilated duct and parenchymal atrophy (fig. 7-5). The double duct sign, which is dilatation of both the pancreatic and bile ducts, is a feature of pancreatic cancer arising in the head of the gland. Early findings on CT include dilatation of the pancreatic duct and abrupt cut-off of the duct (88).

Pancreatic cancers usually appear as hypointense masses on T1-weighted MRIs, and they have variable signal intensities on T2-weighted images, but are usually isointense to hyperintense relative to the normal pancreatic parenchyma (31,205,258). Magnetic resonance cholangiopancreatography (MRCP) can be used to visualize the pancreatic duct and can therefore demonstrate the location of any duct lesions, while magnetic resonance angiography (MRA) can be used to visualize the vascular anatomy and help determine the resectability of pancreatic neoplasms.

EUS is also very accurate for the diagnosis and locoregional staging of pancreatic neoplasms (209,243,282). Most (80 percent) pancreatic cancers are hypoechoic, although they can also be hyperechoic, and invasion of the major peripancreatic vessels can often be ascertained. Fine needle aspiration biopsy can be performed in conjunction with EUS (EUS/FNA), allowing for a definitive tissue diagnosis. Concomitant aspiration of peripancreatic nodes can provide nodal

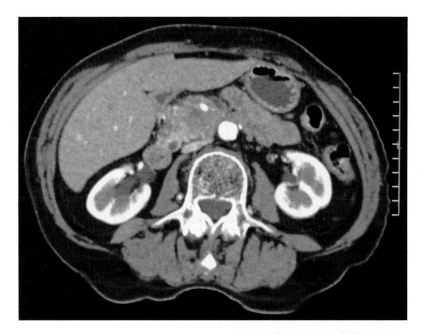

Figure 7-4

DUCTAL ADENOCARCINOMA

Computerized tomography (CT) of an adenocarcinoma in the head of the pancreas. The low attenuation mass encases the superior mesenteric artery. (Courtesy of Dr. S. S. Siegelman, Baltimore, MD.)

Figure 7-5

DUCTAL ADENOCARCINOMA

CT reveals a low attenuation mass in the body of the pancreas and dilatation of the pancreatic duct upstream from the mass. (Courtesy of Dr. S. S. Siegelman, Baltimore, MD.) (Figs. 7-5 and 7-6 are from the same patient.)

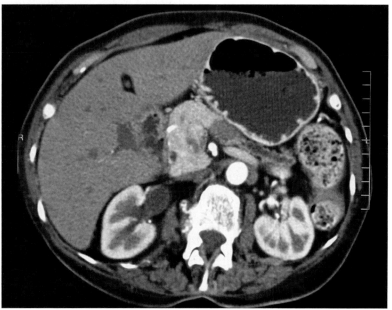

staging as well. EUS is, however, operator dependent and is best performed at specialized centers.

ERCP visualizes the pancreatic duct system. Pancreatic neoplasms can be diagnosed indirectly through the interpretation of changes to the duct architecture, including obstruction and displacement of the ducts. ERCP is more invasive than the other techniques, and is associated with a 2 percent complication rate, making it a less attractive first-line modality for the evaluation of pancreatic neoplasms.

While each of these modalities has its limitations, the rapid progress in imaging technology seen in the last decade suggests that smaller lesions will be detectable in the near future and that the radiologic diagnosis and staging of pancreatic neoplasms will continue to improve. As this happens, the importance of carefully correlating pathologic findings with radiologic abnormalities will only grow.

As exciting as the improvements in imaging technology for patients with known pancreatic

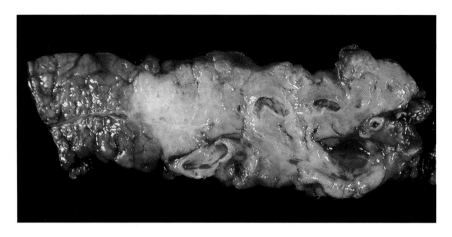

Figure 7-6

DUCTAL ADENOCARCINOMA

Note the normal caliber of the pancreatic duct (left), the carcinoma (center), and the upstream dilation of the pancreatic duct (right).

disease are, the central problem with pancreatic cancer remains the lack of an effective screening test for early asymptomatic disease. Serum carcinoembryonic antigen (CEA) and carbohydrate antigen (CA) 19-9 levels have proven to be ineffective screening tests for pancreatic cancer due to a lack of sufficient sensitivity and specificity (89,256). Nonetheless, CA19-9 levels have been used to prognosticate and to monitor the effectiveness of therapy, and are useful in conjunction with other diagnostic tests (89,233). Some pancreatic cancers produce human chorionic gonadotropin, resulting in elevated serum levels of this hormone.

A great deal of effort has gone into developing new screening tests for early pancreatic cancer. These include the identification of differentially expressed genes using global assays of gene expression, screening for mutant DNA shed from the cancers, identification of genes specifically hypermethylated in pancreatic cancer, and proteomics technologies to identify novel proteins or groups of proteins differentially overexpressed by pancreatic cancers.

PATHOLOGIC FEATURES

Gross Findings

The majority (60 to 70 percent) of pancreatic cancers arise in the head of the gland; cancers also arise in the body (5 to 15 percent), or tail (10 to 15 percent), and 5 to 15 percent diffusely involve the gland (60,145,161a,273,279). Carcinomas that arise in the head of the gland are more often resectable than are carcinomas that involve the body or tail, and carcinomas of the head are therefore overrepresented in

most surgical series. The vast majority of pancreatic cancers are solitary, but multifocal disease can occur. Rare instances of a pancreatic carcinoma arising in ectopic pancreatic tissue have been reported (16).

Pancreatic cancer can range in size from microscopic disease to large, bulky masses over 10 cm (60). The average size of surgically resected carcinomas of the head of the pancreas is 3 cm, while surgically resected carcinomas of the tail of the gland tend to be larger (mean, 5 cm) (178,278). Pancreatic cancer usually enlarges the gland. On cut section, most are firm, stellate, poorly defined, and white-yellow, and obscure the normal lobular architecture of the pancreas (figs. 7-6–7-10). In some cases, the carcinoma may be nearly impossible to distinguish grossly from adjacent areas of fibrosing chronic pancreatitis, making the dimensions of the carcinoma difficult to assess. The regions involved by the carcinoma may have a more gritty texture than the foci of pancreatitis.

Most pancreatic cancers are solid, but some, particularly larger carcinomas, can focally form cysts (168a). Cystic change may be due to necrosis, in which case a large degenerative cyst is found in the center of the neoplasm; in other cases, cysts are found adjacent to the carcinoma due to localized dilatation of obstructed ducts (retention cysts) (fig. 7-6). Finally, some pancreatic carcinomas contain dilated invasive glands large enough to be seen grossly as small cysts.

The non-neoplastic pancreatic parenchyma upstream from the carcinoma is usually firm and atrophic secondary to chronic pancreatitis, and the pancreatic duct can be dilated. In some cases this dilatation is dramatic and

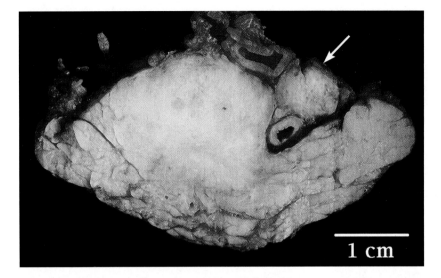

Figure 7-7

DUCTAL ADENOCARCINOMA

The small nodule (arrow) adjacent to the main mass is a lymph node metastasis.

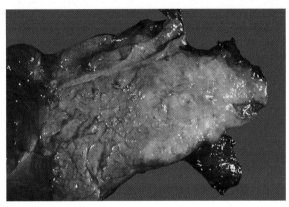

Figure 7-8

DUCTAL ADENOCARCINOMA

A firm, sclerotic, poorly defined mass is seen in the head of the pancreas. The bile duct traverses the top edge of the specimen.

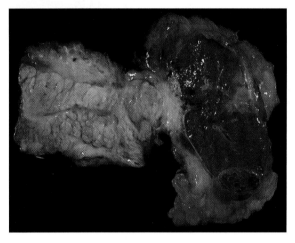

Figure 7-9

DUCTAL ADENOCARCINOMA

Carcinoma in the tail of the gland extends into the spleen. Note the associated splenic infarcts.

associated with prominent haustration of the duct. In contrast to intraductal papillary mucinous neoplasms, pancreatic ducts dilated secondary to an obstructive pancreatic cancer have a smooth lining and contain watery fluid rather than thick tenacious mucin. Carcinomas of the head of the gland almost always cause stenosis of the distal common bile duct and the bile duct proximal to this area of stenosis is dilated and thickened. Diffuse carcinomas can mimic chronic pancreatitis and some small carcinomas are not apparent grossly.

Most carcinomas of the pancreas grossly extend beyond the gland (60). Large vessel invasion with vascular stenosis and thrombosis is common, as is invasion into the ampulla of Vater or the wall of the duodenum (figs. 7-11, 7-12) (222). Because periampullary carcinomas often involve multiple anatomic structures, a careful gross examination to establish the epicenter of the neoplasm is invaluable in determining the organ of origin. Most pancreatic cancers infiltrate into retroperitoneal structures, and larger pancreatic cancers can invade the duodenum, peritoneum, stomach, transverse colon, jejunum, adrenal gland, kidney, ureter, and even the gallbladder (60). Carcinomas of the tail of the pancreas, because of their more

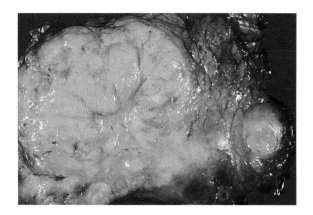

Figure 7-10

DUCTAL ADENOCARCINOMA

Relatively well-demarcated carcinoma.

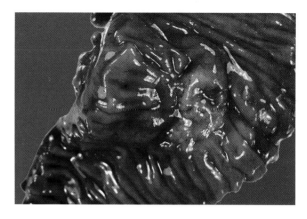

Figure 7-11

DUCTAL ADENOCARCINOMA

Puckering of the duodenum associated with duodenal invasion.

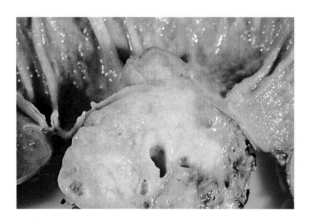

Figure 7-12

DUCTAL ADENOCARCINOMA

Invasion of the cancer into the duodenum.

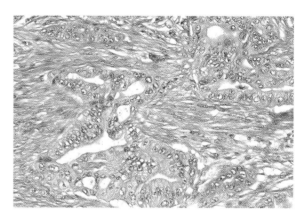

Figure 7-13

DUCTAL ADENOCARCINOMA

Intense desmoplastic reaction to the invasive carcinoma.

advanced stage at presentation, often infiltrate into the peritoneum, spleen, left adrenal gland, and intestines (60).

Microscopic Findings

Infiltrating adenocarcinomas of the pancreas are invasive, gland-forming, mucin-producing epithelial neoplasms that elicit an intense desmoplastic reaction (fig. 7-13) (57,60,145,161a, 279). The degree of gland formation is proportional to the degree of differentiation, and varies from well-formed glands, to partially formed glands, to focal intracellular mucin production by poorly oriented cells infiltrating singly or forming solid sheets.

The neoplastic glands in infiltrating adenocarcinoma are distributed in a disorganized fashion. This can be appreciated in several ways. First, normal pancreatic ducts and atrophic benign pancreatic ducts have a well-developed branching lobular appearance that is generally preserved even in the presence of chronic pancreatitis (fig. 7-14). By contrast, the invasive glands of a pancreatic adenocarcinoma grow in a haphazard fashion, violating the predictable branching of benign glands (fig. 7-15). Second, in the normal pancreas the small and medium-sized ducts are present in the center of the lobules, while the muscular blood vessels run in the connective tissues at the periphery of the lobules (fig.

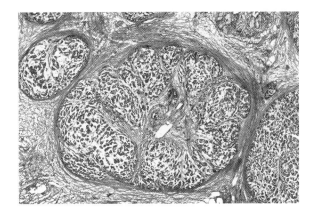

Figure 7-14

ATROPHIC CHRONIC PANCREATITIS

Even, markedly atrophic glands retain a lobular growth pattern.

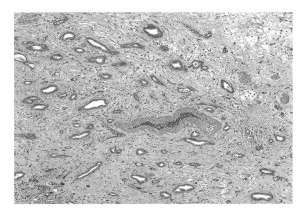

Figure 7-15

DUCTAL ADENOCARCINOMA

Invasive ducts produce a haphazard growth pattern.

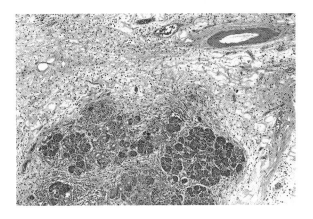

Figure 7-16

ATROPHIC CHRONIC PANCREATITIS

The muscular arteries (upper right) normally are present at the periphery of the lobules, separated from larger glands.

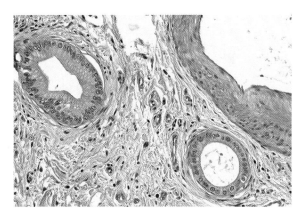

Figure 7-17

DUCTAL ADENOCARCINOMA

A gland is adjacent to a muscular blood vessel, without intervening acini or stroma.

7-16). Therefore, in the normal pancreas the ducts are surrounded by acini and anatomically separated from the muscular vessels (274). The neoplastic glands of an invasive adenocarcinoma of the pancreas violate this architectural organization and can be found immediately adjacent to muscular blood vessels, without intervening acini or stroma (figs. 7-15, 7-17) (274).

Virtually all adenocarcinomas of the pancreas elicit an intense non-neoplastic desmoplastic stromal reaction consisting of collagen, myofibroblasts, lymphocytes, and other inflammatory cells (fig. 7-13) (59,145,161a,279). This desmoplastic reaction accounts for the firm consistency of most pancreatic cancers. Normal pancreatic structures, including islets of Langerhans, are often trapped within the desmoplastic reaction. As a result, the neoplastic epithelial cells in most pancreatic cancers comprise only a small portion of the cells in the tumor. Focal hemorrhage, central necrosis, and cystic degeneration can be seen, particularly in larger carcinomas.

Infiltrating adenocarcinomas of the pancreas are extraordinarily invasive neoplasms. They not only infiltrate into the connective tissue stroma of the pancreas, but they also typically infiltrate into and along a variety of preexisting structures. Most (70 percent) infiltrating adenocarcinomas grow into and along benign pancreatic ducts, particularly the large branch ducts

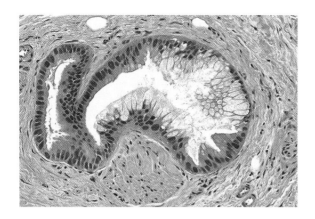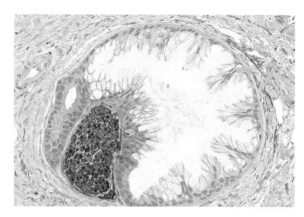

Figure 7-18

DUCTAL ADENOCARCINOMA

Perineural invasion (left) can be highlighted by immunolabeling of nerves with S-100 protein (right).

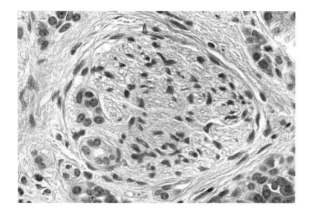

Figure 7-19

CHRONIC PANCREATITIS

Extremely rare benign glandular inclusions in a nerve.

(332). In so doing, infiltrating carcinomas extend beyond the main neoplastic mass, and this intraductal extension of an invasive cancer can mimic pancreatic intraepithelial neoplasia.

The majority of infiltrating adenocarcinomas of the pancreas also infiltrate into and grow along nerves (fig. 7-18) (121). Perineural invasion is seen in over 75 percent of pancreatic cancers (121,219, 224,293). Perineural invasion is often present along the leading edge of the carcinoma and, in the substance of the pancreas, is associated with extension of the carcinoma into the retroperitoneal nerves beyond the gland (121,219, 294). Exceedingly rare examples of benign glandular inclusions in a nerve have been reported (fig. 7-19), but this phenomenon is so rare that

the presence of glands within a nerve is virtually diagnostic of invasive adenocarcinoma (52).

Infiltrating adenocarcinomas of the pancreas also frequently infiltrate into lymphatics and blood vessels (figs. 7-20–7-22) (60,145,161a, 279). The normal lymphatics in the pancreas run together with the blood vessels, and lymphatic invasion is seen in the majority of surgically resected pancreatic cancers. Lymphatic invasion is associated with lymph node metastases. Pancreatic cancers also infiltrate larger blood vessels (fig. 7-20). This vascular invasion can cause thrombosis of the vessels. In some instances, infiltrating adenocarcinomas appear to replace the endothelial cells of the vessels, and a layer of neoplastic epithelial cells can uniformly line the vessel lumen (fig. 7-22). This finding can mimic a non-neoplastic gland until it is realized that there is an elastic lamina or muscular wall surrounding the otherwise benign-appearing epithelial cells.

Most infiltrating adenocarcinomas of the pancreas obstruct the pancreatic duct, and the pancreatic parenchyma upstream from such obstructions show marked atrophy and chronic pancreatitis. In some cases, the pancreatic parenchyma is so scarred that only a few residual atrophic ducts and islets of Langerhans remain. The islets of Langerhans in the areas of atrophy and chronic pancreatitis become clustered and fuse, and are significantly larger than normal islets of Langerhans (60). These changes represent a reactive, not a neoplastic, process and should not be mistaken for a small well-differentiated

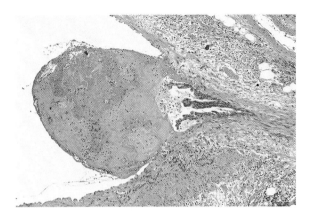

Figure 7-20

DUCTAL ADENOCARCINOMA

Large vessel invasion.

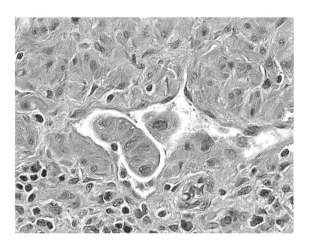

Figure 7-21

DUCTAL ADENOCARCINOMA

Invasion of a small lymphatic vessel.

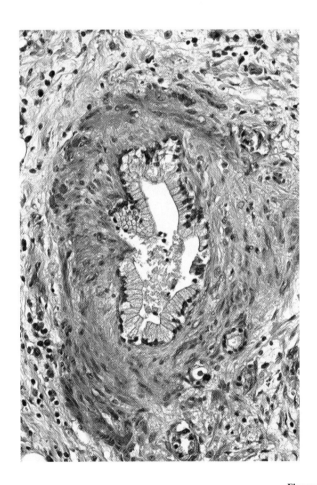

Figure 7-22

DUCTAL ADENOCARCINOMA

Invasive carcinoma growing along the inner lining of a blood vessel (left) is highlighted with the Verhoeff stain (right).

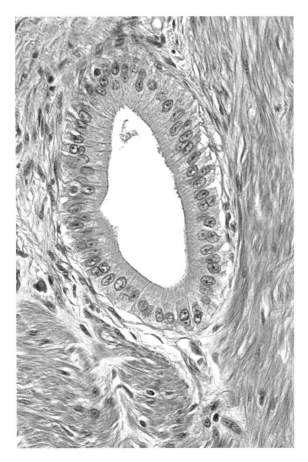

Figure 7-23

DUCTAL ADENOCARCINOMA

Invasion into the muscularis propria of the duodenum.

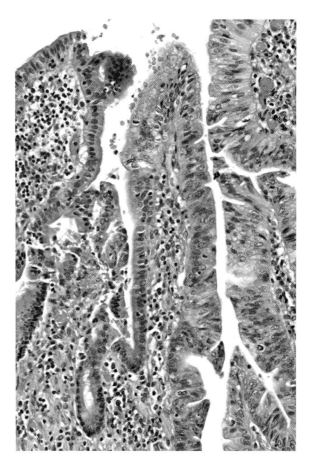

Figure 7-24

DUCTAL ADENOCARCINOMA

Invasion into the mucosa of the duodenum can mimic a primary neoplasm of the duodenum.

endocrine neoplasm. Infiltrating adenocarcinomas of the pancreas can invade into islets of Langerhans, but non-neoplastic glands can be found intimately associated with islets as well, and the finding of glands within an islet is, therefore, entirely nonspecific. Invasion into the duodenum and into peripancreatic fat is common (fig. 7-23).

When infiltrating adenocarcinomas of the pancreas invade into a preexisting epithelium, such as the bile duct or duodenum, the neoplastic cells often grow along the epithelial basement membrane, a pattern of growth that can mimic an in situ carcinoma in the bile duct or an adenoma in the duodenum or ampulla. In some instances, the intramucosal portion of the carcinoma is better differentiated and has a more intestinal appearance than the carcinoma

within the duodenal wall or pancreas (fig. 7-24). In these cases, an abrupt transition from normal to highly atypical epithelium is a clue to the diagnosis of an invasive cancer.

The nuclear morphology of pancreatic carcinoma is helpful in establishing a malignant diagnosis. The nuclei typically vary in size, shape, and intracellular location from cell to cell within the individual gland. A four-fold variation in nuclear area between adjacent cells in a single gland is virtually diagnostic of carcinoma, although well-differentiated examples may still have relatively uniform nuclei. Loss of nuclear polarity may be pronounced, but is also seen in pancreatic intraepithelial neoplasia. Nuclear enlargement is usually present in carcinomas; comparison with adjacent benign ducts may facilitate the recognition of the uniform nuclear

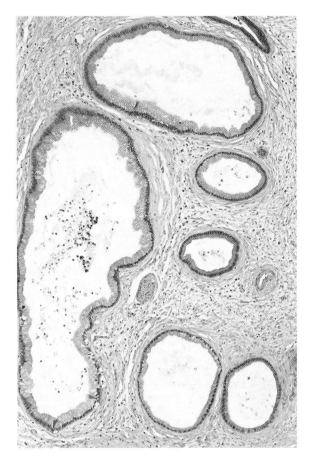

Figure 7-25

DUCTAL ADENOCARCINOMA

Low magnification of a well-differentiated ductal adenocarcinoma.

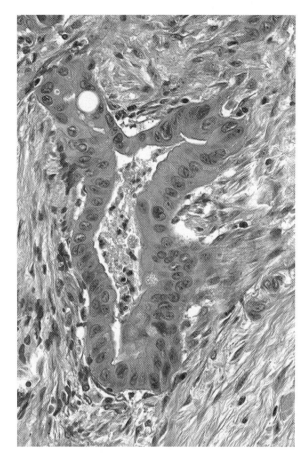

Figure 7-26

DUCTAL ADENOCARCINOMA

High magnification of a moderately differentiated ductal adenocarcinoma.

enlargement of well-differentiated adenocarcinomas. Many ductal adenocarcinomas have abundant mucinous cytoplasm, and, as a result, the nuclear to cytoplasmic ratio may not be significantly increased.

The neoplastic epithelial cells of invasive *well-differentiated adenocarcinoma* form well-defined glands (figs. 7-23, 7-25) (145,161a,279). Occasionally, incomplete gland formation is seen, as well as cribriforming and micropapillary projections. The cuboidal to columnar neoplastic cells have basally oriented, uniform round to oval nuclei with evenly dispersed chromatin. Only minimal nuclear pleomorphism is seen. These nuclei typically contain one or two relatively inconspicuous nucleoli. The cytoplasm is abundant and can be slightly basophilic, clear, or slightly eosinophilic. Mitotic

figures are seen, but are not numerous, nor are they atypical.

Moderately differentiated adenocarcinoma has a more disorganized growth pattern and gland formation is less well-defined (fig. 7-26) (145,161a, 279). Incomplete glandular lumens and rupture of mucin into the stroma are common. Nuclear pleomorphism is more prominent and the nucleoli are larger and more irregular. Mitoses are more common, and some may be atypical.

Poorly differentiated adenocarcinomas have small poorly formed glands, individual infiltrating cells, and solid areas (fig. 7-27) (145,161a,279). The neoplastic cells produce significantly less mucin than the better-differentiated examples. Nuclear pleomorphism is more prominent, with occasional large, somewhat bizarre nuclei. The nucleoli are large, multiple, and more irregular.

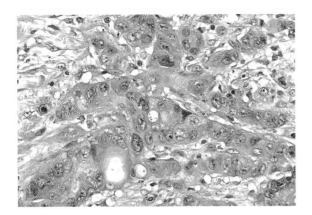

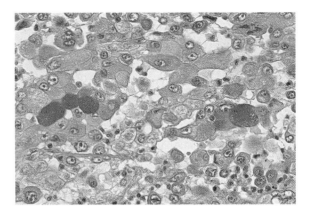

Figure 7-27

DUCTAL ADENOCARCINOMA

Poorly differentiated ductal adenocarcinoma.

Figure 7-28

DUCTAL ADENOCARCINOMA

Mucicarmine stain highlights intracytoplasmic and extracellular mucin.

Table 7-2

HISTOLOGIC GRADING OF PANCREATIC CANCER[a]

Tumor Grade	Glandular Differentiation	Mucin Production	Mitoses (per 10 hpf[b])	Nuclear Atypia
1	Well-differentiated duct-like glands	Intensive	≤5	Polar arrangement, little pleomorphism
2	Moderately differentiated duct-like structures and tubular glands	Irregular	6-10	Moderate pleomorphism
3	Poorly differentiated glands, muco-epidermoid and pleomorphic structures	Abortive	>10	Marked pleomorphism and increased nuclear size

[a]Data from reference 162.
[b]hpf = high-power fields.

Mitoses are common and often atypical. Hemorrhage and necrosis are often present.

Several systems have been developed to grade infiltrating adenocarcinomas of the pancreas. Klöppel (162) developed a well-defined system that incorporates the degree of glandular differentiation, mucin production, and nuclear atypia, along with the mitotic count (Table 7-2). While this system has been shown to have prognostic significance, it is somewhat complex and time consuming to implement in daily practice (99). Simpler grading systems, such as the TMN grading system (see chapter 3), correlate well with the system proposed by Klöppel and may be more practical to use.

It is relatively common in pancreatic carcinomas to have a combination of well-formed glands as well as individual cells and clusters, resulting in the appearance of both well-differentiated and poorly differentiated elements in the same carcinoma. In these cases, the carcinoma should be assigned a grade that reflects the worst degree of differentiation present in a significant portion of the carcinoma.

Conventional special stains confirm the expression of mucin in the majority of pancreatic cancers. The mucicarmine stain reveals both intracellular apical and extracellular mucin (fig. 7-28), and a periodic acid–Schiff (PAS) stain will be positive, even after digestion with diastase. The mucins produced by adenocarcinomas of the pancreas are primarily sialo-type and sulfated (acid)-type mucins; high-iron diamine and Alcian blue (pH 2.5) stains are therefore usually positive. Grimilius/Cherukian-Schenk (argyrophilic) and Fontana-Masson (argentaffin) stains highlight scattered endocrine cells at the base of the neoplastic epithelium in 25 percent of carcinomas.

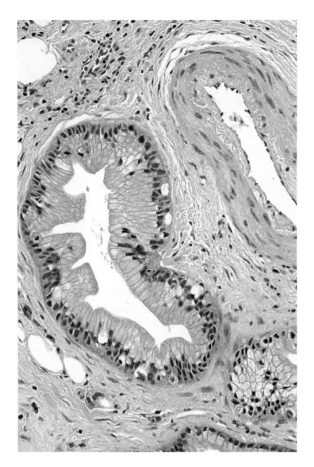

Figure 7-29

DUCTAL ADENOCARCINOMA

Foamy gland pattern.

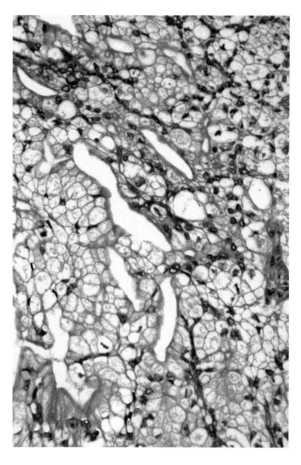

Figure 7-30

DUCTAL ADENOCARCINOMA

Prominent clear cell change can mimic a metastasis of a renal cell carcinoma.

Histologic Types

Histologic variants include the adenosquamous, colloid (mucinous noncystic), hepatoid, medullary, signet ring cell, undifferentiated, and undifferentiated carcinoma with osteoclast-like giant cells. These are described in detail in chapter 8.

A *foamy gland* pattern of adenocarcinoma of the pancreas has been described (3). These deceptively bland, benign-appearing cells have a prominent microvesicular cytoplasm that gives them a "foamy" appearance (fig. 7-29). In addition, the luminal aspect of these cells has a distinctive cytoplasmic condensation, called a "brush border–like zone." This morphologic pattern does not have prognostic significance, but it is important to recognize because it can mimic benign glands (3).

Other ductal adenocarcinomas have abundant clear cytoplasm that is not due to the accumulation of mucin granules as in foamy gland adenocarcinomas; the clear cytoplasm resembles that of renal cell carcinomas (fig. 7-30) (152,190,254). Some of these neoplasms also have a predominantly solid growth pattern, furthering the resemblance to kidney primaries. Often designated *clear cell carcinoma* of the pancreas, these neoplasms produce mucin and immunolabel for other markers of ductal adenocarcinomas; furthermore, they harbor mutations in the *KRAS* oncogene (190,254). Thus, they are now regarded as *ductal adenocarcinomas with clear cell features*, a cytoplasmic change that is not uncommon as a focal finding in many ductal adenocarcinomas.

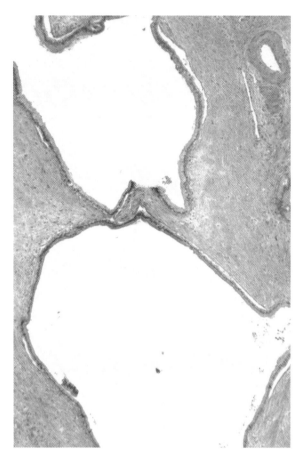

Figure 7-31

DUCTAL ADENOCARCINOMA

Large duct type can be very well differentiated, as in this example.

A *microadenocarcinoma* pattern of pancreatic cancer, characterized by small uniform cells arranged in small microglandular structures, was described by Cubilla and Fitzgerald in 1975 (59). Recent reanalysis of these carcinomas using modern immunolabeling techniques has demonstrated that the microadenocarcinoma pattern, in fact, represents a mix of ductal adenocarcinoma, endocrine neoplasm, and acinar cell carcinoma (183). This pattern of growth should be considered an aggressive growth pattern and not a distinct entity.

Some ductal adenocarcinomas are composed of large, dilated invasive glands that are usually architecturally simple. These glands can be sufficiently dilated to be seen as microcysts grossly. This variant has been designated the *large duct adenocarcinoma* (fig. 7-31), and the

Table 7-3
FEATURES USEFUL IN ESTABLISHING A DIAGNOSIS OF INFILTRATING ADENOCARCINOMA ON FROZEN SECTION
Haphazard growth pattern
Glands adjacent to muscular vessels
Perineural or vascular invasion
Incomplete lumens
Four to one rule
Huge irregular nucleoli
Glandular necrotic debris
Mitoses, particularly atypical mitoses

individual invasive glands may simulate pancreatic intraepithelial neoplasia. Recognition that the normal lobular arrangement of the pancreatic ducts is lost, or finding dilated glands in abnormal locations such as in the muscularis propria of the duodenum, will help confirm the invasive nature of these carcinomas. This pattern of growth does not appear to have prognostic significance.

Frozen Section

Frozen section evaluation of the pancreas can be extremely difficult. Infiltrating well-differentiated adenocarcinoma can look essentially benign, and, conversely, the reactive glands of chronic pancreatitis can mimic an invasive cancer. This treacherous landscape can be safely navigated with the consistent application of well-defined diagnostic criteria (Table 7-3), a familiarity with diagnostic clues, and good communication between the surgeon and the pathologist.

A number of investigators have defined the histologic features that are most useful in establishing the diagnosis of infiltrating adenocarcinoma on frozen section (48,135,321). These features include: 1) a haphazard pattern of growth. Benign glands have a structured lobular growth pattern, while infiltrating carcinomas grow haphazardly (see fig. 7-15); 2) the finding of a gland immediately adjacent to a muscular vessel without intervening stroma or acini (fig. 7-32). As discussed earlier, glands and muscular blood vessels normally do not run together in the pancreas; 3) the finding of perineural or vascular invasion (fig. 7-33).

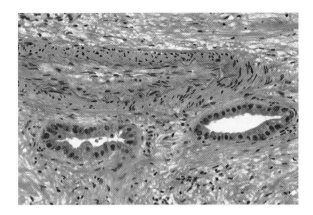

Figure 7-32

DUCTAL ADENOCARCINOMA

Frozen section reveals a gland immediately adjacent to a muscular vessel, without intervening stroma or acini, supporting a diagnosis of malignancy.

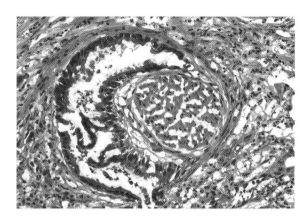

Figure 7-33

DUCTAL ADENOCARCINOMA

Perineural invasion demonstrated on frozen section.

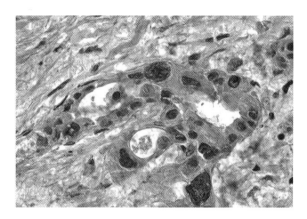

Figure 7-34

DUCTAL ADENOCARCINOMA

Anisonucleosis of ≥4:1 (the "four to one" rule) on frozen section supports the diagnosis of cancer.

While virtually diagnostic features, perineural and vascular invasion are often not present in smaller biopsies; 4) incomplete lumens of infiltrating adenocarcinoma instead of complete lumens of non-neoplastic glands. Single cells infiltrating into stroma represent the extreme of this; 5) the finding that the area of one nucleus is four or more times larger than the area of another nucleus within a single gland (fig. 7-34). This has been called the four to one rule; the nuclei in non-neoplastic glands do not vary in size significantly; 6) huge, irregular nucleoli one quarter to one third the diameter of the nucleus; 7) necrotic glandular debris (fig. 7-35); and 8) the presence of numerous or abnormal mitotic figures, although mitoses can be seen in benign processes. When these criteria are rigorously applied, frozen section evaluation of the pancreas can have false positive and false negative rates of less than 2 percent, particularly when frozen sections are interpreted in the light of clinical information from the surgeon (48).

Due to the frequent coexistence of pancreas cancer and chronic pancreatitis, and the difficulty of distinguishing the two processes based on inspection or palpation of the pancreas, it is common for core needle biopsies from a pancreas with a ductal adenocarcinoma to reveal only chronic pancreatitis. Furthermore, the infiltrating glands at the periphery of an adenocarcinoma may be widely spaced, and a single core biopsy may contain too few glands to appreciate the overall architecture. Thus, it may be necessary to obtain several core biopsies for frozen section to identify unequivocal evidence of carcinoma.

Immunohistochemical Findings

A distinct pattern of immunohistochemical labeling is emerging for pancreatic cancer, and it is anticipated that more markers of ductal adenocarcinoma will be discovered through newer technologies that allow for global analyses of gene expression in cancer. It is unlikely that one single marker will be 100 percent sensitive and specific. Instead, it is much more likely that

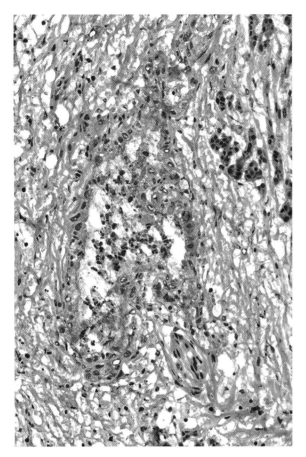

Figure 7-35

DUCTAL ADENOCARCINOMA

Necrotic glandular debris on frozen section.

Table 7-4
IMMUNOHISTOCHEMICAL LABELING OF INFILTRATING DUCTAL ADENOCARCINOMA
Cytokeratins 7, 8, 18, 19
MUC1, MUC3, MUC4, and MUC5AC
CEA[a], CA19-9, B72.3, CA125, DUPAN-2
Mesothelin, PSCA[b], claudin 4
Fascin, S-100A4, S-100A6, S-100P
Loss of Dpc4, p16
Nuclear accumulation of p53
Scattered endocrine cells at base of epithelial cells

[a]CEA = carcinoembryonic antigen.
[b]PSCA = prostate stem cell antigen.

cinoma or high-grade pancreatic intraepithelial neoplasia from reactive glands (161).

Adenocarcinomas of the pancreas express several high molecular weight glycoproteins (mucins) including MUC1 (a panepithelial mucin), MUC3, MUC4, and MUC5AC (a gastric foveolar mucin) (15,157,174,192,213,292). About 25 percent of ductal adenocarcinomas express MUC6 (a pyloric gland mucin) and less than 10 percent, MUC2. By contrast, the majority of intraductal papillary mucinous neoplasms (IPMNs) and mucinous cystic neoplasms (MCNs) express MUC2 but not MUC1 (340). Similarly, only a minority of ductal adenocarcinomas express trefoil factor-2, while this trefoil peptide is expressed in over 90 percent of IPMNs and MCNs. Most infiltrating adenocarcinomas also express the mucin associated carbohydrate antigen sialyl Tn.

Several glycosylphosphatidyl inositol–anchored proteins are expressed in pancreatic cancer, including mesothelin (expressed in 90 to 100 percent) and prostate stem cell antigen (expressed in 60 percent) (17,18,292). Claudin 4 is overexpressed in close to 100 percent of pancreatic cancers, sea urchin fascin homolog in 95 percent, and ADAM9 in over 95 percent (201,230, 292). A number of the S-100 proteins (so named because they are soluble in 100 percent ammonium sulfate) are overexpressed in pancreatic cancer, including S-100A4, S-100A6, and S-100P (56,262, 319). The antiapoptotic protein survivin, associated with a lower apoptotic rate in pancreatic cancer, is expressed in 75 percent of cases (150,253). The potential therapeutic/chemoprevention target

panels of markers will be developed which, when taken together, will be useful tools in identifying and classifying cancers of the pancreas.

Most adenocarcinomas of the pancreas express the cytokeratins (CKs) 7, 8, 13, 18 and 19 (Table 7-4) (70,106,174). CK7, CK8, CK18, and CK19 are expressed in 90 to 100 percent of pancreatic cancers; CK17 in 50 percent; and CK20 in less than 20 percent. This pattern of immunolabeling can be diagnostically useful, as most endocrine and acinar neoplasms of the pancreas do not express CK7, and most colorectal cancers express CK20 and not CK7. Ductal adenocarcinomas of the pancreas also express a variety of glycoprotein tumor antigens including CEA, CA19-9, B72.3 (TAG-72), CA125, and DUPAN-2. The expression of CEA, B72.3, and CA125 may be useful in distinguishing infiltrating adenocar-

cyclooxygenase-2 is expressed in 70 to 90 percent, and 5-lipoxygenase and leukotriene B4 receptor are expressed in the majority of pancreatic cancers (238,309).

Scattered endocrine cells expressing chromogranin A, leu-7, synaptophysin, and neuron-specific enolase can be found at the base of the neoplastic epithelial cells in a quarter to a third of pancreatic cancers (151,250). Rarely, labeling with these markers is more diffuse, although this labeling pattern raises the possibility of a poorly differentiated endocrine carcinoma (see chapter 12).

Many growth factors and receptors are overexpressed in pancreatic cancers. These include epidermal growth factor and its receptor, c-erbB-2; erbB-3; transforming growth factors alpha and beta and their receptors; nerve growth factor and its receptor, TrkA; platelet-derived growth factors A and B and their receptors, (PDGFR); fibroblast growth factors and their receptors; connective tissue growth factor and its receptor, alpha-2 macroglobulin; vascular endothelial growth factor and its receptors; and the neurokinin-1 receptor (NK-1R) and its ligand, substance P (71,80–82,139,143,165–167, 175,186,297,303,342). Most ductal adenocarcinomas of the pancreas do not express vimentin, trypsin, chymotrypsin, or lipase.

The desmoplastic stroma associated with almost all infiltrating adenocarcinomas of the pancreas expresses a variety of inflammatory and stromal markers. The inflammatory cells are mostly T cells (CD3 positive); CD8-positive cells predominate slightly over CD4-positive lymphocytes (1). Scattered B cells (CD20 positive) and macrophages (MAC387 and KP1 positive) are also usually present. The macrophages usually express osteopontin, and osteopontin can be detected in the serum of patients with pancreatic cancer (164). The spindle cells in the desmoplastic stroma express alpha-smooth muscle actin, smooth muscle myosin heavy chain, and collagen IV, markers of myofibroblastic differentiation (333). The stroma almost always labels for heat shock protein 47 and fibronectin, as well as for proteins associated with tissue remolding such as urokinase-type plasminogen activator, the matrix metalloproteinases (including MMP-1, MMP-2, MMP-3, MMP-7 [matrilysin], MMP-9, MMP-10, and MMP-13), and the

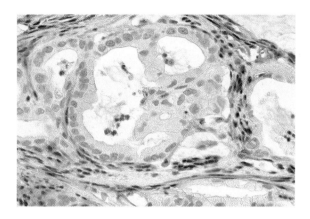

Figure 7-36

DUCTAL ADENOCARCINOMA

Immunohistochemical labeling demonstrates a complete loss of Dpc4 expression in the neoplastic glands.

tissue inhibitors of metalloproteinases (TIMP-1 and TIMP-2) (168,201,328,341).

Antibodies that are sensitive and specific for the gene products of a number of the cancer-associated genes inactivated in pancreatic cancer have been developed. These antibodies are useful in evaluating tissue samples from the pancreas. Immunolabeling for the Dpc4 protein mirrors the *DPC4/MADH4* gene status; 55 percent of infiltrating adenocarcinomas show complete loss of Dpc4 immunolabeling (fig. 7-36) (327). Almost all benign processes in the pancreas express Dpc4 at an immunohistochemically detectable level, therefore, the evaluation of Dpc4 expression may be a useful adjunct in the interpretation of difficult biopsies of the pancreas (298,317). Abnormal nuclear labeling for the protein product of the *TP53* gene, p53, occurs in 50 to 75 percent of pancreatic cancers, and immunolabeling for the protein product of the *p16/CDKN2A* gene shows loss of p16 expression in over 90 percent of the cancers (69,317,324). Immunolabeling for the p53 protein is, however, not specific for a *TP53* gene mutation, and immunolabeling for the p16 protein can be difficult to interpret because of high background labeling with most antibodies.

Global analyses of gene expression using serial analysis of gene expression, cDNA arrays, and oligonucleotide arrays have been used to identify literally hundreds of genes that are overexpressed in pancreatic cancer (55,68,112,

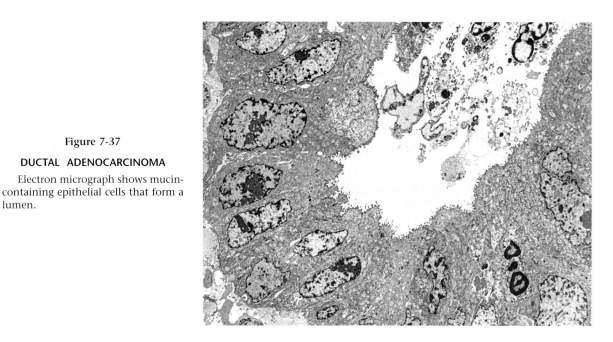

Figure 7-37

DUCTAL ADENOCARCINOMA

Electron micrograph shows mucin-containing epithelial cells that form a lumen.

116,136–138,182,210,266,339). These genes encode for proteins with cytoskeletal (CK7, CK17, and CK19, fascin, and pleckstrin), DNA transcription (topoisomerase II-alpha and acute myelogenous leukemia [AML]1), DNA repair (ataxia-telangiectasia group D-complementing [ATDC]), cell cycle regulation (p21 and cyclin D), secretory (e.g., HE4), cell surface (e.g., mesothelin, PSCA), transmembrane (e.g., CEACAM6), growth factors (MIC1), tight junction related (e.g., claudins 1, 3, 4, and 7, and connexin), cell matrix interactions (e.g., integrin-α3 and -α6), serine proteases (kallikrein 6 and 10), and calcium homeostasis (e.g., S-100A4, S-100A6, S-100A10, S-100A11, S-100 calcium-binding protein P, Trop-2, and ALG-2) functions.

Global analyses of gene expression have also helped define the gene expression profile of the desmoplastic reaction associated with almost all pancreatic cancers (139,267). These "invasion-specific" genes encode for collagens (type 1α1 and 1β2), heat shock protein 47, growth factors (connective tissue growth factor and IGFBP7), matrix metalloproteinases (MMP-2, MMP-7, MMP-11, and MMP-14), and markers of specific cell types (hevin). Similarly, proteomics-based analyses have demonstrated that hepatocarcinoma-intestine-pancreas/pancreatitis-associated protein-1 (HIP/PAP-1) is overexpressed by the non-neoplastic tissues adjacent to infiltrating adenocarcinomas (260). The identification of genes

differentially overexpressed by pancreatic cancer will increase. The challenge will be to identify and develop a panel of markers that is both sensitive and specific for pancreatic cancer.

Ultrastructural Findings

Given the battery of immunohistochemical markers currently available, ductal adenocarcinomas are only rarely examined ultrastructurally. Ductal adenocarcinomas, as expected, are composed of epithelial cells that form lumens, apical mucin granules (0.4 to 2.0 µm), microvilli, intermediate filaments, and tight junctions (fig. 7-37) (156,162,234). Ductal adenocarcinomas with the foamy gland pattern have an apical concentration of smaller mucin granules (corresponding to the brush border–like zone) that are distinct from the large mucin granules that fill the remainder of the cytoplasm and produce the foamy appearance (3).

Cytologic Findings

The interpretation of aspiration cytology smears is influenced by the technique used to obtain the specimen. Most solid masses of the pancreas clinically suspicious for adenocarcinoma are sampled using CT-guided percutaneous fine needle aspiration biopsy. EUS-guided aspiration biopsy, however, is increasingly used in both major academic centers and large community hospitals. In contrast to percutaneous biopsies, EUS-guided biopsies traverse the stomach or duodenal wall and can contain epithelial contamination from these sites. The challenge of identifying gastrointestinal epithelial contamination is generally not an issue with poorly differentiated carcinomas, however, it can be a significant issue with well-differentiated adenocarcinomas. The criteria of overall cellularity and number of glandular groups associated with malignancy in percutaneous biopsies are less useful in interpreting EUS-guided biopsies. The use of brush cytology of a stenotic main pancreatic duct or intrapancreatic common bile duct results in a higher false negative rate than does fine needle aspiration biopsy (120). The initial approach to all aspiration cytology smears should include a low-power evaluation of the overall cellularity of the smears, the cellular composition, the architectural arrangement, the cohesiveness of the cells, and the background elements such as the presence of inflammation, mucin, and necrosis.

In contrast to benign and reactive processes such as pancreatitis, the primary entity in the differential diagnosis, percutaneous aspiration biopsy of carcinoma produces cellular smears in which glandular epithelial cells are predominant and cover a large area of the glass slide. Overall cellularity, however, is directly related to the experience of the interventional radiologist, the method of biopsy, and the composition of the neoplasm. The technical difficulty of EUS-guided biopsy relative to percutaneous biopsy often leads to fewer individual punctures and thus a lower cellular yield. The characteristic desmoplastic reaction associated with many invasive carcinomas may also lead to paucicellular smears.

Gastrointestinal contamination can contribute to what appears to be a highly cellular specimen on EUS-guided biopsy and care must be taken to carefully distinguish epithelium from the stomach or duodenum from epithelium from the pancreas. High cellularity is not as important a criterion for poorly differentiated carcinoma as it is for well-differentiated carcinoma, and there is no established minimum number of malignant cells or groups of cells for the diagnosis of poorly differentiated carcinoma (49,180,257).

The composition of the cellular elements on the slide is important for distinguishing benign

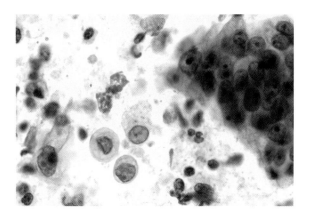

Figure 7-38

DUCTAL ADENOCARCINOMA

Poorly differentiated carcinoma with high nuclear to cytoplasmic ratios and markedly irregular nuclei, nuclear membranes, and chromatin distribution (direct smear; Papanicolaou stain).

from malignant. Smears of carcinoma should be relatively pure with only ductal cells. Smears composed of both acinar and ductal cells should be interpreted with caution. Similarly, the presence of granulation tissue and fibrous tissue fragments with inflammation is associated more with active pancreatitis than carcinoma.

The architectural arrangement of carcinoma cells ranges from large crowded sheets, to small three-dimensional clusters and balls, to single cells. The arrangement of the cells in groups and sheets is important, especially for well-differentiated carcinomas. Single intact cells are common in poorly differentiated carcinomas and their presence is directly related to the loss of cellular cohesion. Single malignant cells may be scattered in the smear background but are also seen at the edge of more cohesive groups. The presence of single atypical intact epithelial cells in a well-differentiated carcinoma is significant and supports a malignant interpretation.

In poorly differentiated carcinomas, the cellular features of malignancy are overt. The cells have a high nuclear to cytoplasmic ratio that is best appreciated in the single cells (fig. 7-38). This high nuclear to cytoplasmic ratio yields an increased nuclear density in cell clusters and sheets relative to benign ductal groups (fig. 7-39), and dense nucleation leads to cellular crowding, nuclear overlapping, and loss of nuclear polarity. In well-differentiated carcinomas that have

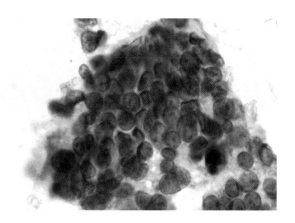

Figure 7-39

DUCTAL ADENOCARCINOMA

Poorly differentiated carcinoma forms a densely nucleated cluster of crowded hyperchromatic cells (direct smear; Papanicolaou stain).

Table 7-5

MAJOR AND MINOR CRITERIA FOR THE CYTOLOGIC DIAGNOSIS OF ADENOCARCINOMA[a,b]

Major Criteria	Minor Criteria
Nuclear crowding and over-lapping	Nuclear enlargement
Irregular chromatin distribution	Single malignant cells
Irregular nuclear contour	Necrosis; mitoses

[a]Two or more major or one major plus three minor criteria = adenocarcinoma with 100% sensitivity and specificity.
[b]Data from reference 257.

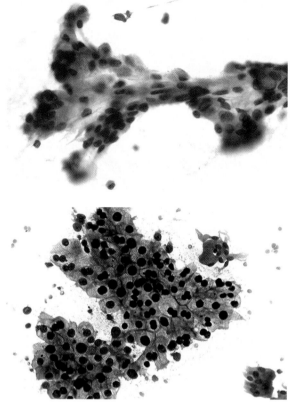

Figure 7-40

DUCTAL ADENOCARCINOMA

The "drunken honeycomb" pattern of well-differentiated adenocarcinoma can be appreciated on fixed (top) and air-dried (bottom) smears (direct smears; Papanicolaou [top] and Romanowsky [bottom] stains).

more abundant, often mucinous cytoplasm, the variation in cell size and cytoplasmic volume leads to irregular and uneven spacing of the nuclei that has been termed "drunken honeycomb" (66); this pattern can be appreciated in both fixed (fig. 7-40, top) and air-dried smears (fig. 7-40, bottom). This is in contrast to the generally regular and even nuclear spacing seen in benign ductal groups and in epithelial cells from the stomach and duodenum (fig. 7-41).

Nuclear features are the key to a diagnosis of carcinoma (7,49,78,180,211,257). In poorly differentiated carcinomas, the nuclei are overtly malignant and enlarged, usually at least 2 to 3 times the size of a normal ductal cell nucleus (about 15 μm), with anisonucleosis of at least four times within a single sheet of tumor cells ("four to one" rule) (fig. 7-42). These two features, coupled with

nuclear molding, have, by regression analysis, a sensitivity of 98 percent and specificity of 100 percent for poorly differentiated carcinomas (49). Using a combination of the major and minor criteria listed in Table 7-5, the sensitivity and specificity for a cytologic diagnosis of carcinoma reach 100 percent (257). All three major criteria relate to the nucleus: nuclear overlapping, nuclear contour irregularity, and nuclear chromatin clearing and/or clumping. Combining any two major or one major and three minor criteria improves prospective diagnostic accuracy from 70 to 90 percent.

Unfortunately, nuclear atypia is subtle in well-differentiated carcinomas. Nuclei are not as large (at least 2.5 times the size of an erythrocyte on air-dried smears) (fig. 7-43) (257), the nuclear chromatin demonstrates more clearing

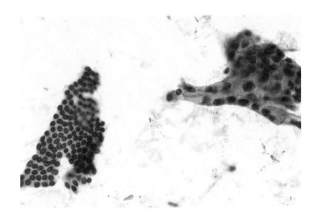

Figure 7-41

BENIGN DUCTAL EPITHELIUM AND ADENOCARCINOMA

The even distribution of round, regular nuclei differentiates benign ducts (left) from well-differentiated carcinoma (right) (direct smear; Papanicolaou stain).

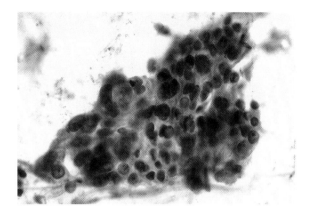

Figure 7-42

DUCTAL ADENOCARCINOMA

Poorly differentiated carcinoma displays marked anisonucleosis (direct smear; Papanicolaou stain).

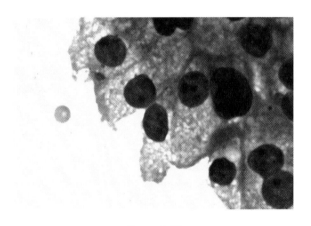

Figure 7-43

DUCTAL ADENOCARCINOMA

Well-differentiated carcinoma with nuclei enlarged at least 2.5 times the size of a red blood cell (left) on an air-dried smear (direct smear; Romanowsky stain).

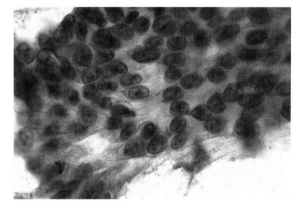

Figure 7-44

DUCTAL ADENOCARCINOMA

The cells of well-differentiated carcinoma display chromatin clearing and subtle nuclear atypia (direct smear; Papanicolaou stain).

than clumping, and the nuclear membrane irregularities are subtle, with nuclear grooves and slightly odd nuclear shapes (fig. 7-44) (180, 257). These subtle nuclear changes, coupled with slight nuclear crowding and overlapping or uneven nuclear distribution (drunken honeycomb), are the key to a diagnosis of well-differentiated carcinoma. Although more prominent in carcinoma, nucleoli and mitotic figures are not distinguishing features from reactive atypia. Frequent or abnormal mitotic figures, however, support a malignant interpretation.

The smear background can also contain helpful clues to the diagnosis. Coagulative necrosis is suspicious for, but not independently diagnostic of, carcinoma. Coagulative necrosis needs to be distinguished from fat necrosis, which is a feature of pancreatitis. Coagulative necrosis is cellular necrosis with visible ghost tumor cells (fig. 7-45, left), which contrasts with fat necrosis, in which saponification and liquefactive necrosis are present in association with foamy histiocytes (fig. 7-45, right). Fibrous tissue fragments are not specific for carcinoma since they may represent

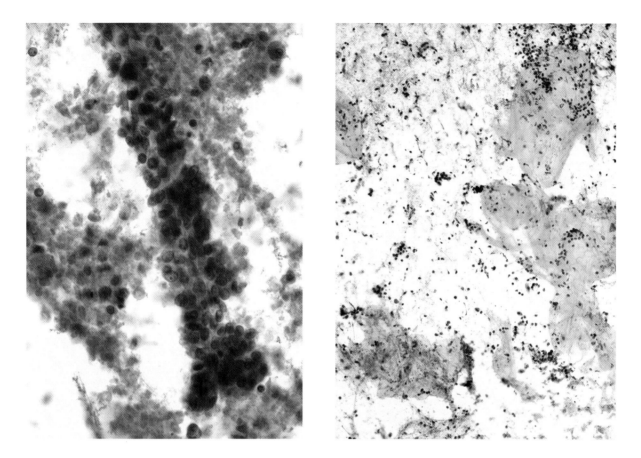

Figure 7-45

DUCTAL ADENOCARCINOMA AND CHRONIC PANCREATITIS

Coagulative tissue necrosis in adenocarcinoma (left) is distinct from fat necrosis in chronic pancreatitis (right) (direct smears; Papanicolaou stain).

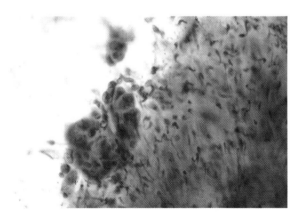

Figure 7-46

DUCTAL ADENOCARCINOMA

Poorly differentiated adenocarcinoma cells adjacent to a fragment of sclerotic stroma (direct smear; Papanicolaou stain).

the fibrosis of chronic pancreatitis or the desmoplasia of carcinoma. Atrophic acinar cells may be noted in chronic pancreatitis, and occasionally, clusters of carcinoma cells are seen within or at the edge of the sclerosis (fig. 7-46).

The recognition of gastric and duodenal epithelial contamination is critical for the accurate interpretation of EUS-guided biopsies. Gastritis and duodenitis with injury and repair of the epithelium can lead to a false positive interpretation of carcinoma, and neoplastic groups of well-differentiated adenocarcinoma can be disregarded as gastrointestinal contamination.

Duodenal epithelium is recognized by the large, folded, sheet-like arrangement of evenly spaced cells studded with goblet cells. The luminal edges of contiguous nonmucinous cytoplasm have a brush border (fig. 7-47) (220). Difficulty arises when folds in sheets appear "papillary,"

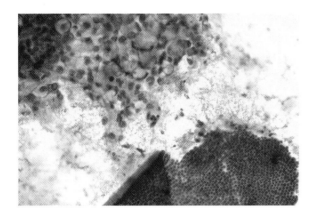

Figure 7-47

**DUCTAL ADENOCARCINOMA
AND DUODENAL EPITHELIUM**

The anisonucleosis of the enlarged, unevenly spaced nuclei in the cluster of adenocarcinoma cells (top) is easily distinguished from the orderly, monolayered sheet of duodenal epithelial cells with a luminal edge (bottom) (direct smear; Papanicolaou stain).

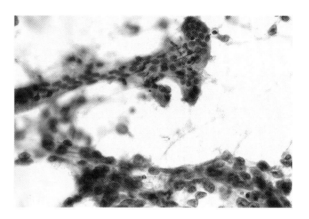

Figure 7-48

**DUCTAL ADENOCARCINOMA
AND GASTRIC EPITHELIUM**

Attention to nuclear size, uniformity, and spacing helps to differentiate gastric epithelium (top) from adenocarcinoma (bottom) (direct smear; Papanicolaou stain).

the nuclear chromatin appears somewhat cleared, or the epithelium fragments into smaller groups. Attention to nuclear size is important. Duodenal nuclei are generally uniformly small, round, and regular whereas the nuclei of well-differentiated adenocarcinoma cells are at least twice as large and not as round or evenly spaced.

Gastric epithelial contamination may also occur as large sheets, but more commonly occurs as smaller, flat monolayered groups of cells. The luminal edges are not as common as with duodenal epithelium and a brush border is absent. Foveolar cells may display apical cytoplasmic mucin, but the epithelium is predominantly nonmucinous (220). Foveolar hyperplasia and regenerative atypia can cause diagnostic difficulty. The epithelial atypia, however, is not significant enough for a diagnosis of poorly differentiated carcinoma, and the nuclear membrane irregularities and chromatin clearing necessary for a diagnosis of well-differentiated carcinoma should be absent or focal at best (fig. 7-48). A summary of the cytologic features of gastrointestinal contamination, chronic pancreatitis, and low- and high-grade carcinoma are presented in Table 7-6.

Molecular and Other Special Techniques

The genetic alterations in infiltrating adenocarcinomas of the pancreas have been well characterized. It is clear that specific cancer-associated genes are targeted in pancreatic cancer and that multiple genes are often mutated in a single cancer (Table 7-7). The discovery of the genes that are altered in pancreatic cancer is exciting because this knowledge can be used to develop new screening tests and new diagnostic tests to aid in the interpretation of difficult biopsies, and to design new therapies.

The first clue that pancreatic cancers harbor significant genetic alterations came from measurements of tumor ploidy using image and flow cytometry. These analyses demonstrated that most pancreatic cancers are aneuploid (9,33,249). Measurements of tumor ploidy cannot, however, be used to identify the specific genes targeted by these genetic alterations. Karyotyping can be used to identify the chromosomes lost or gained in a cancer, and cytogenetic analyses of large series of resected pancreatic cancers has revealed recurrent patterns of alterations in specific chromosomes (111,147). These include losses of whole copies of chromosomes 18, 13, 12, 17, and 6; gains of whole copies of chromosomes 20, 11, 2, and 7; and structural rearrangements involving 1p, 1q, 3p, 3p, 6q, 7q, 8p, 11p, 17p, and 19q (111,147). More poorly differentiated carcinomas often have more complex karyotypes than better differentiated carcinomas. Chromosome arms 1p, 8p, 17p, and 19p frequently have structural abnormalities that include translocations and breakpoints

Table 7-6

CYTOLOGIC FEATURES OF GASTROINTESTINAL CONTAMINATION, CHRONIC PANCREATITIS, AND WELL- AND POORLY DIFFERENTIATED ADENOCARCINOMA

Cytologic Feature	Gastrointestinal Contaminant	Chronic Pancreatitis	Well-Differentiated Adenocarcinoma	Poorly Differentiated Adenocarcinoma
Overall cellularity	Variable	Low	Variable	Variable, usually high
Cellular composition	glandular epithelium, +/– mucin	Ductal cells, acini, inflammation	Ductal cells only	Ductal cells only
Epithelial group architecture	Large, folded, cohesive sheets (duo), smaller groups (gastric)	Cohesive, flat, monolayered	Cohesive, flat, mostly monolayered, rare single cells	3D groups and balls, many single cells
Nuclear enlargement	None	None to mild	Mild, 2.5X RBC[a] on air-dried smear	Significant, >2–3X normal ductal cells
Nuclear crowding	None	Minimal	Mild	Marked
Anisonucleosis	None	Minimal	Mild	Marked and four-fold in a single group
Loss of polarity	None	None	Mild	Marked
Nuclear membrane abnormalities	None	Minimal	Mild	Marked
Chromatin pattern	Euchromatic, occasionally cleared	Variable, but not cleared	Hypochromatic	Hyperchromatic
Mitoses	None	Rare	Rare	Variable, but more common
Cytoplasm	Nonmucinous, gastric can have apical mucin	Nonmucinous	Variable, but frequently mucinous	Variable, but occasionally mucinous
Background mucin	Present, thin and focal	Absent	Variable	Variable
Necrosis	Absent	Fat necrosis	Rare, coagulative	Common, coagulative

[a]RBC = red blood cell; duo = duodenum; 3D = three-dimensional.

(111,147). These analyses demonstrate that most pancreatic cancers are genetically very complex; that is, most pancreatic cancers harbor multiple karyotypic abnormalities, and many cytogenetically distinct clones can be present in a single carcinoma (109).

Comparative genomic hybridization (CGH), array CGH, and allelotyping using microsatellite markers are used to localize more precisely the genetic losses in a cancer (22,235). CGH and array CGH analyses have confirmed the losses observed using standard karyotyping techniques (losses of 18q, 13q, 6q, and 9p), and, importantly, these techniques have been used to identify a number of amplifications including gains of 1p, 3q, 5p, 6p, 6q (the site of the *MYB* gene), 7p (*EGFR*), 7q, 8p, 8q (*MYC*), 12p (*KRAS*), 12q (*MDM2*), 16q, 17q (*HER2*), 18q, 19q (*AKT2*), 20q (*AIB1*), and 22q (5,19,62,83,94,124, 197,280).

Several large series of pancreatic cancers have been allelotyped using microsatellite markers. The highest frequencies of allelic loss (over 60 percent of the cancers) are found on chromosome arms 1p, 9p, 17p, and 18q (115). These losses suggest that the *p16/CDKN2A* tumor suppressor gene on chromosome 9p, the *TP53* tumor suppressor gene on 17p, and the *MADH4/DPC4* tumor suppressor gene on 18q are all targeted for inactivation in pancreatic cancer (115). Chromosome arms 3p, 6p, 6q, 8p, 10q, 12q, 13q, 18p, 21q, and 22q show a moderate (40 to 60 percent) degree of allelic loss, and the genes targeted by these losses have not yet been identified (115,330). Metastases have been shown to harbor slightly more, but otherwise similar, genetic losses as the primary cancers from which they were derived.

While these allelic losses suggest a number of genes that may be targeted in pancreatic

Table 7-7

SOMATIC GENETIC ALTERATIONS IN PANCREATIC CANCER

Type of Gene	Gene	Chromo-some	Mechanism of Alteration	% of Cases
Oncogenes	*KRAS*	12p	Point mutations in codon 12	>90
	BRAF	7q	Point mutations	Tumors with wild-type KRAS
	MYB	6q	Amplification	10
	AKT2	19q	Amplification	10–20
	AIB1	20q	Amplification	60
	HER2/neu	17q	Overexpression	Large range
Tumor suppressor genes	*p16 /CDKN2A*	9p	LOH+IM[a], HD, Meth	>95
	TP53	17p	LOH+IM	50–75
	MAD4/DPC4	18q	LOH+IM, HD	55
	MKK4	17p	LOH+IM, HD	4
	STK11/LKB1	19p	Germline, LOH+IM	4–6
	TGFβR1 (ALK5)	9q	HD	2
	TGFβR2	3p	HD, Bi-IM	4-7 (tumors with MSI)
	ACVR1β (ALK4)	12q	HD, LOH+IM	2
	ACVR2	2q	Bi-IM, LOH+IM	Tumors with MSI
	FBXW7	4q	LOH+IM	<5
	EP300	22q	LOH+IM	25
DNA mismatch repair	*MLH1*	3p	Germline, Meth	3-15
	BRCA2	13q	Germline	7
	FANC-C	9q	HD, LOH+IM	<5
	FANC-G	9p	LOH+IM	<5
Mitochondrial genome	Multiple	Mitochon-drial DNA	IM	100

[a]LOH = loss of heterozygosity; IM = intragenic mutation; HD=homozygous mutation; Meth = hypermethylation; Bi-IM = bi-allelic intragenic mutations, usually in a poly A tract in MSI cases; MSI = microsatellite instability.

cancer, the functional inactivation of a tumor suppressor gene in a cancer is best established with the demonstration that both copies (alleles) of the gene are inactivated. To do this usually requires gene sequencing. When this has been done in pancreatic cancer, a number of tumor suppressor genes have been shown to be biallelically inactivated (Table 7-7). These genes include *p16/CDKN2A* (inactivated in 95 percent of cases), *TP53* (50 to 75 percent), *SMADH4/DPC4* (55 percent), and a large number of lower mutational frequency targets including the *MKK4, STK11/LKB1, TGFβR1 (ALK5), TGFβR2, ACVR1β (ALK4), ACVR2, FBXW7,* and *EP300* genes (38,40,90,103,114,119,140,181,225,255, 263,271,285–287,300,313,314). Remarkably, multiple tumor suppressor genes are often inactivated in a single carcinoma (263).

The discovery of the genes targeted for inactivation in pancreatic cancer has diagnostic implications. For example, the *MADH4/DPC4* gene is inactivated in 55 percent of pancreatic cancers but not in normal tissues. As mentioned earlier, immunolabeling with antibodies to the Dpc4 protein has been shown to mirror *MADH4/DPC4* gene status, so immunolabeling is a useful adjunct to the interpretation of difficult biopsies (see fig. 7-36) (298,317). The complete loss of Dpc4 protein expression in atypical cells in a biopsy favors the diagnosis of cancer (298). Similarly, the complete loss of Dpc4 protein expression in a metastasis favors a pancreatic primary (fig. 7-49), although *MADH4/DPC4* gene inactivation does occur in carcinomas of other organs.

Genes are made nonfunctional by epigenetically silencing their expression by methylation of promoter CpG islands. Methylation appears to be a common mechanism for gene silencing in pancreatic cancer (203). The genes methylated in pancreatic cancer include *UCHL1* (methylated in 100 percent of cases), *NPTX2* (98 percent), *SARP2* (95 percent), *ppENK* (93 percent), *CLDN5* (93 percent), *REPRIMO* (86 percent), *LHX1* (76 percent), *WNT7A* (71 percent), *FOXE1* (69

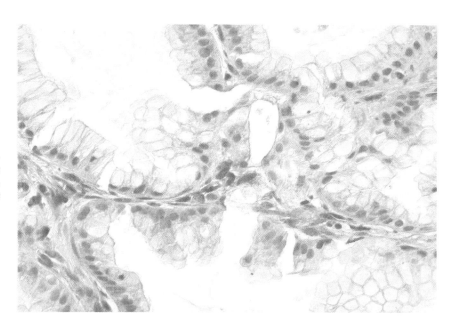

Figure 7-49

DUCTAL ADENOCARCINOMA

Complete loss of immuno-labeling for Dpc4 in a pancreatic cancer metastatic to the lungs. Note the intact labeling of the stroma.

percent), *CYCLIN D2* (65 percent), *RARbeta* (20 percent), *CDH3* (19 percent), *p16/CDKN2A* (18 percent), *CACNA1G* (16 percent), *TIMP-3* (11 percent), *E-CAD* (7 percent), *THBS1* (7 percent), *MLH1* (4 percent), *CYCLIN G* (3 percent), and *DAP kinase* (2 percent) (203,268,310,311). Since methylation leads to gene silencing, hypo-methylation would be expected to increase gene expression, and, indeed, a number of the genes that are overexpressed in pancreatic cancer are hypomethylated in the cancers relative to normal cells.

Microsatellite instability (MSI) is present in about 4 percent of pancreatic cancers and such cancers appear to have a distinct morphology (101,325,329). They are poorly differentiated, have pushing borders, and have a syncytial growth pattern. This morphology has been called the "medullary" histology (see chapter 8). MSI-high pancreatic cancers usually have wild-type *KRAS* genes and they do not have anaphase bridges, and patients appear to have an improved survival rate relative to those with conventional ductal adenocarcinomas (101, 214,325,329). As discussed earlier, these cancers may arise in patients with the hereditary non-polyposis colorectal cancer syndrome (HNPCC), or they may arise sporadically (329). The *MLH1* gene is often inactivated in MSI-high pancreatic cancers that arise sporadically, either by mutation or hypermethylation.

The oncogene most frequently activated in pancreatic cancer is the *KRAS* oncogene on chromosome 12 (10). Activating point mutations in this oncogene are present in 90 to 95 percent of pancreatic cancers. The mutations are primarily limited to codon 12 of the gene and are therefore relatively easy to detect. *KRAS* mutational analysis has been used as a supplement for the interpretation of difficult fine needle aspiration biopsies, and in tests to screen pancreatic juice, stool, and even plasma for DNA shed from a pancreatic cancer (27,39,85,141, 163,236,275,317).

A number of other oncogenes can be activated in pancreatic cancer including *AKT2* (amplified in 10 to 20 percent), *AIB1* (amplified in 60 percent), *BRAF* (mutated in one third of the small minority of cancers with wild-type *KRAS*), *HER2/neu*, *c-MYC*, and *c-MYB* (5,40,44,212,265,320).

Mutations in the mitochondrial genome are found in almost all pancreatic cancers (148, 200). Because there are so many more copies of the mitochondrial genome per cell than there are copies of the nuclear genome, mitochondrial mutations may be useful in the development of new screening tests (200).

Although not strictly a molecular genetic abnormality, the enzyme telomerase is over-expressed in the vast majority (over 90 percent) of infiltrating adenocarcinomas of the pancreas (122,288). Telomerase activity has been used as a diagnostic supplement in the interpretation of difficult biopsies and to screen for pancreatic cancer (144,248,289).

DIFFERENTIAL DIAGNOSIS

The diagnosis of pancreatic cancer has great clinical significance, and yet, well-differentiated pancreatic cancer can closely mimic a variety of completely benign processes. Added to this, the retroperitoneal location of the pancreas makes the organ difficult to biopsy and, as a result, biopsies of the pancreas are often scanty or even inadequate. The meticulous application of well-established diagnostic criteria is the only way to avoid making critical errors.

Chronic pancreatitis tops the list of entities in the differential diagnosis (2). Chronic pancreatitis can be clinically, grossly, and microscopically confused with pancreatic cancer, and yet the prognosis and treatment of these two diseases couldn't be further apart. Clinically, age less than 40 years favors the diagnosis of chronic pancreatitis. Grossly, chronic pancreatitis usually diffusely scars the gland and does not form a discrete mass. Microscopically, acinar tissue in a pancreas with chronic pancreatitis is lost and replaced by inflammation and scar tissue. Although the epithelial cells in the remaining glands can show mild nuclear enlargement, these glands retain their branching, lobular architecture. Although the glands of chronic pancreatitis can involve islets of Langerhans, they do not infiltrate into nerves or blood vessels. Fatty infiltration of the pancreas may occur in chronic pancreatitis, but individual glands remain surrounded by some stromal tissue. In contrast, pancreatic cancer is more likely in patients over the age of 50, and it usually forms a mass. Carcinomas of the head of the pancreas often cause dramatic focal stenosis of the bile duct, while chronic pancreatitis, if it does narrow the duct, will do so more diffusely.

The microscopic pattern of growth is the single most helpful finding in distinguishing between chronic pancreatitis and pancreatic cancer (see Table 7-3). Even well-differentiated pancreatic cancer grows in a haphazard pattern. The normal growth pattern of a larger duct surrounded by nests of smaller glands is lost, and neoplastic glands grow in an unpredictable pattern. As discussed in the section on frozen section diagnosis, the presence of glands immediately adjacent to a muscular blood vessel is an indication of an abnormal pattern of growth and therefore supports the diagnosis of carcinoma. The glands of ductal adenocarcinoma also may be closely apposed to adipocytes ("naked glands" in the fat). In addition, the findings of perineural invasion, invasion into vascular spaces, and invasion into other organs such as the muscularis propria of the duodenum, all strongly support the diagnosis of pancreatic cancer. In contrast to the complete round to oval lumens of benign glands, the glands of pancreatic cancer often have an abnormal shape. They form incomplete lumens, which can contain necrotic debris, and single cells can be found infiltrating in the stroma. Nuclear features can also help. Large irregular nuclei, prominent and multiple nucleoli, mitoses (particularly abnormal mitoses), and nuclear pleomorphism all favor the diagnosis of pancreatic cancer. Immunohistochemical labeling is usually not needed, but can supplement the histologic diagnosis. Most reactive glands do not express CEA, B72.3, CA125, or p53 at immunohistochemically detectable levels, and they all label for the Dpc4 protein. By contrast, most pancreatic cancers express CEA, 75 percent express B72.3, 50 to 75 percent express p53, 45 percent express CA125, and 55 percent show complete loss of Dpc4 expression.

Several features of the islets of Langerhans in chronic pancreatitis should be noted, because they can confuse even the experienced pathologist. Islets can normally contain non-neoplastic glands, and the endocrine cells in an islet can show significant nuclear pleomorphism. Glands and nuclear pleomorphism in an islet should not be mistaken for a carcinoma. In cases of severe chronic pancreatitis the islets can become enlarged or, in other areas, disrupted so that small groups of endocrine cells are embedded in dense stroma or even demonstrate perineural invasion. These non-neoplastic endocrine cells should not be confused with carcinoma.

One form of chronic pancreatitis that deserves special mention is lymphoplasmacytic sclerosing pancreatitis (LPSP) (see chapter 15). LPSP is characterized by a duct-centric inflammatory infiltrate composed of a mixture of lymphocytes and plasma cells. There is often venulitis. LPSP can clinically and grossly mimic pancreatic cancer, but the histologic appearance of LPSP is usually obvious as long as the entity is kept in mind.

Other exocrine neoplasms of the pancreas should be included in the differential diagnosis of ductal adenocarcinoma. Features that favor the diagnosis of acinar cell carcinoma in histologic sections include a highly cellular neoplasm with the formation of acini, basally polarized nuclei, eosinophilic granular cytoplasm, and single prominent nucleoli. In cytologic material, the cells of poorly differentiated carcinoma demonstrate more nuclear atypia than the cells of acinar cell carcinoma. The cells of poorly differentiated carcinoma show significant convolution of nuclei and marked hyperchromasia. This is in contrast to the rounder, centrally located and less convoluted nuclei of acinar cell carcinoma. Nucleoli may be prominent in both, but in acinar cell carcinoma they tend to be more uniform and central in the nucleus. The cytoplasmic differences are also important as acinar cells tend to have granular cytoplasm in contrast to the mucinous cytoplasm of adenocarcinoma, but both granules and mucin may be sparse. In some cases, particularly when there is a diffuse pattern of growth, strong and diffuse immunolabeling for the enzyme markers trypsin and chymotrypsin and lack of expression of CK7 point to an acinar cell carcinoma. Glycoprotein markers (e.g., CEA) are usually negative in acinar cell carcinomas. Immunolabeling can be applied to cell blocks in difficult cytology cases.

Although most pancreatoblastomas occur in children and most ductal adenocarcinomas occur in the elderly, up to a third of pancreatoblastomas occur in adults and ductal adenocarcinomas can on rare occasion occur in children. Pancreatoblastomas should, therefore, be part of the differential diagnosis. While both entities can show ductal differentiation, the presence of squamoid nests and significant acinar differentiation are features of pancreatoblastomas.

Solid-pseudopapillary neoplasms are included in the differential diagnosis of ductal adenocarcinomas. The majority of solid-pseudopapillary neoplasms occur in women in their twenties, distinguishing this neoplasm from ductal adenocarcinoma. In addition, although solid-pseudopapillary neoplasms can grow in solid sheets, they at least focally form pseudopapillae and do not form true lumens. Uniform polygonal cells, eosinophilic globules, and cholesterol crystals all favor the diagnosis of a solid-pseudopapillary neoplasm. In problematic cases, immunohistochemical labeling readily distinguishes these two neoplasms: solid-pseudopapillary neoplasms express vimentin, CD10, and alpha-1-antitrypsin, and they show an abnormal nuclear accumulation of the beta-catenin protein.

Pancreatic cancers arising in association with an IPMN, or in association with an MCN, need to be distinguished from ductal adenocarcinomas that do not arise in association with one of these cystic neoplasms (340). Patients with adenocarcinomas that arise in association with MCNs or IPMNs may have a better prognosis. Careful examination of the gross specimen and adequate sampling of any cystic areas are needed to make this distinction. The distinction of well-differentiated ductal adenocarcinoma from pancreatic intraepithelial neoplasia is discussed later in this chapter.

Well-differentiated endocrine neoplasms of the pancreas should also be in the differential diagnosis of ductal adenocarcinomas. In histologic sections, well-differentiated endocrine neoplasms grow in nests and trabeculae, and often are accompanied by a hyalinized stroma. The nuclei of well-differentiated endocrine neoplasms are usually centrally placed, uniform, and have "salt and pepper" chromatin. Pancreatic endocrine neoplasms can also be confused with adenocarcinoma in cytology preparations. Smears of pancreatic endocrine neoplasms, however, typically produce a more noncohesive pattern, with a monomorphic, relatively small cell population. The cytoplasm is nonmucinous and often very scant and ill-defined, or eccentric yielding a plasmacytoid appearance to the cells. Although the light microscopic features may be helpful in suggesting the correct diagnosis, there are cases in which immunohistochemical labeling for the general endocrine markers chromogranin and synaptophysin are needed to rule out a well-differentiated endocrine neoplasm. In contrast to ductal adenocarcinomas, most well-differentiated endocrine neoplasms do not express CK7. Immunolabeling can be performed on cell block preparations or destained smears in difficult cases.

The other periampullary cancers, ampullary carcinoma, bile duct cancer, and duodenal carcinoma, also need to be distinguished from ductal adenocarcinomas of the pancreas. All four of these carcinomas can have a similar morphologic appearance. The correct classification relies on two findings: the gross epicenter of the neoplastic mass and the presence of an in situ or preinvasive neoplastic component.

Finally, metastases to the pancreas from an extrapancreatic neoplasm, although rare, should be considered in the differential diagnosis. The patient's history and the morphology of the carcinoma can be used to establish the diagnosis. Clear cells should suggest a renal cell carcinoma metastatic to the pancreas (305, 322). In cytologic preparations, renal cell carcinoma is recognized by the large polygonal shape of the neoplastic cells, which may be single, in small clusters, or loosely attached to traversing vessels. The nuclei are usually round and central with large macronucleoli, frequently surrounded by a clear halo ("owl's eye" appearance). The cytoplasm is distinguished from ductal adenocarcinoma by the presence of multiple fine vacuoles (in the most common clear cell type) in contrast to the often large single vacuoles of adenocarcinoma. Signet ring cells suggest a gastric carcinoma; noncohesive individual cells, a lobular carcinoma of the breast; and brown pigment, a melanoma.

SPREAD AND METASTASES

As noted earlier, by the time most pancreatic cancers are clinically diagnosed, they have already spread beyond the pancreas. Only 10 to 20 percent of pancreatic carcinomas are surgically resectable, and at the time of resection, most have already metastasized to regional lymph nodes (50,51,218,232,273). Clearly, pancreatic cancer is an extraordinarily aggressive neoplasm.

Perineural and lymphatic invasion are present in the majority of cases. Perineural invasion is seen in three quarters of surgically resected pancreatic carcinomas, and is associated with the presence of perineural invasion in the extrapancreatic retroperitoneal nerve plexus (121,219, 224,293,294). This latter finding is present in about 60 percent of surgically resected carcinomas of the head of the pancreas; involvement of the retroperitoneal margin is a greatly under-appreciated basis for the failure of surgery to cure patients with pancreatic cancer (155,191).

Lymphatic invasion is also identified in most pancreatic cancers and is associated with metastases to lymph nodes (60,145,279,340). Lymph node metastases are present in about 70 percent of resected carcinomas of the head of the pancreas and in about 80 percent of resected carcinomas of the body or tail of the gland. Lymph node metastases are usually present even when the primary carcinoma is small (under 2 cm) (86). The lymph nodes around the pancreas are divided into groups and metastatic pancreatic cancer most often involves the superior head, anterior pancreaticoduodenal, and posterior pancreaticoduodenal lymph node groups (61, 142,153,204). Less frequently involved groups include the lymph nodes around the common hepatic artery, those around the hepatoduodenal ligament, those around the superior mesenteric artery, and the perigastric and paraaortic lymph nodes (154,204). Involvement of the perigastric and paraaortic lymph nodes suggests that some lymph node metastases are not resected in the standard pancreatoduodenectomy, a possibility that has been used by some surgeons to advocate for more radical lymph node resections (154). Micrometastases in lymph nodes that appear negative on initial histologic examination can be found with additional histologic sections, molecular analyses for *KRAS* gene mutations, and immunohistochemical labeling for epithelial antigens. The clinical significance of such micrometastases is, however, unproven (37,67,126,231).

Pancreatic cancers often extend beyond the gland into the adjacent large vessels. These include the vessels of the celiac axis and the superior mesenteric artery. Portal vein invasion is seen in a quarter of pancreatic cancers. Large vessel invasion can make a pancreatic cancer unresectable.

Most pancreatic cancers invade into the peritoneum, and peritoneal cytology is positive in 15 percent of patients with radiologically resectable pancreatic cancers (206). As discussed earlier, pancreatic cancer can also directly infiltrate into adjacent organs, including the duodenum, stomach, colon, spleen, gallbladder, and adrenal glands (60).

Distant metastases are all too common in pancreatic cancer. The most frequent sites of

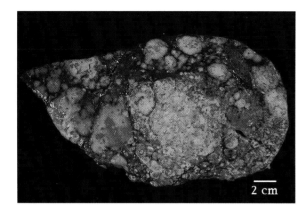

Figure 7-50

DUCTAL ADENOCARCINOMA

Multiple liver metastases.

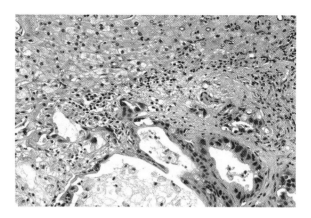

Figure 7-51

DUCTAL ADENOCARCINOMA

Metastasis to the liver.

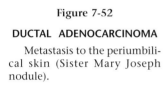

Figure 7-52

DUCTAL ADENOCARCINOMA

Metastasis to the periumbilical skin (Sister Mary Joseph nodule).

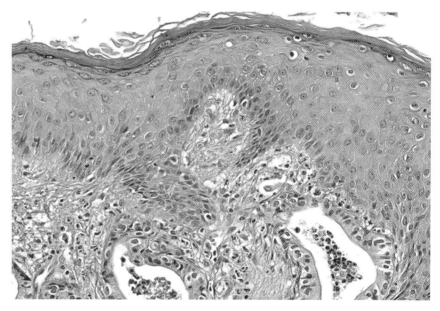

metastases, in decreasing order, are the liver (figs. 7-50, 7-51), the lungs, the adrenal glands, and the skin (fig. 7-52) (60). Metastatic pancreatic cancer has been reported in almost every organ, including the bone, brain, diaphragm, dura, gallbladder, heart, intestines, kidneys, muscles, ovaries, pericardium, pleura, salivary gland, seminal vesicles, spleen, testis, thyroid gland, urinary bladder, and uterus (60). Even small (under 2 cm) pancreatic cancers can distantly metastasize (86). Liver metastases are found in two thirds of patients with pancreatic cancer at autopsy, and pulmonary metastases in a third (60). Calculations based on estimates of tumor doubling times have suggested that occult liver metastases are often present at the time of pancreatectomy (12).

Small metastases to the liver need to be distinguished from benign epithelial lesions, including bile duct adenomas and bile duct hamartomas (von Meyenberg complexes). Bile duct adenomas are small (under 1 cm), subcapsular, circumscribed, solitary lesions composed of uniform cuboidal cells that form tubules (fig. 7-53) (45, 110). Bile duct hamartomas are usually multiple, contain bile, and are lined by flattened uniform epithelial cells (fig. 7-54) (47). Metastases can be distinguished from these two benign processes by the disorganized pattern of growth, nuclear

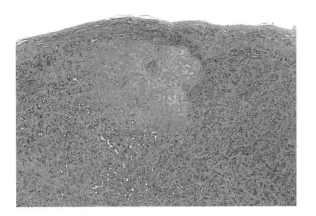 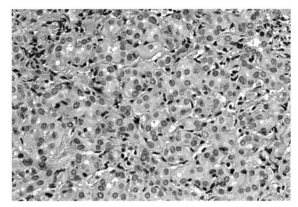

Figure 7-53

BILE DUCT ADENOMA

Low- (left) and high- (right) magnification views show a well-demarcated lesion composed of well-differentiated glands lined by uniform cuboidal epithelial cells.

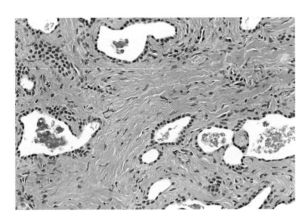 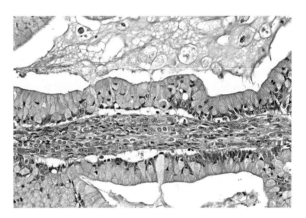

Figure 7-54	**Figure 7-55**
BILE DUCT HAMARTOMA	**DUCTAL ADENOCARCINOMA**
The glands have a flattened epithelial lining and luminal bile.	Pancreatic cancer metastatic to the ovary mimics a primary mucinous neoplasm of the ovary.

atypia, and mitoses. While most benign bile duct proliferations can be morphologically distinguished from metastases, molecular analyses may help in difficult cases. For example, *KRAS* gene mutations are present in over 90 percent of metastatic pancreatic cancers, but in less than 7 percent of benign bile duct proliferations (132). Abnormal expression patterns for glycoprotein markers (CEA, B72.3 [TAG-72], and CA125) as well as p53, mesothelin, and Dpc4 favor a metastasis (125,290).

When pancreatic cancer metastasizes to the ovary it can mimic a primary mucinous neoplasm (fig. 7-55) (272,338). Features that suggest metastatic pancreatic cancer over an ovarian primary include bilaterality, surface desmoplastic implants, size over 10 cm, and extraovarian spread (272,338).

Immunohistochemical labeling for epithelial markers and molecular analyses for genetic mutations can identify micrometastases in the peritoneal cavity, as well as circulating neoplastic cells in the bone marrow of patients with pancreatic cancer (149,259,306,316). Remarkably, a quarter to a half of patients with surgically resectable pancreatic cancer have epithelial cells in their bone marrow, and the presence of cells labeling for cytokeratin in the bone marrow is a poor prognostic sign (149,259).

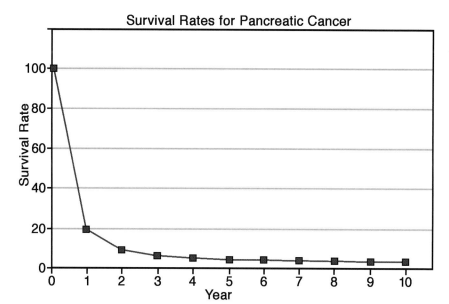

Figure 7-56

DUCTAL ADENOCARCINOMA

SEER data on survival. (Modified from SEER Fast Stats: www. seer.cancer.gov.)

Autopsy studies of patients who died following surgical resection of pancreatic cancer have helped define the patterns of recurrence after surgery (155). Eighty percent of these patients have recurrence in the local retroperitoneum, two thirds have liver metastases, half have peritoneal dissemination, and half have lymph node recurrence.

STAGING, TREATMENT, AND PROGNOSIS

Staging

The staging of carcinomas of the pancreas is presented in detail in chapter 3.

Treatment

Surgical resection is the treatment of choice for pancreatic cancer (178,278). Unfortunately, the majority of cancers are not resectable. At the time of diagnosis, only 10 to 20 percent of carcinomas of the head of the gland are surgically resectable, and the number is even lower for carcinoma of the body or tail (50,51,273, 281). Pancreatoduodenectomies are usually performed for carcinomas of the head of the gland. These are complex operations and best performed at high volume centers with experience. The operative mortality rate varies from 16 percent at low volume centers to 1 percent at high volume centers (29,41,108). Surgical resection of carcinomas of the body or tail of the gland is called a distal pancreatectomy.

Pancreatic cancer is singularly unresponsive to most forms of chemotherapy and radiation therapy. It is generally agreed that adjuvant chemotherapy has a survival benefit in patients with resected pancreatic cancer, however, the role of adjuvant combined chemoradiotherapy is controversial (227,334). Ten to 25 percent of patients with unresectable pancreatic cancer achieve a partial response with gemcitabine combined with a second agent such as 5-fluorouracil, cisplatin, oxaliplatin, Erbitux, avastin, exatecan, pemetrexed, or Irinotecan; 1-year survival rates are between 18 and 35 percent with combination therapy (25,171,176).

Prognosis

The 5-year survival rate for patients diagnosed with pancreatic cancer between 1992 and 1999 was 4 percent (fig. 7-56) (146). This represents only a trivial improvement over the 3 percent 5-year survival rate for patients diagnosed in the 1950s (fig. 7-57) (146).

The most important factor in determining patient prognosis is resectability (50,170,188, 204,226,273,323). Most pancreatic cancers are not surgically resectable because of distant metastases or involvement of large vessels. The median survival period for patients with nonresectable tumors is only 5 months and the 5-year survival rate close to 0 percent. By contrast, the median survival period for patients with carcinoma of the head of the gland who

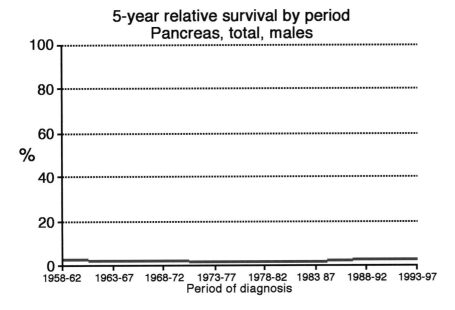

5-year relative survival by period
Pancreas, total, males

Figure 7-57

DUCTAL ADENOCARCINOMA

Five-year survival rate by decade. (Data from Cancer Registry of Norway. http://www.kreft-registeret.no.)

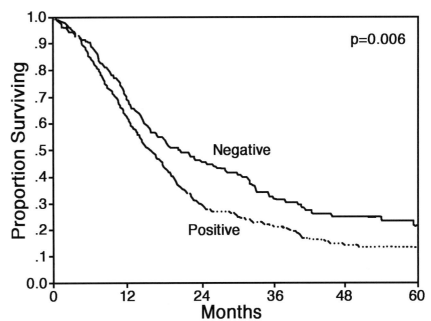

Figure 7-58

DUCTAL ADENOCARCINOMA

Kaplan-Meier actuarial survival curves comparing pancreaticoduodenectomy patients with negative lymph notes to pancreaticoduodenectomy patients with positive lymph nodes. (Fig. 4B from Sohn TA, Yeo CJ, Cameron JL, et al. Resected adenocarcinoma of the pancreas-616 patients: results, outcomes, and prognostic indicators. J Gastrointest Surg 2000; 4:574.)

undergo a pancreatoduodenectomy is 15 months, and the 1-, 2-, 3-, and 5-year survival rates are 45 percent, 30 percent, 25 percent, and 15 to 20 percent, respectively (50,179,273). The 10-year survival rate following surgical resection was 5 percent in one series, demonstrating that some patients die of their disease more than 5 years after apparently curative surgical resection (50,337).

The stage and the status of the margins are the main prognostic indicators for patients with surgically resected tumors (23,222). Patients with grossly and microscopically negative margins have a median survival period close to 20 months, compared to 10 to 12 months for patients with positive margins (336). Other important prognosticators include tumor size, major vessel involvement, degree of differentiation, and lymph node status (figs. 7-58, 7-59) (23,65,91,142,170,179,196,204,221,336). Patients with surgically resected cancer and negative lymph nodes have a 25 to 40 percent 5-

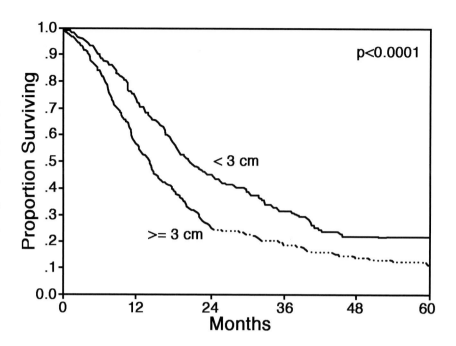

Figure 7-59

DUCTAL ADENOCARCINOMA

Kaplan-Meier actuarial survival curves comparing pancreaticoduodenectomy patients with carcinomas over 3 cm to pancreaticoduodenectomy patients with carcinomas 3 cm or smaller. (Fig. 4C from Sohn TA, Yeo CJ, Cameron JL, et al. Resected adenocarcinoma of the pancreas-616 patients: results, outcomes, and prognostic indicators. J Gastroentest Surg 2000; 4:574.)

year survival rate compared to 0 to 8 percent for patients with lymph node metastases.

Other reported poor prognostic indicators for patients with surgically resected carcinomas of the pancreas include high mitotic rate, perineural invasion (particularly involvement of extrapancreatic nerves), aneuploidy, positive peritoneal cytology, loss of Dpc4 expression, nuclear labeling for S100A6, and vascular invasion (206,222,223,241,264,295,299,319,335).

Patients with a carcinoma in the body or tail of the gland do worse than patients with carcinomas in the head (273,281). Carcinomas arising in the body or tail tend to present at a more advanced stage and even when resected, the 5-year survival rate is only 12.5 percent (281). Small pancreatic carcinomas, particularly those in the tail of the gland, can metastasize to distant organs. Therefore, a pancreatic primary, and in particular a primary carcinoma in the tail of the pancreas, should be considered in patients with metastatic adenocarcinoma of unknown primary.

PANCREATIC INTRAEPITHELIAL NEOPLASIA

Most infiltrating adenocarcinomas of the pancreas are associated with noninvasive epithelial proliferations within the smaller pancreatic ducts, called *pancreatic intraepithelial neoplasia* (PanIN) (130). These lesions have been

recognized for close to a century, and a growing body of evidence now suggests that PanIN is neoplastic and can progress to infiltrating ductal adenocarcinoma (35,36,131,134). This evidence includes the morphologic association of PanIN with infiltrating adenocarcinomas, anecdotal case reports in which patients with histologically documented PanIN later develop an infiltrating adenocarcinoma of the pancreas, and molecular analyses which demonstrate that PanIN harbors many of the same genetic alterations as are found in infiltrating adenocarcinoma. Older terms for PanIN include *duct hyperplasia, hypertrophy, metaplasia, dysplasia, duct lesion*, and *carcinoma in situ* (130).

As described in detail in chapter 1, the epithelium lining the pancreatic ducts is normally cuboidal to low columnar without atypia (fig. 7-60). PanIN lesions have been classified into three grades, one of which is subdivided into A and B subcategories (130). PanIN-1A consists of flat epithelial lesions composed of uniform columnar cells, with basally located, uniform round to oval uniform nuclei (fig. 7-61) (130). The nuclei are oriented perpendicular to the basement membrane and the cells may contain abundant supranuclear mucin. While molecular analyses have demonstrated that many lesions with this morphology are neoplastic, it is recognized that some may be non-neoplastic. Therefore, the

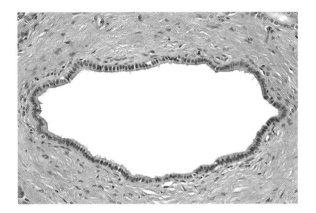

Figure 7-60

NORMAL PANCREATIC DUCT

Uniform epithelium without atypia.

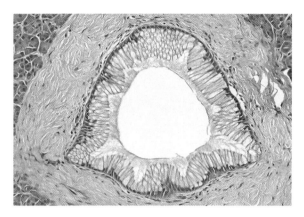

Figure 7-61

PANCREATIC INTRAEPITHELIAL NEOPLASIA-1A

The epithelium in pancreatic intraepithelial neoplasia (PanIN)-1A is flat and has only minimal architectural and cytologic atypia.

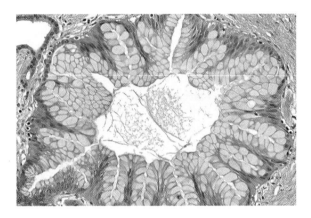

Figure 7-62

PANCREATIC INTRAEPITHELIAL NEOPLASIA-1B

The epithelium in PanIN-1B is papillary and has only minimal architectural and cytologic atypia.

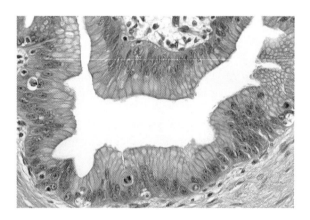

Figure 7-63

PANCREATIC INTRAEPITHELIAL NEOPLASIA-2

The epithelium in PanIN-2 is usually papillary and has moderate architectural and cytologic atypia.

addition of the modifier "L" for lesion (PanIN-1A/L) is acceptable. PanIN-1B is morphologically identical to PanIN-1A, but PanIN-1B has a papillary or micropapillary, rather than flat, architecture (fig. 7-62).

PanIN-2 lesions, by definition, have some nuclear abnormalities (130). Most PanIN-2 lesions are papillary, but some may be flat. The nuclear abnormalities in PanIN-2 include some loss of polarity, crowding, enlargement, pseudostratification, and hyperchromasia (fig. 7-63). Mitoses are only rarely seen, and when present, are basal and morphologically normal.

PanIN-3 lesions are characterized by the presence of significant architectural and cytologic atypia (fig. 7-64) (130). These lesions are usually papillary or micropapillary, although rarely, they are flat. True cribriforming, the budding off of clusters of cells, and luminal necrosis are features of PanIN-3. These architectural changes are matched by cytologic abnormalities. The nuclei are enlarged and hyperchromatic, and show a loss of orientation such that they are no longer perpendicular to the basement membrane; the nuclear to cytoplasmic ratio is increased (87). Dystrophic goblet cells with nuclei oriented towards the lumen may be seen. Nucleoli can be prominent, and mitoses, some of which may be luminal or atypical, may be present.

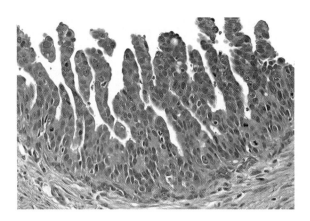

Figure 7-64

PANCREATIC INTRAEPITHELIAL NEOPLASIA-3

The epithelium in PanIN-3 is usually papillary and has significant architectural and cytologic atypia.

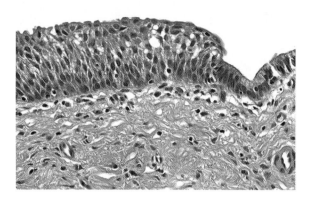

Figure 7-65

SQUAMOUS METAPLASIA

The normal glandular epithelium (right) has been replaced by mature squamous epithelium (left).

PanINs, even low-grade PanINs, can be associated with lobular parenchymal atrophy (37a,68a). This atrophy can range from subtle thinning of the acinar cells with loss of apical granular cytoplasm, to marked acinar drop-out (37a,68a).

Oncocytic and intestinal variants of PanIN have been proposed. It has been suggested that the oncocytic variant can progress to intraductal oncocytic papillary neoplasms, and the intestinal variant to IPMN (8). These lesions, however, are not well-described in the absence of a concurrent intraductal papillary mucinous or intraductal oncocytic papillary neoplasm. Oncocytic epithelium also may be found in the smaller ducts (see chapter 1) but has not been shown to have the genetic abnormalities of a neoplasm and has been designated oncocytic metaplasia.

PanIN should be distinguished from other lesions in the pancreatic ducts including squamous metaplasia (fig. 7-65), reactive changes, cancerization of the ducts, and IPMNs (130). Squamous metaplasia of the pancreatic ducts is a reactive process associated with repeated injury to the epithelium. The normal cuboidal cells are replaced by mature stratified squamous or pseudostratified transitional epithelium. This epithelium lacks significant atypia. Significant inflammation in the ducts can induce other reactive changes including nuclear and nucleolar enlargement. Caution should be exercised before diagnosing a PanIN in the setting of inflammation. In gen-

eral, the nuclear and nucleolar enlargement seen in reactive change is much more uniform than that seen in PanIN.

As discussed earlier, infiltrating ductal adenocarcinoma of the pancreas often grows along preexisting benign ducts. This "cancerization of the ducts" can also mimic PanIN. Two features are helpful in diagnosing cancerization of the ducts (130). First, the presence of an invasive carcinoma in the connective tissue immediately adjacent to a duct should raise the possibility of cancerization, as should an abrupt transition from a morphologically normal epithelium to an epithelium with significant atypia. High-grade PanIN often transitions to lower-grade PanIN rather than normal ductal epithelium.

PanIN is distinguished from IPMN on the basis of size and the morphology of the papillae (133). The majority of PanIN lesions cannot be appreciated grossly and are smaller than 0.5 cm; conversely, the majority of IPMNs are larger than 1 cm and can be appreciated grossly and radiographically. A size cut-off of 0.5 to 1.0 cm is a useful point of differentiation. Most lesions smaller than 0.5 cm in greatest dimension are PanIN, while those greater than 1.0 cm are usually IPMN. In addition, the papillae in IPMN, even those of small neoplasms, are taller and more complex than the papillae of PanIN (fig. 7-66). Abundant luminal mucin and the expression of MUC2 should suggest the diagnosis of IPMN (133).

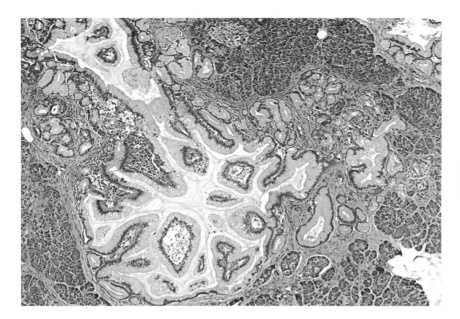

Figure 7-66

INTRADUCTAL PAPILLARY MUCINOUS NEOPLASM

Long complex papillae are typical, even in small neoplasms, in contrast to the short papillae of PanINs.

There are several clinical parallels between PanIN and infiltrating carcinomas. PanIN, particularly high-grade lesions (PanIN-2 and PanIN-3), are more common in pancreata with an infiltrating carcinoma than they are in pancreata without a cancer (13,58,169,251). In addition, just as is true for infiltrating adenocarcinoma of the pancreas, the prevalence of PanIN increases with age and PanIN is reported to be more common in the head of the gland than in the tail (13,58,169,251). Low-grade PanIN is actually common, being reported in up to 45 percent of the pancreata of older adults at autopsy (216). Low-grade PanIN is also a common incidental finding adjacent to pancreatic neoplasms other than ductal adenocarcinomas, including those for which no association between the PanIN and the established neoplasm has been suggested (e.g., well-differentiated pancreatic endocrine neoplasms and serous cystadenomas) (281a).

PanIN harbors many of the same genetic alterations as are found in infiltrating adenocarcinomas. While these genetic alterations do not occur in a specific sequence, their prevalence tends to increase from PanIN-1 to PanIN-2 to PanIN-3. Telomere shortening and activating point mutations in codon 12 of the *KRAS* gene occur early (in PanIN-1A and PanIN-1B), while there is a tendency for inactivating mutations in the *p16/CDKN2A* gene to occur in intermediate lesions (PanIN-2), and for inactivation of *SMAD4, TP53,* and *BRCA2* in late lesions (PanIN-

3) (34,100,117,187,198,215,261,301,315,324, 326,331). In addition, the hypermethylation of the *ppENK, TSLC1,* and *p16* genes has been demonstrated in PanIN, and the prevalance of hypermethylation increases from low-grade to high-grade lesions (84). The proliferation rate, as measured by immunolabeling for Ki-67, increases with increasing grade of PanIN (160).

Molecular analyses of PanIN has not only demonstrated that these lesions are neoplasms (they have clonal mutations in cancer associated genes) and that they can progress (the prevalence of mutations increases with increasing grade of PanIN), but in some instances they have also shown genetic divergence (215,331). This latter finding suggests that PanINs can sustain multiple genetic alterations and that only some progress to infiltrating cancer.

The immunohistochemical labeling pattern of PanIN parallels that of infiltrating duct carcinoma. Almost all PanIN lesions do not express MUC2, but most, and particularly the high-grade PanINs (PanIN-3) express MUC1, MUC4, MUC5AC, and MUC6 (4,157,198,291). The expression of mucin-associated carbohydrate antigen (sialyl Tn) is markedly increased only in PanIN-3 and infiltrating adenocarcinoma (157). The patterns of gene expression observed in PanIN, including the expression of MUCs, suggest that PanIN, particularly low-grade PanIN, shows gastric differentiation. One third of PanINs express cyclooxygenase-2 (199). Global analyses of gene expression have revealed the expression of multiple gastric epithelial markers as well as the effects of Hedgehog-mediated signaling activity (252).

The most appropriate therapy for PanIN is not known. While some progress to infiltrating carcinoma, it is not known how often or how rapidly they progress. Evidence-based decisions on treatment cannot be made without these two critical pieces of information. Nonetheless, it is generally agreed that no therapy is needed for PanIN-1 or PanIN-2 at a margin. There have been anecdotal case reports of PanIN-3 lesions progressing to invasive ductal adenocarcinoma (35,36). Therefore, the resection of additional pancreatic parenchyma to achieve a margin free of PanIN-3 may be warranted in some instances. The patient's clinical situation must be taken into account when making the decision to resect additional pancreatic parenchyma. If the patient has a large invasive cancer with multiple lymph node metastases, then their invasive cancer poses a significantly greater threat to their life than a PanIN-3 lesion ever will. In these instances it is reasonable to recommend that no additional pancreas be resected. By contrast, if the patient is young and has a small invasive cancer or a benign lesion, the resection of additional parenchyma to achieve a margin free of PanIN-3 may be justified.

Not all precursor lesions in the pancreas fall into a well-defined pathologic group (e.g., IPMN, MCN, and PanIN). Some small foci of carcinoma in situ involve larger nondilated ducts (296). While it is often difficult to definitively classify these small foci, it is probably best to simply grade the degree of dysplasia and comment on the size of the lesion.

REFERENCES

1. Ademmer K, Ebert M, Muller-Ostermeyer F, et al. Effector T lymphocyte subsets in human pancreatic cancer: detection of CD8+CD18+ cells and CD8+CD103+ cells by multi-epitope imaging. Clin Exp Immunol 1998;112:21-6.
2. Adsay NV, Bandyopadhyay S, Basturk O, et al. Chronic pancreatitis or pancreatic ductal adenocarcinoma? Semin Diagn Pathol 2004;21:268-76.
3. Adsay NV, Logani S, Sarkar F, Crissman J, Vaitkevicius V. Foamy gland pattern of pancreatic ductal adenocarcinoma: a deceptively benign-appearing variant. Am J Surg Pathol 2000; 24:493-504.
4. Adsay NV, Merati K, Andea A, et al. The dichotomy in the preinvasive neoplasia to invasive carcinoma sequence in the pancreas: differential expression of MUC1 and MUC2 supports the existence of two separate pathways of carcinogenesis. Mod Pathol 2002;15:1087-95.
5. Aguirre AJ, Brennan C, Bailey G, et al. High-resolution characterization of the pancreatic adenocarcinoma genome. Proc Natl Acad Sci U S A 2004;101:9067-72.
6. Ahlgren JD. Epidemiology and risk factors in pancreatic cancer. Semin Oncol 1996;23:241-50.
7. Al-Kaisi N, Siegler EE. Fine needle aspiration cytology of the pancreas. Acta Cytol 1989;33: 145-52.
8. Albores-Saavedra J, Wu J, Crook T, Amirkhan RH, Jones L, Hruban RH. Intestinal and oncocytic variants of pancreatic intraepithelial neoplasia (PanIN): a morphologic and immunohistochemical study. Mod Pathol 2005; 18(Suppl 1):273A.
9. Allison DC, Piantadosi S, Hruban RH, et al. DNA content and other factors associated with ten-year survival after resection of pancreatic carcinoma. J Surg Oncol 1998;67:151-9.
10. Almoguera C, Shibata D, Forrester K, Martin J, Arnheim N, Perucho M. Most human carcinomas of the exocrine pancreas contain mutant c-K-ras genes. Cell 1988;53:549-54.
11. Amikura K, Kobari M, Matsuno S. The time of occurrence of liver metastasis in carcinoma of the pancreas. Int J Pancreatol 1995;17:139-46.
12. Amundadottir LT, Thorvaldsson S, Gudbjartsson DF, et al. Cancer as a complex phenotype: pattern of cancer distribution within and beyond the nuclear family. PLoS Med 2004;1:e65. Epub 2004 Dec 28.
13. Andea A, Sarkar F, Adsay NV. Clinicopathological correlates of pancreatic intraepithelial neoplasia: a comparative analysis of 82 cases with and 152 cases without pancreatic ductal adenocarcinoma. Mod Pathol 2003;16:996-1006.
14. Anderson KE, Johnson TW, Lazovich D, Folsom AR. Association between nonsteroidal anti-inflammatory drug use and the incidence of pancreatic cancer. J Natl Cancer Inst 2002;94:1168-71.

15. Andrianifahanana M, Moniaux N, Schmied BM, et al. Mucin (MUC) gene expression in human pancreatic adenocarcinoma and chronic pancreatitis: a potential role of MUC4 as a tumor marker of diagnostic significance. Clin Cancer Res 2001;7:4033-40.

16. Arao J, Fukui H, Hirayama D, et al. A case of aberrant pancreatic cancer in the jejunum. Hepatogastroenterology 1999;46:504-7.

17. Argani P, Iacobuzio-Donahue CA, Ryu B, et al. Mesothelin is overexpressed in the vast majority of ductal adenocarcinomas of the pancreas: identification of a new pancreatic cancer marker by serial analysis of gene expression (SAGE). Clin Cancer Res 2001;7:3862-8.

18. Argani P, Rosty C, Reiter RE, et al. Discovery of new markers of cancer through serial analysis of gene expression: prostate stem cell antigen is overexpressed in pancreatic adenocarcinoma. Cancer Res 2001;61:4320-4.

19. Armengol G, Knuutila S, Lluís F, Capella G, Miro R, Caballin MR. DNA copy number changes and evaluation of MYC, IGF1R, and FES amplification in xenografts of pancreatic adenocarcinoma. Cancer Genet Cytogenet 2000;116:133-41.

20. Bartsch DK, Kress R, Sina-Frey M, et al. Prevalence of familial pancreatic cancer in Germany. Int J Cancer 2004;110:902-6.

21. Bartsch DK, Sina-Frey M, Lang S, et al. CDKN2A germline mutations in familial pancreatic cancer. Ann Surg 2002;236:730-7.

22. Bashyam MD, Bair R, Kim YH, et al. Array-based comparative genomic hybridization identifies localized DNA amplifications and homozygous deletions in pancreatic cancer. Neoplasia 2005;7: 556-62.

23. Benassai G, Mastrorilli M, Quarto G, et al. Factors influencing survival after resection for ductal adenocarcinoma of the head of the pancreas. J Surg Oncol 2000;73:212-8.

24. Bergman W, Watson P, de Jong J, Lynch HT, Fusaro RM. Systemic cancer and the FAMMM syndrome. Br J Cancer 1990;61:932-6.

25. Berlin JD, Adak S, Vaughn DJ, et al. A phase II study of gemcitabine and 5-fluorouracil in metastatic pancreatic cancer: an Eastern Cooperative Oncology Group Study (E3296). Oncology 2000;58:215-8.

26. Berman DB, Costalas J, Schultz DC, Grana G, Daly M, Godwin AK. A common mutation in BRCA2 that predisposes to a variety of cancers is found in both Jewish Ashkenazi and non-Jewish individuals. Cancer Res 1996;56:3409-14.

27. Berndt C, Haubold K, Wenger F, et al. K-ras mutations in stools and tissue samples from patients with malignant and nonmalignant pancreatic diseases. Clin Chem 1998;44:2103-7.

28. Berrington de Gonzalez A, Sweetland S, Spencer E. A meta-analysis of obesity and the risk of pancreatic cancer. Br J Cancer 2003;89:519-23.

29. Birkmeyer JD, Siewers AE, Finlayson EV, et al. Hospital volume and surgical mortality in the United States. N Engl J Med 2002;346:1128-37.

30. Bluemke DA, Cameron JL, Hruban RH, et al. Potentially resectable pancreatic adenocarcinoma: spiral CT assessment with surgical and pathologic correlation. Radiology 1995;197:381-5.

31. Bluemke DA, Fishman EK. CT and MR evaluation of pancreatic cancer. Surg Oncol Clin N Am 1998;7:103-24.

32. Bocsi J, Berczi C, Balazs G, Lapis K. Flow cytometric studies on the relationship between DNA content and clinicopathologic features of pancreatic cancers. Anticancer Res 1998;18:1839-43.

33. Borg A, Sandberg T, Nilsson K, et al. High frequency of multiple melanomas and breast and pancreas carcinomas in CDKN2A mutation-positive melanoma families. J Natl Cancer Inst 2000;92:1260-6.

34. Boschman CR, Stryker S, Reddy JK, Rao MS. Expression of p53 protein in precursor lesions and adenocarcinoma of human pancreas. Am J Pathol 1994;145:1291-5.

35. Brat DJ, Lillemoe KD, Yeo CJ, Warfield PB, Hruban RH. Progression of pancreatic intraductal neoplasias to infiltrating adenocarcinoma of the pancreas. Am J Surg Pathol 1998;22:163-9.

36. Brockie E, Anand A, Albores-Saavedra J. Progression of atypical ductal hyperplasia/carcinoma in situ of the pancreas to invasive adenocarcinoma. Ann Diagn Pathol 1998;2:286-92.

37. Brown HM, Ahrendt SA, Komorowski RA, Doffek KM, Wilson SD, Demeure MJ. Immunohistochemistry and molecular detection of nodal micrometastases in pancreatic cancer. J Surg Res 2001;95:141-6.

37a. Brune KA, Abe T, Canto MI, et al. Multifocal neoplastic precursor lesions associated with lobular atrophy of the pancreas in patients having a strong family history of pancreatic cancer. Am J Surg Pathol 2006;30:1067-76.

38. Caldas C, Hahn SA, da Costa LT, et al. Frequent somatic mutations and homozygous deletions of the p16 (MTS1) gene in pancreatic adenocarcinoma. Nat Genet 1994;8:27-32.

39. Caldas C, Hahn SA, Hruban RH, Redston MS, Yeo CJ, Kern SE. Detection of K-ras mutations in the stool of patients with pancreatic adenocarcinoma and pancreatic ductal hyperplasia. Cancer Res 1994;54:3568-73.

40. Calhoun ES, Jones JB, Ashfaq R, et al. BRAF and FBXW7 (CDC4, FBW7, AGO, SEL10) mutations in distinct subsets of pancreatic cancer: potential therapeutic targets. Am J Pathol 2003;163: 1255-60.

41. Cameron JL, Riall TS, Coleman J, Belcher KA. One thousand consecutive pancreaticoduodenectomies. Ann Surg 2006;244:10-5.

41a. Cancer risks in BRCA2 mutation carriers. The Breast Cancer Linkage Consortium. J Natl Cancer Inst 1999;91:1310-6.

42. Carney CP, Jones L, Woolson RF, Noyes R Jr, Doebbeling BN. Relationship between depression and pancreatic cancer in the general population. Psychosom Med 2003;65:884-8.

43. Chari ST, Mohan V, Pitchumoni CS, Viswanathan M, Madanagopalan N, Lowenfels AB. Risk of pancreatic carcinoma in tropical calcifying pancreatitis: an epidemiologic study. Pancreas 1994;9:62-6.

44. Cheng JQ, Ruggeri B, Klein WM, et al. Amplification of AKT2 in human pancreatic cells and inhibition of AKT2 expression and tumorgenicity by antisense RNA. Proc Natl Acad Sci 1996;93:3636-41.

45. Cho C, Rullis I, Rogers LS. Bile duct adenomas as liver nodules. Arch Surg 1978;113:272-4.

46. Chow WH, Gridley G, Nyren O, et al. Risk of pancreatic cancer following diabetes mellitus: a nationwide cohort study in Sweden. J Natl Cancer Inst 1995;87:930-1.

47. Chung EB. Multiple bile-duct hamartomas. Cancer 1970;26:287-96.

48. Cioc AM, Ellison EC, Proca DM, Lucas JG, Frankel WL. Frozen section diagnosis of pancreatic lesions. Arch Pathol Lab Med 2002;126: 1169-73.

49. Cohen MB, Egerter DP, Holly EA, Ahn DK, Miller TR. Pancreatic adenocarcinoma: regression analysis to identify improved cytologic criteria. Diagn Cytopathol 1991;7:341-5.

50. Conlon KC, Klimstra DS, Brennan MF. Long-term survival after curative resection for pancreatic ductal adenocarcinoma. Clinicopathologic analysis of 5-year survivors. Ann Surg 1996;223:273-9.

51. Connolly MM, Dawson PJ, Michelassi F, Moossa AR, Lowenstein F. Survival in 1001 patients with carcinoma of the pancreas. Ann Surg 1987;206: 366-73.

52. Costa J. Benign epithelial inclusions in pancreatic nerves. Am J Clin Pathol 1977;67:306-7.

53. Couch FJ, Johnson MR, Rabe K, et al. Germ line Fanconi anemia complementation group C mutations and pancreatic cancer. Cancer Res 2005;65:383-6.

54. Coughlin SS, Calle EE, Patel AV, Thun MJ. Predictors of pancreatic cancer mortality among a large cohort of United States adults. Cancer Causes Control 2000;11:915-23.

55. Crnogorac-Jurcevic T, Efthimiou E, Nielsen T, et al. Expression profiling of microdissected pancreatic adenocarcinomas. Oncogene 2002;21: 4587-94.

56. Crnogorac-Jurcevic T, Missiaglia E, Blaveri E, et al. Molecular alterations in pancreatic carcinoma: expression profiling shows that dysregulated expression of S100 genes is highly prevalent. J Pathol 2003;201:63-74.

57. Cubilla AL, Fitzgerald PJ. Classification of pancreatic cancer (nonendocrine). Mayo Clin Proc 1979;54:449-58.

58. Cubilla AL, Fitzgerald PJ. Morphological lesions associated with human primary invasive nonendocrine pancreas cancer. Cancer Res 1976;36: 2690-8.

59. Cubilla AL, Fitzgerald PJ. Morphological patterns of primary nonendocrine human pancreas carcinoma. Cancer Res 1975;35:2234-48.

60. Cubilla AL, Fitzgerald PJ. Pancreas cancer. I. Duct adenocarcinoma. A clinical-pathologic study of 380 patients. Pathol Annu 1978;13(Pt 1):241-89.

61. Cubilla AL, Fortner JG, Fitzgerald PJ. Lymph node involvement in carcinoma of the head of the pancreas area. Cancer 1978;41:880-7.

62. Curtis LJ, Li Y, Gerbault-Seureau M, et al. Amplification of DNA sequences from chromosome 19q13.1 in human pancreatic cell lines. Genomics 1998;53:42-55.

63. Cuzick J, Babiker AG. Pancreatic cancer, alcohol, diabetes mellitus and gall-bladder disease. Int J Cancer 1989;43:415-21.

64. de vos tot Nederveen Cappel WH, Offerhaus GJ, van Puijenbroek M, et al. Pancreatic carcinoma in carriers of a specific 19 base pair deletion of CDKN2A/p16 (p16-leiden). Clin Cancer Res 2003;9:3598-605.

65. Delcore R, Rodriguez FJ, Forster J, Hermreck AS, Thomas JH. Significance of lymph node metastases in patients with pancreatic cancer undergoing curative resection. Am J Surg 1996;172:463-8.

66. DeMay RM. Pancreas. In: DeMay RM. The art and science of cytopathology, vol 2. Chicago, Ill: ASCP Press; 1996:1053-1078.

67. Demeure MJ, Doffek KM, Komorowski RA, Wilson SD. Adenocarcinoma of the pancreas: detection of occult metastases in regional lymph nodes by a polymerase chain reaction-based assay. Cancer 1998;83:1328-34.

68. Dennis JL, Vass JK, Wit EC, Keith WN, Oien KA. Identification from public data of molecular markers of adenocarcinoma characteristic of the site of origin. Cancer Res 2002;62:5999-6005.

68a. Detlefsen S, Sipos B, Feyerabend B, Klöppel G. Pancreatic fibrosis associated with age and ductal papillary hyperplasia. Virchows Arch 2005;447:800-5.

69. DiGiuseppe JA, Hruban RH, Goodman SN, et al. Overexpression of p53 protein in adenocarcinoma of the pancreas. Am J Clin Pathol 1994;101:684-8.

70. Duval JV, Savas L, Banner BF. Expression of cytokeratins 7 and 20 in carcinomas of the extrahepatic biliary tract, pancreas, and gallbladder. Arch Pathol Lab Med 2000;124:1196-200.

71. Ebert M, Yokoyama M, Friess H, Kobrin MS, Buchler MW, Korc M. Induction of platelet-derived growth factor A and B chains and overexpression of their receptors in human pancreatic cancer. Int J Cancer 1995;62:529-35.

72. Ekbom A, McLaughlin JK, Karlson BM, et al. Pancreatitis and pancreatic cancer: a population-based study. J Natl Cancer Inst 1994;86: 625-7.

73. Eriguchi N, Aoyagi S, Hara M, et al. Synchronous or metachronous double cancers of the pancreas and other organs: report on 12 cases. Surg Today 2000;30:718-21.

74. Eriguchi N, Aoyagi S, Imayama H, et al. Resectable carcinoma of the pancreatic head developing 7 years and 4 months after distal pancreatectomy for carcinoma of the pancreatic tail. J Hepatobiliary Pancreat Surg 2000;7:316-20.

75. Everhart J, Wright D. Diabetes mellitus as a risk factor for pancreatic cancer. A meta-analysis. JAMA 1995;273:1605-9.

76. Falk RT, Pickle LW, Fontham ET, Correa P, Fraumeni JF. Life-style risk factors for pancreatic cancer in Louisana: a case-control study. Am J Epidemiol 1988;128:324-36.

77. Farrow DC, Davis S. Diet and the risk of pancreatic cancer in men. Am J Epidemiol 1990;132:423-31.

78. Fekete PS, Nunez C, Pitlik DA. Fine-needle aspiration biopsy of the pancreas: a study of 61 cases. Diagn Cytopathol 1986;2:301-6.

79. Fernandez E, La Vecchia C, D'Avanzo B, Negri E, Franceschi S. Family history and the risk of liver, gallbladder, and pancreatic cancer. Cancer Epidemiol Biomarkers Prev 1994;3:209-12.

80. Friess H, Yamanaka Y, Buchler M, et al. Enhanced expression of transforming growth factor beta isoforms in pancreatic cancer correlates with decreased survival. Gastroenterology 1993;105:1846-56.

81. Friess H, Yamanaka Y, Kobrin MS, Do DA, Buchler MW, Korc M. Enhanced erbB-3 expression in human pancreatic cancer correlates with tumor progression. Clin Cancer Res 1995;1: 1413-20.

82. Friess H, Zhu Z, Liard V, et al. Neurokinin-1 receptor expression and its potential effects on tumor growth in human pancreatic cancer. Lab Invest 2003;83:731-42.

83. Fukushige S, Waldman FM, Kimura M, et al. Frequent gain of copy number on the long arm of chromosome 20 in human pancreatic adenocarcinoma. Genes Chromosomes Cancer 1997;19:161-9.

84. Fukushima N, Sato N, Ueki T, et al. Aberrant methylation of preproenkephalin and p16 genes in pancreatic intraepithelial neoplasia and pancreatic ductal adenocarcinoma. Am J Pathol 2002;160:1573-81.

85. Fukushima N, Suzuki M, Fukayama M. Analysis of K-ras oncogene mutation directly applied to atypical cell clusters on cytologic smear slides of bile and pancreatic juice. Pathol Int 1998;48: 33-40.

86. Furukawa H, Okada S, Saisho H, et al. Clinicopathologic features of small pancreatic adenocarcinoma. A collective study. Cancer 1996;78: 986-90.

87. Furukawa T, Chiba R, Kobari M, Matsuno S, Nagura H, Takahashi T. Varying grades of epithelial atypia in the pancreatic ducts of humans. Classification based on morphometry

88. Gangi S, Fletcher JG, Nathan MA, et al. Time interval between abnormalities seen on CT and the clinical diagnosis of pancreatic cancer: retrospective review of CT scans obtained before diagnosis. AJR Am J Roentgenol 2004;182:897-903.

89. Gattani AM, Mandeli J, Bruckner HW. Tumor markers in patients with pancreatic carcinoma. Cancer 1996;78:57-62.

90. Gayther SA, Batley SJ, Linger L, et al. Mutations truncating the EP300 acetylase in human cancers. Nat Genet 2000;24:300-3.

91. Gebhardt C, Meyer W, Reichel M, Wunsch PH. Prognostic factors in the operative treatment of ductal pancreatic carcinoma. Langenbecks Arch Surg 2000;385:14-20.

92. Gerdes B, Ziegler A, Ramaswamy A, Wild A, Langer P, Bartsch DK. Multiple primaries in pancreatic cancer patients: indicator of a genetic predisposition? Int J Epidemiol 2000;29:999-1003.

93. Gerstenkorn C, Thomusch O. Transmission of a pancreatic adenocarcinoma to a renal transplant recipient. Clin Transplant 2003;17:473-6.

94. Ghadimi BM, Schröck E, Walker RL, et al. Specific chromosomal aberrations and amplification of the AIB1 nuclear receptor coactivator gene in pancreatic carcinomas. Am J Pathol 1999;154:525-36.

95. Ghadirian P, Liu G, Gallinger S, et al. Risk of pancreatic cancer among individuals with a family history of cancer of the pancreas. Int J Cancer 2002;97:807-10.

96. Ghadirian P, Simard A, Baillargeon J. Tobacco, alcohol, and coffee and cancer of the pancreas. A population-based, case-control study in Quebec, Canada. Cancer 1991;67:2664-70.

97. Giardiello FM, Brensinger JD, Tersmette AC, et al. Very high risk of cancer in familial Peutz-Jeghers syndrome. Gastroenterology 2000;119: 1447-53.

98. Giardiello FM, Offerhaus GJ, Lee DH, et al. Increased risk of thyroid and pancreatic carcinoma in familial adenomatous polyposis. Gut 1993;34:1394-6.

99. Giulianotti PC, Boggi U, Fornaciari G, et al. Prognostic value of histological grading in ductal adenocarcinoma of the pancreas. Klöppel vs TNM grading. Int J Pancreatol 1995;17:279-89.

100. Goggins M, Hruban RH, Kern SE. BRCA2 is inactivated late in the development of pancreatic intraepithelial neoplasia: evidence and implications. Am J Pathol 2000;156:1767-71.

101. Goggins M, Offerhaus GJ, Hilgers W, et al. Pancreatic adenocarcinomas with DNA replication errors (RER+) are associated with wild-type K-ras and characteristic histopathology. Poor differentiation, a syncytial growth pattern, and pushing borders suggest RER+. Am J Pathol 1998;152:1501-7.

102. Goggins M, Schutte M, Lu J, et al. Germline BRCA2 gene mutations in patients with apparently sporadic pancreatic carcinomas. Cancer Res 1996;56:5360-4.

103. Goggins M, Shekher M, Kenan T, Yeo CJ, Hruban RH, Kern SE. Genetic alterations of the transforming growth factor beta receptor genes in pancreatic and biliary adenocarcinomas. Cancer Res 1998;58:5329-32.

104. Gold EB, Goldin SB. Epidemiology of and risk factors for pancreatic cancer. Surg Oncol Clin N Am 1998;7:67-91.

105. Goldstein AM, Fraser MC, Struewing JP, et al. Increased risk of pancreatic cancer in melanoma-prone kindreds with p16INK4 mutations. N Engl J Med 1995;333:970-4.

106. Goldstein NS, Bassi D. Cytokeratins 7, 17, and 20 reactivity in pancreatic and ampulla of Vater adenocarcinomas. Percentage of positivity and distribution is affected by the cut-point threshold. Am J Clin Pathol 2001;115:695-702.

107. Gordis L. Consumption of methylxanthine-containing beverages and risk of pancreatic cancer. Cancer 1990;52:1-12.

108. Gordon TA, Bowman HM, Tielsch JM, Bass EB, Burleyson GP, Cameron JL. Statewide regionalization of pancreaticoduodenectomy and its effect on in-hospital mortality. Ann Surg 1998;228:71-8.

109. Gorunova L, Johansson B, Dawiskiba S, et al. Massive cytogenetic heterogeneity in a pancreatic carcinoma: fifty-four karyotypically unrelated clones. Genes Chromosomes Cancer 1995;14: 259-66.

110. Govindarajan S, Peters RL. The bile duct adenoma. A lesion distinct from Meyenburg complex. Arch Pathol Lab Med 1984;108:922-4.

111. Griffin CA, Hruban RH, Morsberger L, et al. Consistent chromosome abnormalities in adenocarcinoma of the pancreas. Cancer Res 1995;55:2394-9.

112. Grutzmann R, Foerder M, Alldinger I, et al. Gene expression profiles of microdissected pancreatic ductal adenocarcinoma. Virchows Arch 2003;443:508-17.

113. Hahn SA, Greenhalf B, Ellis I, et al. BRCA2 germline mutations in familial pancreatic carcinoma. J Natl Cancer Inst 2003;95:214-21.

114. Hahn SA, Schutte M, Hoque AT, et al. DPC4, a candidate tumor suppressor gene at human chromosome 18q21.1. Science 1996;271:350-3.

115. Hahn SA, Seymour AB, Hoque AT, et al. Allelotype of pancreatic adenocarcinoma using xenograft enrichment. Cancer Res 1995;55:4670-5.

116. Han H, Bearss DJ, Browne LW, Calaluce R, Nagle RB, Von Hoff DD. Identification of differentially expressed genes in pancreatic cancer cells using cDNA microarray. Cancer Res 2002;62:2890-6.

117. Heinmöller E, Dietmaier W, Zirngibl H, et al. Molecular analysis of microdissected tumors and preneoplastic intraductal lesions in pancreatic carcinoma. Am J Pathol 2000;157:83-92.

118. Hemminki K, Li X. Familial and second primary pancreatic cancers: a nationwide epidemiologic study from Sweden. Int J Cancer 2003;103:525-30.

119. Hempen PM, Zhang L, Bansal RK, et al. Evidence of selection for clones having genetic inactivation of the activin A type II receptor (ACVR2) gene in gastrointestinal cancers. Cancer Res 2003;63:994-9.

120. Henke AC, Jensen CS, Cohen MB. Cytologic diagnosis of adenocarcinoma in biliary and pancreatic duct brushings. Adv Anat Pathol 2002;9:301-8.

121. Hirai I, Kimura W, Ozawa K, et al. Perineural invasion in pancreatic cancer. Pancreas 2002;24: 15-25.

122. Hiyama E, Kodama T, Shinbara K, et al. Telomerase activity is detected in pancreatic cancer but not in benign tumors. Cancer Res 1997; 57:326-31.

123. Holly EA, Eberle CA, Bracci PM. Prior history of allergies and pancreatic cancer in the San Francisco Bay area. Am J Epidemiol 2003;158:432-41.

124. Holzmann K, Kohlhammer H, Schwaenen C, et al. Genomic DNA-chip hybridization reveals a higher incidence of genomic amplifications in pancreatic cancer than conventional comparative genomic hybridization and leads to the identification of novel candidate genes. Cancer Res 2004;64:4428-33.

125. Hornick JL, Lauwers GY, Odze RD. Immunohistochemistry can help distinguish metastatic pancreatic adenocarcinomas from bile duct adenomas and hamartomas of the liver. Am J Surg Pathol 2005;29:381-9.

126. Hosch SB, Knoefel WT, Metz S, et al. Early lymphatic tumor cell dissemination in pancreatic cancer: frequency and prognostic significance. Pancreas 1997;15:154-9.

127. Howard JM, Hess W. History of the pancreas: mysteries of a hidden organ. New York: Kluwer Academic/Plenum Publishers; 2002.

128. Howe GR, Ghadirian P, DeMesquita HB, et al. A collaborative case-control study of nutrient intake and pancreatic cancer within the search programme. Int J Cancer 1992;51:365-72.

129. Howe GR, Jain M, Burch JD, Miller AB. Cigarette smoking and cancer of the pancreas: evidence from a population-based case-control study in Toronto, Canada. Int J Cancer 1991;47: 323-8.

130. Hruban RH, Adsay NV, Albores-Saavedra J, et al. Pancreatic intraepithelial neoplasia: a new nomenclature and classification system for pancreatic duct lesions. Am J Surg Pathol 2001; 25:579-86.

131. Hruban RH, Goggins M, Parsons JL, Kern SE. Progression model for pancreatic cancer. Clin Cancer Res 2000;6:2969-72.

132. Hruban RH, Sturm PD, Slebos RJ, et al. Can K-ras codon 12 mutations be used to distinguish benign bile duct proliferations from metastases in the liver? A molecular analysis of 101 liver lesions from 93 patients. Am J Pathol 1997;151:943-9.

133. Hruban RH, Takaori K, Klimstra DS, et al. An illustrated consensus on the classification of pancreatic intraepithelial neoplasia and intraductal papillary mucinous neoplasms. Am J Surg Pathol 2004;28:977-87.

134. Hulst SP. Zur kenntnis der Genese des Adenokarzinoms und Karzinoms des Pankreas. Virchows Arch [B] 1905;180:288-316.

135. Hyland C, Kheir SM, Kashlan MB. Frozen section diagnosis of pancreatic carcinoma: a prospective study of 64 biopsies. Am J Surg Pathol 1981;5:179-91.

136. Iacobuzio-Donahue CA, Ashfaq R, Maitra A, et al. Highly expressed genes in pancreatic ductal adenocarcinomas: a comprehensive characterization and comparison of the transcription profiles obtained from three major technologies. Cancer Res 2003;63:8614-22.

137. Iacobuzio-Donahue CA, Maitra A, Olsen M, et al. Exploration of global gene expression patterns in pancreatic adenocarcinoma using cDNA microarrays. Am J Pathol 2003;162:1151-62.

138. Iacobuzio-Donahue CA, Maitra A, Shen-Ong GL, et al. Discovery of novel tumor markers of pancreatic cancer using global gene expression technology. Am J Pathol 2002;160:1239-49.

139. Iacobuzio-Donahue CA, Ryu B, Hruban RH, Kern SE. Exploring the host desmoplastic response to pancreatic carcinoma: gene expression of stromal and neoplastic cells at the site of primary invasion. Am J Pathol 2002;160:91-9.

140. Iacobuzio-Donahue CA, Song J, Parmiagiani G, Yeo CJ, Hruban RH, Kern SE. Missense mutations of MADH4: characterization of the mutational hot spot and functional consequences in human tumors. Clin Cancer Res 2004;10:1597-604.

141. Iguchi H, Sugano K, Fukayama N, et al. Analysis of Ki-ras codon 12 mutations in the duodenal juice of patients with pancreatic cancer. Gastroenterology 1996;110:221-6.

142. Ishikawa O, Ohigashi H, Sasaki Y, et al. Practical grouping of positive lymph nodes in pancreatic head cancer treated by an extended pancreatectomy. Surgery 1997;121:244-9.

143. Itakura J, Ishiwata T, Shen B, Kornmann M, Korc M. Concomitant over-expression of vascular endothelial growth factor and its receptors in pancreatic cancer. Int J Cancer 2000;85:27-34.

144. Iwao T, Hiyama E, Yokoyama T, et al. Telomerase activity for the preoperative diagnosis of pancreatic cancer. J Natl Cancer Inst 1997;89:1621-3.

145. Japanese Pancreas Society. Classification of pancreatic carcinoma, 2nd English ed. Tokyo: Kanehara & Co; 2003.

146. Jemal A, Siegel R, Ward E, et al. Cancer statistics, 2004. CA Cancer J Clin 2006;56:8-106-30.

147. Johansson B, Bardi G, Pandis N, et al. Karyotypic pattern of pancreatic adenocarcinomas correlates with survival and tumour grade. Int J Cancer 1994;58:8-13.

148. Jones JB, Song JJ, Hempen PM, Parmigiani G, Hruban RH, Kern SE. Detection of mitochondrial DNA mutations in pancreatic cancer offers a "mass"-ive advantage over detection of nuclear DNA mutations. Cancer Res 2001;61:1299-304.

149. Juhl H, Stritzel M, Wroblewski A, et al. Immunocytological detection of micrometastatic cells: comparative evaluation of findings in the peritoneal cavity and the bone marrow of gastric, colorectal and pancreatic cancer patients. Int J Cancer 1994;57:330-5.

150. Kami K, Doi R, Koizumi M, et al. Survivin expression is a prognostic marker in pancreatic cancer patients. Surgery 2004;136:443-8.

151. Kamisawa T, Fukayama M, Tabata I, et al. Neuroendocrine differentiation in pancreatic duct carcinoma: special emphasis on duct-endocrine cell carcinoma of the pancreas. Pathol Res Pract 1996;192:901-8.

152. Kanai N, Nagaki S, Tanaka T. Clear cell carcinoma of the pancreas. Acta Pathol Jpn 1987;37:1521-6.

153. Kayahara M, Nagakawa T, Kobayashi H, et al. Lymphatic flow in carcinoma of the head of the pancreas. Cancer 1992;70:2061-6.

154. Kayahara M, Nagakawa T, Ohta T, et al. Analysis of paraaortic lymph node involvement in pancreatic carcinoma: a significant indication for surgery? Cancer 1999;85:583-90.

155. Kayahara M, Nagakawa T, Ueno K, Ohta T, Takeda T, Miyazaki I. An evaluation of radical resection for pancreatic cancer based on the mode of recurrence as determined by autopsy and diagnostic imaging. Cancer 1993;72:2118-23.

156. Kern HF, Roher HD, von Bulow M, Klöppel G. Fine structure of three major grades of malignancy of human pancreatic adenocarcinoma. Pancreas 1987;2:2-13.

157. Kim GE, Bae HI, Park HU, et al. Aberrant expression of MUC5AC and MUC6 gastric mucins and sialyl Tn antigen in intraepithelial neoplasms of the pancreas. Gastroenterology 2002;123:1052-60.

158. Klein AP, Beaty TH, Bailey-Wilson JE, Brune KA, Hruban RH, Petersen GM. Evidence for a major gene influencing risk of pancreatic cancer. Genet Epidemiol 2002;23:133-49.

159. Klein AP, Brune K, Petersen GM, et al. Prospective risk of pancreatic cancer in familial pancreatic cancer kindreds. Cancer Res 2004;64:2634-8.

160. Klein WM, Hruban RH, Klein-Szanto AJ, Wilentz RE. Direct correlation between proliferative activity and dysplasia in pancreatic intraepithelial neoplasia (PanIN): additional evidence for a recently proposed model of progression. Mod Pathol 2002;15:441-7.

161. Klimstra DS, Hameed MR, Marrero AM, Conlon KC, Brennan MF. Ductal proliferative lesions associated with infiltrating ductal adenocarcinoma of the pancreas. Int J Pancreatol 1994; 16:224-5.

161a. Klöppel G, Hruban RH, Longnecker DS, Adler G, Kern SE, Partanen TJ. Ductal adenocarcinoma of the pancreas. In Hamilton SR, Aaltonen LA, eds. World Health Organization Classification of Tumours. Pathology and genetics of tumours of the digestive system. Lyon: IARC Press; 2000:221-30.

162. Klöppel G, Lingenthal G, von Bulow M, Kern HF. Histological and fine structural features of pancreatic ductal adenocarcinomas in relation to growth and prognosis: studies in xenografted tumors and clinico-histopathological correlation in a series of 75 cases. Histopathology 1985;9:841-56.

163. Kondo H, Sugano K, Fukayama N, et al. Detection of point mutations in the K-ras oncogene at codon12 in pure pancreatic juice for diagnosis of pancreatic carcinoma. Cancer 1994;73:1589-94.

164. Koopmann J, Fedarko NS, Jain A, et al. Evaluation of osteopontin as biomarker for pancreatic adenocarcinoma. Cancer Epidemiol Biomarkers Prev 2004;13:487-91.

165. Korc M. Role of growth factors in pancreatic cancer. Surg Oncol Clin N Am 1998;7:25-41.

166. Korc M, Chandrasekar B, Yamanaka Y, Friess H, Buchier M, Beger HG. Overexpression of the epidermal growth factor receptor in human pancreatic cancer is associated with concomitant increases in the levels of epidermal growth factor and transforming growth factor alpha. J Clin Invest 1992;90:1352-60.

167. Kornmann M, Beger HG, Korc M. Role of fibroblast growth factors and their receptors in pancreatic cancer and chronic pancreatitis. Pancreas 1998;17:169-75.

168. Koshiba T, Hosotani R, Wada M, et al. Involvement of matrix metalloproteinase-2 activity in invasion and metastasis of pancreatic carcinoma. Cancer 1998;82:642-50.

168a. Kosmahl M, Pauser U, Anlauf M, Klöppel G. Pancreatic ductal adenocarcinomas with cystic features: neither rare nor uniform. Mod Pathol 2005;18:1157-64.

169. Kozuka S, Sassa R, Taki T, et al. Relation of pancreatic duct hyperplasia to carcinoma. Cancer 1979;43:1418-28.

170. Kuhlmann KF, de Castro SM, Wesseling JG, et al. Surgical treatment of pancreatic adenocarcinoma; actual survival and prognostic factors in 343 patients. Eur J Cancer 2004;40:549-58.

171. Kulke MH. Advanced pancreatic cancer: is there a role for combination therapy? Expert Rev Anticancer Ther 2003;3:729-39.

172. Lal G, Liu G, Schmocker B, et al. Inherited predisposition to pancreatic adenocarcinoma: role of family history and germ-line p16, BRCA1, and BRCA2 mutations. Cancer Res 2000;60: 409-16.

173. Launois B, Franci J, Bardaxoglou E, et al. Total pancreatectomy for ductal adenocarcinoma of the pancreas with special reference to resection of the portal vein and multicentric cancer. World J Surg 1993;17:122-7.

174. Lee MJ, Lee HS, Kim WH, Choi Y, Yang M. Expression of mucins and cytokeratins in primary carcinomas of the digestive system. Mod Pathol 2003;16:403-10.

175. Leung HY, Gullick WJ, Lemoine NR. Expression and functional activity of fibroblast growth factors and their receptors in human pancreatic cancer. Int J Cancer 1994;59:667-75.

176. Li D, Xie K, Wolff R, Abbruzzese JL. Pancreatic cancer. Lancet 2004;363:1049-57.

177. Liede A, Karlan BY, Narod SA. Cancer risks for male carriers of germline mutations in BRCA1 or BRCA2: a review of the literature. J Clin Oncol 2004;22:735-42.

178. Lillemoe KD, Kaushal S, Cameron JL, Sohn TA, Pitt HA, Yeo CJ. Distal pancreatectomy: indications and outcomes in 235 patients. Ann Surg 1999;229:693-8.

179. Lim JE, Chien MW, Earle CC. Prognostic factors following curative resection for pancreatic adenocarcinoma: a population-based, linked database analysis of 396 patients. Ann Surg 2003;237:74-85.

180. Lin F, Staerkel G. Cytologic criteria for well differentiated adenocarcinoma of the pancreas in fine-needle aspiration biopsy specimens. Cancer 2003;99:44-50.

181. Liu Q, Yan YX, McClure M, Nakagawa H, Fujimura F, Rustgi AK. MTS-1 (CDKN2) tumor suppressor gene deletions are a frequent event in esophagus squamous cancer and pancreatic adenocarcinoma cell lines. Oncogene 1995;10: 619-22.

182. Logsdon CD, Simeone DM, Binkley C, et al. Molecular profiling of pancreatic adenocarcinoma and chronic pancreatitis identifies multiple genes differentially regulated in pancreatic cancer. Cancer Res 2003;63:2649-57.

183. Lonardo F, Cubilla AL, Klimstra DS. Microadenocarcinoma of the pancreas—morphologic pattern or pathologic entity? A reevaluation of the original series. Am J Surg Pathol 1996;20: 1385-93.

184. Lowenfels AB, Maisonneuve EP, Dimagno YE, et al. Hereditary pancreatitis and the risk of pancreatic cancer. International Hereditary Pancreatitis Study Group. J Natl Cancer Inst 1997;89:442-6.

185. Lowenfels AB, Maisonneuve P, Cavallini G, et al. Pancreatitis and the risk of pancreatic cancer. International Hereditary Pancreatitis Study Group. N Engl J Med 1993;328:1433-7.

186. Lu Z, Friess H, Graber HU, et al. Presence of two signaling TGF-beta receptors in human pancreatic cancer correlates with advanced tumor stage. Dig Dis Sci 1997;42:2054-63.

187. Lüttges J, Galehdari H, Brocker V, et al. Allelic loss is often the first hit in the biallelic inactivation of the p53 and DPC4 genes during pancreatic carcinogenesis. Am J Pathol 2001;158: 1677-83.

188. Lüttges J, Schemm S, Vogel I, Hedderich J, Kremer B, Klöppel G. The grade of pancreatic ductal carcinoma is an independent prognostic factor and is superior to the immunohistochemical assessment of proliferation. J Pathol 2000;191:154-61.

189. Lüttges J, Stigge C, Pacena M, Klöppel G. Rare ductal adenocarcinoma of the pancreas in patients younger than age 40 years. Cancer 2004;100:173-82.

190. Lüttges J, Vogel I, Menke M, Henne-Bruns D, Kremer B, Klöppel G. Clear cell carcinoma of the pancreas: an adenocarcinoma with ductal phenotype. Histopathology 1998;32:444-8.

191. Lüttges J, Vogel I, Menke M, Henne-Bruns D, Kremer B, Klöppel G. The retroperitoneal resection margin and vessel involvement are important factors determining survival after pancreaticoduodenectomy for ductal adenocarcinoma of the head of the pancreas. Virchows Arch 1998;433:237-42.

192. Lüttges J, Zamboni G, Longnecker DS, Klöppel G. The immunohistochemical mucin expression pattern distinguishes different types of intraductal papillary mucinous neoplasms of the pancreas and determines their relationship to mucinous noncystic carcinoma and ductal adenocarcinoma. Am J Surg Pathol 2001;25: 942-8.

193. Lynch HT, Brand RE, Hogg D, et al. Phenotypic variation in eight extended CDKN2A germline mutation familial atypical multiple mole melanoma-pancreatic carcinoma-prone families: the familial atypical mole melanoma-pancreatic carcinoma syndrome. Cancer 2002;94:84-96.

194. Lynch HT, Deters CA, Snyder CL, et al. BRCA1 and pancreatic cancer: pedigree findings and their causal relationships. Cancer Genet Cytogenet 2005;158:119-25.

195. Lynch HT, Voorhees GJ, Lanspa SJ, McGreevy PS, Lynch J. Pancreatic carcinoma and hereditary nonpolyposis colorectal cancer: a family study. Br J Cancer 1985;52:271-3.

196. Magistrelli P, Antinori A, Crucitti A, et al. Prognostic factors after surgical resection for pancreatic carcinoma. J Surg Oncol 2000;74:36-40.

197. Mahlamaki EH, Hoglund M, Gorunova L, et al. Comparative genomic hybridization reveals frequent gains of 20q, 8q, 11q, 12p, and 17q, and losses of 18q, 9p, and 15q in pancreatic cancer. Genes Chromosomes Cancer 1997;20: 383-91.

198. Maitra A, Adsay NV, Argani P, et al. Multicomponent analysis of the pancreatic adenocarcinoma progression model using a pancreatic intraepithelial neoplasia tissue microarray. Mod Pathol 2003;16:902-12.

199. Maitra A, Ashfaq R, Gunn CR, et al. Cyclooxygenase 2 expression in pancreatic adenocarcinoma and pancreatic intraepithelial neoplasia: an immunohistochemical analysis with automated cellular imaging. Am J Clin Pathol 2002;118:194-201.

200. Maitra A, Cohen Y, Gillespie SE, et al. The human MitoChip: a high-throughput sequencing microarray for mitochondrial mutation detection. Genome Res 2004;14:812-9.

201. Maitra A, Iacobuzio-Donahue CA, Rahman A, et al. Immunohistochemical validation of a novel epithelial and a novel stromal marker of pancreatic ductal adenocarcinoma identified by global expression microarrays: sea urchin fascin homolog and heat shock protein 47. Am J Clin Pathol 2002;118:52-9.

202. Mao C, Domenico DR, Kim K, Hanson DJ, Howard JM. Observations on the developmental patterns and the consequences of pancreatic exocrine adenocarcinoma. Findings of 154 autopsies. Arch Surg 1995;130:125-34.

203. Matsubayashi H, Sato N, Fukushima N, et al. Methylation of cyclin D2 is observed frequently in pancreatic cancer but is also an age-related phenomenon in gastrointestinal tissues. Clin Cancer Res 2003;9:1446-52.

204. Matsuno S, Egawa S, Fukuyama S, et al. Pancreatic Cancer Registry in Japan: 20 years of experience. Pancreas 2004;28:219-30.

205. Megibow AJ, Zhou XH, Rotterdam H, et al. Pancreatic adenocarcinoma: CT versus MR imaging in the evaluation of resectability—report of the Radiology Diagnostic Oncology Group. Radiology 1995;195:327-32.

206. Merchant NB, Conlon KC, Saigo P, Dougherty E, Brennan MF. Positive peritoneal cytology predicts unresectability of pancreatic adenocarcinoma. J Am Coll Surg 1999;188:421-6.

207. Michaud DS, Giovannucci E, Willett WC, Colditz GA, Stampfer MJ, Fuchs CS. Physical activity, obesity, height, and the risk of pancreatic cancer. JAMA 2001;286:921-9.

208. Michaud DS, Liu S, Giovannucci E, Willett WC, Colditz GA, Fuchs CS. Dietary sugar, glycemic load, and pancreatic cancer risk in a prospective study. J Natl Cancer Inst 2002;94:1293-300.

209. Midwinter MJ, Beveridge CJ, Wilsdon JB, Bennett MK, Baudouin CJ, Charnley RM. Correlation between spiral computed tomography, endoscopic ultrasonography and findings at operation in pancreatic and ampullary tumours. Br J Surg 1999;86:189-93.

210. Missiaglia E, Blaveri E, Terris B, et al. Analysis of gene expression in cancer cell lines identifies candidate markers for pancreatic tumorigenesis and metastasis. Int J Cancer 2004;112:100-12.

211. Mitchell ML, Carney CN. Cytologic criteria for the diagnosis of pancreatic carcinoma. Am J Clin Pathol 1985;83:171-6.

212. Miwa W, Yasuda J, Murakami Y, et al. Isolation of DNA sequences amplified at chromosome 19q13.1-q13.2 including the AKT2 locus in human pancreatic cancer. Biochem Biophys Res Commun 1996;225:968-74.

213. Monges GM, Mathoulin-Portier MP, Acres RB, et al. Differential MUC 1 expression in normal and neoplastic human pancreatic tissue. An immunohistochemical study of 60 samples. Am J Clin Pathol 1999;112:635-40.

214. Montgomery E, Wilentz RE, Argani P, et al. Analysis of anaphase figures in routine histologic sections distinguishes chromosomally unstable from chromosomally stable malignancies. Cancer Biol Ther 2003;2:248-52.

215. Moskaluk CA, Hruban RH, Kern SE. p16 and K-ras gene mutations in the intraductal precursors of human pancreatic adenocarcinoma. Cancer Res 1997;57:2140-3.

216. Mukada T, Yamada S. Dysplasia and carcinoma in situ of the exocrine pancreas. Tohoku J Exp Med 1982;137:115-24.

217. Murphy KM, Brune KA, Griffin CA, et al. Evaluation of candidate genes MAP2K4, MADH4, ACVR1B, and BRCA2 in familial pancreatic cancer: deleterious BRCA2 mutations in 17%. Cancer Res 2002;62:3789-93.

218. Nagakawa T, Konishi I, Ueno K, Ohta T, Kayahara M. A clinical study on lymphatic flow in carcinoma of the pancreatic head area—peripancreatic regional lymph node grouping. Hepatogastroenterology 1993;40:457-62.

219. Nagakawa T, Mori K, Nakano T, et al. Perineural invasion of carcinoma of the pancreas and biliary tract. Br J Surg 1993;80:619-21.

220. Nagle N, Wibur DC, Pitman MB. The cytomorphology of gastric and duodenal epithelium and reactivity to B72.3: a baseline for comparison to pancreatic neoplasms apirated by EUS-FNAB. Diagn Cytopathol 2005;33:381-6.

221. Nakao A, Harada A, Nonami T, et al. Lymph node metastasis in carcinoma of the body and tail of the pancreas. Br J Surg 1997;84:1090-2.

222. Nakao A, Harada A, Nonami T, Kaneko T, Inoue S, Takagi H. Clinical significance of portal invasion by pancreatic head carcinoma. Surgery 1995;117:50-5.

223. Nakao A, Harada A, Nonami T, Kaneko T, Takagi H. Clinical significance of carcinoma invasion of the extrapancreatic nerve plexus in pancreatic cancer. Pancreas 1996;12:357-61.

224. Nakao A, Oshima K, Nomoto S, et al. Clinical usefulness of CA-19-9 in pancreatic carcinoma. Semin Surg Oncol 1998;15:15-22.

225. Naumann M, Savitskaia N, Eilert C, Schramm A, Kalthoff H, Schmiegel W. Frequent codeletion of p16/MTS1 and p15/MTS2 and genetic alterations in p16/MTS1 in pancreatic tumors. Gastroenterology 1996;110:1215-24.

226. Neoptolemos JP, Stocken DD, Dunn JA, et al. Influence of resection margins on survival for patients with pancreatic cancer treated by adjuvant chemoradiation and/or chemotherapy in the ESPAC-1 randomized controlled trial. Ann Surg 2001;234:758-68.

227. Neoptolemos JP, Stocken DD, Friess H, et al. A randomized trial of chemoradiotherapy and chemotherapy after resection of pancreatic cancer. N Engl J Med 2004;350:1200-10.

228. Neugut AI, Ahsan H, Robinson E. Pancreas cancer as a second primary malignancy. A population-based study. Cancer 1995;76:589-92.

229. Newill VA. Distribution of cancer mortality among ethnic subgroups of the white population in New York City, 1953-1958. J Natl Cancer Inst 1961;26:405-17.

230. Nichols LS, Ashfaq R, Iacobuzio-Donahue CA. Claudin 4 protein expression in primary and metastatic pancreatic cancer: support for use as a therapeutic target. Am J Clin Pathol 2004;121:226-30.

231. Niedergethmann M, Rexin M, Hildenbrand R, et al. Prognostic implications of routine, immunohistochemical, and molecular staging in resectable pancreatic adenocarcinoma. Am J Surg Pathol 2002;26:1578-87.

232. Niederhuber JE, Brennan MF, Menck HR. The National Cancer Data Base report on pancreatic cancer. Cancer 1995;76:1671-7.

233. Nishida K, Kaneko T, Yoneda M, et al. Doubling time of serum CA 19-9 in the clinical course of patients with pancreatic cancer and its significant association with prognosis. J Surg Oncol 1999;71:140-6.

234. Nonomura A, Kono N, Mizukami Y, Nakanuma Y, Matsubara F. Duct-acinar-islet cell tumor of the pancreas. Ultrastruct Pathol 1992;16:317-29.

235. Nowak NJ, Gaile D, Conroy JM, et al. Genome-wide aberrations in pancreatic adenocarcinoma. Cancer Genet Cytogenet 2005;161:36-50.

236. Ochi K, Hasuoka H, Mizushima T, Matsumura N, Harada H. A case of small pancreatic cancer diagnosed by serial follow-up studies promptly by a positive K-ras point mutation in pure pancreatic juice. Am J Gastroenterol 1998;93:1366-8.

237. Offerhaus GJ, Tersmette AC, Tytgat GN, Hoedemaeker PJ, Vandenbroucke JP. Gastric, pancreatic, and colorectal carcinogenesis following remote peptic ulcer surgery. Review of the literature with the emphasis on risk assessment and underlying mechanism. Mod Pathol 1988;1(5):352-6.

238. Okami J, Yamamoto H, Fujiwara Y, et al. Overexpression of cyclooxygenase-2 in carcinoma of the pancreas. Clin Cancer Res 1999;5:2018-24.

239. Okusaka T, Okada S, Ueno H, et al. Abdominal pain in patients with resectable pancreatic cancer with reference to clinicopathologic findings. Pancreas 2001;22:279-84.

240. O'Malley ME, Boland GW, Wood BJ, Fernandez-del Castillo C, Warshaw AL, Mueller PR. Adenocarcinoma of the head of the pancreas: determination of surgical unresectability with thin-section pancreatic-phase helical CT. AJR Am J Roentgenol 1999;173:1513-8.

241. Ozaki H, Hiraoka T, Mizumoto R, et al. The prognostic significance of lymph node metastasis and intrapancreatic perineural invasion in pancreatic cancer after curative resection. Surg Today 1999;29:16-22.

242. Ozcelik H, Schmocker B, DiNicola N, et al. Germline BRCA2 6174delT mutations in Ashkenazi Jewish pancreatic cancer patients. Nat Genet 1997;16:17-8.

243. Palazzo L, Roseau G, Gayet B, et al. Endoscopic ultrasonography in the diagnosis and staging of pancreatic adenocarcinoma. Results of a prospective study with comparison to ultrasonography and CT scan. Endoscopy 1993;25:143-50.

244. Park DI, Lee JK, Kim JE, et al. The analysis of resectability and survival in pancreatic cancer patients with vascular invasion. J Clin Gastroenterol 2001;32:231-4.

245. Parker JF, Florell SR, Alexander A, DiSario JA, Shami PJ, Leachman SA. Pancreatic carcinoma surveillance in patients with familial melanoma. Arch Dermatol 2003;139:1019-25.

246. Parkin DM, Bray F, Ferlay J, Pisani P. Estimating the world cancer burden: Globocan 2000. Int J Cancer 2001;94:153-6.

247. Passik SD, Breitbart WS. Depression in patients with pancreatic carcinoma. Diagnostic and treatment issues. Cancer 1996;78:615-26.

248. Pearson AS, Chiao P, Zhang L, et al. The detection of telomerase activity in patients with adenocarcinoma of the pancreas by fine needle aspiration. Int J Oncol 2000;17:381-5.

248a. Pogue-Geile KL, Chen R, Bronner MP, et al. Palladin mutation causes familial pancreatic cancer and suggests a new cancer mechanism. PLoS Medicine 2006;3:1-13.

249. Porschen R, Remy U, Bevers G, Schauseil S, Hengels KJ, Borchard F. Prognostic significance of DNA ploidy in adenocarcinoma of the pancreas. A flow cytometric study of paraffin-embedded specimens. Cancer 1993;71:3846-50.

250. Pour PM, Permert J, Mogaki M, Fujii H, Kazakoff K. Endocrine aspects of exocrine cancer of the pancreas. Their patterns and suggested biologic significance. Am J Clin Pathol 1993;100:223-30.

251. Pour PM, Sayed S, Sayed G. Hyperplastic, preneoplastic and neoplastic lesions found in 83 human pancreases. Am J Clin Pathol 1982;77:137-52.

252. Prasad NB, Biankin AV, Fukushima N, et al. Gene expression profiles in pancreatic intraepithelial neoplasia reflect the effects of Hedgehog signaling on pancreatic ductal epithelial cells. Cancer Res 2005;65:1619-26.

253. Qiao JG, Zhang YQ, Yin YC, Tan Z. Expression of survivin in pancreatic cancer and its correlation to expression of Bcl-2. World J Gastroenterol 2004;10:2759-61.

254. Ray S, Lu Z, Rajendiran S. Clear cell ductal adenocarcinoma of pancreas: a case report and review of the literature. Arch Pathol Lab Med 2004;128:693-6.

255. Redston MS, Caldas C, Seymour AB, et al. p53 mutations in pancreatic carcinoma and evidence of common involvement of homocopolymer tracts in DNA microdeletions. Cancer Res 1994;54:3025-33.

256. Ritts RE, Pitt HA. CA 19-9 in pancreatic cancer. Surg Oncol Clin N Am 1998;7:93-101.

257. Robins DB, Katz RL, Evans DB, Atkinson EN, Green L. Fine needle aspiration of the pancreas. In quest of accuracy. Acta Cytol 1995;39:1-10.

258. Robinson PA. The role of MRI in pancreatic cancer. Eur Radiol 2002;12:267-9.

259. Roder JD, Thorban S, Pantel K, Siewert JR. Micrometastases in bone marrow: prognostic indicators for pancreatic cancer. World J Surg 2003;23:888-91.

260. Rosty C, Christa L, Kuzdzal S, et al. Identification of hepatocarcinoma-intestine-pancreas/pancreatitis-associated protein I as a biomarker for pancreatic ductal adenocarcinoma by protein biochip technology. Cancer Res 2002;62:1868-75.

261. Rosty C, Geradts J, Sato N, et al. p16 inactivation in pancreatic intraepithelial neoplasias (PanINs) arising in patients with chronic pancreatitis. Am J Surg Pathol 2003;27:1495-501.

262. Rosty C, Ueki T, Argani P, et al. Overexpression of S100A4 in pancreatic ductal adenocarcinomas is associated with poor differentiation and DNA hypomethylation. Am J Pathol 2002;160:45-50.

263. Rozenblum E, Schutte M, Goggins M, et al. Tumor-suppressive pathways in pancreatic carcinoma. Cancer Res 1997;57:1731-4.

264. Rugge M, Sonego F, Leandro G, et al. Nuclear DNA content and pathology in radically treated pancreatic carcinoma. The prognostic significance of DNA ploidy, histology and nuclear grade. Cancer 1996;77:459-66.

265. Ruggeri BA, Huang L, Wood M, Cheng JQ, Testa JR. Amplification and overexpression of the AKT2 oncogene in a subset of human pancreatic ductal adenocarcinomas. Mol Carcinog 1998;21:81-6.

266. Ryu B, Jones JB, Blades NJ, et al. Relationships and differentially expressed genes among pancreatic cancers examined by large-scale serial analysis of gene expression. Cancer Res 2002; 62:819-26.

267. Ryu B, Jones JB, Hollingsworth MA, Hruban RH, Kern SE. Invasion-specific genes in malignancy: serial analysis of gene expression comparisons of primary and passaged cancers. Cancer Res 2001;61:1833-8.

268. Sato N, Fukushima N, Maitra A, et al. Discovery of novel targets for aberrant methylation in pancreatic carcinoma using high-throughput microarrays. Cancer Res 2003;63:3735-42.

269. Sato N, Rosty C, Jansen M, et al. STK11/LKB1 Peutz-Jeghers gene inactivation in intraductal papillary-mucinous neoplasms of the pancreas. Am J Pathol 2001;159:2017-22.

270. Schenk M, Schwartz AG, O'Neal E, et al. Familial risk of pancreatic cancer. J Natl Cancer Inst 2001;93:640-4.

271. Schutte M, Hruban RH, Geradts J, et al. Abrogation of the Rb/p16 tumor-suppressive pathway in virtually all pancreatic carcinomas. Cancer Res 1997;57:3126-30.

272. Seidman JD, Kurman RJ, Ronnett BM. Primary and metastatic mucinous adenocarcinomas in the ovaries: incidence in routine practice with a new approach to improve intraoperative diagnosis. Am J Surg Pathol 2003;27:985-93.

273. Sener SF, Fremgen A, Menck HR, Winchester DP. Pancreatic cancer: a report of treatment and survival trends for 100,313 patients diagnosed from 1985-1995, using the National Cancer Database. J Am Coll Surg 1999;189:1-7.

274. Sharma S, Green KB. The pancreatic duct and its arteriovenous relationship: an underutilized aid in the diagnosis and distinction of pancreatic adenocarcinoma from pancreatic intraepithelial neoplasia. A study of 126 pancreatectomy specimens. Am J Surg Pathol 2004;28: 613-20.

275. Shibata D, Almoguera C, Forrester K, et al. Detection of c-K-ras mutations in fine needle aspirates from human pancreatic adenocarcinomas. Cancer Res 1990;50:1279-83.

276. Silverman DT, Hoover RN, Brown LM, et al. Why do black Americans have a higher risk of pancreatic cancer than white Americans? Epidemiology 2003;14:45-54.

277. Silverman DT, Schiffman M, Everhart J, et al. Diabetes mellitus, other medical conditions and familial history of cancer as risk factors for pancreatic cancer. Br J Cancer 1999;80:1830-7.

278. Sohn TA, Yeo CJ, Cameron JL, et al. Resected adenocarcinoma of the pancreas-616 patients: results, outcome, and prognostic indications. J Gastrointest Surg 2000;4:567-79.

279. Solcia E, Capella C, Klöppel G. Tumors of the pancreas. AFIP tlas of Tumor Pathology, 3rd Series, Fascicle 20. Washington, DC: American Registry of Pathology; 1997.

280. Solinas-Toldo S, Wallrapp C, Muller-Pillasch F, Bentz M, Gress TM, Lichter P. Mapping of chromosomal imbalances in pancreatic carcinoma by comparative genomic hybridization. Cancer Res 1996;56:3803-7.

281. Sperti C, Pasquali C, Pedrazzoli S. Ductal adenocarcinoma of the body and tail of the pancreas. J Am Coll Surg 1997;185:255-9.

281a. Stelow EB, Adams RB, Moskaluk CA. The prevalence of pancreatic intraepithelial neoplasia in pancreata with uncommon types of primary neoplasms. Am J Surg Pathol 2006;30:36-41.

282. Stevens PD, Lightdale CJ. The role of endosonography in the diagnosis and management of pancreatic cancer. Surg Oncol Clin N Am 1998;7:125-33.

283. Stolzenberg-Solomon RZ, Albanes D, Nieto FJ, et al. Pancreatic cancer risk and nutrition-related methyl-group availability indicators in male smokers. J Natl Cancer Inst 1999;91:535-41.

284. Stolzenberg-Solomon RZ, Pietinen P, Barrett MJ, Taylor PR, Virtamo J, Albanes D. Dietary and other methyl-group availability factors and pancreatic cancer risk in a cohort of male smokers. Am J Epidemiol 2001;153:680-7.

285. Su GH, Bansal RK, Murphy KM, et al. ACVR1B (ALK4, activin receptor type 1B) gene mutation in pancreatic carcinoma. Proc Natl Acad Sci U S A 2001;98:3254-7.

286. Su GH, Hilgers W, Shekher M, et al. Alterations in pancreatic, biliary, and breast carcinomas support MKK4 as a genetically targeted tumor-suppressor gene. Cancer Res 1998;58:2339-42.

287. Su GH, Hruban RH, Bova GS, et al. Germline and somatic mutations of the STK11/LKB1 Peutz-Jeghers gene in pancreatic and biliary cancers. Am J Pathol 1999;154:1835-40.

288. Suehara N, Mizumoto K, Muta T, et al. Telomerase elevation in pancreatic ductal carcinoma compared to nonmalignant pathological states. Clin Cancer Res 1997;3:993-8.

289. Suehara N, Mizumoto K, Tanaka M, et al. Telomerase activity in pancreatic juice differentiates ductal carcinoma from adenoma and pancreatitis. Clin Cancer Res 1997;3:2479-83.

290. Suriawinata A, Klimstra DS. Distinguishing bile duct adenoma, hamartoma and ductular proliferation from metastatic pancreatic adenocarcinoma in the liver by immunohistochemistry. Mod Pathol 2002;15:294A.

291. Swartz MJ, Batra SK, Varshney GC, et al. MUC4 expression increases progressively in pancreatic intraepithelial neoplasia. Am J Clin Pathol 2002;117:791-6.

292. Swierczynski SL, Maitra A, Abraham SC, et al. Analysis of novel tumor markers in pancreatic and biliary carcinomas using tissue microarrays. Hum Pathol 2004;35:357-66.

293. Takahashi S, Hasebe T, Oda T, et al. Extra-tumor perineural invasion predicts postoperative development of peritoneal dissemination in pancreatic ductal adenocarcinoma. Anticancer Res 2001;21:1407-12.

294. Takahashi T, Ishikura H, Kato H, Tanabe T, Yoshiki T. Intra-pancreatic, extra-tumoral perineural invasion (nex). An indicator for the presence of retroperitoneal neural plexus invasion by pancreas carcinoma. Acta Pathol Jpn 1992;42:99-103.

295. Takahashi T, Ishikura H, Motohara T, Okushiba S, Dohke M, Katoh H. Perineural invasion by ductal adenocarcinoma of the pancreas. J Surg Oncol 1997;65:164-70.

296. Takaori K, Matsusue S, Fujikawa T, et al. Carcinoma in situ of the pancreas associated with localized fibrosis: a clue to early detection of neoplastic lesions arising from pancreatic ducts. Pancreas 1998;17:102-5.

297. Tang RF, Itakura J, Aikawa T, et al. Over-expression of lymphangiogenic growth factor VEGF-C in human pancreatic cancer. Pancreas 2001;22:285-92.

298. Tascilar M, Offerhaus GJ, Altink R, et al. Immunohistochemical labeling for the Dpc4 gene product is a specific marker for adenocarcinoma in biopsy specimens of the pancreas and bile duct. Am J Clin Pathol 2001;116:831-7.

299. Tascilar M, Skinner HG, Rosty C, et al. The SMAD4 protein and prognosis of pancreatic ductal adenocarcinoma. Clin Cancer Res 2001; 7:4115-21.

300. Teng DH, Perry WL, Hogan JK, et al. Human mitogen-activated protein kinase kinase 4 as a candidate tumor suppressor. Cancer Res 1997;57:4177-82.

301. Terhune PG, Phifer DM, Tosteson TD, Longnecker DS. K-ras mutation in focal proliferative lesions of human pancreas. Cancer Epidemiol Biomarkers Prev 1998;7:515-21.

302. Tersmette AC, Petersen GM, Offerhaus GJ, et al. Increased risk of incident pancreatic cancer among first-degree relatives of patients with familial pancreatic cancer. Clin Cancer Res 2001;7:738-44.

303. Tezel E, Kawase Y, Takeda S, Oshima K, Nakao A. Expression of neural cell adhesion molecule in pancreatic cancer. Pancreas 2001;22:122-5.

304. Thompson D, Easton DF. Cancer Incidence in BRCA1 mutation carriers. J Natl Cancer Inst 2002;94:1358-65.

305. Thompson LD, Heffess CS. Renal cell carcinoma to the pancreas in surgical pathology material. Cancer 2000;89:1076-88.

306. Thorban S, Roder JD, Pantel K, Siewert JR. Immunocytochemical detection of isolated epithelial tumor cells in bone marrow of patients with pancreatic carcinoma. Am J Surg 1996;172:297-8.

307. Thorlacius S, Olafsdottir GH, Tryggvadottir L, et al. A single BRCA2 mutation in male and female breast cancer families from Iceland with varied cancer phenotypes. Nat Genet 1996;13: 117-9.

308. Tryka AF, Brooks JR. Histopathology in the evaluation of total pancreatectomy for ductal carcinoma. Ann Surg 1979;190:373-81.

309. Tucker ON, Dannenberg AJ, Yang EK, et al. Cyclooxygenase-2 expression is up-regulated in human pancreatic cancer. Cancer Res 1999;59:987-90.

310. Ueki T, Toyota M, Skinner H, et al. Identification and characterization of differentially methylated CpG islands in pancreatic carcinoma. Cancer Res 2001;61:8540-6.

311. Ueki T, Toyota M, Sohn TA, et al. Hypermethylation of multiple genes in pancreatic adenocarcinoma. Cancer Res 2000;60:1835-9.

312. Valls C, Andia E, Sanchez A, et al. Dual-phase helical CT of pancreatic adenocarcinoma: assessment of resectability before surgery. AJR Am J Roentgenol 2002;178:821-6.

313. van der Heijden MS, Brody JR, Gallmeier E, et al. Functional defects in the Fanconi anemia pathway in pancreatic cancer cells. Am J Pathol 2004;165:651-7.

314. van der Heijden MS, Yeo CJ, Hruban RH, Kern SE. Fanconi anemia gene mutations in young-onset pancreatic cancer. Cancer Res 2003;63: 2585-8.

315. van Heek NT, Meeker AK, Kern SE, et al. Telomere shortening is nearly universal in pancreatic intraepithelial neoplasia. Am J Pathol 2002;161:1541-7.

316. van Heek NT, Tascilar M, van Beekveld JL, Drillenburg P, Offerhaus GJ, Gouma DJ. Micrometastases in bone marrow of patients with suspected pancreatic and ampullary cancer. Eur J Surg Oncol 2001;27:740-5.

317. van Heek T, Rader AE, Offerhaus GJ, et al. K-ras, p53, and DPC4 (MAD4) alterations in fine-needle aspirates of the pancreas: a molecular panel correlates with and supplements cytologic diagnosis. Am J Clin Pathol 2002;117: 755-65.

318. Vasen HF, Gruis NA, Frants RR, van der Velden PA, Hille ET, Bergman W. Risk of developing pancreatic cancer in families with familial atypical multiple mole melanoma associated with a specific 19 deletion of p16 (p16-Leiden). Int J Cancer 2000;87:809-11.

319. Vimalachandran D, Greenhalf W, Thompson C, et al. High nuclear S100A6 (Calcyclin) is significantly associated with poor survival in pancreatic cancer patients. Cancer Res 2005;65: 3218-25.

320. Wallrapp C, Müeller-Pillasch F, Solinas-Toldo S, et al. Characterization of a high copy number amplification at 6q24 in pancreatic cancer identifies c-myb as a candidate oncogene. Cancer Res 1997;57:3135-9.

321. Weiland LH. Frozen section diagnosis in tumors of the pancreas. Semin Diagn Pathol 1984;1:54-8.

322. Weir M, Pitman MB. The vascular architecture of renal cell carcinoma in fine-needle aspiration biopsies. An aid in its distinction from hepatocellular carcinoma. Cancer 1997;81:45-50.

323. Whipple AO, Parsons WB, Mullins CR. Treatment of carcinoma of the ampulla of Vater. Ann Surg 1935;102:763-79.

324. Wilentz RE, Geradts J, Maynard R, et al. Inactivation of the p16 (INK4A) tumor-suppressor gene in pancreatic duct lesions: loss of intranuclear expression. Cancer Res 1998;58:4740-4.

325. Wilentz RE, Goggins M, Redston M, et al. Genetic, immunohistochemical, and clinical features of medullary carcinoma of the pancreas: a newly described and characterized entity. Am J Pathol 2000;156:1641-51.

326. Wilentz RE, Iacobuzio-Donahue CA, Argani P, et al. Loss of expression of Dpc4 in pancreatic intraepithelial neoplasia: evidence that DPC4 inactivation occurs late in neoplastic progression. Cancer Res 2000;60:2002-6.

327. Wilentz RE, Su GH, Dai JL, et al. Immunohistochemical labeling for Dpc4 mirrors genetic status in pancreatic adenocarcinomas: a new marker of DPC4 inactivation. Am J Pathol 2000;156:37-43.

328. Yamamoto H, Itoh F, Iku S, et al. Expression of matrix metalloproteinases and tissue inhibitors of metalloproteinases in human pancreatic adenocarcinomas: clinicopathologic and prognostic significance of matrilysin expression. J Clin Oncol 2001;19:1118-27.

329. Yamamoto H, Itoh F, Nakamura H, et al. Genetic and clinical features of human pancreatic ductal adenocarcinomas with widespread microsatellite instability. Cancer Res 2001;61:3139-44.

330. Yamanaka S, Sunamura M, Furukawa T, et al. Chromosome 12, frequently deleted in human pancreatic cancer, may encode a tumor-suppressor gene that suppresses angiogenesis. Lab Invest 2004;84:1339-51.

331. Yamano M, Fujii H, Takagaki T, Kadowaki N, Watanabe H, Shirai T. Genetic progression and divergence in pancreatic carcinoma. Am J Pathol 2000;156:2123-33.

332. Yamasaki S, Suda K, Nobukawa B, Sonoue H. Intraductal spread of pancreatic cancer. Clinicopathologic study of 54 pancreatectomized patients. Pancreatology 2002;2:407-12.

333. Yen TW, Aardal NP, Bronner MP, et al. Myofibroblasts are responsible for the desmoplastic reaction surrounding human pancreatic carcinomas. Surgery 2002;131:129-34.

334. Yeo CJ, Abrams RA, Grochow LB, et al. Pancreaticoduodenectomy for pancreatic adenocarcinoma: postoperative adjuvant chemoradiation improves survival. A prospective, single-institution experience. Ann Surg 1997;225:621-33.

335. Yeo CJ, Cameron JL, Lillemoe KD, et al. Pancreaticoduodenectomy for cancer of the head of the pancreas. 201 patients. Ann Surg 1995;221:721-33.

336. Yeo CJ, Cameron JL, Sohn TA, et al. Six hundred fifty consecutive pancreaticoduodenectomies in the 1990s: pathology, complications, and outcomes. Ann Surg 1997;226:248-57.

337. Yeo CJ, Sohn TA, Cameron JL, Hruban RH, Lillemoe KD, Pitt HA. Periampullary adenocarcinoma: analysis of 5-year survivors. Ann Surg 1998;227:821-31.

338. Young RH, Hart WR. Metastases from carcinomas of the pancreas simulating primary mucinous tumors of the ovary. A report of seven cases. Am J Surg Pathol 1989;13:748-56.

339. Yousef GM, Borgono CA, Popalis C, et al. In-silico analysis of kallikrein gene expression in pancreatic and colon cancers. Anticancer Res 2004;24:43-51.

340. Zamboni G, Klöppel G, Hruban RH, Longnecker DS, Adler G. Mucinous cystic neoplasms of the pancreas. In: Hamilton SR, Aaltonen LA, eds. World Health Organization Classification of Tumours. Pathology and genetics of tumours of the digestive system. Lyon: IARCPress; 2000:234-6.

341. Zhou W, Sokoll LJ, Bruzek DJ, et al. Identifying markers for pancreatic cancer by gene expression analysis. Cancer Epidemiol Biomarkers Prev 1998;7:109-12.

342. Zhu Z, Friess H, diMola FF, et al. Nerve growth factor expression correlates with perineural invasion and pain in human pancreatic cancer. J Clin Oncol 1999;17:2419-28.

8 ADENOCARCINOMA VARIANTS

Although over 90 percent of carcinomas of the pancreas are ductal adenocarcinomas with conventional tubular morphology, rare variants of adenocarcinoma are important to recognize because, depending on the type, they can confer a significantly better or worse prognosis than conventional ductal adenocarcinoma. For example, colloid and medullary carcinomas of the pancreas are associated with a better prognosis, while the adenosquamous and undifferentiated carcinomas confer a worse prognosis. In addition, the study of variants of adenocarcinoma has shed light on the mechanisms underlying the development of pancreatic neoplasia. For example, the characterization of hepatoid carcinomas of the pancreas has demonstrated that the direction of differentiation of a neoplasm cannot be equated with the cell of origin. The following sections describe seven variants of adenocarcinoma of the pancreas. These include adenosquamous carcinoma, colloid carcinoma, hepatoid carcinoma, medullary carcinoma, signet ring cell carcinoma, undifferentiated carcinoma, and undifferentiated carcinoma with osteoclast-like giant cells.

ADENOSQUAMOUS CARCINOMA

Definition. *Adenosquamous carcinoma* is a malignant epithelial neoplasm of the pancreas with significant components of both glandular and squamous differentiation (39,44,68). The squamous component should comprise at least 30 percent of the neoplasm.

General Features. The first recognized report of an adenosquamous carcinoma of the pancreas was by G. Herxheimer in 1907 (29). He used the term *cancroide;* today close to 200 adenosquamous carcinomas have been reported under a variety of names including *adenoacanthoma, adenocarcinoma with squamous metaplasia,* and *mucoepidermoid carcinoma.* Adenosquamous carcinoma is the preferred term because both components are malignant. A few cases of pure squamous cell carcinoma of the pancreas have

been reported in which there are no glandular elements (2), but when thoroughly sampled, most primary pancreatic neoplasms with a predominantly squamous appearance prove to have focal glandular differentiation (and thus represent adenosquamous carcinomas). Adenosquamous carcinomas are important to recognize for two reasons. First, they need to be distinguished from squamous cell carcinoma metastatic to the pancreas, and second, patients appear to have a very poor prognosis, few surviving beyond 1 year.

Adenosquamous carcinomas have not been associated with any specific clinical syndromes, although a squamous cell carcinoma of the pancreas has been reported in a patient with the familial atypical multiple mole melanoma (FAMMM) syndrome associated with a germline *p16/CDKN2A* gene mutation (77). A case of an adenosquamous carcinoma arising in association with a mucinous cystic neoplasm has also been reported (11).

Clinical Features. Adenosquamous carcinomas account for 3 to 4 percent of the malignancies of the exocrine pancreas (36,49). The clinical presentation and gross appearance of adenosquamous carcinomas are similar to those of conventional ductal adenocarcinomas. Most patients present with weight loss, anorexia, painless jaundice, abdominal discomfort, or back pain. A single patient had an elevated serum calcium level secondary to the ectopic production of parathyroid hormone-releasing protein by an adenosquamous carcinoma of the pancreas (35). The mean age at diagnosis is 63 years (range, 28 to 86), and men slightly outnumber women, with a male to female ratio of 1.5 to 1.0 (41,49).

Gross Findings. Most adenosquamous carcinomas arise in the head of the pancreas; however, they can also arise in the body or the tail, or even diffusely involve the entire gland. In one study they constituted 23.5 percent of carcinomas arising in the pancreatic tail (9). Adenosquamous carcinomas are large (mean,

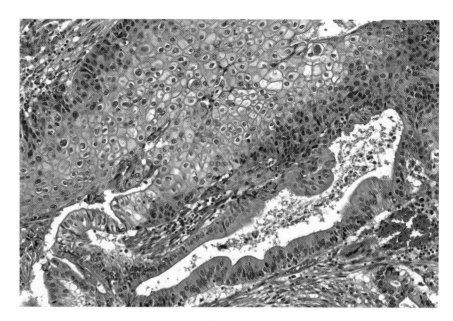

Figure 8-1

ADENOSQUAMOUS CARCINOMA

Both glandular and squamous differentiation are present.

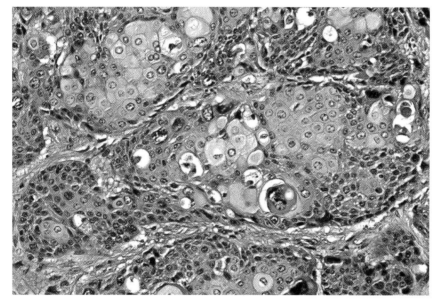

Figure 8-2

ADENOSQUAMOUS CARCINOMA

There is prominent squamous differentiation with keratin pearls.

about 6 cm), firm, poorly defined, tan to yellow masses; they can be cystic.

Microscopic Findings. Two neoplastic components are present on light microscopic examination (fig. 8-1). The adenocarcinoma component resembles a conventional ductal adenocarcinoma. This component can be variably differentiated, with infiltrating columnar to cuboidal cells showing glandular differentiation including extracellular and intracellular mucin production. Goblet cells may also be present and are highlighted by histochemical stains for mucins. The squamous component, if it is kera-

tinizing, is composed of nests of large polygonal cells with opaque eosinophilic cytoplasm (fig. 8-2). Nonkeratinizing squamous differentiation is recognized by the sheet-like and often swirling arrangement of the neoplastic squamous cells. Intercellular bridges are present, and, in the well-differentiated areas, there are keratohyaline granules and squamous pearls.

The two components can be intimately admixed, or they can be topographically separate within the neoplasm. Intermediate cells, of the type seen in mucoepidermoid carcinoma of the salivary gland, are not seen. The squamous

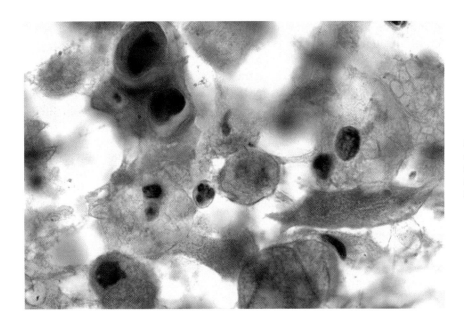

Figure 8-3

ADENOSQUAMOUS CARCINOMA

This aspirate smear demonstrates both a malignant squamous component (upper left) and a malignant glandular component (lower right) (direct smear; Papanicolaou stain).

component may predominate, to the extent that some adenosquamous carcinomas appear to consist solely of squamous elements. Thorough sampling, along with staining for mucin, generally reveals at least focal glandular differentiation. Any glandular differentiation is sufficient to designate the neoplasm as an adenosquamous carcinoma, and the term *squamous cell carcinoma* should only be applied if no glandular elements or mucin production is detected (2). Although definitions vary, the squamous component should comprise at least 30 percent of the neoplasm. This somewhat arbitrary cut-off avoids designating adenocarcinomas with only trivial squamous differentiation as adenosquamous carcinomas, and, as discussed later, has prognostic significance. In some cases, the squamous component occupies the leading edge of the neoplasm, while the glandular component predominates in most metastases (36). A mucicarmine stain will highlight the glandular component.

Immunohistochemical Findings. The immunohistochemical labeling pattern of adenosquamous carcinoma is similar to that of ductal adenocarcinoma. Most express carcinoembryonic antigen (CEA), epithelial membrane antigen (EMA), cytokeratins (AE1/AE3, CAM5.2 [CK8, CK18, and CK19], and CK1, CK7, CK8, CK18, and CK19), and carbohydrate antigen (CA) 19-9 (41,82). The two components of the neoplasm show distinctive labeling patterns. Antibodies to CK5/6, CK13, and CD44(s) pre-

dominantly label the squamous component, while the expression of CK7 and CK20 is often restricted to the glandular elements, as is labeling for CA19-9 and B72.3 (2,41).

Ultrastructural Findings. Electron microscopy confirms both directions of differentiation. The neoplastic cells with glandular differentiation have basal lamina, abundant endoplasmic reticulum, well-developed Golgi complexes, and secretory vesicles (45). By contrast, the neoplastic cells with squamous differentiation have scant endoplasmic reticulum, prominent aggregates of tonofilaments, and well-formed desmosomes.

Cytologic Findings. The two malignant cellular components of adenosquamous carcinoma are recognized in aspirate smears. When both the glandular and squamous components are prominent (fig. 8-3), the diagnosis is straightforward. If, however, either component comprises a minority of the cellular material in the biopsy sample, the diagnosis can be challenging (59). A careful search for glandular differentiation is warranted when the squamous component predominates, particularly given the virtual nonexistence of primary squamous cell carcinoma of the pancreas.

Molecular and Other Special Techniques. Not much is known about the molecular alterations in adenosquamous carcinomas. Most of these neoplasms have activating point mutations in codon 12 of the *KRAS* gene, and the majority are aneuploid (41,49).

Differential Diagnosis. The most important lesion to consider in the differential diagnosis of adenosquamous carcinoma of the pancreas is a metastatic squamous cell carcinoma from another organ. Pure squamous cell carcinomas of the pancreas are extremely rare. A clinical history of an extrapancreatic squamous cell carcinoma and the absence of glandular differentiation should raise the suspicion that a lesion is a metastasis to the pancreas and not a pancreatic primary. Pancreatoblastomas have squamoid nests and may contain glandular elements, but they have a predominant acinar component that labels immunohistochemically for exocrine pancreatic enzymes.

Staging. The staging of adenosquamous carcinomas should follow the staging of carcinomas of the exocrine pancreas (see chapter 3).

Prognosis. Adenosquamous carcinoma of the pancreas is an extremely aggressive neoplasm. Most patients have metastases at the time of diagnosis, and even most resectable carcinomas will have perineural invasion, lymphatic invasion, and lymph node metastases (41,49). The adenocarcinoma component, the squamous component, or both can be found in metastases; however, most metastases contain only the adenocarcinoma component. The median survival period is only 6 months, and few patients survive beyond a year (37,41,49,59,79). Even patients with surgically resectable neoplasms do poorly, with a mean survival of 11 months in one series.

COLLOID CARCINOMA
(MUCINOUS NONCYSTIC CARCINOMA)

Definition. *Colloid carcinoma* of the pancreas is an infiltrating adenocarcinoma characterized by the presence of mucin-producing neoplastic epithelial cells suspended ("floating") in large pools of extracellular mucin (39,44,68). Elements of conventional tubular adenocarcinoma may also be present, but the colloid component should comprise at least 80 percent of the neoplasm (6). The World Health Organization (WHO) classification uses the designation *mucinous noncystic carcinoma* for these neoplasms. We feel this term is too easily confused with mucinous cystic neoplasm, and could lead to the awkward diagnosis of "mucinous noncystic carcinoma arising in association with a mucinous cystic neoplasm." We prefer to use the more distinct and simpler term, colloid carcinoma. Other names for colloid carcinoma include *gelatinous carcinoma* and *pure mucinous carcinoma.*

The term mucinous adenocarcinoma often has been applied to ductal adenocarcinomas that exhibit abundant intracellular or luminal mucin accumulation. Although such neoplasms are indeed mucin-producing, the neoplastic cells are not suspended in large stromal mucin pools. These neoplasms do not have the more favorable prognosis associated with colloid carcinomas, and they are properly classified as conventional tubular-type ductal adenocarcinomas (most of which do produce mucin).

General Features. Colloid carcinomas are relatively rare, accounting for 1 to 3 percent of the malignancies of the exocrine pancreas. The average age at diagnosis is 65 years (range, 35 to 78 years), and 55 percent arise in men (6,63).

Clinical Features. Presenting manifestations include abdominal pain, diarrhea and light stools, jaundice, weight loss, and pancreatitis (6). Several patients with colloid carcinomas have developed migratory thrombophlebitis (Trousseau's syndrome) and some have died of thromboembolism, all of whom had undergone incisional (open) biopsies of the neoplasm (6). Computerized tomography (CT) scans usually demonstrate a well-demarcated low attenuation mass (fig. 8-4).

The majority of colloid carcinomas arise in the head of the gland, but occasional cases have been reported in the body or tail. When carefully examined, almost all colloid carcinomas of the pancreas can be shown to arise in association with an intraductal papillary mucinous neoplasm (IPMN) (63). The association with IPMN may explain the propensity of colloid carcinoma to arise in the head of the pancreas. A case of a mucinous cystic neoplasm in which the invasive component was a colloid carcinoma has also been reported (6).

Gross Findings. Colloid carcinomas are larger, on average, than infiltrating ductal (tubular) adenocarcinomas of the pancreas (6). The mean size of surgically resected colloid carcinomas is 4.5 cm (range, 1 to 16 cm). On cross section they are usually well-demarcated and have a soft gelatinous appearance (figs. 8-5, 8-6). Usually the mucin is thick and tenacious, and is retained in the stroma when incised, in

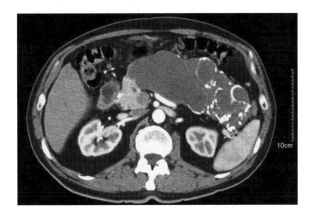

Figure 8-4

COLLOID CARCINOMA

Computerized tomography (CT) scan of a large colloid carcinoma. The low attenuation mass replaces almost the full length of the pancreas and is associated with circular calcifications. (Courtesy of Dr. S. S. Siegelman, Baltimore, MD.) (Figs. 8-4 and 8-5 are from the same patient.)

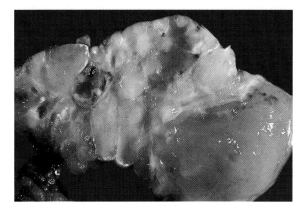

Figure 8-5

COLLOID CARCINOMA

Cross section of a large colloid carcinoma shows large gelatinous areas.

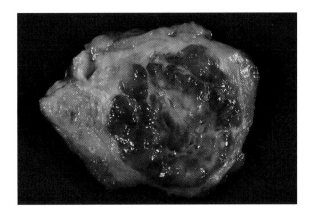

Figure 8-6

COLLOID CARCINOMA

Gelatinous colloid carcinoma in the head of the pancreas.

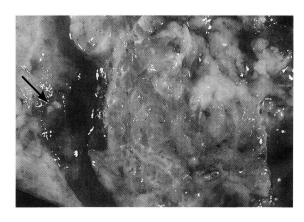

Figure 8-7

COLLOID CARCINOMA

This example arose in association with an intraductal papillary mucinous neoplasm (arrow).

contrast to the thinner secretions within the cysts of mucinous cystic neoplasms. True cysts are not commonly found within colloid carcinomas. Careful gross examination of the adjacent pancreatic tissue often reveals dilated ducts filled with papillary masses, characteristic of an associated noninvasive IPMN (fig. 8-7).

Microscopic Findings. Colloid carcinomas are composed of large pools of extracellular mucin in connective tissue stroma, an appearance that has been referred to as a "muconodular growth pattern." The neoplastic mucin-produc-

ing epithelial cells are suspended within these pools of mucin (fig. 8-8). The epithelial cells are usually well-differentiated and cuboidal to columnar; they often are present at the edges of the pools of mucin (fig. 8-9) and form clusters floating near the center of the mucin pools (fig. 8-8) (6). Signet ring cells can also be seen within the mucin pools. In some cases, the neoplastic epithelial cells form strips that incompletely line the periphery of the mucin pools. Perineural invasion and lymphatic invasion are seen (fig. 8-10), but are not as common as in infiltrating ductal adenocarcinomas (6).

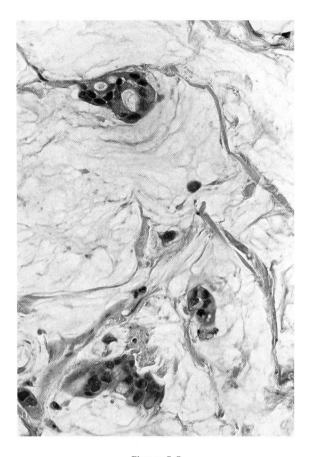

Figure 8-8

COLLOID CARCINOMA

Neoplastic epithelium is suspended in large pools of extracellular mucin.

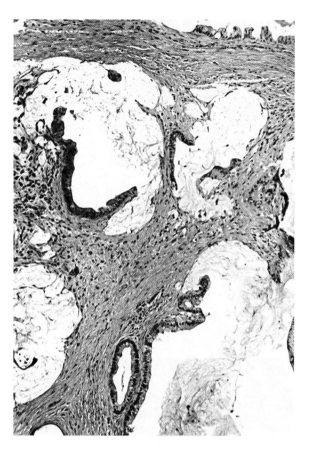

Figure 8-9

COLLOID CARCINOMA

The neoplastic epithelial cells rim the large pools of extracellular mucin.

As noted earlier, most colloid carcinomas arise in association with an IPMN, and these IPMNs usually have significant dysplasia (IPMN with carcinoma in situ) (63). Almost all of these IPMNs exhibit intestinal-type papillae, although a rare colloid carcinoma is associated with pancreatobiliary-type IPMN or intraductal oncocytic papillary neoplasms (see chapter 6) (1,3).

Colloid differentiation in an invasive carcinoma can be focal or extensive. A more favorable prognosis is associated with colloid differentiation of 80 percent or more and, therefore, the designation of a colloid carcinoma should be reserved for those neoplasms in which 80 percent or more of the infiltrating carcinoma shows colloid differentiation (6).

Special stains are usually not needed to establish a diagnosis. When performed, however, they confirm the presence of copious amounts of in-tracellular and extracellular mucin. Mucicarmine and Alcian blue stains are strongly positive, and the high iron diamine stain turns the mucin blue, suggesting that it is acidic-sialated mucin (6).

Immunohistochemical Findings. Immunohistochemical labeling is strongly positive for cytokeratin, CEA, CA19-9, MUC2, and CDX2 (6). By contrast, labeling for MUC1 is negative in most cases. MUC2 and CDX2 are also expressed in intestinal-type IPMNs, suggesting that both the preinvasive and the invasive components of these neoplasms have intestinal differentiation (4). Scattered neuroendocrine cells within the neoplastic epithelium label for chromogranin or synaptophysin.

Ultrastructural Findings. By electron microscopy, the cells of colloid carcinomas appear to have abnormal polarity (5). Mucin secretory vacuoles are found at the stroma-facing (basal)

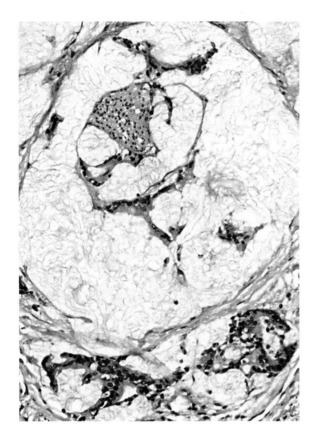

Figure 8-10

COLLOID CARCINOMA

The presence of perineural invasion establishes that this is an invasive carcinoma.

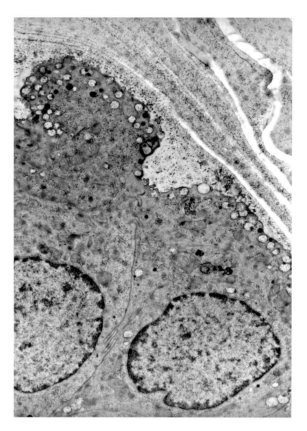

Figure 8-11

COLLOID CARCINOMA

Electron micrograph shows polarization of the neoplastic cells towards the stroma.

surface of the cells (fig. 8-11), explaining the accumulation of mucin between the cells and the fibrous stroma. It has been speculated that this mucin, which contains abundant MUC2, may act as a containment factor, limiting the spread of the carcinoma and contributing to its relatively favorable prognosis (see below) (5,47).

Cytologic Findings. The features of the neoplasm on aspiration cytology are similar to those of IPMN and mucinous cystic neoplasm (see chapters 5 and 6) as well as the cytologic appearance of colloid carcinomas of other sites, such as the breast. Thick viscous mucin, with or without an identifiable epithelial component, is obtained. The issue of gastrointestinal contamination should not be of concern given the abundance of mucin characteristic of colloid carcinoma. Recognition of malignant cells in the thick "colloid-like" mucin is necessary for the diagnosis of a malignant mucin-producing

neoplasm. The correlation of the cytologic findings with the clinical and radiologic features determines whether the mass is associated with a cyst and the exact location of the biopsy, e.g., a biopsy of the cyst contents versus a biopsy of a mass in the wall of a cyst.

Molecular and Other Special Techniques. The genetic alterations identified to date in colloid carcinomas are similar to those identified in conventional infiltrating ductal adenocarcinomas, but they occur at a lower prevalence. One third of colloid carcinomas harbor activating point mutations in codon 12 of the *KRAS* oncogene, and a quarter have inactivating *TP53* gene mutations (6). The vast majority are microsatellite stable, and have intact expression of the DNA mismatch repair proteins MLH1, MSH2, and MSH6 (48). The expression of Dpc4 is intact in almost all cases (33). A fraction of colloid carcinomas harbor mutations in the

171

PIK3CA gene (A. Maitra, Baltimore, MD; personal communication).

Differential Diagnosis. Colloid carcinomas should be distinguished from mucinous cystic neoplasms. Most colloid carcinomas are not grossly cystic, although the associated IPMN component may appear as a cyst. Mucinous cystic neoplasms almost always arise in women, and by definition, have a distinctive ovarian-type stroma not found in colloid carcinomas. Confusion can arise when the invasive component of a mucinous cystic neoplasm shows colloid differentiation. In these cases we prefer to designate each component separately: "invasive well-differentiated colloid carcinoma (3 cm) arising in association with a mucinous cystic neoplasm with high-grade dysplasia (5 cm)."

Colloid carcinomas also need to be distinguished from mucin extravasated from a noninvasive IPMN. Mucin extravasated from an IPMN produces mucous lakes without suspended neoplastic cells and is usually located in the periductal stroma, while the pools of mucin containing neoplastic epithelial cells in colloid carcinomas are in a location incompatible with the normal ductal system (fig. 8-10). Extravasated mucin due to ductal rupture often elicits an intense inflammatory reaction, whereas the mucin of colloid carcinomas dissects through the stroma without inducing inflammation.

Staging. The staging of colloid carcinomas should follow the staging of carcinomas of the exocrine pancreas (see chapter 3).

Prognosis. When a cut-off of 80 percent or more of mucinous noncystic differentiation for the invasive carcinoma is used, the prognosis for patients with surgically resected colloid carcinomas is significantly better than for patients with surgically resected infiltrating ductal adenocarcinomas. In one series, the 2- and 5-year survival rates for patients with surgically resected colloid carcinomas were 70 and 57 percent, compared to only 28 and 12 percent for a comparable group of patients with infiltrating ductal adenocarcinomas (6). The survival rates for patients with colloid carcinomas are remarkable considering that the resected colloid carcinomas in this series were larger than the infiltrating ductal adenocarcinomas; also, 40 percent of those alive without disease had lymph node metastases and another 40 percent had perineural or vascular invasion at the time of surgical resection. One patient developed pseudomyxoma peritonei as a complication of a colloid carcinoma (12).

HEPATOID CARCINOMA

Definition. *Hepatoid carcinoma* of the pancreas is a malignant epithelial neoplasm in which a significant component shows hepatocellular differentiation. Only a handful of neoplasms with hepatocellular differentiation have been reported in the pancreas (16,31,57,58,81). As is true in other gastrointestinal organs, these neoplasms usually also have areas with a more common direction of differentiation, particularly ductal adenocarcinoma. Thus, although the term hepatoid carcinoma is applied to these neoplasms, it is probably more informative to describe all of the directions of differentiation in the neoplasm (e.g., invasive carcinoma with hepatocellular and ductal differentiation).

Gross Findings. These neoplasms are grossly nondescript. Most are large, infiltrative, and gray-white to yellow (31,32,81). Some hepatoid carcinomas are tan to red-brown, and some even have a green hue (fig. 8-12).

Microscopic Findings. Well-differentiated hepatoid carcinomas are composed of large polygonal cells with abundant eosinophilic cytoplasm (fig. 8-13). The cells form trabeculae and may even have a sinusoidal vascularity. Nuclei tend to be centrally placed and nucleoli are prominent. Bile production has been described and can be highlighted with a bile stain such as the Hall bile stain (Fouchet reagent) (16, 57). Periodic acid–Schiff (PAS)-positive, diastase-resistant, intracytoplasmic hyaline globules are sometimes present (57). Less well-differentiated hepatoid carcinomas are composed of haphazardly arranged pleomorphic cells.

Immunohistochemical Findings. Immunohistochemical labeling for hepatocyte paraffin-1 (Hep Par-1), polyclonal CEA, CD10, and alpha-fetoprotein can help establish the presence of hepatocellular differentiation (fig. 8-14) (16, 57,81). Polyclonal CEA and CD10 produce a canalicular pattern of labeling in some cases.

Other directions of differentiation reported in hepatoid carcinomas include ductal differentiation with gland formation and mucin production, acinar differentiation with lipase

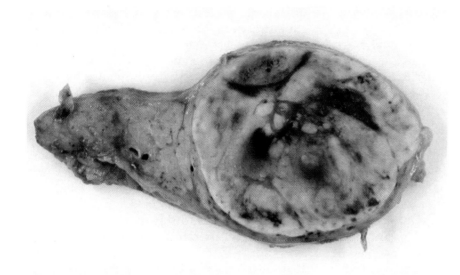

Figure 8-12

HEPATOID CARCINOMA

A relatively well-demarcated tan-brown mass with focal green hues. (Courtesy of Dr. J. Imura, Ibaraki, Japan.)

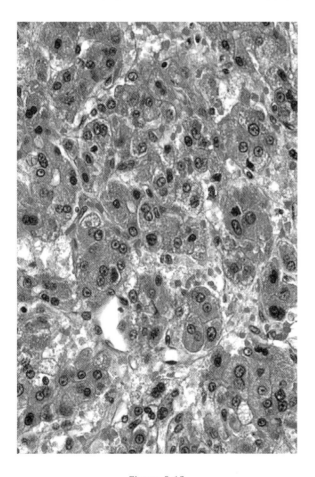

Figure 8-13

HEPATOID CARCINOMA

This example was composed of polygonal cells with abundant eosinophilic cytoplasm. (Courtesy of Dr. J. Imura, Ibaraki, Japan.)

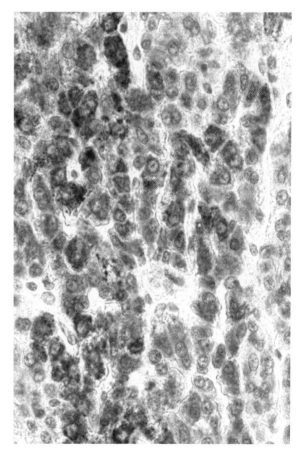

Figure 8-14

HEPATOID CARCINOMA

Immunolabeling for Hep Par-1. (Courtesy of Dr. J. Imura, Ibaraki, Japan.)

production, and endocrine differentiation with glucagon production.

Differential Diagnosis. The differential diagnosis should include metastases from a liver primary, germ cell neoplasms, acinar cell carcinomas, and pancreatoblastomas. Metastasis from a liver primary is best ruled out clinically; germ cell tumors may have trophoblastic elements or Schiller-Duval bodies; acinar cell carcinomas diffusely express lipase, trypsin, or chymotrypsin; and pancreatoblastoma is recognized by the presence of squamoid nests. Pancreatic neoplasms with acinar differentiation (both acinar cell carcinoma and pancreatoblastoma) can produce alpha-fetoprotein, sometimes resulting in markedly elevated serum levels (14). In addition, these neoplasms may contain polygonal cells with eosinophilic cytoplasm, resembling hepatocytes. Thus, the production of alpha-fetoprotein alone is not sufficient to qualify a pancreatic neoplasm as a hepatoid carcinoma if the neoplastic cells are acinar in nature.

Staging. The staging of hepatoid carcinoma should follow the staging of carcinomas of the exocrine pancreas (see chapter 3).

Prognosis. Too few pancreatic neoplasms with hepatocellular differentiation have been reported to make definitive comments on clinical outcome (57). Patients with extrapancreatic gastrointestinal hepatoid carcinomas tend to have a poor prognosis. When elevated, serum alpha-fetoprotein levels can be used to monitor response to therapy.

MEDULLARY CARCINOMA

Definition. *Medullary carcinoma* of the pancreas is a malignant epithelial neoplasm characterized by poor differentiation, well-defined borders, a syncytial growth pattern, and necrosis (24). This carcinoma was only recently recognized through a study of microsatellite instability in pancreatic carcinoma (24).

General Features. Medullary carcinomas are slightly more common in men than in women, and the average age at diagnosis is 68 years (24,78). The clinical presentation is similar to that of infiltrating ductal adenocarcinoma. Patients with medullary carcinomas of the pancreas are more likely to have a first-degree relative with cancer than are patients with conventional infiltrating ductal adenocarcinomas, al-

though the cancers are not necessarily pancreatic primaries (78). Some patients with medullary carcinoma of the pancreas have synchronous and metachronous colon carcinomas, and some of these patients presumably have the hereditary nonpolyposis colorectal cancer (HNPCC) syndrome (78,80).

Gross Findings. Grossly, medullary carcinomas are better circumscribed than most infiltrating ductal adenocarcinomas, and they are often softer. Indeed, the term "medullary" comes from the Latin "medulla" for center, and it has the connotation of soft.

Microscopic Findings. Four features characterize medullary carcinomas at the microscopic level (figs. 8-15, 8-16): they are poorly differentiated; they have pushing rather than infiltrating borders; they have a syncytial growth pattern in which individual cell borders are not distinct; and they usually have at least focal necrosis (24,78). In some reports, intratumoral lymphocytes are prominent. These histologic features are very similar to those of another neoplasm associated with microsatellite instability, medullary carcinoma of the colon. In contrast to medullary carcinoma of the colon, medullary carcinoma of the pancreas usually does not have a prominent Crohn-like lymphoid infiltrate, and there are no associated mucinous adenocarcinoma components. Molecular analyses have demonstrated that, in contrast to medullary carcinomas, most colloid (mucinous noncystic) carcinomas of the pancreas are microsatellite stable and have intact expression of the DNA mismatch repair proteins MLH1, MSH2, and HMSH6 (48). Special stains reveal rare intracytoplasmic mucin vacuoles in some cases.

Immunohistochemical Findings. Immunohistochemical labeling demonstrates the expression of cytokeratin, while immunolabeling for chromogranin, synaptophysin, lipase, chymotrypsin, and trypsin is usually negative. Immunolabeling for MLH1 and MSH2 reveals loss of expression of one of these DNA mismatch repair proteins in many of the cancers. Immunostains for lymphocytes highlight the presence of numerous intratumoral T lymphocytes (CD3 positive) in some cases. In situ hybridization for Epstein-Barr virus RNA was positive in a single medullary carcinoma with prominent lymphoepithelial features (78).

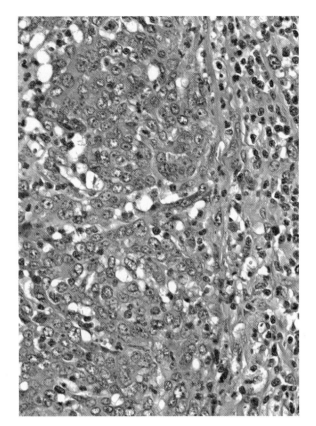

Figure 8-15

MEDULLARY CARCINOMA

Well-defined border and associated lymphocytes.

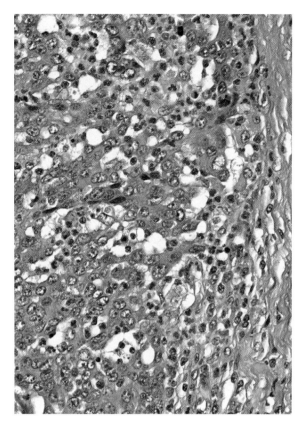

Figure 8-16

MEDULLARY CARCINOMA

Syncytial growth of poorly differentiated cells with a well-defined border.

Molecular and Other Special Techniques. As mentioned earlier, medullary carcinomas of the pancreas were first recognized because of their association with microsatellite instability. Goggins et al. (24) examined a series of 82 carcinomas of the pancreas using a panel of microsatellite markers and found that 3 of the 82 (4 percent) had microsatellite instability. These three had a medullary histology, and all had wild-type *KRAS* genes. Conversely, Wilentz et al. (78) showed that some, but not all, carcinomas with medullary histology have microsatellite instability (78). Microsatellite instability in medullary carcinomas in patients with HNPCC syndrome is caused by an inherited mutation in one of the mismatch repair genes (*MLH1, MSH2,* etc.), coupled with an acquired loss of the wild-type allele in the carcinoma (80). Microsatellite instability in sporadic medullary carcinomas is usually caused by somatic hyper-

methylation of the *MLH1* promoter (73). Inactivation of one of these DNA mismatch repair genes leads to mutations in polyadenine tracts in other genes. Mutations in polyadenine tracts in the activin A type II receptor (*ACVR2*) and transforming growth factor beta-receptor 2 (*TGFβR2*) genes have been demonstrated in medullary carcinomas of the pancreas (25,28). As noted earlier, most medullary carcinomas have wild-type *KRAS* genes; Calhoun et al. (10) identified mutations in another member of the KRAS pathway, the *BRAF* gene, in a third of *KRAS* wild-type pancreatic cancers, including medullary carcinomas.

The association of a histologically distinct pancreatic cancer with specific genetic abnormalities provides an opportunity for the diagnostic pathologist to suggest, based on morphologic findings, that a specific genetic pathway has been targeted in a carcinoma. Because the

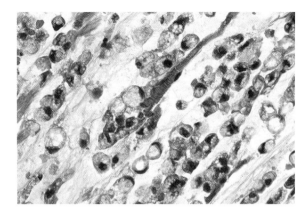

Figure 8-17
SIGNET RING CELL CARCINOMA
Noncohesive cells with intracellular mucin.

DNA mismatch repair pathway can be inactivated by inherited genetic alterations (HNPCC), genetic counseling may be indicated for patients with pancreatic medullary carcinoma (78).

Differential Diagnosis. The two entities to consider in the differential diagnosis are acinar cell carcinoma and poorly differentiated ductal adenocarcinoma. Acinar cell carcinoma can grow in solid sheets and, if poorly differentiated, can mimic medullary carcinoma (42). In these instances, immunolabeling for trypsin, MLH1, and MSH2 helps establish the diagnosis. Acinar cell carcinomas label with trypsin and show intact labeling for MLH1 and for MSH2, while medullary carcinomas do not label for trypsin and frequently show loss of either MLH1 or MSH2 expression. The borders of poorly differentiated ductal adenocarcinomas are more infiltrative and less well-defined than those of medullary carcinomas. The presence of necrosis and intratumoral lymphocytes suggests the diagnosis of medullary carcinoma.

Staging. The staging of medullary carcinoma should follow the staging of carcinomas of the exocrine pancreas (see chapter 3).

Treatment and Prognosis. Surgical resection is the treatment of choice for medullary carcinomas. Insufficient data are available on specific chemotherapies and radiation therapies. In some, but not all, of the early series of medullary carcinomas there was a trend towards longer survival in patients with medullary carcinoma of the pancreas as compared to patients with infiltrating ductal adenocarcinoma (24,78).

More recent larger series have shown that patients with surgically resected microsatellite unstable pancreatic cancers (not necessarily of medullary type) live a mean of 62 months compared to 10 months for patients with surgically resected ductal adenocarcinomas (53,54).

SIGNET RING CELL CARCINOMA

Definition. As the name suggests, *signet ring cell carcinoma* is a malignant epithelial neoplasm in which the predominant component is composed of infiltrating, round, noncohesive (isolated) cells containing intracytoplasmic mucin (39,44,68). Signet-ring cell carcinomas of the pancreas are very rare, with only a handful of case reports in the literature (13). A separate component of conventional tubular type ductal adenocarcinoma may be present; in fact, most pancreatic carcinomas with a signet ring cell component consist predominantly of ductal adenocarcinoma elements. It is recommended that at least half of the neoplasm consist of signet ring cells before that term is applied to a pancreatic neoplasm.

Pathologic Findings. Microscopically, signet ring cell carcinoma is characterized by small collections of cells or individual cells with abundant intracellular mucin (fig. 8-17). The multivacuolated mucin typically impinges on the nucleus, creating a scalloped indentation, which imparts the classic signet ring cell appearance. This feature of nuclear indentation by the cytoplasmic vacuole is helpful both histologically and cytologically (fig. 8-18) in separating what may be relatively bland-appearing malignant epithelial cells from histiocytes. Although the neoplastic cells may be associated with extracellular mucin, they do not form the large nodular pools of mucin seen in colloid (mucinous noncystic) carcinomas. Instead, signet ring cell carcinomas are much more infiltrative and linear groups of cells dissect between bands of collagen. Some cells lack obvious intracellular mucin but maintain the individual cell growth pattern, as seen in signet ring cell carcinomas of the stomach (Lauren's diffuse type of gastric adenocarcinoma).

Special stains for mucin are strongly positive, as is immunolabeling for cytokeratin and CEA (71). Dramatically elevated serum CEA levels have been reported in some patients (71).

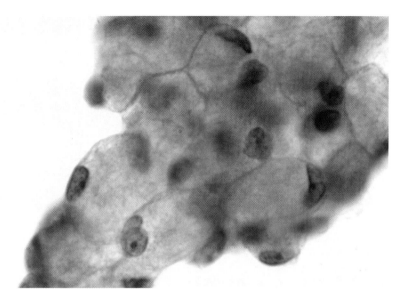

Figure 8-18

**SIGNET RING
CELL CARCINOMA**

Large cytoplasmic mucin vacuoles indent the hyperchromatic nuclei (direct smear; Papanicolaou stain).

Differential Diagnosis. The differential diagnosis for signet ring cell carcinoma of the pancreas is broad. Metastases to the pancreas from
a gastric or mammary primary are probably
more common than primary pancreatic signet
ring cell carcinoma and need to be ruled out
before the diagnosis of a pancreatic primary is
established.

An important primary pancreatic neoplasm
to exclude is colloid (mucinous noncystic) carcinoma. Colloid carcinomas often contain signet ring cells floating within large stromal mucin pools. In contrast to signet ring cell carcinomas, however, these neoplasms do not have
individual neoplastic cells infiltrating the
stroma, and the pools of extracellular mucin
also contain strips and cribriformed nests of
neoplastic glandular cells. In addition, most colloid carcinomas are associated with an intraductal papillary mucinous neoplasm, while signet ring cell carcinomas are not.

Other entities to consider in the differential
include well-differentiated pancreatic endocrine
neoplasm with rhabdoid features, acinar carcinoma with signet ring cell change, and signet
ring cell lymphoma (69). None of these neoplasms typically contain intracellular mucin (the
signet ring cell change being due to other accumulated cytoplasmic materials) and all have
highly characteristic immunohistochemical labeling patterns. Although not as invasive as the
typical signet ring cell carcinoma, the neoplastic cells of the solid-pseudopapillary neoplasm

of the pancreas can have vacuolated cytoplasm
that results in a signet ring cell appearance. In
contrast to signet ring cell carcinomas, solid-
pseudopapillary neoplasms lack intracellular
mucin, express CD10, and have a nuclear pattern of labeling for beta-catenin.

Staging. The staging of signet ring cell carcinoma should follow the staging of carcinomas
of the exocrine pancreas (see chapter 3).

Prognosis. Because of the rarity of this entity,
it is hard to make definitive statements about
prognosis. The survival period of most reported
patients has only been a few months (13,71).

UNDIFFERENTIATED CARCINOMA

Definition. *Undifferentiated carcinoma* is a
malignant epithelial neoplasm with a significant
component showing no glandular structures or
other features to indicate a definite direction of
differentiation. Undifferentiated carcinomas
have a spectrum of morphologies ranging from
pleomorphic epithelioid mononuclear cells
containing abundant eosinophilic cytoplasm
admixed with bizarre frequently multinucleated
giant cells, to relatively monomorphic spindle
cells (39,44,68), and individual cases may contain more than one pattern. Because this entity
includes a spectrum of morphologies, it would
be wise to include pertinent descriptors when
diagnosing an undifferentiated carcinoma.

Synonyms include *pleomorphic carcinoma,
pleomorphic large cell carcinoma,* and *pleomorphic
giant cell carcinoma.* The term *carcinosarcoma* can

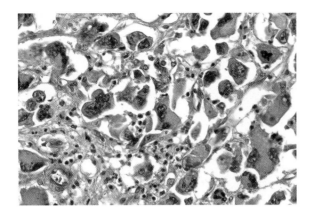

Figure 8-19

UNDIFFERENTIATED CARCINOMA

The anaplastic giant cell variant is composed of bizarre giant cells without a clear direction of differentiation.

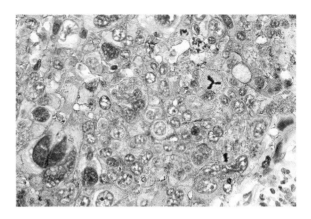

Figure 8-20

UNDIFFERENTIATED CARCINOMA

The epithelial nature of these neoplasms can sometimes be established with immunolabeling for cytokeratin.

be used for undifferentiated carcinomas containing separate recognizable epithelial (glandular) and spindle cell (undifferentiated carcinoma) components.

General Features. Undifferentiated carcinomas arise de novo or occur in association with mucinous cystic or other pancreatic neoplasms. Undifferentiated carcinomas containing osteoclast-like giant cells constitute a distinct type of pancreatic neoplasm, and are discussed separately (see below).

The reported incidence of undifferentiated carcinoma ranges from 0.3 percent of pancreatic neoplasms submitted to a referral center, to about 10 percent of nonendocrine pancreatic neoplasms seen at autopsy (30,56,72). Men are affected more often than women, with a male to female ratio of 3 to 1. The mean age at diagnosis is 63 years (range, 25 to 96 years).

Clinical Features. The most common presenting signs and symptoms are weight loss, abdominal pain, fatigue, nausea and vomiting, anorexia, a palpable abdominal mass, and, infrequently, jaundice. A case of a parathyroid hormone–related protein-producing anaplastic carcinoma associated with humoral hypercalcemia of malignancy has been reported (40). Radiologic imaging demonstrates an aggressive pancreatic mass but is not specific for undifferentiated carcinoma.

Gross Findings. These are usually very large aggressive neoplasms. The average size in most series is 9 or 10 cm (range, 2.5 to 20.0 cm), and any portion of the pancreas can be involved.

On cross section, undifferentiated carcinomas are usually rubbery or fleshy, and often show central cystic degeneration with hemorrhage and extensive necrosis (30,56,72). Frequently, these neoplasms grossly infiltrate into adjacent organs including the stomach, duodenum, spleen, and adrenal gland.

Microscopic Findings. Undifferentiated carcinoma can have a variety of microscopic appearances. Most are *anaplastic giant cell carcinomas*, composed of relatively noncohesive, pleomorphic mononuclear cells admixed with bizarre, frequently multinucleated giant cells that contain abundant eosinophilic cytoplasm (fig. 8-19). The nuclei are large, hyperchromatic, sharply angulated, and pleomorphic, and contain variable numbers and sizes of nucleoli. Numerous mitoses are easily identified, including bizarre mitoses (fig. 8-20). In some anaplastic giant cell carcinomas the neoplastic cells are suspended in a sea of neutrophils. Neoplastic cells engulfing other neoplastic cells ("cannibalism," or "emperipolesis"), erythrocytes, and inflammatory cells are seen (56). In contrast to infiltrating ductal adenocarcinomas, the stroma between the neoplastic cells is usually scant. Necrosis and hemorrhage are usually extensive.

A spindle cell component may also be present (figs. 8-21, 8-22) (7,56). When the spindle cell morphology is predominant, the neoplasm may resemble a sarcoma and is often designated *sarcomatoid carcinoma*. Sarcomatoid carcinomas contain relatively minimal stroma and have

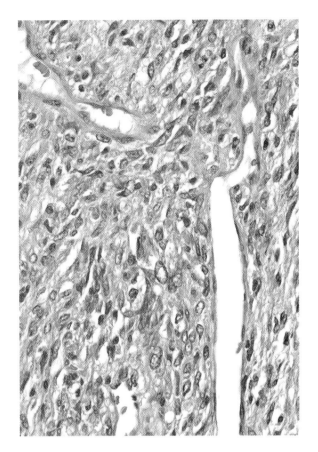

Figure 8-21

UNDIFFERENTIATED CARCINOMA

The sarcomatoid variant has prominent spindle cell differentiation.

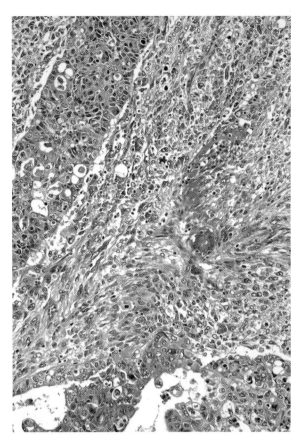

Figure 8-22

UNDIFFERENTIATED CARCINOMA

The carcinosarcomatous variant is composed of a mixture of poorly differentiated glandular and spindle cell differentiation.

cells arranged in fascicles, sometimes in a herringbone pattern. The nuclei are usually plump, elongated, and rounded at the ends. Although there is less pleomorphism than in anaplastic giant cell carcinomas, significant atypia is common. Necrosis is usually extensive and may have a peritheliomatous pattern, leaving viable cells only in the regions surrounding the vessels. Sometimes there is sufficient mesenchymal differentiation to result in heterologous stromal elements such as bone, cartilage, or striated muscle. Again, individual cases of undifferentiated carcinoma may contain a variety of patterns, including both anaplastic and sarcomatoid elements. An undifferentiated carcinoma with rhabdoid features also has been reported (46).

As evidence of their relationship to ductal adenocarcinomas, more than half of undifferentiated carcinomas contain an infiltrating ductal adenocarcinoma component, and as such, these neoplasms are designated *carcinosarcomas.* The ductal carcinoma component may occur prior to the development of an undifferentiated carcinoma, or synchronously (fig. 8-22) (30,56). Focal squamous differentiation is seen in a quarter to a third of undifferentiated carcinomas.

Undifferentiated carcinomas are typically widely invasive. Extensive intrapancreatic, extrapancreatic, vascular, lymphatic, and perineural invasion are present in the majority.

Stains for mucin, including mucicarmine and PAS, demonstrate mucin in the glandular components of carcinosarcomas. They also occasionally stain intracytoplasmic vacuoles in anaplastic or sarcomatoid carcinomas.

Immunohistochemical Findings. Cytokeratin is expressed in over 80 percent of these

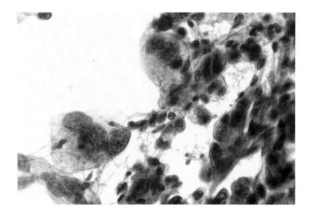

Figure 8-23

UNDIFFERENTIATED CARCINOMA

There is a combination of malignant mononuclear cells and malignant pleomorphic giant cells (direct smear; Papanicolaou stain).

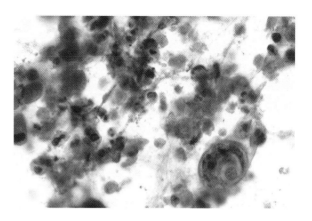

Figure 8-24

UNDIFFERENTIATED CARCINOMA

Cellular cannibalism is common in this neoplasm (direct smear; Papanicolaou stain).

carcinomas, although the labeling may be very focal, especially in sarcomatoid carcinomas (30, 56). The cytokeratins expressed include CK7, CK8, CK18, and CK19. Most of these neoplasms also express vimentin, CEA, MUC1, CA19-9, and DUPAN-2. Immunolabeling for chromogranin, synaptophysin, neuron-specific enolase, CK20, and B72.3 is negative in the majority of cases. The spindle cells of sarcomatoid carcinomas often label for actin, although desmin is not commonly expressed. In undifferentiated carcinomas with heterologous stromal elements, there may be immunolabeling consistent with the line of mesenchymal differentiation expressed in these cells (e.g., myoglobin or myogenin in striated muscle, S-100 protein in chondroid elements). Scattered neoplastic cells are occasionally positive for CD68 and CD45, but most of the cells labeling with these markers are reactive inflammatory cells (30).

Ultrastructural Findings. Electron microscopy may reveal microvilli and, occasionally, mucin granules in some of the neoplastic cells. Other undifferentiated carcinomas show minimal evidence of epithelial differentiation (intercellular junctions and cytoplasmic keratin filaments) even at the ultrastructural level.

Cytologic Findings. The cytologic diagnosis of this neoplasm depends upon the recognition of the large, bizarre, mononuclear and multinuclear anaplastic tumor giant cells that are present in small clusters and singly (fig. 8-23) (27, 66). As noted histologically, there is generally high cellularity, with a more typical high-grade malignant mononuclear glandular proliferation untethered by the sclerotic stroma common in conventional ductal adenocarcinoma. The malignant cells may appear spindled and sarcomatoid, and they may display frequent mitotic activity and cellular cannibalism (fig. 8-24). Background necrosis is also commonly present. Squamous differentiation may be seen focally, but, in contrast to adenosquamous carcinomas, cells with squamous differentiation are associated with anaplastic giant cells.

Molecular and Other Special Techniques. The genetic alterations identified in undifferentiated carcinomas parallel those seen in ductal adenocarcinomas (30,56). Most undifferentiated carcinomas harbor activating point mutations in codon 12 of the *KRAS* oncogene. In carcinosarcomas with both ductal adenocarcinoma and undifferentiated carcinoma elements, both components harbor identical *KRAS* gene mutations, supporting the hypothesis that undifferentiated carcinomas arise from ductal adenocarcinomas. Accumulation of the p53 protein, suggesting *TP53* gene mutations, has been reported in 70 percent of these carcinomas (56).

Differential Diagnosis. The differential diagnosis for undifferentiated carcinoma is wide and varies depending upon the specific morphologic patterns of a given undifferentiated carcinoma. Broadly, the differential diagnosis includes undifferentiated carcinoma with osteoclast-like giant cells, metastatic melanoma, and poorly differentiated epithelial, mesenchymal, germ cell, and hematopoietic neoplasms.

In contrast to the dramatic pleomorphism seen in the larger cells in undifferentiated carcinomas, the multinucleated giant cells in undifferentiated carcinoma with osteoclast-like giant cells have abundant cytoplasm and uniform oval nuclei without atypia, and they immunolabel intensely for CD68 and KP1 (27). Sarcomatoid carcinomas are often difficult to distinguish from true sarcomas. Since primary pancreatic sarcomas are extremely rare, an undifferentiated spindle cell neoplasm is more likely to be a sarcomatoid carcinoma than a sarcoma, especially when no specific line of mesenchymal differentiation is present. Immunolabeling for keratin, even if focal, favors an epithelial neoplasm (sarcomatoid carcinoma), although rare primary pancreatic synovial sarcomas have been described and exhibit keratin labeling. Both sarcomas and sarcomatoid carcinomas express vimentin, and focal actin labeling is also common in sarcomatoid carcinomas, but positivity for other mesenchymal lineage markers favors the diagnosis of sarcoma.

Other entities in the differential diagnosis are also excluded by immunolabeling: melanomas express S-100 protein, HMB-45, and melan-A; lymphomas express CD45 and other lymphocyte markers. Undifferentiated carcinoma resembles choriocarcinoma, with its syncytiotrophoblasts, but choriocarcinoma expresses human chorionic gonadotropin-beta and generally affects a younger age group. The immunolabeling pattern for an undifferentiated carcinoma metastatic to the pancreas and a primary undifferentiated carcinoma of the pancreas is the same. These two entities can be distinguished by identifying a significant intraductal component (pancreatic intraepithelial neoplasia [PanIN-3]) or other preinvasive neoplastic precursors such as a mucinous cystic neoplasm within the pancreatic primary, or, more likely, on clinical grounds.

Spread and Metastasis. Metastases are present at the time of diagnosis in most undifferentiated carcinomas. The most common sites of metastases, in decreasing order, are the lymph nodes, liver, lung, peritoneum, adrenal gland, kidney, heart, spleen, brain, bone, pleura, and thyroid gland (30,56,72). Metastases of carcinosarcomas may contain only the undifferentiated component, or they may show glandular or squamous differentiation.

Staging. The staging of undifferentiated carcinomas should follow the staging of carcinomas of the exocrine pancreas (see chapter 3).

Treatment. Surgical resection is the treatment of choice for undifferentiated carcinomas. Unfortunately, the majority of these neoplasms have metastasized by the time of diagnosis. Radiation and chemotherapy are of unproven benefit.

Prognosis. Reported survival rates are extremely poor (30,56,72). In one of the largest reported series, 29 of 35 patients died of disease at a mean of 5.2 months after diagnosis (56).

UNDIFFERENTIATED CARCINOMA WITH OSTEOCLAST-LIKE GIANT CELLS

Definition. *Undifferentiated carcinoma with osteoclast-like giant cells* is a malignant epithelial neoplasm composed of benign-appearing multinucleated giant cells admixed with atypical neoplastic mononuclear cells (39,44,68). These neoplasms can focally form osteoid and may arise in association with an intraductal carcinoma (PanIN-3), an invasive ductal adenocarcinoma, or a mucinous cystic neoplasm.

Synonyms include *giant cell tumor of the pancreas*, *giant cell carcinoma of the pancreas* (epulisosteoid type), *osteoclastoma of the pancreas*, *osteoclast-like giant cell tumor of the pancreas*, and *osteoclastoid type of giant cell tumor* (8,51). A neoplasm reported as giant cell malignant fibrous histiocytoma of the pancreas (70) also appears to represent the same entity. In the previous edition of this Fascicle these neoplasms were designated "giant cell tumor of the pancreas." The current terminology reflects recent molecular findings that demonstrate that the atypical mononuclear cells are neoplastic and of epithelial origin, while the osteoclast-like giant cells are non-neoplastic reactive cells.

General Features. Although rare, over 75 undifferentiated carcinomas with osteoclast-like giant cells have been reported in the English literature (17,19,20,30,51,62,76). There is a slight female predominance, with 55 percent of the reported cases occurring in women. The average age at diagnosis is 62 years (range, 32 to 93 years).

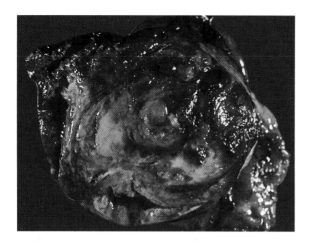

Figure 8-25

**UNDIFFERENTIATED CARCINOMA
WITH OSTEOCLAST-LIKE GIANT CELLS**

Cross section reveals a soft, fleshy, somewhat hemorrhagic tumor.

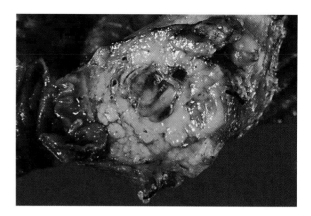

Figure 8-26

**UNDIFFERENTIATED CARCINOMA
WITH OSTEOCLAST-LIKE GIANT CELLS**

A small tumor in the head of the pancreas.

Clinical Features. The most common presenting signs and symptoms are those of an aggressive pancreatic neoplasm: abdominal pain (often radiating to the back), jaundice, weight loss, nausea and vomiting, and fatigue (17,19, 20,30,51,62,76). Rarely, patients are asymptomatic and diagnosed by physical examination or during imaging for another indication (60). CT and ultrasound studies usually demonstrate a solid, or a solid and cystic mass in the pancreas (22,64). Some undifferentiated carcinomas with osteoclast-like giant cells are almost completely cystic and can mimic a pseudocyst or mucinous cystic neoplasm of the pancreas (64). Administration of contrast enhances some tumors, whereas others have areas with low attenuation secondary to necrosis (22). Serum CA19-9 levels are elevated in some patients.

Gross Findings. Half of undifferentiated carcinomas with osteoclast-like giant cells involve the head of the pancreas, a quarter the body, and a quarter the tail (17,19,20,30,51,62,76). They range in size from 3 to 17 cm (mean, 10 cm). On cut section, carcinomas may be solid, firm, and white, but most are soft, yellow-tan, and partially cystic with friable red-brown hemorrhagic or necrotic areas (figs. 8-25, 8-26) (50,51,61). Gross invasion into large blood vessels and into adjacent organs, including the duodenum and stomach, is common (50,61). When they arise in association with a mucinous

cystic neoplasm, the mucinous cystic component is often grossly appreciable (fig. 8-27).

Microscopic Findings. As the name suggests, undifferentiated carcinomas with osteoclast-like giant cells have at least two distinct cell populations. Large, benign-appearing, multinucleated osteoclast-like giant cells are scattered among undifferentiated, round to spindle-shaped, atypical mononuclear cells (figs. 8-28, 8-29) (8,51,61). The osteoclast-like giant cells are often more numerous in areas adjacent to hemorrhage or necrosis. They contain multiple, small uniform nuclei and abundant eosinophilic cytoplasm. Mitotic figures are not seen in the giant cells. Some of the osteoclast-like giant cells are phagocytically active and, as a result, they can contain hemosiderin as well as engulfed neoplastic mononuclear cells (fig. 8-30) (51,76). The osteoclast-like giant cells are seen in both primary lesions and in metastases (15,51).

The atypical mononuclear cells are round to spindle shaped, contain scant to moderate amounts of eosinophilic cytoplasm, and, in contrast to the multinucleated giant cells, can show dramatic nuclear pleomorphism and hyperchromasia (8). Mitotic figures are common and bizarre mitoses are seen (fig. 8-31) (8). The mononuclear cells appear somewhat noncohesive and generally lack fibrous stroma.

Mononuclear cells without significant atypia may also been seen. These presumably represent non-neoplastic histiocytes and have regular oval nuclei (62).

Forty percent of undifferentiated carcinomas with osteoclast-like giant cells are associated with a gland-forming epithelial neoplasm (26,51,75, 76). These include mucinous cystic neoplasm, invasive ductal adenocarcinoma, and even PanIN-3. Examples with a ductal adenocarcinoma component show a sharp separation between the two elements; the osteoclast-like giant cells are usually restricted to areas with undifferentiated mononuclear cells, and even when malignant glands are distributed throughout the neoplasm, a transition between the two components is not seen. A significant minority of these neoplasms contain osteoid, and a case with focal chondroid differentiation has been reported (20,21,50,51). When metastases are present, they may consist of the undifferentiated carcinoma component, the glandular component or, in those with an associated adenocarcinoma, both components.

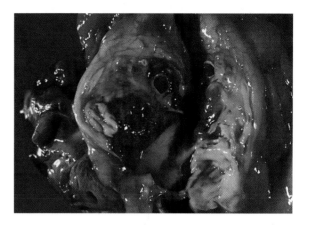

Figure 8-27

UNDIFFERENTIATED CARCINOMA WITH OSTEOCLAST-LIKE GIANT CELLS

This neoplasm arose in association with a mucinous cystic neoplasm. Note the solid, somewhat hemorrhagic mass in the center surrounded by well-defined cysts.

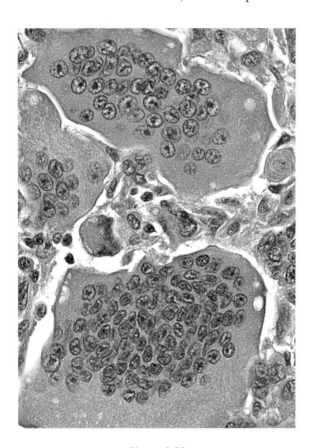

Figure 8-28

UNDIFFERENTIATED CARCINOMA WITH OSTEOCLAST-LIKE GIANT CELLS

Atypical mononuclear cells are interspersed between large multinucleated giant cells without atypia.

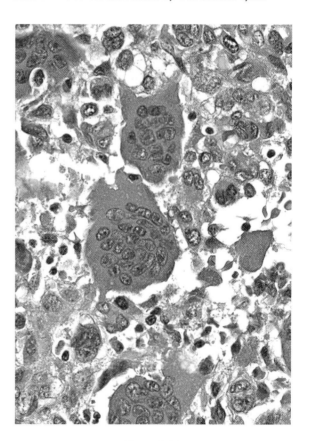

Figure 8-29

UNDIFFERENTIATED CARCINOMA WITH OSTEOCLAST-LIKE GIANT CELLS

In contrast to the giant cells, significant nuclear atypia can be appreciated in the mononuclear cells.

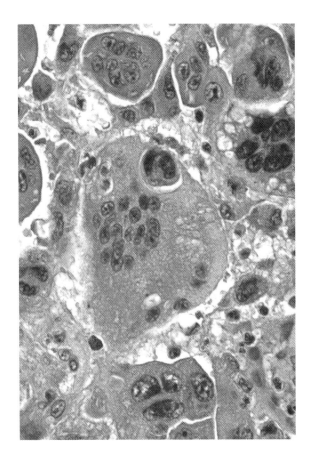

Figure 8-30

**UNDIFFERENTIATED CARCINOMA
WITH OSTEOCLAST-LIKE GIANT CELLS**

A multinucleated giant cell is phagocytizing an atypical mononuclear cell.

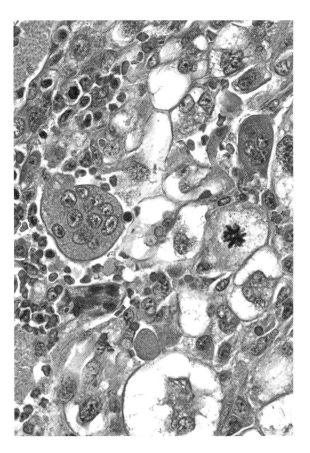

Figure 8-31

**UNDIFFERENTIATED CARCINOMA
WITH OSTEOCLAST-LIKE GIANT CELLS**

Mononuclear cell with a bizarre mitosis.

Immunohistochemical Findings. The literature on immunohistochemical labeling has been confusing and, at times, conflicting (50). A growing consensus is emerging that the atypical mononuclear cells variably express markers of epithelial differentiation, while the osteoclast-like giant cells express markers of histiocytic differentiation. The atypical mononuclear cells almost always express vimentin, while only a minority express cytokeratin (CAM5.2, CK7, or AE1/AE3), CEA, and EMA (fig. 8-32) (8,17,18,21,30,47a,51,62). In some cases, all of the epithelial markers are negative. The atypical mononuclear cells have a high proliferation rate as demonstrated by immunolabeling for Ki-67 or proliferating cell nuclear antigen (PCNA) (17,51).

The osteoclast-like giant cells express CD68, KP1, common leukocyte antigen (CD45), vimen-

tin, and alpha-1-antichymotrypsin (fig. 8-33) (17, 18,21,30,47a,51,62,65). In contrast to the atypical mononuclear cells, the osteoclast-like giant cells do not express cytokeratin, EMA, or CEA, and they have a low proliferation rate as assessed by Ki-67 or PCNA labeling (17). The osteoclast-like giant cells have been reported to express cathepsin K and, in an area of osteoid formation, osteonectin (20). The expression of cathepsin K suggests true osteoclastic differentiation by the multinucleated giant cells.

Ultrastructural Findings. The ultrastructural findings parallel the differentiation seen with immunolabeling. The atypical mononuclear cells have been reported to show evidence of epithelial differentiation, including well-formed desmosomes, zona occludens, and microvilli, however this may reflect selective reporting of the better-differentiated glandular components

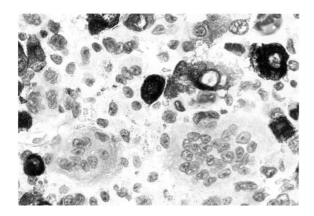

Figure 8-32

**UNDIFFERENTIATED CARCINOMA
WITH OSTEOCLAST-LIKE GIANT CELLS**

Immunolabeling for pancytokeratin marks the atypical mononuclear cells but not the osteoclast-like giant cells.

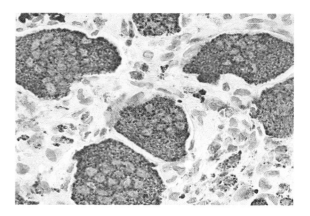

Figure 8-33

**UNDIFFERENTIATED CARCINOMA
WITH OSTEOCLAST-LIKE GIANT CELLS**

Immunolabeling for CD68 marks the osteoclast-like giant cells.

(8,15,60). More typically, only very primitive cells with rudimentary cell junctions are seen. Numerous mitochondria and prominent rough endoplasmic reticulum are usually present. Some contain electron-dense granules initially thought to represent zymogen granules (8,38,61); subsequent studies have failed to confirm the suggestion of acinar differentiation, however. The neoplastic cells can contain phagocytosed debris.

The osteoclast-like giant cells contain numerous mitochondria, free ribosomes, dilated endoplasmic reticulum, and, in some instances, filopodia (15,50,60). The giant cells do not have desmosomes.

Cytologic Findings. This neoplasm should be considered for any pancreatic aspirate composed of an obviously malignant cellular proliferation containing benign-appearing osteoclast-like giant cells. Smears are typically hypercellular because most undifferentiated carcinomas with osteoclast-like giant cells are large and are not associated with significant desmoplasia. Two cell populations are present: atypical mononuclear cells and the osteoclast-like giant cells. Most of the limited reports of the cytologic features of this neoplasm describe the mononuclear cell component as predominant (15,52,67), but the giant cells are dominant in some cases (50,74).

The mononuclear cells appear singly or in small clusters and can range from medium-sized polygonal epithelioid cells with clear cytoplasm to large bizarre sarcomatoid cells with dense and/

or spindled cytoplasm (fig. 8-34). The mononuclear cells are intimately intermingled with the osteoclast-type giant cells, which may be few in number or numerous. The giant cells often contain 10 or more bland-appearing, centrally clustered and slightly overlapping nuclei, with even chromatin and occasionally prominent nucleoli (fig. 8-35). The cytoplasm is abundant and dense, and may contain phagocytic material.

Molecular and Other Special Techniques. Molecular analyses have helped elucidate the nature of the atypical mononuclear cells and the osteoclast-like giant cells. Activating point mutations in codon 12 of the *KRAS* oncogene are present in about 90 percent of these neoplasms (17,23,30,34,47a,62). Genetic analyses of microdissected tumors have demonstrated that it is the atypical mononuclear cells that harbor these mutations. In addition, when there is an associated neoplastic epithelial component, identical *KRAS* gene mutations are found in the atypical mononuclear and the neoplastic epithelial cells (62,76). By contrast, when the osteoclast-like giant cells have been microdissected and analyzed genetically they either do not harbor *KRAS* gene mutations, or, if they do, these apparent mutations are believed to represent phagocytosed mutant DNA and not genetic alterations in the genome of the giant cells themselves (62,76). Immunohistochemical labeling for the p53 protein, a surrogate marker for *TP53* gene mutations, demonstrates

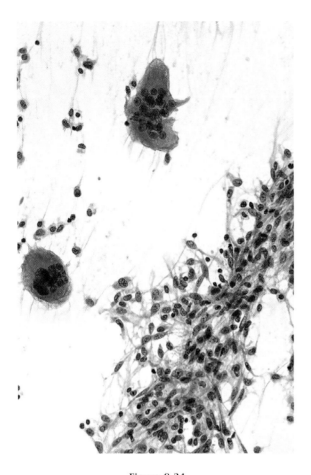

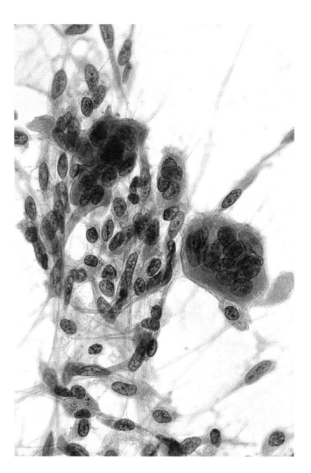

Figure 8-34

**UNDIFFERENTIATED CARCINOMA
WITH OSTEOCLAST-LIKE GIANT CELLS**

The mononuclear cells appear as a loose sheet of atypical spindled to epithelioid cells. Osteoclast-type giant cells are seen at 9 and 12 o'clock (direct smear; Papanicolaou stain).

Figure 8-35

**UNDIFFERENTIATED CARCINOMA
WITH OSTEOCLAST-LIKE GIANT CELLS**

The giant cells often contain 10 or more bland-appearing, centrally clustered and slightly overlapping nuclei with even chromatin and occasionally prominent nucleoli (direct smear; Papanicolaou stain).

abnormal labeling in the atypical mononuclear cells in half of the neoplasms, while the osteoclast-like giant cells do not show abnormal labeling (fig. 8-36) (17,51). Genetic analyses of a single case failed to demonstrate inactivation of the *SMAD4/DPC4, TP53, APC,* or *p16/CDKN2A* tumor suppressor genes (34).

Ploidy studies using image analysis techniques have shown that individual nuclei in the osteoclast-like giant cells are diploid, while the atypical mononuclear cells are often aneuploid (17).

Pathogenesis. The currently accepted name for these neoplasms, undifferentiated carcinomas with osteoclast-like giant cells, reflects the belief that these are fundamentally epithelial

malignancies with reactive osteoclast-like giant cells of histiocytic derivation. At least three lines of evidence suggest that the atypical mononuclear cells are neoplastic and that these neoplasms are fundamentally epithelial: the atypical mononuclear cells are aneuploid, these neoplasms are often associated with intraductal and infiltrating epithelial neoplasms, and identical *KRAS* gene mutations are seen in the epithelial and mononuclear components (62,76). Conversely, the observations that the osteoclast-like giant cells do not harbor *TP53* mutations, that they are diploid, and that they have a low proliferation rate, all suggest that the giant cells are non-neoplastic reactive cells (17,51).

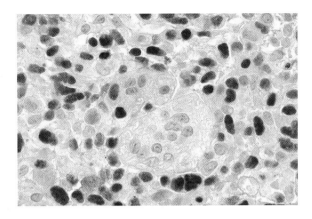 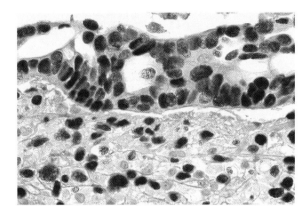

Figure 8-36

UNDIFFERENTIATED CARCINOMA WITH OSTEOCLAST-LIKE GIANT CELLS

Antibodies to p53 label the atypical mononuclear cells (left) and the glandular component (right), but not the osteoclast-like giant cells (left).

It has been speculated that the neoplastic epithelial cells may produce substances that attract histiocytes to form osteoclast-like giant cells within the neoplasm (43). Histologically similar carcinomas occur in other organs, and even sarcomas and melanomas may have osteoclast-like giant cell components with similar undifferentiated neoplastic cells that lack immunohistochemical evidence of cell lineage. The exact origin of the osteoclast-like giant cells within these neoplasms, however, remains a mystery.

Differential Diagnosis. Multinucleated histiocytic giant cells are seen in a variety of non-neoplastic and neoplastic conditions in the pancreas. The non-neoplastic conditions include pseudocysts, abscesses, fat necrosis, tuberculosis, sarcoidosis, and fungal infections (52,55). The absence of atypical cells distinguishes these lesions from undifferentiated carcinoma with osteoclast-like giant cells. The neoplastic conditions include Hodgkin's disease, large cell lymphoma, trophoblastic neoplasms, malignant fibrous histiocytoma, anaplastic carcinoma, and giant cell reaction to a degenerating conventional duct adenocarcinoma (52). The benign appearance and uniform distribution of the giant cells helps distinguish undifferentiated carcinoma with osteoclast-like giant cells from most of these other neoplasms in which the giant cells are neoplastic and atypical. Immunohistochemical labeling using a panel of markers that includes vimentin, cytokeratin (CAM5.2, CK7, or AE1/AE3), CD68, leu-M1, common leukocyte antigen (CD45), human chorionic gonadotropin, actin, and desmin can be used to establish the diagnosis (52). In some undifferentiated carcinomas with osteoclast-like giant cells there is considerable cytologic atypia in the mononuclear cell component, resembling anaplastic giant cell carcinomas. A careful evaluation reveals the two different types of giant cells.

Spread and Metastasis. Undifferentiated carcinomas with osteoclast-like giant cells are locally invasive neoplasms (50). Vascular invasion and perineural invasion are common, and invasion into adjacent organs including the duodenum and stomach can be seen (50).

Approximately half of the patients have metastases at the time of diagnosis. The most common sites of metastases are regional lymph nodes, liver, and lung (15,50,62).

Staging. Undifferentiated carcinomas with osteoclast-like giant cells are staged according to the system employed for other carcinomas of the exocrine pancreas (see chapter 3).

Treatment. Surgical resection is the treatment of choice. The effectiveness of radiation and chemotherapy has not been established (50).

Prognosis. It was initially thought that undifferentiated carcinoma with osteoclast-like giant cells was not as aggressive as infiltrating ductal adenocarcinoma. While occasional long-term survival has been reported, it has become clear that this is, in fact, a highly aggressive neoplasm with a mean survival of only 12 months (19,50).

REFERENCES

1. Adsay NV, Conlon KC, Zee SY, Brennan MF, Klimstra DS. Intraductal papillary-mucinous neoplasms of the pancreas: an analysis of in situ and invasive carcinomas in 28 patients. Cancer 2002;94:62-77.
2. Adsay NV, Hasteh F, Sarkar F, Cheng J, Klimstra DS. Squamous cell and adenosquamous carcinomas of the pancreas: a clinicopathologic analysis of 11 cases. Mod Pathol 2000;13:179A.
3. Adsay NV, Merati K, Andea A, et al. The dichotomy in the preinvasive neoplasia to invasive carcinoma sequence in the pancreas: differential expression of MUC1 and MUC2 supports the existence of two separate pathways of carcinogenesis. Mod Pathol 2002;15:1087-95.
4. Adsay NV, Merati K, Basturk O, et al. Pathologically and biologically distinct types of epithelium in intraductal papillary mucinous neoplasms: delineation of an "intestinal" pathway of carcinogenesis in the pancreas. Am J Surg Pathol 2004;28:839-48.
5. Adsay NV, Merati K, Nassar H, et al. Pathogenesis of colloid (pure mucinous) carcinoma of exocrine organs: coupling of gel-forming mucin (MUC2) production with altered cell polarity and abnormal cell-stroma interaction may be the key factor in the morphogenesis and indolent behavior of colloid carcinoma in the breast and pancreas. Am J Surg Pathol 2003;27:571-8.
6. Adsay NV, Pierson C, Sarkar F, et al. Colloid (mucinous noncystic) carcinoma of the pancreas. Am J Surg Pathol 2001;25:26-42.
7. Alguacil-Garcia A, Weiland LH. The histologic spectrum, prognosis, and histogenesis of the sarcomatoid carcinoma of the pancreas. Cancer 1977;39:1181-9.
8. Berendt RC, Shnitka TK, Wiens E, Manickavel V, Jewell LD. The osteoclast-type giant cell tumor of the pancreas. Arch Pathol Lab Med 1987;111:43-8.
9. Brennan MF, Moccia RD, Klimstra DS. Management of adenocarcinoma of the body and tail of the pancreas. Ann Surg 1996;223:506-11.
10. Calhoun ES, Jones JB, Ashfaq R, et al. BRAF and FBXW7 (CDC4, FBW7, AGO, SEL10) mutations in distinct subsets of pancreatic cancer: potential therapeutic targets. Am J Pathol 2003;163:1255-60.
11. Campman SC, Fajardo MA, Rippon MB, Kraegel SA, Ruebner BH. Adenosquamous carcinoma arising in a mucinous cystadenoma of the pancreas. J Surg Oncol 1997;64:159-62.
12. Chejfec G, Rieker WJ, Jablokow VR, Gould VE. Pseudomyxoma peritonei associated with colloid carcinoma of the pancreas. Gastroenterology 1986;90:202-5.
13. Chow LT, Chow WH. Signet-ring mucinous adenocarcinoma of the pancreas. Chin Med Sci J 1994;9:176-8.
14. Cingolani N, Shaco-Levy R, Farruggio A, Klimstra DS, Rosai J. Alpha-fetoprotein production by pancreatic tumors exhibiting acinar cell differentiation: study of five cases, one arising in a mediastinal teratoma. Hum Pathol 2000;31:938-44.
15. Combs SG, Hidvegi DF, Ma Y, Rosen ST, Radosevich JA. Pleomorphic carcinoma of the pancreas with osteoclast-like giant cells expressing an epithelial-associated antigen detected by monoclonal antibody 44-3A6. Diagn Cytopathol 1988;4:316-22.
16. Cuilliere P, Lazure T, Bui M, et al. Solid adenoma with exclusive hepatocellular differentiation: a new variant among pancreatic benign neoplasms? Virchows Arch 2002;441:519-22.
17. Deckard-Janatpour K, Kragel S, Teplitz RL, et al. Tumors of the pancreas with osteoclast-like and pleomorphic giant cells: an immunohistochemical and ploidy study. Arch Pathol Lab Med 1998;122:266-72.
18. Dizon MA, Multhaupt HA, Paskin DL, Warhol MJ. Osteoclastic giant cell tumor of the pancreas: an immunohistochemical study. Arch Pathol Lab Med 1996;120:306-9.
19. Dworak O, Wittekind C, Koerfgen HP, Gall FP. Osteoclastic giant cell tumor of the pancreas. An immunohistological study and review of the literature. Pathol Res Pract 1993;189:228-31.
20. Fischer HP, Altmannsberger M, Kracht J. Osteoclast-type giant cell tumour of the pancreas. Virchows Arch A Pathol Anat Histopathol 1988;412:247-53.
21. Gatteschi B, Saccomanno S, Bartoli FG, Salvi S, Liu G, Pugliese V. Mixed pleomorphic-osteoclast-like tumor of the pancreas. Light microscopical, immunohistochemical, and molecular biological studies. Int J Pancreatol 1995;18:169-75.
22. Gil-Garcia I, Valls C, Sanchez-Marquez A, Catala I. Osteoclast-type giant-cell tumor of the pancreas. AJR Am J Roentgenol 1992;159:1128.
23. Gocke CD, Dabbs DJ, Benko FA, Silverman JF. K-ras oncogene mutations suggest a common histogenetic origin for pleomorphic giant cell tumor of the pancreas, osteoclastoma of the pancreas, and pancreatic duct adenocarcinoma. Hum Pathol 1997;28:80-3.
24. Goggins M, Offerhaus GJ, Hilgers W, et al. Pancreatic adenocarcinomas with DNA replication errors (RER+) are associated with wild-type K-ras and characteristic histopathology. Poor differentiation, a syncytial growth pattern, and pushing borders suggest RER+. Am J Pathol 1998;152:1501-7.

25. Goggins M, Shekher M, Kenan T, Yeo CJ, Hruban RH, Kern SE. Genetic alterations of the transforming growth factor beta receptor genes in pancreatic and biliary adenocarcinomas. Cancer Res 1998;58:5329-32.

26. Goldberg RD, Michelassi F, Montag AG. Osteoclast-like giant cell tumor of the pancreas: immunophenotypic similarity to giant cell tumor of bone. Hum Pathol 1991;22:618-22.

27. Gupta RK, Wakefield SJ. Needle aspiration cytology, immunocytochemistry, and electron microscopic study of unusual pancreatic carcinoma with pleomorphic giant cells. Diagn Cytopathol 1992;8:522-7.

28. Hempen PM, Zhang L, Bansal RK, et al. Evidence of selection for clones having genetic inactivation of the activin A type II receptor (ACVR2) gene in gastrointestinal cancers. Cancer Res 2003;63:994-9.

29. Herxheimer G. Über heterologe Cancroide. Beitr Pathol Anat 1907;41:348-412.

30. Hoorens A, Prenzel K, Lemoine NR, Klöppel G. Undifferentiated carcinoma of the pancreas: analysis of intermediate filament profile and Ki-ras mutations provides evidence of a ductal origin. J Pathol 1998;185:53-60.

31. Hruban RH, Molina JM, Reddy MN, Boitnott JK. A neoplasm with pancreatic and hepatocellular differentiation presenting with subcutaneous fat necrosis. Am J Clin Pathol 1987;88:639-45.

32. Hughes K, Kelty S, Martin R. Hepatoid carcinoma of the pancreas. Am Surg 2004;70:1030-3.

33. Iacobuzio-Donahue CA, Klimstra DS, Adsay NV, et al. Dpc-4 protein is expressed in virtually all human intraductal papillary mucinous neoplasms of the pancreas: comparison with conventional ductal carcinomas. Am J Pathol 2000;157:755-61.

34. Imai Y, Morishita S, Ikeda Y, et al. Immunohistochemical and molecular analysis of giant cell carcinoma of the pancreas: a report of three cases. Pancreas 1999;18:308-15.

35. Inoue T, Nagao S, Tajima H, et al. Adenosquamous pancreatic cancer producing parathyroid hormone-related protein. J Gastroenterol 2004;39: 176-80.

36. Ishikawa O, Matsui Y, Aoki I, Iwanaga T, Terasawa T, Wada A. Adenosquamous carcinoma of the pancreas: a clinicopathologic study and report of three cases. Cancer 1980;46:1192-6.

37. Itani KM, Karni A, Green L. Squamous cell carcinoma of the pancreas. J Gastrointest Surg 1999;3:512-5.

38. Jalloh SS. Giant cell tumour (osteoclastoma) of the pancreas—an epithelial tumour probably of pancreatic acinar origin. J Clin Pathol 1983;36: 1171-5.

39. Japanese Pancreas Society. Classification of pancreatic carcinoma, 2nd English ed. Tokyo: Kanehara & Co, Ltd; 2003.

40. Kakizaki S, Ohya N, Yoshinaga T, et al. Undifferentiated pancreatic cancer associated with humoral hypercalcemia of malignancy. Jpn J Clin Oncol 1998;28:563-6.

41. Kardon DE, Thompson LD, Przygodzki RM, Heffess CS. Adenosquamous carcinoma of the pancreas: a clinicopathologic series of 25 cases. Mod Pathol 2001;14:443-51.

42. Klimstra DS, Heffess CS, Oertel JE, Rosai J. Acinar cell carcinoma of the pancreas. A clinicopathologic study of 28 cases. Am J Surg Pathol 1992;16:815-37.

43. Klimstra DS, Rosai J. Osteoclastic giant cell tumor of the pancreas. Critical commentary. Path Res Pract 2005;189:232-3.

44. Klöppel G, Hruban RH, Longnecker DS, Adler G, Kern SE, Partanen TJ. Ductal adenocarcinoma of the pancreas. In: Hamilton SR, Aaltonen LA, eds. World Health Organization Classification of Tumours. Pathology and genetics of tumours of the digestive system. Lyon: IARC Press; 2000: 221-30.

45. Kovi J. Adenosquamous carcinoma of the pancreas: a light and electron microscopic study. Ultrastruct Pathol 1982;3:17-23.

46. Kuroda N, Sawada T, Miyazaki E, et al. Anaplastic carcinoma of the pancreas with rhabdoid features. Pathol Int 2000;50:57-62.

47. Levi E, Klimstra DS, Andea A, Basturk O, Adsay NV. MUC1 and MUC2 in pancreatic neoplasia. J Clin Pathol 2004;57:456-62.

47a. Lukas Z, Dvorak K, Kroupova I, Valaskova I, Habanec B. Immunohistochemical and genetic analysis of osteoclastic giant cell tumor of the pancreas. Pancreas 2006;32:325-9.

48. Lüttges J, Beyser K, Pust S, Paulus A, Ruschoff J, Klöppel G. Pancreatic mucinous noncystic (colloid) carcinomas and intraductal papillary mucinous carcinomas are usually microsatellite stable. Mod Pathol 2003;16:537-42.

49. Madura JA, Jarman BT, Doherty MG, Yum MN, Howard TJ. Adenosquamous carcinoma of the pancreas. Arch Surg 1999;134:599-603.

50. Manci EA, Gardner LL, Pollock WJ, Dowling EA. Osteoclastic giant cell tumor of the pancreas. Aspiration cytology, light microscopy, and ultrastructure with review of the literature. Diagn Cytopathol 1985;1:105-10.

51. Molberg KH, Heffess CS, Delgado R, Albores-Saavedra J. Undifferentiated carcinoma with osteoclast-like giant cells of the pancreas and periampullary region. Cancer 1998;82:1279-87.

52. Mullick SS, Mody DR. "Osteoclastic" giant cell carcinoma of the pancreas. Report of a case with aspiration cytology. Acta Cytol 1996;40:975-9.

53. Nakata B, Wang YQ, Yashiro M, et al. Negative hMSH2 protein expression in pancreatic carcinoma may predict a better prognosis of patients. Oncol Rep 2003;10:997-1000.

54. Nakata B, Wang YQ, Yashiro M, et al. Prognostic value of microsatellite instability in resectable pancreatic cancer. Clin Cancer Res 2002;8: 2536-40.

55. Oehler U, Jurs M, Klöppel G, Helpap B. Osteoclast-like giant cell tumour of the pancreas presenting as a pseudocyst-like lesion. Virchows Arch 1997;431:215-8.

56. Paal E, Thompson LD, Frommelt RA, Przygodzki RM, Heffess CS. A clinicopathologic and immunohistochemical study of 35 anaplastic carcinomas of the pancreas with a review of the literature. Ann Diagn Pathol 2001;5:129-40.

57. Paner GP, Thompson KS, Reyes CV. Hepatoid carcinoma of the pancreas. Cancer 2000;88: 1582-9.

58. Priesel A. Über ein ungewöhnliches Gewächs der Bauchspeicheldrüse. Virchows Arch 1928;354-62.

59. Rahemtullah A, Misdraji J, Pitman MB. Adenosquamous carcinoma of the pancreas: cytologic features in 14 cases. Cancer 2003;99:372-8.

60. Robinson L, Damjenov I, Brezina P. Multinucleated giant cell neoplasm of pancreas: light and electron microscopy features. Arch Pathol Lab Med 1977;101:590-3.

61. Rosai J. Carcinoma of pancreas simulating giant cell tumor of bone. Electron-microscopic evidence of its acinar cell origin. Cancer 1968;22: 333-44.

62. Sakai Y, Kupelioglu AA, Yanagisawa A, et al. Origin of giant cells in osteoclast-like giant cell tumors of the pancreas. Hum Pathol 2000;31: 1223-9.

63. Seidel G, Zahurak M, Iacobuzio-Donahue CA, et al. Almost all infiltrating colloid carcinomas of the pancreas and periampullary region arise from in situ papillary neoplasms: a study of 39 cases. Am J Surg Pathol 2002;26:56-63.

64. Shindoh N, Ozaki Y, Kyogoku S, Nakanishi A, Sumi Y, Katayama H. Osteoclast-type giant cell tumor of the pancreas: helical CT scans. AJR Am J Roentgenol 1998;170:653-4.

65. Shiozawa M, Imada T, Ishiwa N, et al. Osteoclast-like giant cell tumor of the pancreas. Int J Clin Oncol 2002;7:376-80.

66. Silverman JF, Dabbs DJ, Finley JL, Geisinger KR. Fine-needle aspiration biopsy of pleomorphic (giant cell) carcinoma of the pancreas. Cytologic, immunocytochemical, and ultrastructural findings. Am J Clin Pathol 1988;89:714-20.

67. Silverman JF, Finley JL, Berns L, Unverferth M. Significance of giant cells in fine-needle aspiration biopsies of benign and malignant lesions of the pancreas. Diagn Cytopathol 1989;5:388-91.

68. Solcia E, Capella C, Klöppel G. Tumors of the pancreas. AFIP Atlas of Tumor Pathology, 3rd Series, Fascicle 20. Washington, DC: American Registry of Pathology; 1997.

69. Stokes MB, Kumar A, Symmans WF, Scholes JV, Melamed J. Pancreatic endocrine tumor with signet ring cell features: a case report with novel ultrastructural observations. Ultrastruct Pathol 1998;22:147-52.

70. Suster S, Phillips M, Robinson MJ. Malignant fibrous histiocytoma (giant cell type) of the pancreas. A distinctive variant of osteoclast-type giant cell tumor of the pancreas. Cancer 1989;64:2303-8.

71. Tracey KJ, O'Brien MJ, Williams LF, et al. Signet ring carcinoma of the pancreas, a rare variant with very high CEA values. Immunohistologic comparison with adenocarcinoma. Dig Dis Sci 1984;29:573-6.

72. Tschang T, Garza-Garza R, Kissane JM. Pleomorphic carcinoma of the pancreas: an analysis of 15 cases. Cancer 1977;39:2114-26.

73. Ueki T, Toyota M, Sohn T, et al. Hypermethylation of multiple genes in pancreatic adenocarcinoma. Cancer Res 2000;60:1835-9.

74. Walts AE. Osteoclast-type giant-cell tumor of the pancreas. Acta Cytol 1983;27:500-4.

75. Watanabe M, Miura H, Inoue H, et al. Mixed osteoclastic/pleomorphic-type giant cell tumor of the pancreas with ductal adenocarcinoma: histochemical and immunohistochemical study with review of the literature. Pancreas 1997;15: 201-8.

76. Westra WH, Sturm PJ, Drillenburg P, et al. K-ras oncogene mutations in osteoclast-like giant cell tumors of the pancreas and liver: genetic evidence to support origin from the duct epithelium. Am J Surg Pathol 1998;22:1247-54.

77. Whelan AJ, Bartsch D, Goodfellow PJ. Brief report: a familial syndrome of pancreatic cancer and melanoma with a mutation in the CDKN2 tumor-suppressor gene. N Engl J Med 1995;333: 975-7.

78. Wilentz RE, Goggins M, Redston M, et al. Genetic, immunohistochemical, and clinical features of medullary carcinoma of the pancreas: a newly described and characterized entity. Am J Pathol 2000;156:1641-51.

79. Yamaguchi K, Enjoji M. Adenosquamous carcinoma of the pancreas: a clinicopathologic study. J Surg Oncol 1991;47:109-16.

80. Yamamoto H, Itoh F, Nakamura H, et al. Genetic and clinical features of human pancreatic ductal adenocarcinomas with widespread microsatellite instability. Cancer Res 2001;61: 3139-44.

81. Yano T, Ishikura H, Wada T, et al. Hepatoid adenocarcinoma of the pancreas. Histopathology 1999;35:90-2.

82. Ylagan LR, Scholes J, Demopoulos R. Cd44: a marker of squamous differentiation in adenosquamous neoplasms. Arch Pathol Lab Med 2000;124:212-5.

9 ACINAR NEOPLASMS

Despite the fact that acinar cells make up the bulk of the pancreas, pancreatic neoplasms exhibiting predominantly acinar differentiation are rare. Acinar differentiation in neoplastic cells is defined as the production of zymogen granules that contain pancreatic exocrine enzymes (27). Early reports of acinar cell carcinoma detailed a dramatic clinical syndrome of lipase hypersecretion by the neoplasm (5,41,58) and helped draw attention to the histologic differences between acinar cell carcinomas and ductal adenocarcinomas. More recently, the availability of antibodies against trypsin, chymotrypsin, lipase, and other pancreatic exocrine enzymes (27,31,46,67) has helped characterize a group of pancreatic neoplasms with acinar differentiation, including mixed acinar carcinomas, pancreatoblastoma, and cystic acinar neoplasms. Pancreatoblastomas also commonly have endocrine and ductal differentiation as well as other distinctive histologic features; they are discussed in chapter 10.

Almost all acinar neoplasms of the pancreas are malignant. Benign counterparts to acinar cell carcinoma ("acinar cell adenoma") have been proposed (38,78), but no convincing cases have been reported. The only benign acinar neoplasm reported is acinar cell cystadenoma; the remaining entities discussed in this chapter (acinar cell carcinoma, acinar cell cystadenocarcinoma, and mixed acinar carcinoma) are malignant.

ACINAR CELL CYSTADENOMA

Definition. *Acinar cell cystadenoma* is a benign cystic lesion lined by cells with acinar differentiation. The size and complexity of the lesion vary considerably. The nuclei are uniform and lack atypia.

General Features. Only 12 acinar cell cystadenomas have been reported (4,9,80). Because it is a relatively recently recognized entity, it is not clear whether the paucity of reports truly reflects the rarity of the lesion; however, no cases were identified in several large reviews of cystic lesions of the pancreas (3). Patients with acinar cell cystadenoma are usually adults with a mean age of 47 years (range, 16 to 66 years). The majority of patients (67 percent) are women.

Clinical Features. Of the 12 reported acinar cell cystadenomas, 6 caused symptoms and 6 were incidental findings. The symptomatic patients had abdominal pain and, one patient, polyarthralgia (80).

Gross Findings. In symptomatic patients, acinar cell cystadenomas are often large, ranging from 1.5 to 10.0 cm and averaging 6.2 cm in greatest dimension. They may be unilocular or multilocular. Multicentricity is common, and some diffusely involve the entire gland. Acinar cell cystadenomas found incidentally are often microscopic, usually measuring less than 1.0 cm. Both the head and tail of the pancreas may be affected, and some multifocal cases have demonstrated separate lesions in both regions of the gland. Gross communication of the cysts with the pancreatic ducts is rare (80). The individual cysts are well circumscribed and contain clear, watery fluid (fig. 9-1). Smaller acinar cell cystadenomas are usually unilocular. A fibrous pseudocapsule, which is sometimes calcified,

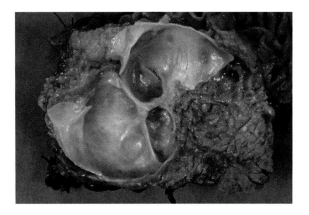

Figure 9-1

ACINAR CELL CYSTADENOMA

Gross appearance. (Fig. 1 from Zamboni G, Terris B, Scarpa A, et al. Acinar cell cystadenoma of the pancreas: a new entity? Am J Surg Pathol 2002;26:700.)

191

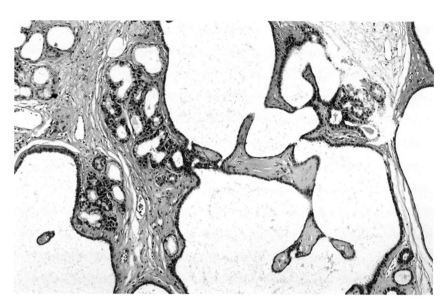

Figure 9-2

ACINAR CELL CYSTADENOMA

Smaller cystic spaces are found between the larger locules, and incomplete septa appear as broad papillary projections.

may surround larger lesions. The lining of the cysts is smooth and shiny, without papillary projections or solid areas.

Microscopic Findings. Both microscopic and grossly evident acinar cell cystadenomas have a similar epithelial lining consisting of one to several layers of cuboidal cells with round, basally oriented nuclei and granular, eosinophilic apical cytoplasm (fig. 9-2). The basal cytoplasm is basophilic. In some areas, the luminal layer is flattened, resembling simple squamous epithelium. The outer nonluminal epithelium contains dilated acinar structures, with lumens among interconnecting cords of cells. Clusters of acinar cells are found adjacent to the cysts. In smaller lesions, the cysts are lined by a single layer of undulating acinar cells (fig. 9-3, left). Mitotic figures are not detected. Some of the cells have a columnar shape, and a transition to mucin-containing ductal epithelium may be found (fig. 9-3, right), as may microscopic continuity with native ducts. This continuity with preexisting ductal epithelium suggests that acinar cell cystadenomas may be metaplastic rather than truly neoplastic processes.

The cyst lumens often contain eosinophilic secretions with concentrically lamellated plugs representing precipitated enzymatic secretions. Incomplete septa between adjacent locules appear as broad pseudopapillae that project into the cysts. A thick fibrous pseudocapsule composed of dense collagen with scattered fibroblasts may surround the larger cysts.

Immunohistochemical Findings. The labeling pattern of acinar cell cystadenomas is almost identical to that of non-neoplastic acinar cells. The apical zymogen granules are positive with the periodic acid–Schiff (PAS) stain and resistant to diastase; no intracellular mucin is found. Immunohistochemical labeling for the enzymes trypsin, chymotrypsin, and lipase is positive (4,9,80), and cytokeratins are detectable, including cytokeratin (CK) 7 (80). The expression of CK7 is the single identifiable difference from normal acinar cells, which are CK7 negative.

Pathogenesis. It is clear that acinar cell cystadenoma comprises a spectrum ranging from large, clinically relevant neoplasms to small, incidental lesions. Whereas the former cases appear to demonstrate neoplastic features, it could be argued that the smaller lesions, some of which appear to involve native ducts, may not be truly neoplastic. The possibility of acinar metaplasia of the ducts has been suggested to explain these small lesions as well as those that diffusely involve the gland (28). Since the smaller lesions are incidental and rather subtle findings, it is possible they are more common than currently recognized. Whether these small, possibly intraductal acinar proliferations may transform into grossly identifiable acinar cystic neoplasms is yet to be determined.

Differential Diagnosis. Smaller acinar cell cystadenomas resemble foci of pancreatic intraepithelial neoplasia (PanIN). The lack of mucin and the focal complexity of the epithelium in

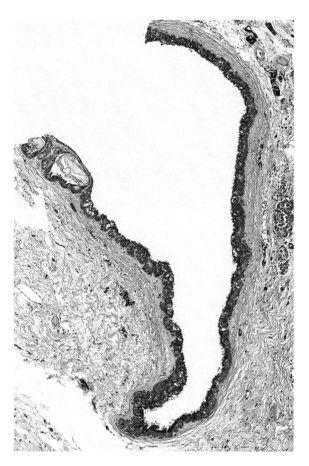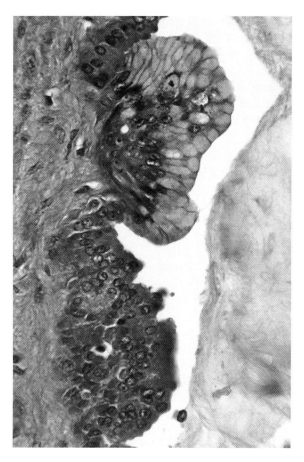

Figure 9-3

ACINAR CELL CYSTADENOMA

Left: Detected incidentally, this unilocular lesion is lined by several layers of undulating acinar cells.

Right: At higher power, the typical cytologic features of the acinar cells are evident, and there is a transition to mucinous ductal epithelium.

acinar cell cystadenomas may even resemble high-grade PanIN. If close attention is paid to the granular, eosinophilic cytoplasm, the acinar nature of the cells is usually apparent.

Larger acinar cell cystadenomas may resemble several other cystic lesions of the pancreas, including ductal retention cysts and serous cystic neoplasms. Again, recognition of the acinar nature of the lining epithelium is essential. The clear cells of serous cystic neoplasms have not been described in acinar cell cystadenomas. In cases where the granular cytoplasm of an acinar tumor is not readily recognized, immunohistochemical labeling for exocrine enzymes can be performed.

Perhaps the most difficult entity to exclude is acinar cell cystadenocarcinoma (7,68). This neoplasm is exceedingly rare. Reported cases have resembled acinar cell cystadenomas (especially the case of Cantrell et al. [7]), but the epithelium of acinar cell cystadenocarcinoma is more complex, the acinar cells are less well polarized, and there is more nuclear atypia, with prominent single nucleoli. Areas of necrosis, solid nests of neoplastic cells, easily identifiable mitotic figures, and infiltration into the surrounding stroma support a malignant diagnosis.

Treatment. As a benign lesion, acinar cell cystadenoma is curable by simple surgical excision. One case was observed for 7 years with only a gradual increase in the size of the cyst, and no examples of malignant transformation have been reported. Whether small, asymptomatic lesions should be removed is unclear,

Table 9-1

ACINAR CELL CARCINOMA: PRESENTING CLINICAL FEATURES[a]

Symptom/Sign	% of Patients
Weight loss	52
Abdominal pain	32
Nausea and vomiting	20
Lipase hypersecretion[b]	16
Jaundice	12
Melena	12
Weakness	12
Anorexia	12
Diarrhea	8

[a]Adapted from reference 31.
[b]Subcutaneous fat necrosis, polyarthralgia, markedly increased serum lipase.

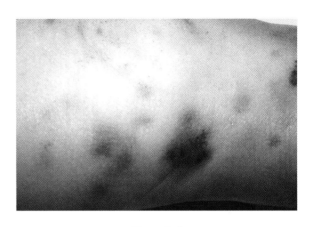

Figure 9-4

ACINAR CELL CARCINOMA

Subcutaneous fat necrosis in a patient with acinar cell carcinoma complicated by the lipase hypersecretion syndrome.

although excision may be necessary to establish the correct benign diagnosis.

ACINAR CELL CARCINOMA

Definition. *Acinar cell carcinoma* is a malignant epithelial neoplasm with evidence of exocrine enzyme production by the neoplastic cells. Significant endocrine or ductal components (not more than 25 percent of the neoplastic cells) are lacking. An alternative term is *acinic cell carcinoma.*

General Features. Approximately 1 to 2 percent of adult pancreatic neoplasms and 15 percent of pediatric neoplasms are acinar cell carcinomas (20,22,31). Pancreatic neoplasms are, however, more common in adults and as a result, most patients with acinar cell carcinoma are adults, with a peak incidence in the 60s and a mean age of 58.3 years (range, 10 to 87 years) (20,22,31). About 6 percent of acinar cell carcinomas occur in children (38,42,57,79), and the entity is uncommon between the ages of 20 and 40 years. In both the pediatric and adult populations, males are affected more frequently than females (male to female ratio, 3.6 to 1.0). There are no racial associations.

Clinical Features. Table 9-1 summarizes the relative frequencies of presenting symptoms for patients with acinar cell carcinoma. Most patients have relatively nonspecific symptoms including abdominal pain, nausea, vomiting, and weight loss (20,22,31,43). In contrast to ductal

adenocarcinoma, acinar cell carcinoma rarely obstructs the common bile duct, so jaundice is infrequent, occurring in only 12 percent of the patients in one study (31).

Some patients develop the *lipase hypersecretion syndrome*, in which massive quantities of lipase are released into the bloodstream, with levels reaching over 10,000 U/dL (6,17,29,35,61). Patients with the lipase hypersecretion syndrome develop multiple nodular foci of subcutaneous fat necrosis (fig. 9-4) associated with polyarthralgia. Peripheral blood eosinophilia can also occur. In almost every instance, these patients have hepatic metastasis at the time the syndrome develops, although occasionally there is an extremely large organ-limited primary carcinoma. Because of the clinically dramatic nature of the lipase hypersecretion syndrome, there are numerous case reports of it in the earlier literature; however, in more recent studies, the lipase hypersecretion syndrome occurs in only 10 to 15 percent of patients with acinar cell carcinoma (20,31).

Radiologic studies, including computerized tomography (CT) and magnetic resonance imaging (MRI), reveal well-marginated, large, round to oval masses that either enhance homogeneously less than the surrounding pancreas or show cystic areas (71).

Serum tumor markers are not consistently elevated in patients with acinar cell carcinomas. A modest elevation in serum lipase levels may be detected even in those patients without the

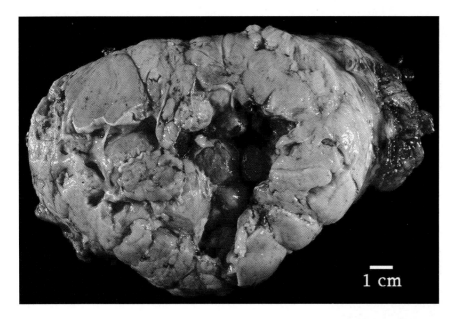

Figure 9-5

ACINAR CELL CARCINOMA

The predominantly solid tumor is soft and fleshy, and composed of tan lobules. Areas of necrosis are present, resulting in the central degenerative cystic change.

lipase hypersecretion syndrome. A number of reports have documented secretion of alpha-fetoprotein, especially in younger adults and children (11,26,48,54,66). Serum glycoprotein markers (such as carbohydrate antigen [CA] 19-9) are usually not elevated.

Gross Findings. Acinar cell carcinomas arise in any portion of the pancreas and are only slightly more common in the head of the gland (20,22,31). At the time they are detected, most are large, averaging 10 cm in diameter; acinar cell carcinomas less than 2 cm are rare. The carcinomas are generally circumscribed, and some appear grossly to be encapsulated. They are usually tan to red, soft and fleshy (fig. 9-5). Some display gross lobulation, with fibrotic stroma separating soft tumor lobules. There are often areas of gross necrosis, and degenerative cystic change may occur. Because of their circumscribed nature, acinar cell carcinomas are more likely to displace adjacent structures with a pushing border rather than to invade them, but invasion of the spleen, duodenum, or other adjacent organs occurs. In rare cases, grossly identifiable finger-like projections extend beyond the periphery of the main tumor into the pancreatic duct (14).

Microscopic Findings. The low-power microscopic appearance of acinar cell carcinoma is characterized by marked cellularity and a paucity of fibrous stroma (fig. 9-6). The periphery of the carcinoma is generally circumscribed, although extension of neoplastic lobules through the pe-

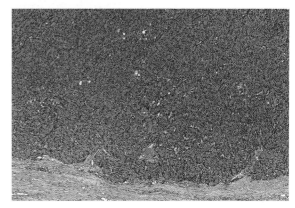

Figure 9-6

ACINAR CELL CARCINOMA

At low power, these carcinomas are often highly cellular and circumscribed, with minimal stroma within the carcinoma itself.

ripheral fibrous capsule is common. Some cases demonstrate more abundant stroma within the main tumor, generally in the form of broad, hypocellular connective tissue bands between cellular nodules of neoplastic cells; stromal desmoplasia is uncommon. In some cases, regions of the carcinoma demonstrate individual neoplastic glands infiltrating a fibrotic stroma. This pattern is unusual, however, and should raise the possibility of ductal differentiation (see Mixed Acinar-Ductal Carcinoma, below). Necrosis is not always present but may be extensive.

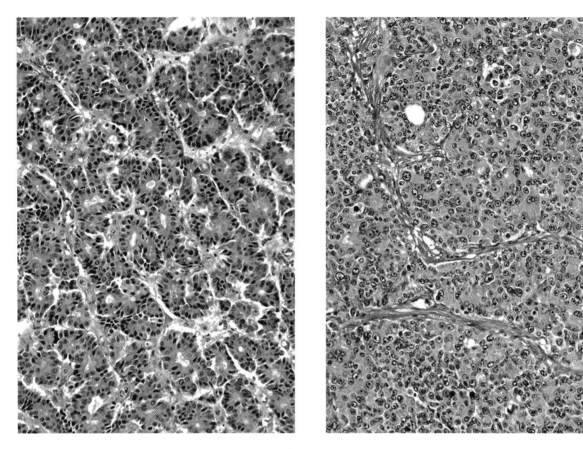

Figure 9-7

ACINAR CELL CARCINOMA

Left: The acinar pattern simulates non-neoplastic acinar parenchyma.
Right: In other areas acini are less organized but have numerous luminal spaces.

The neoplastic cells are arranged in several different architectural patterns, the most prevalent of which are the solid and acinar patterns. In the acinar pattern, the neoplastic cells form minute lumens, similar to non-neoplastic acini. The nuclei are basally located and there is a moderate amount of amphophilic to eosinophilic granular apical cytoplasm (fig. 9-7). The solid pattern is characterized by sheets and nests of cells without evident lumen formation (fig. 9-8). In some solid areas, the nuclei appear randomly distributed within the cells, but there is commonly basal localization at the interface of the solid cell nests with the delicate fibrovascular stroma that separates them, resulting in basal palisading of the nuclei (fig. 9-9). The amount of cytoplasm in solid areas generally varies from minimal to moderate, and it may be more abundant in the cells abutting the stroma.

The pure solid and acinar patterns account for the majority of acinar cell carcinomas, each constituting the bulk of the neoplasm in 30 to 40 percent of cases (31), and an equal mixture of the two patterns is seen in the remaining third. Less common architectural patterns include a glandular pattern, in which acinar structures are dilated, and a trabecular pattern, with interlacing ribbons of cells, each composed of two rows of cells with nuclei oriented toward the periphery of the ribbon (fig. 9-10). Rarely, the trabeculae are tortuous, producing a gyriform pattern similar to that of endocrine neoplasms.

The nuclei in acinar cell carcinomas are relatively uniform, generally with only moderate variability in shape and size (fig. 9-9). Marked nuclear pleomorphism is an uncommon finding. A characteristic feature is the presence of large, central, single nucleoli (fig. 9-11, left).

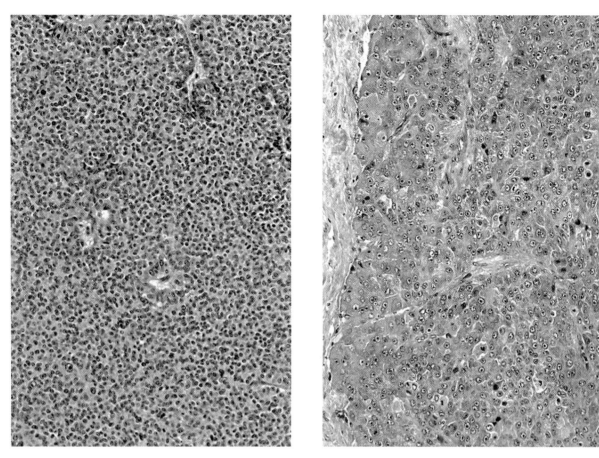

Figure 9-8

ACINAR CELL CARCINOMA: SOLID PATTERN

Left: Solid sheets of cells are punctuated by small blood vessels.
Right: Some cells in the solid regions have more abundant eosinophilic cytoplasm, especially at the interface with the stroma.

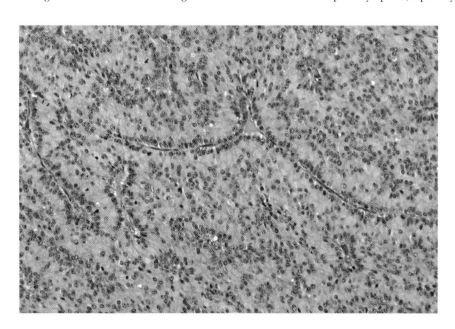

Figure 9-9

ACINAR CELL CARCINOMA

Basal nuclear polarization in the cells adjacent to the vessels results in nuclear palisading.

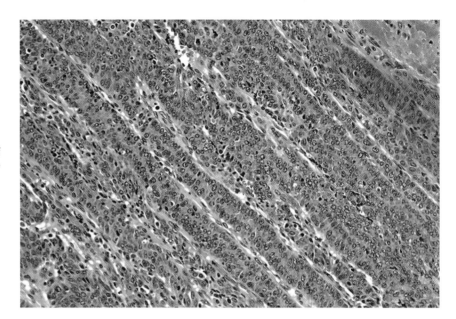

Figure 9-10

ACINAR CELL CARCINOMA: TRABECULAR PATTERN

Each trabecula consists of two rows of cells with peripherally arrayed nuclei.

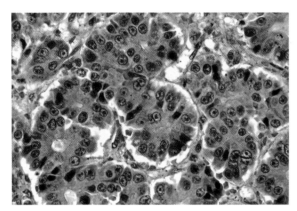
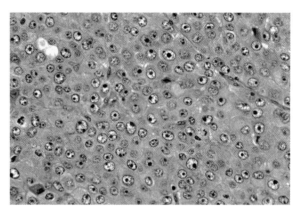

Figure 9-11

ACINAR CELL CARCINOMA

Prominent nucleoli are evident in the acinar (left) and solid (right) growth patterns. Note the relative uniformity of nuclear size and shape.

These nucleoli provide an important clue to the diagnosis in acinar cell carcinomas with a solid growth pattern (fig. 9-11, right). The mitotic rate is variable; although some neoplasms have relatively few mitotic figures, in most mitoses are easy to find, ranging from 5 to 20 (mean, 14) per 10 high-power fields (31). Atypical mitoses are occasionally found.

The striking eosinophilic granularity of the cytoplasm reflects the presence of cytoplasmic zymogen granules. In some well-granulated carcinomas, this feature is readily identifiable in routinely stained sections (fig. 9-12). In most cases, however, the cytoplasmic granularity is not well developed or may be completely inapparent. Thus, special stains are generally required to document the presence of pancreatic exocrine enzymes.

Microscopically, there is nearly always evidence of invasive growth. Vascular invasion within the capsule of the neoplasm is common, and perineural invasion and extension into peripancreatic tissues may be seen (fig. 9-13). Gross intraductal extension is a rare occurrence, but sometimes, microscopic polypoid projections of carcinoma within the lumen of

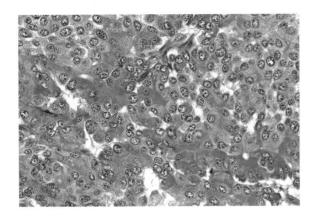

Figure 9-12

ACINAR CELL CARCINOMA

Eosinophilic and granular cytoplasm are seen, especially in the apical regions of well-polarized cells.

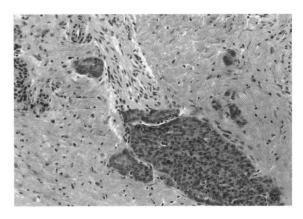

Figure 9-13

ACINAR CELL CARCINOMA

Perineural invasion.

an otherwise normal duct are seen at the periphery of the carcinoma.

Special stains can document the production of exocrine pancreatic enzymes. Zymogen granules in 95 percent of the cancers are positive with the PAS stain, and resistant to diastase digestion (dPAS). In cases with typical histologic features, the finding of granular dPAS positivity in the apical cytoplasm may be sufficient to confirm a diagnosis of acinar cell carcinoma (fig. 9-14). Many acinar cell carcinomas, however, do not contain sufficient quantities of zymogen granules for this stain to provide convincing results. The butyrate esterase stain detects the presence of enzymatically active lipase (6,31,76). This stain demonstrates lipase in the neoplastic cells and is highly specific for acinar differentiation; however, it is not widely utilized and is only positive in 70 to 75 percent of cases (31). Stains for mucins (Alcian blue or mucicarmine) are negative in the cytoplasm, although focal faint reactivity may be noted in the luminal secretions.

Uncommon Histologic Findings. Rarely, acinar cell carcinomas exhibit eosinophilic granularity due to an abundance of mitochondria rather than zymogen granules (fig. 9-15). These oncocytic acinar cell carcinomas are difficult to recognize without electron microscopy. Perhaps because the cytoplasm is largely filled with mitochondria, zymogen granules are less abundant in oncocytic acinar cell carcinomas,

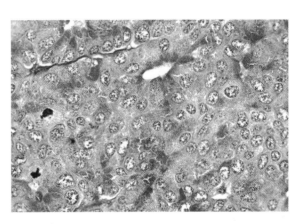

Figure 9-14

ACINAR CELL CARCINOMA

Periodic acid–Schiff with diastase (dPAS) intensely stains a well-granulated carcinoma.

and immunolabeling for trypsin may be focal. Another unusual feature is the appearance of signet ring cells. In these foci, crescentic nuclei are displaced to the cell periphery by abundant granular cytoplasm. These carcinomas can be distinguished from signet ring cell carcinomas of pancreatic ductal (or metastatic) origin by the lack of intracellular mucin in the acinar cell carcinoma and the finding of signet ring cells within larger solid nests rather than infiltrating the stroma individually. Focal papillary formations may also occur. Clear cell change may be found in some acinar cell carcinomas. The etiology of this appearance is not known.

Table 9-2

ACINAR CELL CARCINOMA:
IMMUNOHISTOCHEMICAL FINDINGS

Antigen	% Positive
Trypsin	95
Chymotrypsin	95
Lipase	80
Amylase	15
Chromogranin	35f[a]
Synaptophysin	35f
CEA[b]	20f
CA19-9	20f
Alpha-1-antitrypsin	80
Alpha-1-antichymotrypsin	80
Cytokeratins[c]	95
CK7	10
CK20	10
EMA	40
Alpha-fetoprotein	6

[a]f = focal.
[b]CEA = carcinoembryonic antigen; CA = carbohydrate antigen; CK = cytokeratin; EMA = epithelial membrane antigen.
[c]Cytokeratins 8 and 18.

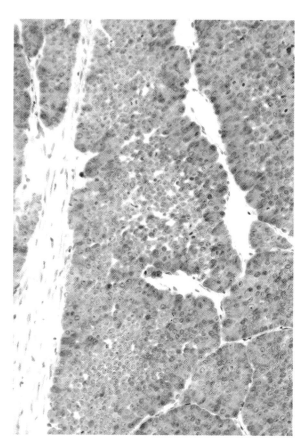

Figure 9-16

ACINAR CELL CARCINOMA

Immunohistochemical labeling for chymotrypsin.

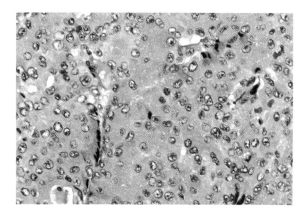

Figure 9-15

ONCOCYTIC ACINAR CELL CARCINOMA

The cells have abundant granular eosinophilic cytoplasm.

Immunohistochemical Findings. Commercial antibodies are available against pancreatic exocrine enzymes including trypsin, chymotrypsin, lipase, and elastase (Table 9-2) (22,24,31,46,67). The first three of these are the most widely employed, and labeling for trypsin and chymotrypsin has the highest degree of sensitivity (55). Trypsin has been detected in more than 95 percent of cases, and although some studies have shown less sensitivity for chymotrypsin (31), we have found current antibodies to chymotrypsin to be nearly equal in sensitivity as those for trypsin. Immunohistochemical labeling for lipase is positive in 75 to 85 percent of the cancers (55). Interestingly, pancreatic amylase is rarely detected in acinar cell carcinomas despite its presence in non-neoplastic acinar cells (22,31). The pattern of immunoreactivity for pancreatic enzymes parallels the distribution of zymogen granules in the neoplastic cells (fig. 9-16). In areas showing well-established cell polarity, the reaction product is generally found in the apical cytoplasm.

Acinar cell carcinomas also commonly have focal endocrine differentiation (22,31,51). Scattered cells in 35 to 54 percent of cases immunolabel for chromogranin or synaptophysin

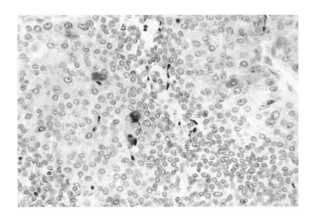

Figure 9-17

ACINAR CELL CARCINOMA

Immunohistochemical labeling for chromogranin shows scattered positive cells.

(fig. 9-17). Carcinomas with greater degrees of endocrine differentiation (more than 25 percent of the neoplastic cells) are classified as mixed acinar-endocrine carcinomas (see below). Rarely, peptide hormones such as glucagon or somatostatin are expressed in acinar cell carcinomas. Glycoproteins characteristic of ductal differentiation (carcinoembryonic antigen [CEA], CA19-9, CA125, and B72.3) may also be found focally.

Other immunohistochemical markers that are reportedly positive in acinar cell carcinoma include pancreatic stone protein, pancreatic secretory trypsin inhibitor, phospholipase A2, alpha-1-antitrypsin, and alpha-1-antichymotrypsin (36,67). The last two markers are, however, much less specific than labeling for trypsin or chymotrypsin. Acinar cell carcinomas produce CK8 and CK18 and are therefore positive for CAM5.2 and AE1/AE3. Immunolabeling for CK7, CK19, and CK20 is generally negative, and epithelial membrane antigen is expressed in only half of the carcinomas (55).

Alpha-fetoprotein (AFP) has been detected by immunohistochemistry in acinar cell carcinomas in patients with and without elevated serum AFP (11,26,46a,48,54,66). In studies not specifically reporting AFP-producing acinar cell carcinomas, about 6 percent of the neoplasms show AFP positivity (31); cases with serum elevations show more diffuse and intense labeling (11).

Ultrastructural Findings. Ultrastructural examination of acinar cell carcinomas (8,23, 31,56,59,74,75) reveals abundant evidence of

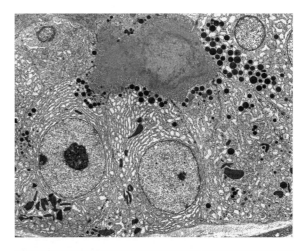

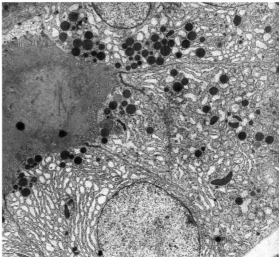

Figure 9-18

ACINAR CELL CARCINOMA

Top: Ultrastructurally, the cells are polarized and rest on a basement membrane. The cytoplasm contains abundant rough endoplasmic reticulum and mitochondria and there are well-formed lumens.

Bottom: Abundant, large (500 to 600 nm), round, and homogeneous zymogen granules are found, principally in the apical cytoplasm.

exocrine secretory function. Well-formed luminal spaces are generally identifiable, and the cells contain basally oriented nuclei, abundant rough endoplasmic reticulum, and numerous mitochondria (fig. 9-18). Most acinar cell carcinomas also contain abundant zymogen granules. These granules are round and homogeneously electron dense, with a closely applied limiting membrane. They range in size from 125 to 1,000 nm, a somewhat broader size range than

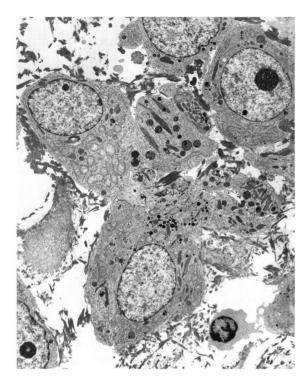

Figure 9-19

ACINAR CELL CARCINOMA

Irregular fibrillary granules are randomly distributed in the cytoplasm and are larger than the zymogen granules.

zymogen granules in non-neoplastic acinar cells (250 to 1,000 nm). In well-polarized cells, the zymogen granules are usually apically located and may fuse with the apical membrane, resulting in secretory products accumulating in the lumens. In less-polarized cells, the zymogen granules are more randomly oriented within the cytoplasm.

A second granule type, the irregular fibrillary granule, is highly characteristic of pancreatic acinar differentiation (8,31,59,75). These granules are generally larger than the round zymogen granules, ranging up to 3,500 nm in size. They are irregularly shaped, and often elongated, angulated, or bilobed (fig. 9-19). The content of fibrillary granules is less homogenously electron dense, and there are parallel fibrillar arrays within the granules. Some irregular fibrillary granules appear to be membrane bound, but others are free within the cytoplasm. In some cases, transitional forms between the irregular fibrillary granules and classic zymogen granules are found, with round membrane-bound granules demonstrating a fibrillary internal matrix (74,75).

The enzymatic content of the round zymogen granules of acinar cell carcinoma can be readily demonstrated by immunoelectron microscopy using antibodies against trypsin or chymotrypsin (32). The nature of the irregular fibrillary granules is less certain. No similar granule type is identifiable in the acinar cells of normal adult pancreata. The acinar cells of the developing fetal pancreas, however, transiently contain granules with the same irregular shape and internal fibrillary content (39). These have been interpreted to represent zymogen granules in the fetal acinar cells, but attempts to demonstrate enzymes within the irregular fibrillary granules of acinar cell carcinomas have been largely unsuccessful (32). In fact, some investigators have suggested that the irregular fibrillary granules contain bundles of intracellular keratin (59). Whatever the nature of the irregular fibrillary granules, they appear to be quite specific for acinar differentiation in pancreatic neoplasms, since they have not been identified in neoplasms of ductal or endocrine nature.

Cytologic Findings. Acinar cell carcinomas are generally sampled cytologically via fine needle aspiration biopsy since they do not typically invade the bile duct or duodenum and are therefore not usually accessible by brush cytology. Aspirate smears of acinar cell carcinoma tend to be moderately cellular. The neoplastic cells are arranged in irregularly shaped groups, solid sheets, and small glandular clusters as well as individually (fig. 9-20). This is in contrast to the organized grape-like clustering of benign acini (see chapter 1). The smear background is generally clean but may contain cytoplasmic granules stripped from the neoplastic cells, the consequence of which is naked tumor nuclei, a helpful diagnostic finding (fig. 9-21). Typically, the individual neoplastic cells are disarmingly bland, with a polygonal cell shape, low nuclear to cytoplasmic ratio, and uniform nuclei. The cells may be pleomorphic, however, and occasionally appear plasmacytoid (24,52,63,68a,77). The striking plasmacytoid appearance of endocrine neoplasms, however, is not present in acinar cell carcinoma (37).

The chromatin is usually coarsely clumped. The presence of one or two prominent nucleoli

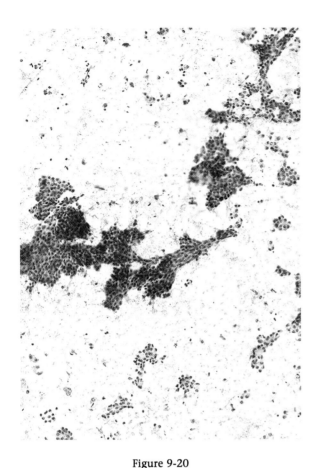

Figure 9-20

ACINAR CELL CARCINOMA

Aspirate smears are generally moderately cellular and composed of neoplastic acinar cells in irregularly shaped groups, sheets, and small glandular clusters. Scattered individual cells and "naked" tumor nuclei are seen in a generally clean background (direct smear; Papanicolaou stain).

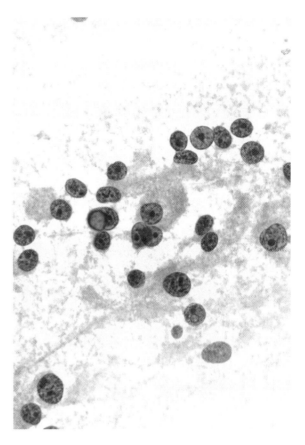

Figure 9-21

ACINAR CELL CARCINOMA

The presence of abundant densely granular cytoplasm, which may be dispersed in an otherwise clean background, and the resulting "naked" tumor nuclei with prominent nucleoli, help identify the cells as neoplastic (direct smear; hematoxylin and eosin [H&E] stain).

coupled with coarsely granular cytoplasm is a helpful diagnostic finding (68a). The cytoplasmic granularity is eosinophilic on hematoxylin and eosin (H&E)-stained smears (fig. 9-22A), where it is more easily seen than on Papanicolaou- (fig. 9-22B) (63) and Romanowsky-stained smears (fig. 9-22C). The last two stains produce cytoplasm that appears denser and more finely granular, making the granules less visible. The absence of striking cytoplasmic granularity and large, prominent nucleoli is common in acinar cell carcinoma, adding to the diagnostic difficulty. Identification of mitotic activity supports a neoplastic process.

Molecular Findings. Due to the rarity of acinar cell carcinoma, there are few studies evaluating the molecular features of this neoplasm.

Initial work focused on the genetic abnormalities characteristic of ductal adenocarcinomas. In fact, acinar cell carcinomas generally lack many of the common abnormalities of ductal carcinomas (Table 9-3) (40,44). Approximately 40 cases have been evaluated for mutations in the *KRAS* oncogene, and only one mutation (at codon 12) was detected (22,45,60,72). Only rare cases have exhibited abnormal nuclear accumulation of the p53 protein, and Dpc4 is normally expressed (1,45). Also, abnormalities in p16 expression are not detected (45). Thus, acinar cell carcinoma has a molecular phenotype quite distinct from that of ductal adenocarcinoma.

Recent work has identified losses on chromosome arm 11p in 50 percent of cases (1). In addition, some acinar cell carcinomas share

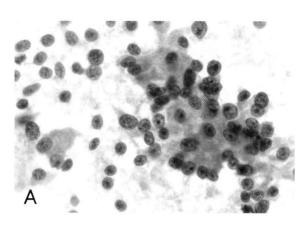

Figure 9-22

ACINAR CELL CARCINOMA

The granularity of the cytoplasm is most pronounced with the H&E stain (A). Routine cytologic stains such as the Papanicolaou (B) and Romanowsky (C) stains demonstrate a finely granular to finely vacuolated cytoplasm (direct smears).

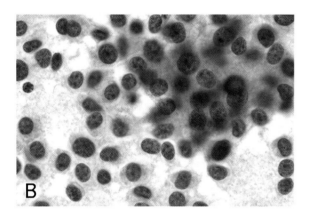

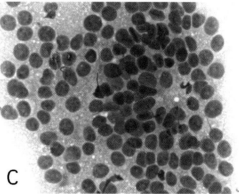

Table 9-3

ACINAR CELL CARCINOMA: MOLECULAR FINDINGS[a]

Gene/Locus	Number Studied	% Abnormal
KRAS	39	3
TP53	71	0
p16/CDKN2A	6	0
SMADH4/DPC4	26	0
11p[b]	12	50
APC	17	6
beta-catenin	17	18

[a]Data from references 1, 22, 45, 60, and 72.
[b]Chromosome 11p losses.

with pancreatoblastomas abnormalities in the APC/beta-catenin pathway, either through activating mutations of the *beta-catenin* gene or truncating mutations of the *APC* gene (1). Although only 24 percent of acinar cell carcinomas have abnormalities in this pathway (compared with 67 percent of pancreatoblastomas [2]), abnormalities in this molecular pathway seem to link pancreatic neoplasms with acinar differentiation.

Other studies of the chromosomal abnormalities in acinar cell carcinoma have revealed gains on chromosomal arms 1q, 12p, and Xq (70) and losses on arms 1p, 4q, 11q, 13q, 15q, 16p, 16q, and 17p (62,70).

Differential Diagnosis. Acinar cell carcinomas share a solid, cellular low-power appearance with a number of other less common pancreatic neoplasms (30). These tumors include well-differentiated pancreatic endocrine neoplasms, solid-pseudopapillary neoplasms, mixed acinar neoplasms, and pancreatoblastomas.

The entity most commonly confused with acinar cell carcinoma is well-differentiated pancreatic endocrine neoplasm. In fact, in one study principally reviewing consultation cases, the original diagnosis for nearly one third of the acinar cell carcinomas was well-differentiated pancreatic endocrine neoplasm (31). With the increased availability of immunohistochemical labeling for pancreatic exocrine enzymes, these two entities can be readily distinguished. A list of the characteristic histologic features of acinar cell carcinomas and pancreatic endocrine neoplasms is presented in Table 9-4. Similarities

Table 9-4

ACINAR CELL CARCINOMA VERSUS
WELL-DIFFERENTIATED PANCREATIC
ENDOCRINE NEOPLASMS: HISTOLOGIC FEATURES

Feature	Acinar Cell Carcinoma	Pancreatic Endocrine Neoplasm
Circumscription	++	++
Cellularity	+++	+++
Amount of stroma	+/-	+/++
Acinar pattern	+++	+
Solid pattern	++	+++
Trabecular pattern	+/-	++
Cellular polarization	++	+/-
Prominent nucleoli	++	+/-
Granular eosinophilic cytoplasm	++	+
Mitosis	+/-	-

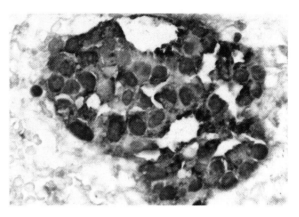

Figure 9-23

ACINAR CELL CARCINOMA

Immunolabeling for trypsin helps to differentiate the neoplastic cells of acinar cell carcinoma from a neuroendocrine neoplasm (destained fixed direct smear).

include a solid, acinar, or glandular architecture; relatively minimal stroma; and nuclear uniformity. Features that favor a diagnosis of acinar cell carcinoma include widespread acinar formations (although pancreatic endocrine neoplasms may also exhibit lumen formation), basal nuclear polarization, eosinophilic cytoplasmic granularity, and single prominent nucleoli. The presence of readily identifiable mitotic figures (greater than 10 per 10 high-power fields) in a neoplasm otherwise showing nuclear uniformity and an overall organoid architecture strongly suggests an acinar cell carcinoma, since most well-differentiated pancreatic endocrine neoplasms have relatively few (if any) mitoses. Features favoring the diagnosis of well-differentiated pancreatic endocrine neoplasm include hyalinized or amyloid-like stroma between nests of neoplastic cells, a trabecular or gyriform growth pattern (particularly when arranged in single cell–thick cords), central nuclear localization, and a coarsely clumped "salt and pepper" chromatin pattern. Although the light microscopic features may be helpful in suggesting the correct diagnosis, there are some cases in which immunohistochemistry for the general endocrine markers chromogranin and synaptophysin and the enzyme markers trypsin and chymotrypsin is absolutely essential to establish the correct diagnosis. Since acinar cell carcinomas may contain scattered endocrine cells, the finding of focal chromogranin

or synaptophysin expression in a solid, cellular pancreatic neoplasm is not sufficient to establish a diagnosis of well-differentiated pancreatic endocrine neoplasm unless the presence of acinar differentiation has been excluded.

Well-differentiated pancreatic endocrine neoplasms are also the most important differential diagnosis of acinar cell carcinomas on cytology preparations (37,68a). Given the overlapping histologic features of these two neoplasms, it is not surprising that they share many cytologic findings as well, including uniform nuclei, numerous individual cells, and a moderate amount of dense cytoplasm. Endocrine neoplasms tend to have a more uniform, noncohesive, single cell smear pattern, with plasmacytoid cells and less well-developed microglandular formations than acinar cell carcinoma. Acinar cell carcinoma also lacks the typical endocrine "salt and pepper" chromatin pattern. Given that endocrine neoplasms can demonstrate prominent nucleoli and acinar cell carcinomas may not demonstrate obviously granular cytoplasm, many cases require immunohistochemical labeling for accurate diagnosis. Studies have documented the utility of labeling for chromogranin, synaptophysin, trypsin, and chymotrypsin in the distinction of acinar cell carcinoma from pancreatic endocrine neoplasm on cytologic smears (fig. 9-23) (37).

Distinguishing mixed acinar neoplasms from pure acinar cell carcinoma is rarely possible on the basis of routine histology alone. This is particularly true for the most common mixed acinar neoplasm, mixed acinar-endocrine carcinoma (32). Because of the overlapping histologic features between acinar and endocrine neoplasms, neoplasms exhibiting both lines of differentiation are particularly hard to recognize. In these instances, comparative immunohistochemical labeling for acinar and endocrine markers is needed to determine the proportion of each cell type. Neoplasms exhibiting more than 25 percent of both cell types are designated mixed acinar-endocrine carcinoma. Likewise, mixed acinar-ductal carcinomas contain more than 25 percent of both acinar and ductal elements, with the ductal differentiation based on the presence of intracellular mucin or immunohistochemical reactivity for glycoproteins such as CEA (using monoclonal antibodies), CA19-9, or B72.3.

Pancreatoblastoma is another solid, cellular pancreatic neoplasm that is closely related to acinar cell carcinoma (21,33). Pancreatoblastomas exhibit extensive acinar differentiation but commonly contain endocrine or ductal cells as well. They also typically have more prominent lobulation and separation of the epithelial components by cellular stromal bands. Finally and most importantly, pancreatoblastomas have squamoid nests: circumscribed aggregates of larger plump to spindled cells that are distinct from the surrounding acinar cells and may show squamous differentiation. Pancreatoblastoma is nearly impossible to distinguish from acinar cell carcinoma on the basis of cytology, since the characteristic squamoid nests of pancreatoblastoma are not reportedly detectable in cytologic smears. Since pancreatoblastomas principally affect children in the first decade of life and most acinar cell carcinomas occur in older adults, the age of the patient is helpful in suggesting the correct diagnosis. Exceptions occur, however, and it may be particularly difficult to distinguish these two entities on the basis of a limited biopsy from a pediatric patient.

Not only is there widespread acinar differentiation and many other morphologic similarities between these two entities, but the genetic features and biologic behavior are similar as well (1,2). Thus, although there may be striking pathologic differences between typical cases of acinar cell carcinoma and pancreatoblastoma, the clini-

cal importance of distinguishing these two tumor types is minimal. In problematic cases, a diagnosis of pancreatoblastoma is favored for neoplasms with acinar differentiation arising in children, especially if a significant component of endocrine or ductal differentiation is detected by immunohistochemistry, unless a careful search of substantial amounts of the neoplasm fails to reveal squamoid nests. Conversely, in the adult patient, a diagnosis of acinar cell carcinoma should be favored unless the classic features of pancreatoblastoma (including squamoid nests) are identified.

A final entity that may be confused with acinar cell carcinoma is solid-pseudopapillary neoplasm (34). These neoplasms can have extensive solid areas with uniform, polygonal cells arranged in nests and sheets separated by small vessels, resembling the solid areas of acinar cell carcinoma. Solid-pseudopapillary neoplasms typically arise in female patients in their twenties, placing them between the pediatric and adult age peaks of acinar cell carcinomas. Histologically, solid-pseudopapillary neoplasms demonstrate characteristic degenerative pseudopapillary formations that have not been described in acinar cell carcinoma. Furthermore, solid-pseudopapillary neoplasms never exhibit true lumen formation, so the presence of an acinar or glandular pattern would exclude this entity. In problematic cases, immunohistochemistry readily distinguishes these two neoplasms. Solid-pseudopapillary neoplasms express vimentin, CD56, CD10, and alpha-1-antitrypsin; show abnormal nuclear labeling for beta-catenin; commonly fail to label with antibodies to cytokeratin; and never express pancreatic enzymes (trypsin or chymotrypsin) or chromogranin. Features helpful in distinguishing solid-pseudopapillary neoplasm from acinar cell carcinoma on cytology include the formation of pseudopapillary structures with the characteristic myxoid stroma, smaller more oval nuclei, the fragility of the cytoplasm (with numerous stripped nuclei without prominent nucleoli), and the presence of longitudinal nuclear grooves in solid-pseudopapillary neoplasm.

Some acinar cell carcinomas are remarkably well differentiated, almost resembling normal acinar cells and raising questions about their malignant nature. Benign solid acinar neoplasms (acinar cell adenomas), however, are not

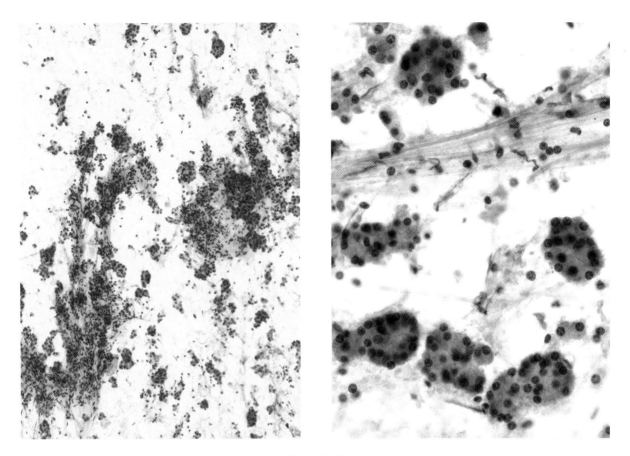

Figure 9-24

BENIGN ACINAR EPITHELIAL CELLS

The pattern of tightly cohesive grape-like clusters of acinar cells with stroma and uniform individual acinar groups without numerous, associated stripped nuclei in the background distinguish these benign acinar cells from acinar cell carcinoma (left and right: direct smears; Papanicolaou stain).

convincingly reported. Prior to the availability of immunohistochemical markers of exocrine enzyme production, a few "acinar adenomas" had been described (78), but it is likely that these represented small pancreatic endocrine neoplasms with an acinar pattern of growth. Other reported cases were considered benign due to the lack of invasive growth and absence of necrosis or conspicuous mitotic activity (38), but not all acinar cell carcinomas exhibit these features, and these neoplasms (which measured 13 and 19 cm) would currently be classified as acinar cell carcinomas.

Acinar cell nodules are microscopic aggregates of acinar cells with altered cytoplasmic or nuclear features (see chapter 1). These non-neoplastic lesions are unlikely to be confused with acinar cell carcinomas.

On occasion, a fine needle aspiration of normal pancreatic parenchyma may produce a smear with many acini that raises the possibility of acinar cell carcinoma. Similarly, a scantily cellular aspirate of an acinar cell neoplasm may be mistaken for normal acini. Benign acini arranged into small, tightly cohesive grape-like clusters and small, uniform individual acinar groups without the associated stripped tumor nuclei, especially admixed with ductal groups and coupled with inconspicuous nucleoli, are features that characterize non-neoplastic pancreatic parenchyma in aspirate smears (fig. 9-24).

Spread and Metastases. Acinar cell carcinomas are highly aggressive neoplasms. Approximately 50 percent of patients have metastatic disease at presentation, and more than half of the remaining patients develop metastases later

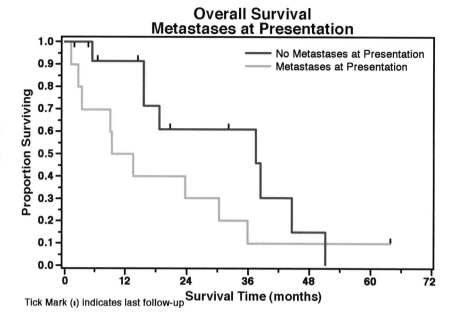

Figure 9-25

ACINAR CELL CARCINOMA

Survival curves for patients with acinar cell carcinoma treated at Memorial Sloan-Kettering Cancer Center. (Modified from fig. 2 from reference 20.)

in their clinical course (31). Most often, metastatic disease is found in regional lymph nodes and liver, although occasional patients develop distant metastases to lung, cervical lymph nodes, and ovary. It is rare for patients to present with distant metastases as the first manifestation of the disease (13,19).

Staging. The staging of acinar cell carcinomas should follow the staging of carcinomas of the exocrine pancreas (see chapter 3).

Prognosis. Although the ultimate survival rate of patients with acinar cell carcinoma is very poor (5-year survival rate, 6 percent [31]), several studies have suggested that this neoplasm is not quite as rapidly lethal as conventional ductal adenocarcinoma. Indeed, the median length of survival for all patients is 18 to 19 months (20,31), and it is not uncommon for patients with distant metastases to survive for 2 to 3 years. The median survival period for 108 patients in the Surveillance Epidemiology and End Results (SEER) program of the National Cancer Institute database was 1.14 years and the 5-year survival rate was 25 percent (www.seer.cancer.gov/seerstat). The survival curve for patients with acinar cell carcinoma treated at Memorial Sloan-Kettering Cancer Center is shown in figure 9-25.

It has been suggested that pediatric patients with acinar cell carcinoma may have a better prognosis than adults (31). Experience with this neoplasm in childhood is limited, precluding an accurate statistical evaluation of this observation, however, long-term survival and cure of pediatric patients have been observed. It should be noted that the pathologic distinction of pediatric acinar cell carcinoma from pancreatoblastoma may be quite difficult, since these two neoplasms are closely related (see Differential Diagnosis). Fortunately, it appears that the biologic behavior of pediatric acinar cell carcinoma is essentially the same as that of pancreatoblastoma (33).

A number of clinical and pathologic variables have been analyzed for prognostic significance in acinar cell carcinoma. Patients presenting with the lipase hypersecretion syndrome have a particularly short survival period, perhaps because most have liver metastases at the time the syndrome develops (31). As such, it may be the strong correlation of tumor stage with outcome, documented in all patients irrespective of symptoms, that dictates the prognosis in these cases. Also likely related to tumor stage is the correlation of improved survival with surgery (versus chemotherapy) as an initial therapeutic approach; only patients with organ-limited disease qualify for resection. Other factors that have been correlated with poor outcome include male gender, age over 60, and tumor size greater than 10 cm (20,31). The extent of the acinar and solid morphologic growth patterns is not prognostically relevant (31).

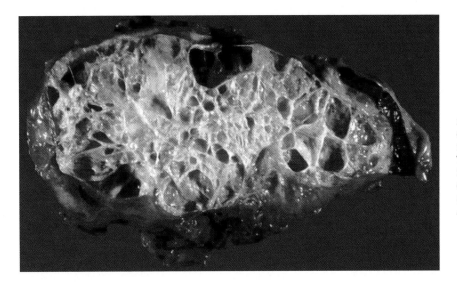

Figure 9-26

ACINAR CELL CYSTADENOCARCINOMA

The 7,000-g carcinoma is multiloculated, with individual cysts ranging from a few millimeters to several centimeters. The septa are thin and the lining is smooth and glistening, without evident papillary projections. (Courtesy of Dr. A. Cubilla, Asuncion, Paraguay.)

Treatment. The treatment for patients with early-stage acinar cell carcinoma is surgical resection. Since many acinar cell carcinomas are quite large at presentation, they may appear to be unresectable. However, these neoplasms, grow in an expansile fashion, rendering even some large carcinomas resectable. In the presence of distant metastases, chemotherapy with or without radiation to the pancreas has been utilized (15,20,46a)). Treated acinar cell carcinomas may show histologic changes including fibrosis and accumulation of histiocytes.

ACINAR CELL CYSTADENOCARCINOMA

Definition. *Acinar cell cystadenocarcinoma* is a rare malignant epithelial neoplasm of the pancreas with a diffusely cystic gross architecture in which the cysts are lined by neoplastic epithelial cells that demonstrate evidence of pancreatic exocrine enzyme production.

General Features. Acinar cell cystadenocarcinoma may be the rarest of the pancreatic acinar neoplasms: only four cases have been reported (7,12,22,68). All four occurred in males (42, 64, 64, and 69 years old). The presenting features were nonspecific and related to the presence of an enlarging mass; none of the patients had the lipase hypersecretion syndrome. Acinar cell cystadenocarcinoma is aggressive, and the three reported cases with available follow-up information showed early dissemination to the peritoneum and liver.

Pathologic Findings. Grossly, acinar cell cystadenocarcinomas are large (mean, 24 cm)

and circumscribed, similar to solid acinar cell carcinomas. In distinction, however, acinar cell cystadenocarcinomas are diffusely cystic, with individual locules ranging from a few millimeters to several centimeters (fig. 9-26). In the case reported by Cantrell (7), the gross appearance resembled that of a large microcystic serous cystadenoma, with a central scar and numerous small cysts imparting a spongy appearance. The other neoplasms had fleshier parenchyma between the cysts.

Microscopically, the cysts are separated by thin fibrous walls and are lined by neoplastic acinar cells with basal basophilic cytoplasm, apical eosinophilic granular cytoplasm, and basally located nuclei with single prominent nucleoli (fig. 9-27). In some regions, the cysts are lined by a single layer of cuboidal to columnar cells, whereas elsewhere there are several layers of epithelial cells, sometimes forming minute lumens within the stratified epithelial lining. Between the larger cysts are clusters of acinar cells, some of which show dilated lumens. There are accumulations of eosinophilic secretions within the luminal spaces and the larger cysts. The nuclei do not show substantial atypia but may be enlarged and somewhat irregular. Invasive growth at the periphery of the neoplasm may be noted.

Special stains can be used to document the presence of acinar differentiation in acinar cell cystadenocarcinomas. The cytoplasmic zymogen granules are positive for PAS, resistant to diastase. As with solid acinar cell carcinomas, immunohistochemistry is much more specific, and

209

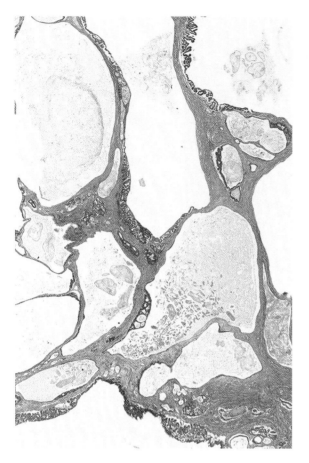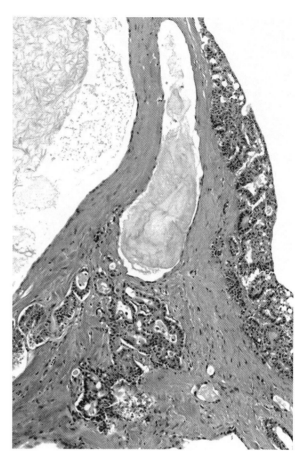

Figure 9-27

ACINAR CELL CYSTADENOCARCINOMA

Left: The cysts are separated by thin fibrous walls.
Right: The lining varies from flattened epithelium to complex, cribriformed structures containing numerous acinar spaces.

immunolabeling for trypsin and chymotrypsin is positive in the neoplastic cells. Presumably, the results of immunohistochemical labeling with other markers would be similar to those in conventional solid acinar cell carcinomas, although the few reported cases have not been studied in detail by immunohistochemistry.

The cases reported by Cantrell et al. (7) and Stamm et al. (68) were examined by electron microscopy. Numerous round, electron-dense, apically situated zymogen granules were identified, in addition to abundant endoplasmic reticulum and numerous mitochondria. Irregular fibrillary granules were not identified in these cases.

Differential Diagnosis. The striking resemblance of the case reported by Cantrell et al. (7) to serous cystadenoma could cause confusion on gross evaluation. Microscopically, however,

acinar cell cystadenocarcinomas lack the clear, glycogen-rich cytoplasm of serous neoplasms. Since some serous neoplasms contain more abundant eosinophilic cytoplasm and smaller, acinar-like glands, immunohistochemical labeling for pancreatic exocrine enzymes may be necessary, in rare instances, to distinguish these two neoplasms. Most other cystic neoplasms of the pancreas are lined by mucinous epithelium, a feature that readily distinguishes them. Focal cystic change may be seen in solid acinar cell carcinomas due to massive dilatation of the neoplastic glands, and gross cystic change may occur due to necrosis (25). The diagnosis of acinar cell cystadenocarcinoma should be reserved for multicystic neoplasms demonstrating widespread cyst formation that is not due simply to central necrosis.

MIXED ACINAR CARCINOMAS

With the increasing use of immunohisto-chemistry to define lines of cellular differentiation, neoplasms exhibiting more than one line of differentiation are being increasingly recognized. Every conceivable combination of acinar, ductal, and endocrine differentiation has been described, and these neoplasms are designated *mixed acinar-endocrine carcinoma, mixed acinar-ductal carcinoma, mixed ductal-endocrine carcinoma* (see chapter 12), and *mixed acinar-endocrine-ductal carcinoma*. Most of these mixed neoplasms are discussed under the heading of acinar neoplasms, not only because an acinar component is present, but because the acinar component usually predominates.

Pancreatic neoplasms with mixed cell lineage are intriguing from a histogenetic standpoint. It is unclear whether the occurrence of more than one line of differentiation reflects origin from relatively primitive precursors that retain the embryologic capacity of multidirectional differentiation (i.e., stem cells) or whether the genetic events triggering neoplasia also influence the lines of differentiation expressed in the resulting neoplasm.

It is somewhat difficult to assess many of the mixed acinar carcinomas reported in the literature. Those reported before the availability of immunohistochemical labeling to identify acinar differentiation were generally less well characterized, and in some instances, definite evidence of each line of differentiation was lacking. In some, only electron microscopic documentation of different types of granules served as evidence for multidirectional differentiation. Other reported mixed neoplasms only contained trivial components of one or more of the cell types.

Although some mixed carcinomas of the pancreas have distinctive histologic features suggesting more than one line of differentiation, many are histologically similar to acinar cell carcinomas, with the mixed differentiation only detected by immunohistochemistry. For this reason and because the acinar elements generally predominate, some authors have argued that these "immunohistochemically defined" entities should not be separated from pure acinar cell carcinomas (51). Indeed, no reproducibly distinctive clinical, molecular, or prognostic features

have been defined for each subtype. Certainly, from a clinical standpoint, it is reasonable to classify these mixed neoplasms with the corresponding predominant cell type (most therefore as acinar cell carcinomas). However, only with careful delineation of the cellular differentiation in additional cases of these unusual tumors will we learn whether significant differences exist between these subtypes. For this reason we recommend a thorough immunohistochemical evaluation of all pancreatic neoplasms exhibiting prominent acinar differentiation.

Mixed Acinar-Endocrine Carcinoma

Definition. *Mixed acinar-endocrine carcinoma* is a malignant epithelial neoplasm exhibiting both endocrine and acinar differentiation. By arbitrary definition, each component must comprise at least 25 percent of the neoplasm for a diagnosis of mixed acinar-endocrine carcinoma.

General Features. Although all pancreatic neoplasms with mixed differentiation are rare, mixed acinar-endocrine carcinoma is probably the most common and certainly the best described in the literature (10,16,18,32,43,47,50, 51,56,65,73). These neoplasms may be difficult to recognize without the aid of immunohistochemistry.

Clinical Features. Patients with mixed acinar-endocrine carcinoma have a demographic spectrum paralleling that of acinar cell carcinoma. Most are adults (mean age, 55 years), and men and women are equally affected (10, 16,18,32,43,47,50,51,56,65,73). Presenting symptoms are nonspecific, usually related to the presence of an expanding mass. Significantly, other than one patient with hypoglycemia (65), none of the reported patients had paraneoplastic syndromes characteristic of either line of differentiation (lipase hypersecretion syndrome or endocrine hormonal hypersecretion syndromes).

The acinar cell component of mixed acinar-endocrine carcinoma almost always predominates. Thus, it is not surprising that the biologic behavior of mixed acinar-endocrine carcinomas parallels that of acinar cell carcinoma, with a relatively aggressive clinical course and uncommon long-term survival, a behavior more aggressive than that of well-differentiated pancreatic endocrine neoplasms.

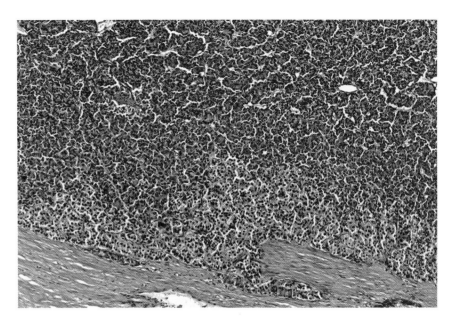

Figure 9-28

MIXED ACINAR-ENDOCRINE
CARCINOMA

Two cell populations are distinguishable histologically. At low power, the peripheral region adjacent to the fibrous pseudo-capsule is composed of a band of endocrine cells, whereas the central portions are acinar.

Pathologic Findings. The gross appearance of mixed acinar-endocrine carcinomas is similar to that of their pure counterparts. Most are circumscribed, solid, and fleshy. Microscopically, two different patterns have been described. One pattern (represented by a single reported case [32]) is characterized by the presence of two sharply segregated, morphologically distinct acinar and endocrine components (fig. 9-28) with minimal intermingling and no individual cells showing both acinar and endocrine differentiation (fig. 9-28). Ultrastructural examination also demonstrated the two distinct cell types, with the acinar cells containing apically located large zymogen granules and the endocrine cells having randomly distributed, small dense core endosecretory granules.

All of the other reported mixed acinar-endocrine carcinomas have displayed less segregation of the two cell types. In fact, in most cases it is not possible to recognize with certainty that two lines of differentiation are present by routine microscopy. Areas of the neoplasm showing more abundant hyalinized stroma and a trabecular architecture without obvious polarization (suggestive of endocrine differentiation) alternate with areas with acinar features including basally located nuclei, prominent nucleoli, and granular eosinophilic cytoplasm. Immunohistochemical labeling, however, shows regions with acinar differentiation and endocrine differentiation diffusely

distributed throughout the entire neoplasm, in some carcinomas not correlating well with the histologic suggestion of different areas of differentiation (fig. 9-29). In these cases, double immunohistochemical labeling for endocrine and acinar markers shows occasional cells that express both markers, a cellular component designated "amphicrine cells." It is rare for mixed acinar-endocrine carcinomas to immunolabel for specific peptide hormones (32,51). Ultrastructural examination of most of these neoplasms has shown primarily acinar differentiation, including both round zymogen granules and irregular fibrillary granules. In some carcinomas, a smaller population of cells with dense core neurosecretory granules has been detected, and rare cells containing both granule types are described (18,32,73).

Mixed Acinar-Ductal Carcinoma

Definition. *Mixed acinar-ductal carcinomas* are malignant epithelial neoplasms with both acinar and ductal differentiation, usually with the acinar component predominating. At least 25 percent of the neoplastic cells must show each line of differentiation, as documented by immunohistochemical labeling for pancreatic exocrine enzymes (acinar component) and by the presence of intracellular mucin or immunohistochemical positivity for glycoproteins such as CEA, CA19-9, B72.3, DUPAN-2, or CA125 (ductal differentiation).

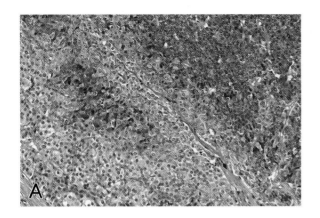

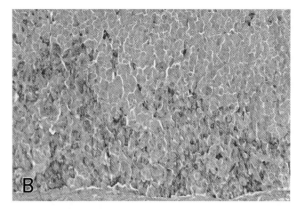

Figure 9-29

MIXED ACINAR-ENDOCRINE CARCINOMA

The dPAS stain (A) highlights the acinar components (top) but is negative in the endocrine cells (bottom). The Grimelius stain (B) shows the opposite pattern of positivity. By immunohistochemistry, the acinar elements are positive for trypsin (C) and the endocrine elements label for chromogranin (D). Simultaneous immunohistochemical staining (E) for trypsin (blue reaction product) and chromogranin (brown reaction product) shows that the two cellular components are entirely separate, without coexpression in individual cells.

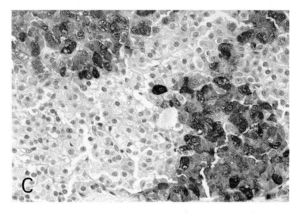

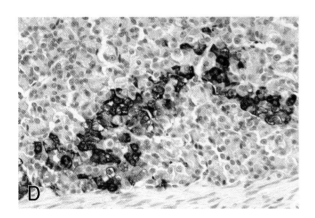

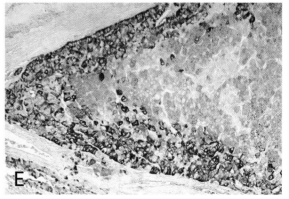

General Features. Only one study has characterized this type of mixed pancreatic carcinoma (64a). The clinical features are nonspecific, and the biologic behavior is aggressive.

Pathologic Findings. Grossly, mixed acinar-ductal carcinomas resemble pure acinar cell carcinomas, although some cases have more fibrosis and lobulation. Histologically, they exhibit a variety of different patterns depending on the proportion and relationship of the different cell types. In some of the neoplasms, there are solid nests of cells as well as individual, infiltrative glands surrounded by a desmoplastic stroma. The solid areas generally contain a predominance of acinar elements, which may be arranged in nests or acinar and glandular formations. In these regions, the cytoplasm is eosinophilic and granular, and lacks detectable mucin. The nuclei are relatively uniform and basally located. Transition to areas with ductal differentiation may be found (fig. 9-30). Ductal elements contain intracellular mucin and generally exhibit a glandular pattern.

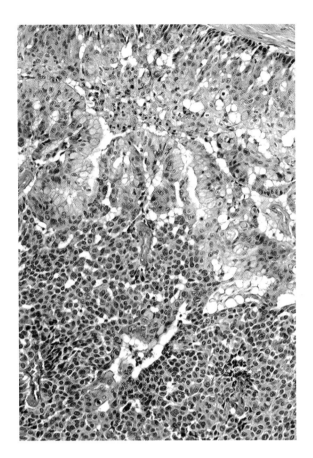

Figure 9-30

MIXED ACINAR-DUCTAL CARCINOMA

Large nests of carcinoma cells have central regions resembling a pure acinar cell carcinoma. The nests are surrounded by columnar glandular cells containing abundant intracellular mucin.

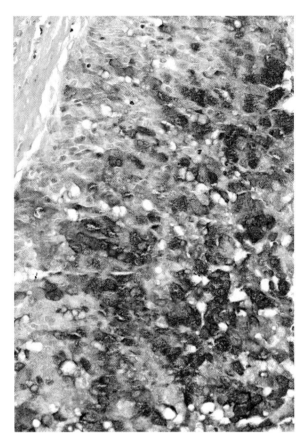

Figure 9-31

MIXED ACINAR-DUCTAL CARCINOMA

Double staining for trypsin (immunohistochemistry, brown reaction product) and mucin (Alcian blue stain) demonstrates the admixture of ductal and acinar elements.

Individual neoplastic glands surrounded by desmoplastic stroma and containing abundant apical mucin (typical of conventional ductal adenocarcinomas) may be found, as may larger cribriformed structures, some of which contain both acinar and ductal cells. Some mixed acinar-ductal carcinomas have solid nests of cells architecturally similar to acinar cell carcinoma but containing intracellular mucin and having marked nuclear atypia.

Histochemical stains for mucins (mucicarmine or Alcian blue) are helpful in detecting the intracellular mucin. The presence of pancreatic enzymes is demonstrated by immunohistochemical labeling, with trypsin or chymotrypsin expressed in more than 25 percent of the neoplastic cells. The ductal elements express glycoprotein markers including CEA, CA19-9, B72.3, or DUPAN-2. Some carcinomas show a relatively sharp distinction between the mucin-positive ductal elements and the enzyme-producing acinar elements, although cells containing both exocrine enzymes and mucin have been found (fig. 9-31). Immunolabeling for chromogranin and synaptophysin may display a minor endocrine cell component that, by definition, should not exceed 25 percent of the neoplastic cellularity.

Mixed Acinar-Endocrine-Ductal Carcinoma

Definition. *Mixed acinar-endocrine-ductal carcinomas* are malignant epithelial neoplasms that demonstrate differentiation towards all three of the normal epithelial cell lines of the pancreas.

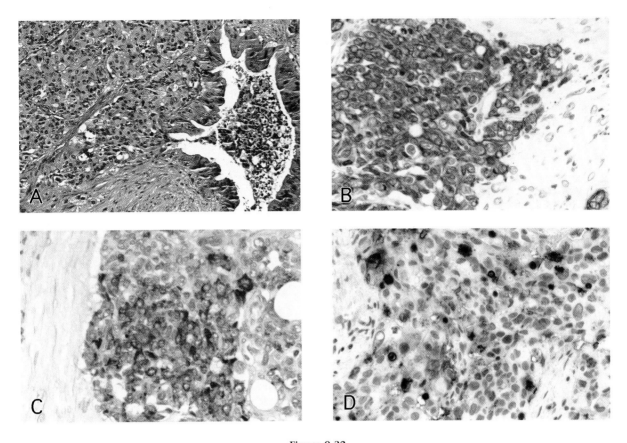

Figure 9-32

MIXED ACINAR-ENDOCRINE-DUCTAL CARCINOMA

The carcinoma is composed of nests of cells with small luminal spaces surrounded by a desmoplastic stroma (A). An adjacent duct demonstrates high-grade pancreatic intraepithelial neoplasia (PanIN). The neoplastic cells are positive for chromogranin (B), trypsin (C), and DUPAN-2 (D).

Histochemical staining and immunohistochemical labeling can be used to document acinar, endocrine, and ductal differentiation, with each component comprising greater than 25 percent of the neoplastic cells.

General and Pathologic Findings. Mixed acinar-endocrine-ductal carcinoma is the least characterized form of pancreatic neoplasm with multiple directions of differentiation (49,53, 64,64a,69). Some reported cases have not quantified the proportion of the neoplasm showing each phenotype, and in some instances, no immunohistochemical proof of trilineage differentiation was presented. The clinical features of the reported cases resemble those of other acinar and mixed pancreatic neoplasms, and the prognosis is equally poor.

Histologically, mixed acinar-endocrine-ductal carcinomas are essentially indistinguishable from mixed acinar-ductal carcinomas, with solid areas reflecting a predominant acinar component and tubular ductal elements containing intracellular mucin accompanied by a desmoplastic stroma (fig. 9-32). The endocrine component was not histologically evident in any of the reported cases but was detected by immunohistochemical labeling for chromogranin or synaptophysin. We have seen one case of mixed acinar-endocrine-ductal carcinoma that also contained a spindle cell sarcomatoid carcinoma component.

REFERENCES

1. Abraham SC, Wu TT, Hruban RH, et al. Genetic and immunohistochemical analysis of pancreatic acinar cell carcinoma: frequent allelic loss on chromosome 11p and alterations in the APC/beta-catenin pathway. Am J Pathol 2002;160: 953-62.

2. Abraham SC, Wu TT, Klimstra DS, Finn L, Hruban RH. Distinctive molecular genetic alterations in sporadic and familial adenomatous polyposis-associated pancreatoblastomas: frequent alterations in the APC/beta-catenin pathway and chromosome 11p. Am J Pathol 2001; 159:1619-27.

3. Adsay NV, Klimstra DS, Compton CC. Cystic lesions of the pancreas. Introduction. Semin Diagn Pathol 2000;17:1-6.

4. Albores-Saavedra J. Acinar cystadenoma of the pancreas: a previously undescribed tumor. Ann Diagn Pathol 2002;6:113-5.

5. Belsky H, Cornell NW. Disseminated focal fat necrosis following radical pancreaticoduodenectomy for acinous carcinoma of head of pancreas. Ann Surg 1955;141:556-62.

6. Burns WA, Matthews MJ, Hamosh M, Weide GV, Blum R, Johnson FB. Lipase-secreting acinar cell carcinoma of the pancreas with polyarthropathy. A light and electron microscopic, histochemical, and biochemical study. Cancer 1974;33:1002-9.

7. Cantrell BB, Cubilla AL, Erlandson RA, Fortner JG, Fitzgerald PJ. Acinar cell cystadenocarcinoma of human pancreas. Cancer 1981;47:410-6.

8. Caruso RA, Inferrera A, Tuccari G, Barresi G. Acinar cell carcinoma of the pancreas. A histologic, immunocytochemical and ultrastructural study. Histol Histopathol 1994;9:53-8.

9. Chatelain D, Paye F, Mourra N, et al. Unilocular acinar cell cystadenoma of the pancreas: an unusual acinar cell tumor. Am J Clin Pathol 2002;118:211-4.

10. Cho KJ, Kim JY, Lee SS, Khang SK, Kim CW. Mixed acinar-endocrine carcinoma of the pancreas—a case report. J Korean Med Sci 1996;11: 188-92.

11. Cingolani N, Shaco-Levy R, Farruggio A, Klimstra DS, Rosai J. Alpha-fetoprotein production by pancreatic tumors exhibiting acinar cell differentiation: study of five cases, one arising in a mediastinal teratoma. Hum Pathol 2000; 31:938-44.

12. Colombo P, Arizzi C, Roncalli M. Acinar cell cystadenocarcinoma of the pancreas: report of rare case and review of the literature. Hum Pathol 2004;35:1568-71.

13. Cubilla AL, Fitzgerald PJ. Tumors of the exocrine pancreas. AFIP Atlas of Tumor Pathology, 2nd Series, Fascicle 19. Washington, DC: American Registry of Pathology; 1984.

14. Fabre A, Sauvanet A, Flejou JF, et al. Intraductal acinar cell carcinoma of the pancreas. Virchows Arch 2001;438:312-5.

15. Feliu J, de la Gandara I, Garrido P, Gonzalez Baron M. Somatostatin analogues and pancreatic acinar cell carcinoma: an alternative in symptomatic treatment? Am J Gastroenterol 1990;85:1539-40.

16. Frank M, Bittinger A, Rothmund M, Arnold R. Immunohistochemical analysis and clinical course of high-malignant composite endocrine-acinar cell carcinoma: a case report. Pancreas 1998;17:210-2.

17. Good AE, Schnitzer B, Kawanishi H, Demetropoulos KC, Rapp R. Acinar pancreatic tumor with metastatic fat necrosis: report of a case and review of rheumatic manifestations. Am J Dig Dis 1976;21:978-87.

18. Hassan MO, Gogate PA. Malignant mixed exocrine-endocrine tumor of the pancreas with unusual intracytoplasmic inclusions. Ultrastruct Pathol 1993;17:483-93.

19. Hewan-Lowe KO. Acinar cell carcinoma of the pancreas: metastases from an occult primary tumor. Arch Pathol Lab Med 1983;107:552-4.

20. Holen KD, Klimstra DS, Hummer A, et al. Clinical characteristics and outcomes from an institutional series of acinar cell carcinoma of the pancreas and related tumors. J Clin Oncol 2002;20:4673-8.

21. Hoorens A, Gebhard F, Kraft K, Lemoine NR, Klöppel G. Pancreatoblastoma in an adult: its separation from acinar cell carcinoma. Virchows Arch 1994;424:485-90.

22. Hoorens A, Lemoine NR, McLellan E, et al. Pancreatic acinar cell carcinoma. An analysis of cell lineage markers, p53 expression, and Ki-ras mutation. Am J Pathol 1993;143:685-98.

23. Horie A, Morohoshi T, Klöppel G. Ultrastructural comparison of pancreatoblastoma, solid cystic tumor and acinar cell carcinoma. J Clin Electron Microscopy 1987;20:353-62.

24. Ishihara A, Sanda T, Takanari H, Yatani R, Liu PI. Elastase-1-secreting acinar cell carcinomas of the pancreas. A cytologic, electron microscopic and histochemical study. Acta Cytol 1989;33:157-63.

25. Ishizaki A, Koito K, Namieno T, Nagakawa T, Murashima Y, Suga T. Acinar cell carcinoma of the pancreas: a rare case of an alpha-fetoprotein-producing cystic tumor. Eur J Radiol 1995; 21:58-60.

26. Itoh T, Kishi K, Tojo M, et al. Acinar cell carcinoma of the pancreas with elevated serum alpha-fetoprotein levels: a case report and a review of 28 cases reported in Japan. Gastroenterol Jpn 1992;27:785-91.

27. Klimstra DS. Cell lineage in pancreatic neoplasms. In: Sarkar FH, Dugan MC, eds. Pancreatic cancer: advances in molecular pathology, diagnosis and clinical management. Natick: BioTechniques Books; 1998:21-47.

28. Klimstra DS. Pancreas. In: Sternberg SS, ed. Histology for pathologists, 2nd ed. Philadelphia: Lippincott-Raven; 1997:613-47.

29. Klimstra DS, Adsay NV. Acinar cell carcinoma of the pancreas. A case associated with the lipase hypersecretion syndrome. Pathol Case Rev 2001;6:121-6.

30. Klimstra DS, Adsay NV. Pancreas cancer: pathology. In: Kelsen DP, Daly JM, Kern SE, Levin B, Tepper JE, eds. Gastrointestinal oncology: principles and practices. Philadelphia: Lippincott, Williams & Wilkins; 2002:459-76.

31. Klimstra DS, Heffess CS, Oertel JE, Rosai J. Acinar cell carcinoma of the pancreas. A clinico-pathologic study of 28 cases. Am J Surg Pathol 1992;16:815-37.

32. Klimstra DS, Rosai J, Heffess CS. Mixed acinar-endocrine carcinomas of the pancreas. Am J Surg Pathol 1994;18:765-78.

33. Klimstra DS, Wenig BM, Adair CF, Heffess CS. Pancreatoblastoma. A clinicopathologic study and review of the literature. Am J Surg Pathol 1995;19:1371-89.

34. Klimstra DS, Wenig BM, Heffess CS. Solid-pseudopapillary tumor of the pancreas: a typically cystic carcinoma of low malignant potential. Semin Diagn Pathol 2000;17:66-80.

35. Kuerer H, Shim H, Pertsemlidis D, Unger P. Functioning pancreatic acinar cell carcinoma: immunohistochemical and ultrastructural analyses. Am J Clin Oncol 1997;20:101-7.

36. Kuopio T, Ekfors TO, Nikkanen V, Nevalainen TJ. Acinar cell carcinoma of the pancreas. Report of three cases. Apmis 1995;103:69-78.

37. Labate AM, Klimstra DS, Zakowski MF. Comparative cytologic features of pancreatic acinar cell carcinoma and islet cell tumor. Diagn Cytopathol 1997;16:112-6.

38. Lack EE, Cassady JR, Levey R, Vawter GF. Tumors of the exocrine pancreas in children and adolescents. A clinical and pathologic study of eight cases. Am J Surg Pathol 1983;7:319-27.

39. Lebenthal E, Lev R, Lee PC. Prenatal and postnatal development of the human exocrine pancreas. In: Go LV, Gardner JD, Brooks FP, DiMagno EP, Lebenthal E, Scheele GA, eds. The exocrine pancreas: biology, pathobiology and diseases. New York: Raven Press; 1986:33-43.

40. Longnecker DS. Molecular pathology of invasive carcinoma. Ann NY Acad Sci 1999;880:74-82.

41. MacMahon HE, Brown PA, Shen EM. Acinar cell carcinoma of the pancreas with subcutaneous fat necrosis. Gastroenterology 1965;49:555-9.

42. Mah P, Loo DC, Tock EP. Pancreatic acinar cell carcinoma in childhood. Am J Dis Child 1974;128:101-4.

43. Mizuta Y, Isomoto H, Futuki Y, et al. Acinar cell carcinoma of the pancreas associated with hypoglycemia: involvement of "big" insulin-like growth factor-II. J Gastroenterol 1998;33:761-5.

44. Moore PS, Beghelli S, Zamboni G, Scarpa A. Genetic abnormalities in pancreatic cancer. Mol Cancer 2003;2:7.

45. Moore PS, Orlandini S, Zamboni G, et al. Pancreatic tumours: molecular pathways implicated in ductal cancer are involved in ampullary but not in exocrine nonductal or endocrine tumorigenesis. Br J Cancer 2001;84:253-62.

46. Morohoshi T, Kanda M, Horie A, et al. Immunocytochemical markers of uncommon pancreatic tumors. Acinar cell carcinoma, pancreatoblastoma, and solid cystic (papillary-cystic) tumor. Cancer 1987;59:739-47.

46a. Mueller SB, Micke O, Herbst H, Schaefer U, Willich N. Alpha-fetoprotein-positive carcinoma of the pancreas: a case report. Anticancer Res 2005;25:1671-4.

47. Muramatsu T, Kijima H, Tsuchida T, et al. Acinar-islet cell tumor of the pancreas: report of a malignant pancreatic composite tumor. J Clin Gastroenterol 2000;31:175-8.

48. Nojima T, Kojima T, Kato H, Sato T, Koito K, Nagashima K. Alpha-fetoprotein-producing acinar cell carcinoma of the pancreas. Hum Pathol 1992;23:828-30.

49. Nonomura A, Kono N, Mizukami Y, Nakanuma Y, Matsubara F. Duct-acinar-islet cell tumor of the pancreas. Ultrastruct Pathol 1992;16:317-29.

50. Ogawa T, Isaji S, Yabana T. A case of mixed acinar-endocrine carcinoma of the pancreas discovered in an asymptomatic subject. Int J Pancreatol 2000;27:249-57.

51. Ohike N, Kosmahl M, Klöppel G. Mixed acinar-endocrine carcinoma of the pancreas. A clinicopathological study and comparison with acinar-cell carcinoma. Virchows Arch 2004;445: 231-5.

52. Ohori NP, Khalid A, Etemad B, Finkelstein SD. Multiple loss of heterozygosity without K-ras mutation identified by molecular analysis on fine-needle aspiration cytology specimen of acinar cell carcinoma of pancreas. Diagn Cytopathol 2002;27:42-6.

53. Okada Y, Mori H, Tsutsumi A. Duct-acinar-islet cell tumor of the pancreas. Pathol Int 1995;45: 669-76.

54. Ono J, Sakamoto H, Sakoda K, et al. Acinar cell carcinoma of the pancreas with elevated serum alpha-fetoprotein. Int Surg 1984;69:361-4.

55. Ordonez NG. Pancreatic acinar cell carcinoma. Adv Anat Pathol 2001;8:144-59.

56. Ordonez NG, Mackay B. Acinar cell carcinoma of the pancreas. Ultrastruct Pathol 2000;24:227-41.

57. Osborne BM, Culbert SJ, Cangir A, Mackay B. Acinar cell carcinoma of the pancreas in a 9-year-old child: case report with electron microscopic observations. South Med J 1977;70:370-2.

58. Osborne RR. Functioning acinous cell carcinoma of the pancreas accompanied with widespread focal fat necrosis. Arch Intern Med 1950;85:933-43.

59. Pasquinelli G, Preda P, Martinelli GN, Galassi A, Santini D, Venza E. Filamentous inclusions in nonneoplastic and neoplastic pancreas: an ultrastructural and immunogold labeling study. Ultrastruct Pathol 1995;19:495-500.

60. Pellegata NS, Sessa F, Renault B, et al. K-ras and p53 gene mutations in pancreatic cancer: ductal and nonductal tumors progress through different genetic lesions. Cancer Res 1994;54:1556-60.

61. Radin DR, Colletti PM, Forrester DM, Tang WW. Pancreatic acinar cell carcinoma with subcutaneous and intraosseous fat necrosis. Radiology 1986;158:67-8.

62. Rigaud G, Moore PS, Zamboni G, et al. Allelotype of pancreatic acinar cell carcinoma. Int J Cancer 2000;88:772-7.

63. Samuel LH, Frierson HF Jr. Fine needle aspiration cytology of acinar cell carcinoma of the pancreas: a report of two cases. Acta Cytol 1996;40:585-91.

64. Schron DS, Mendelsohn G. Pancreatic carcinoma with duct, endocrine, and acinar differentiation. A histologic, immunocytochemical, and ultrastructural study. Cancer 1984;54:1766-70.

64a. Shaco-Levy R, Klimstra DS. Pancreatic carcinomas showing acinar and ductal differentiation: mixed acinar-ductal carcinomas and mixed acinar-endocrine-ductal carcinomas. Am J Surg Pathol 2006. (In press).

65. Shimoike T, Goto M, Nakano I, et al. Acinar-islet cell carcinoma presenting as insulinoma. J Gastroenterol 1997;32:830-5.

66. Shinagawa T, Tadokoro M, Maeyama S, et al. Alpha fetoprotein-producing acinar cell carcinoma of the pancreas showing multiple lines of differentiation. Virchows Arch 1995;426:419-23.

67. Solcia E, Capella C, Klöppel G. Tumors of the pancreas. AFIP Atlas of Tumor Pathology, 3rd Series, Fascicle 20. Washington, DC: American Registry of Pathology; 1997.

68. Stamm B, Burger H, Hollinger A. Acinar cell cystadenocarcinoma of the pancreas. Cancer 1987;60:2542-7.

68a. Stelow EB, Bardales RH, Shami VM, et al. Cytology of pancreatic acinar cell carcinoma. Diagn Cytopathol 2006;34:367-72.

69. Tanakaya K, Teramoto N, Konaga E, et al. Mixed duct-acinar-islet cell tumor of the pancreas: report of a case. Surg Today 2001;31:177-9.

70. Taruscio D, Paradisi S, Zamboni G, Rigaud G, Falconi M, Scarpa A. Pancreatic acinar carcinoma shows a distinct pattern of chromosomal imbalances by comparative genomic hybridization. Genes Chromosomes Cancer 2000;28:294-9.

71. Tatli S, Mortele KJ, Levy AD, et al. CT and MRI features of pure acinar cell carcinoma of the pancreas in adults. AJR Am J Roentgenol 2005;184:511-9.

72. Terhune PG, Heffess CS, Longnecker DS. Only wild-type c-Ki-ras codons 12, 13, and 61 in human pancreatic acinar cell carcinomas. Mol Carcinog 1994;10:110-4.

73. Tobita K, Kijima H, Chino O, et al. Pancreatic acinar cell carcinoma with endocrine differentiation: immunohistochemical and ultrastructural analyses. Anticancer Res 2001;21:2131-4.

74. Toyota N, Takada T, Ammori BJ, Toida S, Haebara H. Acinar cell carcinoma of the pancreas showing finger-print-like zymogen granules by electron microscopy: immunohistochemical study. J Hepatobiliary Pancreat Surg 2000;7:102-6.

75. Tucker JA, Shelburne JD, Benning TL, Yacoub L, Federman M. Filamentous inclusions in acinar cell carcinoma of the pancreas. Ultrastruct Pathol 1994;18:279-86.

76. Ulich T, Cheng L, Lewin KJ. Acinar-endocrine cell tumor of the pancreas. Report of a pancreatic tumor containing both zymogen and neuroendocrine granules. Cancer 1982;50:2099-105.

77. Villanueva RR, Nguyen-Ho P, Nguyen GK. Needle aspiration cytology of acinar-cell carcinoma of the pancreas: report of a case with diagnostic pitfalls and unusual ultrastructural findings. Diagn Cytopathol 1994;10:362-4.

78. Webb JN. Acinar cell neoplasms of the exocrine pancreas. J Clin Pathol 1977;30:103-12.

79. Wilander E, Sundstrom C, Meurling S, Grotte G. A highly differentiated exocrine pancreatic tumour in a young boy. Acta Paediatr Scand 1976;65:769-72.

80. Zamboni G, Terris B, Scarpa A, et al. Acinar cell cystadenoma of the pancreas: a new entity? Am J Surg Pathol 2002;26:698-704.

10 PANCREATOBLASTOMA

DEFINITION

Pancreatoblastoma is a malignant epithelial neoplasm of the pancreas showing multiple lines of differentiation including acinar differentiation and squamoid nests (23,28,47). Endocrine and ductal differentiation, and a distinct mesenchymal component, can also be seen. Previous terms for this neoplasm include *pancreaticoblastoma, infantile pancreatic carcinoma,* and *pancreatic carcinoma of childhood.*

GENERAL FEATURES

The first recognized report of a pancreatoblastoma was by Becker in 1957 (4). A detailed histopathologic description was provided by Frable et al. in 1971 (12). Horie (16) was the first to use the term pancreatoblastoma for two pancreatic neoplasms that arose in children in his presentation to the 20th Annual Meeting of the Japanese Pathological Society (16,19). Horie introduced the term pancreatoblastoma to highlight the histologic resemblance of this neoplasm to the fetal pancreas and to emphasize parallels to other solid embryonic neoplasms of childhood such as nephroblastoma and hepatoblastoma.

Although very rare, pancreatoblastoma is the most common malignant pancreatic neoplasm of childhood (22,45). The exact incidence is difficult to estimate because most reports are of isolated cases. There was only one pancreatoblastoma in Cubilla and Fitzgerald's series of 645 pancreatic neoplasms in patients of all ages; however, in the pediatric population, pancreatoblastoma accounts for approximately 25 percent of pancreatic neoplasms (8,22,45). The other common childhood pancreatic neoplasms are solid-pseudopapillary neoplasm, acinar cell carcinoma, and well-differentiated pancreatic endocrine neoplasm.

Two thirds of pancreatoblastomas occur in children and one third in adults (7,9,11,15–17, 26,29,32). The mean age at diagnosis of the over

100 cases reported to date is 9.8 years (range, neonate to 68 years), but this mean age is somewhat misleading because the age distribution for pancreatoblastoma is bimodal, with a peak in childhood and a separate peak in adults. In the series of 14 pancreatoblastomas reported by Klimstra et al. (29), the mean age in the pediatric age group was 2.4 years (range, newborn to 4 years), and in adults it was 40 years (range, 19 to 56 years). In some series, pancreatoblastomas are reported to be more common in males than in females, with a male to female ratio of 1.3–2.0 to 1.0 (7,11,15–17,26,29,32). When all cases reported to date are tallied, however, males and females are essentially equally represented.

Approximately half of the reported cases have been in Asians, suggesting that this neoplasm is more common in Asians than Caucasians (7,11, 15–17,26,29,32). While some of the Asian predominance may represent an emphasis to report these neoplasms in the Asian literature, Asian patients also appear to be overrepresented in Klimstra's series of pancreatoblastomas from a medical center in the United States (29).

Pancreatoblastomas have been reported in patients with Beckwith-Wiedemann syndrome (10,25,30,43). Beckwith-Wiedemann syndrome is characterized by somatic gigantism, omphalocele, organomegaly including macroglossia, hemihypertrophy, adrenal cytomegaly, and an increased risk of embryonal neoplasms including Wilms' tumor, hepatoblastoma, neuroblastoma, and rhabdomyosarcoma (33). The pancreatoblastomas reported in these patients were diagnosed at birth and were cystic (10,25,30,43). Pancreatoblastoma has also been reported in a patient with familial adenomatous polyposis (FAP), and there has been a single case report of a pancreatoblastoma in a patient who developed Cushing's syndrome secondary to inappropriate adrenocorticotrophic hormone secretion by the neoplasm (1,43).

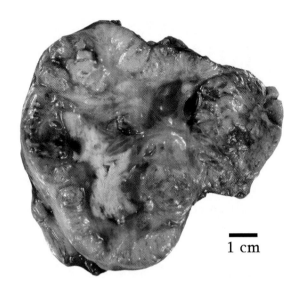

Figure 10-1

PANCREATOBLASTOMA

A soft, solid, well-demarcated mass. (Fig. 1 from Klimstra DS, Wenig BM, Adair CF, Heffess CS. Pancreatoblastoma. A clinicopathologic study and review of the literature. Am J Surg Pathol 1995;19:1371-89.)

CLINICAL FEATURES

Most pancreatoblastomas present as nonspecific upper abdominal masses (7,11,15–17,26,29, 32). The neoplasm can be large and is often palpable in children. Other common presenting symptoms include abdominal pain, diarrhea, weight loss, and vomiting. Jaundice is uncommon and is seen only in association with pancreatoblastomas arising in the head of the pancreas.

Pancreatoblastomas can produce significant amounts of alpha-fetoprotein, and one quarter to one third of patients have elevated serum alpha-fetoprotein levels (5–7,21,26,35,39,40). When elevated, serum alpha-fetoprotein levels can be used to follow the patient's response to therapy.

The radiologic appearance of pancreatoblastomas often suggests the diagnosis (7,31,34,44). Computerized tomography (CT) scanning usually reveals a well-defined pancreatic or peripancreatic mass. Most appear heterogeneous, most enhance, and a minority contain calcifications. Relative to the liver, most pancreatoblastomas have a low to intermediate signal intensity on T1-weighted magnetic resonance images (MRIs), and most have a high signal intensity on T2-weighted images. Vascular encasement or liver metastases have been reported in

one third to half of patients at the time of diagnosis (7,31,34,44).

PATHOLOGIC FEATURES

Gross Findings

Pancreatoblastomas are usually solitary, and arise in the head and the tail of the gland with equal frequency (7,11,15–17,26,29,32). They tend to be large: the mean greatest dimension is 10.6 cm (range, 1.5 to 20.0 cm). In contrast to the highly infiltrative growth of ductal adenocarcinomas, pancreatoblastomas are usually well-circumscribed and at least partially encapsulated (29). On cut section they tend to be soft and fleshy, but some are firm and fibrous, depending on the proportion of stroma to epithelial cells (fig. 10-1). Pancreatoblastomas are usually gray to tan-yellow and grossly lobulated. Necrosis may be present. As noted earlier, pancreatoblastomas are often cystic in patients with the Beckwith-Wiedemann syndrome (10,25,30,43).

Microscopic Findings

Most pancreatoblastomas have a nested or organoid pattern of growth, with lobules separated by distinct fibrous stromal bands (fig. 10-2) (7,11,15–17,26,29,32). The lobules are composed of highly cellular sheets of uniform polygonal cells with distinct borders, pale basophilic cytoplasm, central nuclei, and prominent nucleoli. These sheets merge almost imperceptibly into an acinar component.

Acinar Component. The acinar component predominates in most pancreatoblastomas (fig. 10-3) (7,11,15–17,26,29,32). In a given field, the acinar component may appear identical to an acinar cell carcinoma. The neoplastic cells are polarized around small lumens. The cytoplasm of the cells can be granular and eosinophilic, features highlighted with periodic acid–Schiff diastase (dPAS) staining. The nuclei tend to be basally oriented and often have a single prominent nucleolus. The cells with acinar differentiation merge into distinct squamoid nests.

Squamoid Nests. Squamoid nests are, by definition, present at least focally in every case (23, 28,47). They are usually located in the center of the epithelial lobules, and can vary from small microscopic collections of dozens of cells to collections large enough to be seen grossly

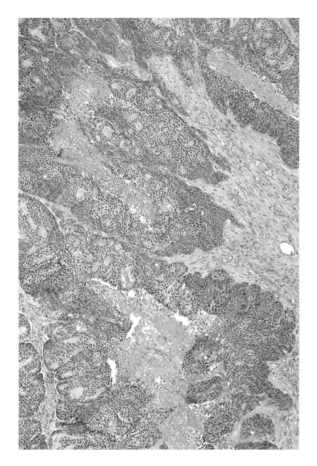

Figure 10-2

PANCREATOBLASTOMA

Lobules and nests are separated by dense fibrous stroma.

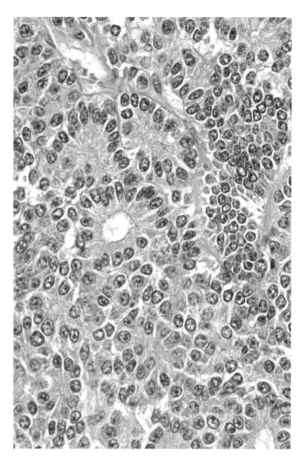

Figure 10-3

PANCREATOBLASTOMA

Acinar differentiation.

as small punctations on the cut surface of the tumor (7,11,15–17,26,29,32). The squamoid nests are composed of whorled, plump spindle-shaped cells (fig. 10-4). These cells have eosinophilic cytoplasm that is more abundant than that of the surrounding cells. Although most squamoid nests are uniform, there can be a gradient of differentiation from less differentiated peripheral cells to mature central cells, some of which may be keratinized (fig. 10-5) (26). The nuclei are large and often clear due to intranuclear biotin; nucleoli are usually absent (48).

Endocrine Component. In addition to an acinar component and squamoid nests, half to two thirds of pancreatoblastomas show evidence of endocrine differentiation (7,11,15–17,26,29, 32). These endocrine cells have a "fried egg" appearance on hematoxylin and eosin (H&E) staining and, as one would expect, have uniform "salt

and pepper" nuclei. The endocrine cells are usually diffusely scattered among the acinar cells, but in some cases, they form trabeculae or solid nests. The Grimelius/Cherukian-Schenk (argyrophilic) stain highlights endocrine cells (20).

Ductal Component. A distinct ductal component is seen in a minority of cases, and when present, is usually very focal. In these areas, columnar cells surround larger lumens, some of which contain concretions (fig. 10-6). A mucicarmine stain is positive in half the cases (fig. 10-7) (29).

Stromal Component. Pancreatoblastomas have a nested or organoid pattern of growth. These nests are separated by a variably cellular stroma (fig. 10-8). The stroma is usually relatively acellular, but it can be quite cellular (particularly in pediatric cases) and may even show osseous and cartilaginous differentiation (fig.

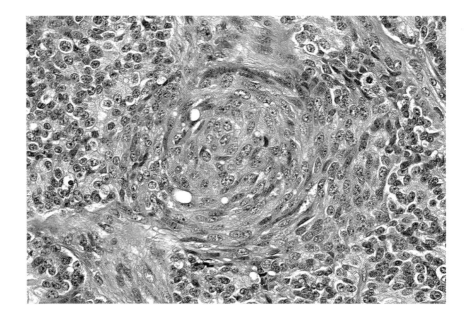

Figure 10-4
PANCREATOBLASTOMA
Squamoid nest.

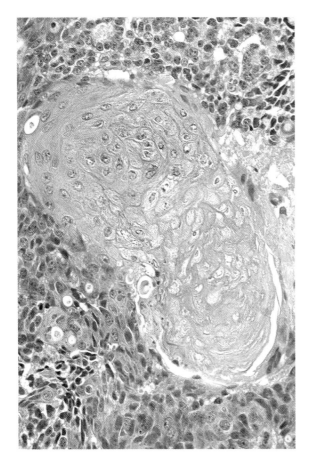

Figure 10-5
PANCREATOBLASTOMA
Squamoid nest with keratinization.

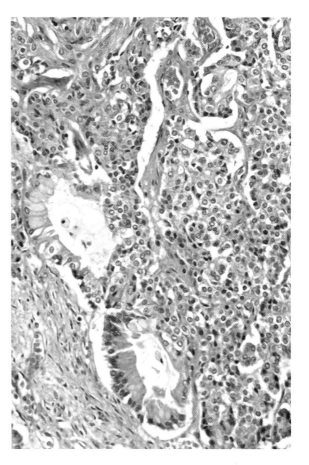

Figure 10-6
PANCREATOBLASTOMA
Focal glandular differentiation.

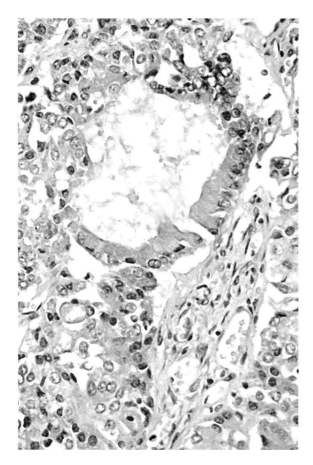

Figure 10-7

PANCREATOBLASTOMA

Foci with glandular differentiation stain with the mucicarmine stain.

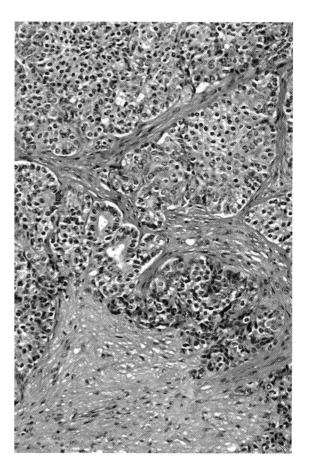

Figure 10-8

PANCREATOBLASTOMA

The stroma is cellular.

10-9) (29). A high-grade spindle cell component is rare, but has been reported.

Primitive Component. Some pancreatoblastomas have a primitive component. The primitive cells appear immature, and are small and monotonous (fig. 10-10).

Thus, pancreatoblastomas in many ways recapitulate the embryologic features of the pancreas (16). Acinar differentiation is the most prominent. Focal squamoid nests are, by definition, present, and endocrine, ductal, and even mesenchymal differentiation can be seen.

Although generally circumscribed, pancreatoblastomas often invade into the adjacent pancreatic parenchyma, and into the duodenum, bile duct, and soft tissue (29). Vascular invasion and perineural invasion are also seen.

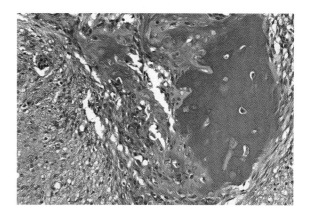

Figure 10-9

PANCREATOBLASTOMA

Focal osseous differentiation.

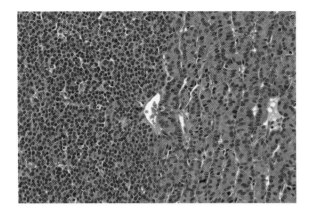

Figure 10-10

PANCREATOBLASTOMA

Round primitive cells (left) and acinar differentiation (right).

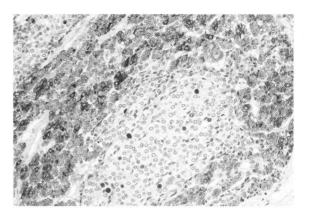

Figure 10-11

PANCREATOBLASTOMA

Immunohistochemical labeling for trypsin. The nonspecific nuclear labeling in the squamoid nest is caused by nuclear biotin.

Frozen Section

The diagnosis of pancreatoblastoma should be considered in the frozen section evaluation of pancreatic tumors from children (29). Acinar differentiation, including the formation of small lumens, and cells with polarized eosinophilic granular cytoplasm and single prominent nucleoli, should suggest pancreatoblastoma as a possible diagnosis. In these cases, the presence of squamoid nests helps establish the correct diagnosis. Pancreatoblastomas can also occur in adults and squamoid nests should be looked for in all cellular pancreatic neoplasms with acinar differentiation.

Immunohistochemical Findings

The immunohistochemical labeling profile of pancreatoblastoma parallels the multiple lines of differentiation seen at the light microscopic level, although the pattern of immunolabeling commonly diverges somewhat from the histologic impression of cellular differentiation. The acinar component labels with antibodies to cytokeratins (CKs) 7, 8, 18, and 19, as well with antibodies to low molecular weight cytokeratin (CAM5.2), high molecular weight cytokeratin (AE1/AE3), trypsin, chymotrypsin, and lipase (fig. 10-11) (14,24,29,38,46). An endocrine component is present in half to two thirds of pancreatoblastomas. The endocrine component expresses chromogranin, synaptophysin and neuron-specific enolase, but, inter-

estingly, usually does not express insulin, glucagon, or somatostatin (fig. 10-12) (29). The ductal component will label with antibodies to cytokeratin, carcinoembryonic antigen (CEA), B72.3, and DUPAN-2 (24,29).

Immunolabeling has not demonstrated a consistent direction of differentiation for the squamoid nests. In most cases, the squamoid nests are not immunoreactive, although they may occasionally label with acinar or endocrine markers, and CEA is positive in 30 percent of the cases (29). In some cases the squamoid nests label with antibodies to epithelial membrane antigen and to CK8, CK18, and CK19, but not CK7 (38). The stroma labels with antibodies to vimentin (35).

As discussed earlier, a quarter to a third of patients with pancreatoblastomas have elevated serum alpha-fetoprotein levels (5–7,21,26,35, 39,40). Immunolabeling usually reveals the cytoplasmic expression of alpha-fetoprotein by the acinar cells.

Immunolabeling for the protein product of the *SMAD4/DPC4* gene, Dpc4, has been shown to be a good surrogate marker for *SMAD4/DPC4* gene status. Abraham et al. (1) reported loss of Dpc4 expression in the epithelial component of two of nine (22 percent) pancreatoblastomas. In one case the loss of Dpc4 expression was diffuse, in the second it was focal. In all nine cases the stromal component showed intact Dpc4 expression. An abnormal nuclear pattern of immunolabeling for the product of the *beta-*

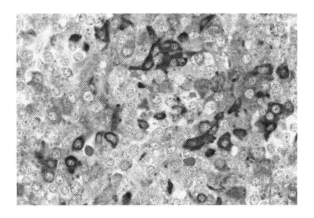

Figure 10-12

PANCREATOBLASTOMA

Immunohistochemical labeling for chromogranin.

catenin gene is seen in 75 percent of pancreatoblastomas (1,49). In general, the abnormal expression is patchy, with the squamoid nests and the areas of sheet-like growth showing abnormal nuclear and cytoplasmic labeling, while the acini and stromal cells show a normal membranous pattern of labeling.

Since the nuclei of the cells in squamoid nests often contain biotin, caution should be exercised in the interpretation of immunohistochemical stains directed against nuclear antigens (48).

Ultrastructural Findings

Ultrastructural examination of pancreatoblastomas has confirmed the acinar differentiation seen by light microscopy and by immunolabeling, and in some cases has also confirmed focal endocrine and ductal differentiation (5,7, 11,18,24,29). All pancreatoblastomas have cells with zymogen granules (400- to 800-nm membrane-bound granules), and the large irregular fibrillary granules characteristic of pancreatic acinar neoplasms have also been identified (28). Dense core neurosecretory (125 to 250 nm) and mucigen granules (500 to 900 nm with flocculent material) have also been reported in a minority of cases. Although the squamoid nests are generally not well demonstrated at the ultrastructural level, Horie et al. (18) reported that squamoid cells contain collections of tonofilaments and desmosome-tonofilament complexes in addition to zymogen-like granules.

Cytologic Findings

The cytologic features of pancreatoblastoma have only rarely been described (14,42,46). Aspirate smears are cellular with both a noncohesive and clustered smear pattern. The appearance of the epithelial cells depends on their direction of differentiation. Cells with acinar differentiation have a polygonal shape, round central to eccentric nuclei, one or more small nucleoli, and a moderate amount of granular, amphophilic to eosinophilic cytoplasm on Papanicolaou stain. The Romanowsky stain highlights basophilic cytoplasm punctuated with granules and tiny small vacuoles (fig. 10-13A) (46). Cells with endocrine differentiation have a more oval to cuboidal shape, a higher nuclear to cytoplasmic ratio, denser, less granular cytoplasm, coarse speckled chromatin, and less conspicuous nucleoli than acinar cells (fig. 10-13B) (14). Squamoid cells, singly or in clusters, have not been described in smears, but have been seen in cell block preparations from fine needle aspiration biopsies (fig. 10-13C) (14,42). Stromal fragments may be scant or prominent, with traversing capillaries (46), depending on the composition of the tumor and the sample collected.

Molecular and Other Special Techniques

A number of genetic alterations have been characterized in pancreatoblastomas. Two pancreatoblastomas have been karyotyped, and both karyotypes were complex (37,52). One included an addition to chromosome 1 [(add(1) (q42)], and the other a translocation involving chromosomes 13 and 22 [t(13, 22)(q10, q10)] (37, 52). Spectral karyotyping and comparative genomic hybridization analyses have also revealed complex karyotypes with multiple regions of chromosomal loss and gain (3).

The molecular alterations present in pancreatoblastoma are similar to those seen in hepatoblastoma and are distinct from those of infiltrating ductal carcinoma of the pancreas (1). The most common genetic alteration identified to date is loss of heterozygosity of the short arm of chromosome 11p near the *WT2* locus (11p15.5) (1,25). Loss of chromosome 11p has also been reported in other embryonal neoplasms that arise in association with the Beckwith-Wiedemann syndrome, including Wilms' tumor and hepatoblastoma (2). As is

Figure 10-13

PANCREATOBLASTOMA

A: Neoplastic cells with acinar differentiation (Romanowsky stain).

B: Neoplastic cells with endocrine differentiation (Papanicolaou stain).

C: Cell block preparation demonstrating a squamoid corpuscle adjacent to cells with acinar differentiation.

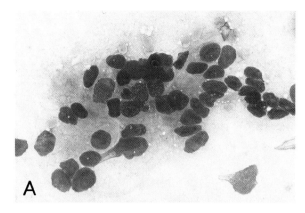

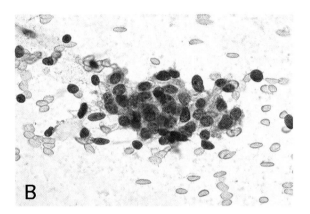

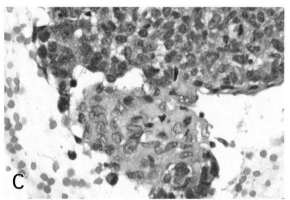

true for these other embryonal neoplasms, the allele lost in pancreatoblastoma in patients with the Beckwith-Wiedemann syndrome is often the maternal allele, a finding suggesting that this chromosome region is highly imprinted (25).

Alterations in the beta-catenin/APC pathway have been reported in 50 to 80 percent of pancreatoblastomas (1,49). Most often these are point mutations in exon 3 of the *beta-catenin* gene, which affect a glycogen synthase kinase-3-beta (GSK-3β) phosphorylation site, and result in the abnormal nuclear accumulation of the *beta-catenin* gene product (1,49). Biallelic inactivation of the *APC* gene has been reported in a pancreatoblastoma that arose in a patient with FAP (1). In this case, a germline intragenic *APC* gene mutation was accompanied by the somatic loss of the remaining wild-type allele in the neoplasm (1).

As noted earlier, the *SMAD4/DPC4* gene is targeted in only a minority (22 percent) of pancreatoblastomas (1). Two other genes commonly altered in infiltrating ductal adenocarcinomas

are not targeted in pancreatoblastomas: most pancreatoblastomas are wild-type for the *KRAS* oncogene and show normal expression of the *TP53* tumor suppressor gene product (1,15,29).

DIFFERENTIAL DIAGNOSIS

Because of the multiple lines of differentiation that can be seen in pancreatoblastomas, the differential diagnosis is broad and includes acinar cell carcinoma, well-differentiated pancreatic endocrine neoplasm, infiltrating ductal adenocarcinoma, and solid-pseudopapillary neoplasm (29).

Pancreatoblastoma and acinar cell carcinoma are closely related neoplasms; in fact, some consider pancreatoblastoma to be the pediatric version of acinar cell carcinoma. Both are characterized by prominent acinar differentiation, and both can show a minor component of endocrine differentiation. The presence of squamoid nests in pancreatoblastoma distinguishes these two entities (27,29). In addition, acinar cell carcinoma tends to occur in older patients (mean age, 61 years) and tends to have a more diffuse, less organoid, pattern of growth than pancreatoblastoma (27,29). The hypercellular stromal component of pancreatoblastoma is lacking in acinar cell carcinoma. The inability to appreciate subtle differences in organoid growth patterns and the absence of squamoid corpuscles in FNAB smears makes the distinction between acinar cell carcinoma and pancreatoblastoma more challenging. Appreciation of more than one cell type and the presence of stromal fragments support the cytologic diagnosis of pancreatoblastoma. The patient's age can help, and care should be taken in making the diagnosis of an acinar cell carcinoma in infants on the basis of a small biopsy, because the squamoid nests can be focal in pancreatoblastomas and may not be sampled in small biopsies, especially FNAB. Nonetheless, it should be remembered that acinar cell carcinomas can occur in infancy, and that a third of pancreatoblastomas occur in adults.

Well-differentiated pancreatic endocrine neoplasms should also be differentiated from pancreatoblastoma (29). While pancreatoblastomas can show endocrine differentiation, it is usually focal and associated with significant acinar differentiation. By contrast, pancreatic endocrine neoplasms show uniform endocrine differentiation, and they typically exhibit, at most, focal acinar differentiation in the form of widely scattered cells immunolabeling for exocrine enzymes (53). Squamoid nests are extremely rare in pancreatic endocrine neoplasms, a feature that by definition should be present for the diagnosis of pancreatoblastoma. The cytologic appearance of a pancreatic endocrine neoplasm is characteristic (see chapter 12), allowing for a distinction of these two entities on morphology alone in most cases. Immunolabeling for chromogranin or synaptophysin and markers of acinar differentiation, including trypsin, chymotrypsin, and lipase, further distinguish these entities.

Solid-pseudopapillary neoplasm should also be considered in the differential diagnosis of pancreatoblastoma (29). While solid-pseudopapillary neoplasms can rarely occur in children, they are seen predominantly in females in their twenties. Solid-pseudopapillary neoplasms have a distinctive pattern of growth with degenerative pseudopapillae that can be appre-

ciated on both histology and cytology. The presence of foamy macrophages, cholesterol crystals, nuclear grooves, and PAS-positive globules should also suggest the diagnosis of solid-pseudopapillary neoplasm. Almost all solid-pseudopapillary neoplasms immunolabel with antibodies to CD10 and none express pancreatic exocrine enzymes. Both pancreatoblastomas and solid-pseudopapillary neoplasms can show abnormal nuclear labeling with antibodies to the beta-catenin protein.

Although pancreatoblastomas can have focal ductal differentiation, ductal adenocarcinoma is usually not in the differential diagnosis. Ductal adenocarcinomas occur in a significantly older population, and they have more pleomorphism, a more invasive pattern of growth, and a much more intense desmoplastic reaction than do pancreatoblastomas (29).

SPREAD AND METASTASES

Although generally well-circumscribed, pancreatoblastomas often invade into adjacent structures including the duodenum, bile duct, stomach, portal vein, peritoneum, and even the transverse colon (7,11,15–17,26,29,32). One third of patients with pancreatoblastomas have metastases at the time of diagnosis, and additional patients develop metastases at the time of local recurrence (7,9,11,15–17,26,29,32). The liver is the most common site of metastases, followed by regional lymph nodes, lung, and peritoneum. Bone metastases have also been reported, but are rare. In general, the histologic appearance of recurrences and metastases is similar to that of the primary pancreatoblastoma, including the presence of squamoid nests and multiple lines of differentiation (29).

STAGING, TREATMENT, AND PROGNOSIS

The staging of pancreatoblastomas should follow the staging employed for other carcinomas of the exocrine pancreas (see chapter 3).

Surgical resection is the treatment of choice for pancreatoblastoma (29). Complete resection is associated with significant long-term survival (29). Radiation and chemotherapy have also been used, primarily to treat unresectable disease or to treat recurrences (13,36,41,50,51). Most reports on the treatment of pancreatoblastomas are anecdotal, and so it is not possible to make definitive evidence-based statements as to the most appropriate nonsurgical treatment; however, clinical responses have been reported with radiation therapy, with chemotherapy, and with combined radiation/chemotherapy.

Pancreatoblastoma is an aggressive malignant neoplasm that tends to present at high stages. Klimstra et al. (29) reviewed the literature on 35 patients with follow-up and found that 37 percent presented with metastases, an additional 15 percent later developed metastases, and 15 of the 35 (43 percent) died from their disease. Half of the more than 100 patients with pancreatoblastoma reported to date had died of their disease at the time their case was reported. A worse prognosis is associated with metastases at presentation and unresectable disease (9,29). It appears that the prognosis is worse in adults than in children (29). Pediatric patients identified prior to the development of metastases have been cured by surgery, whereas almost all adult patients have died of the disease. A similar observation has been made for acinar cell carcinoma (27).

REFERENCES

1. Abraham SC, Wu TT, Klimstra DS, Finn L, Hruban RH. Distinctive molecular genetic alterations in sporadic and familial adenomatous polyposis-associated pancreatoblastomas: frequent alterations in the APC/beta-catenin pathway and chromosome 11p. Am J Pathol 2001; 159:1619-27.

2. Albrecht S, von Schweinitz D, Waha A, Kraus JA, von Deimling A, Pietsch T. Loss of maternal alleles on chromosome arm 11p in hepatoblastoma. Cancer Res 1994;54:5041-4.

3. Barenboim-Stapleton L, Yang X, Tsokos M, et al. Pediatric pancreatoblastoma: histopathologic and cytogenetic characterization of tumor and derived cell line. Cancer Genet Cytogenet 2005; 157:109-17.

4. Becker WF. Pancreatoduodenectomy for carcinoma of the pancreas in an infant; report of a case. Ann Surg 1957;145:864-70.

5. Buchino JJ, Castello FM, Nagaraj HS. Pancreatoblastoma. A histochemical and ultrastructural analysis. Cancer 1984;53:963-9.

6. Chan MH, Shing MM, Poon TC, Johnson PJ, Lam CW. Alpha-fetoprotein variants in a case of pancreatoblastoma. Ann Clin Biochem 2000; 37:681-5.

7. Chun Y, Kim W, Park K, Lee S, Jung S. Pancreatoblastoma. J Pediatr Surg 1997;32:1612-5.

8. Cubilla AL, Fitzgerald PJ. Morphological patterns of primary nonendocrine human pancreas carcinoma. Cancer Res 1975;35:2234-48.

9. Dhebri AR, Connor S, Campbell F, Ghaneh P, Sutton R, Neoptolemos JP. Diagnosis, treatment and outcome of pancreatoblastoma. Pancreatology 2004;4:441-53.

10. Drut R, Jones MC. Congenital pancreatoblastoma in Beckwith-Wiedemann syndrome: an emerging association. Pediatr Pathol 1988; 8:331-9.

11. Dunn JL, Longnecker DS. Pancreatoblastoma in an older adult. Arch Pathol Lab Med 1995;119: 547-51.

12. Frable WJ, Still WJ, Kay S. Carcinoma of the pancreas, infantile type. A light and electron microscopic study. Cancer 1971;27:667-73.

13. Griffin BR, Wisbeck WM, Schaller RT, Benjamin DR. Radiotherapy for locally recurrent infantile pancreatic carcinoma (pancreatoblastoma). Cancer 1987;60:1734-6.

14. Henke AC, Kelley CM, Jensen CS, Timmerman TG. Fine-needle aspiration cytology of pancreatoblastoma. Diagn Cytopathol 2001;25:118-21.

15. Hoorens A, Gebhard F, Kraft K, Lemoine NR, Klöppel G. Pancreatoblastoma in an adult: its separation from acinar cell carcinoma. Virchows Arch 1994;424:485-90.

16. Horie A. Pancreatoblastoma. Histopathologic criteria based upon a review of six cases. In: Humphrey GB, Grindey GB, Dehner LP, Acton RT, Pysher TJ, eds. Pancreatic tumors in children. The Hague: Martinus Nijhoff; 1982:159-66.

17. Horie A, Haratake J, Jimi A, Matsumoto M, Ishii N, Tsutsumi Y. Pancreatoblastoma in Japan, with differential diagnosis from papillary cystic tumor (ductuloacinar adenoma) of the pancreas. Acta Pathol Jpn 1987;37:47-63.

18. Horie A, Morohoshi T, Klöppel G. Ultrastructural comparison of pancreatoblastoma, solid cystic tumor and acinar cell carcinoma. J Clin Electron Microscopy 1987;20:353-62.

19. Horie A, Yano Y, Kotoo Y, Miwa A. Morphogenesis of pancreatoblastoma, infantile carcinoma of the pancreas; report of two cases. Cancer 1977;39:247-54.

20. Hua C, Shu XK, Lei C. Pancreatoblastoma: a histochemical and immunohistochemical analysis. J Clin Pathol 1996;49:952-4.

21. Iseki M, Suzuki T, Koizumi Y, et al. Alpha-fetoprotein-producing pancreatoblastoma. A case report. Cancer 1986;57:1833-5.

22. Jaksic T, Yaman M, Thorner P, Wesson DK, Filler RM, Shandling B. A 20-year review of pediatric pancreatic tumors. J Pediatr Surg 1992;27:1315-7.

23. Japanese Pancreas Society. Classification of pancreatic carcinoma, 2nd English ed. Tokyo: Kanehara & Co, Ltd; 2003.

24. Kawamoto K, Matsuo T, Jubashi T, Ikeda T, Tomita S. Primary pancreatic carcinoma in childhood. Pancreatoblastoma. Acta Pathol Jpn 1985;35:137-43.

25. Kerr NJ, Chun YH, Yun K, Heathcott RW, Reeve AE, Sullivan MJ. Pancreatoblastoma is associated with chromosome 11p loss of heterozygosity and IGF2 overexpression. Med Pediatr Oncol 2002;39:52-4.

26. Kissane JM. Pancreatoblastoma and solid and cystic papillary tumor: two tumors related to pancreatic ontogeny. Semin Diagn Pathol 1994; 11:152-64.

27. Klimstra DS, Heffess CS, Oertel JE, Rosai J. Acinar cell carcinoma of the pancreas. A clinicopathologic study of 28 cases. Am J Surg Pathol 1992;16:815-37.

28. Klimstra DS, Longnecker DS. Pancreatoblastoma. In: Hamilton SR, Aaltonen LA, eds. World Health Organization Classification of Tumours. Pathology and genetics of tumours of the digestive system. Lyon: IARC Press; 2000: 244-5.

29. Klimstra DS, Wenig BM, Adair CF, Heffess CS. Pancreatoblastoma. A clinicopathologic study and review of the literature. Am J Surg Pathol 1995;19:1371-89.

30. Koh TH, Cooper JE, Newman CL, Walker TM, Kiely EM, Hoffmann EB. Pancreatoblastoma in a neonate with Wiedemann-Beckwith syndrome. Eur J Pediatr 1986;145:435-8.

31. Kohda E, Iseki M, Ikawa M, et al. Pancreatoblastoma. Three original cases and review of the literature. Acta Radiol 2000;41:334-7.

32. Levey JM, Banner BF. Adult pancreatoblastoma: a case report and review of the literature. Am J Gastroenterol 1996;91:1841-4.

33. Li M, Squire JA, Weksberg R. Molecular genetics of Wiedemann-Beckwith syndrome. Am J Med Genet 1998;79:253-9.

34. Montemarano H, Lonergan GJ, Bulas DI, Selby DM. Pancreatoblastoma: imaging findings in 10 patients and review of the literature. Radiology 2000;214:476-82.

35. Morohoshi T, Sagawa F, Mitsuya T. Pancreatoblastoma with marked elevation of serum alpha-fetoprotein. Virchows Arch A Pathol Anat Histopathol 1990;416:265-70.

36. Murakami T, Ueki K, Kawakami H, et al. Pancreatoblastoma: case report and review of treatment in the literature. Med Pediatr Oncol 1996;27:193-7.

37. Nagashima Y, Misugi K, Tanaka Y, et al. Pancreatoblastoma: a second report on cytogenetic findings. Cancer Genet Cytogenet 1999;109: 178-9.

38. Nishimata S, Kato K, Tanaka M, et al. Expression pattern of keratin subclasses in pancreatoblastoma with special emphasis on squamoid corpuscles. Pathol Int 2005;55:297-302.

39. Ogawa B, Okinaga K, Obana K, et al. Pancreatoblastoma treated by delayed operation after effective chemotherapy. J Pediatr Surg 2000;35:1663-5.

40. Ohaki Y, Misugi K, Fukuda J, Okudaira M, Hirose M. Immunohistochemical study of pancreatoblastoma. Acta Pathol Jpn 1987;37:1581-90.

41. Palosaari D, Clayton F, Seaman J. Pancreatoblastoma in an adult. Arch Pathol Lab Med 1986;110:650-2.

42. Pitman MB, Faquin WC. The fine-needle aspiration biopsy cytology of pancreatoblastoma. Diagn Cytopathol 2004;31:402-6.

43. Potts SR, Brown S, O'Hara MD. Pancreoblastoma in a neonate associated with Beckwith-Wiedemann syndrome. Z Kinderchir 1986;41:56-7.

44. Roebuck DJ, Yuen MK, Wong YC, Shing MK, Lee CW, Li CK. Imaging features of pancreatoblastoma. Pediatr Radiol 2001;31:501-6.

45. Shorter NA, Glick RD, Klimstra DS, Brennan MF, Laquaglia MP. Malignant pancreatic tumors in childhood and adolescence: The Memorial Sloan-Kettering experience, 1967 to present. J Pediatr Surg 2002;37:887-92.

46. Silverman JF, Holbrook CT, Pories WJ, Kodroff MB, Joshi VV. Fine needle aspiration cytology of pancreatoblastoma with immunocytochemical and ultrastructural studies. Acta Cytol 1990;34:632-40.

47. Solcia E, Capella C, Klöppel G. Tumors of the pancreas. AFIP Atlas of Tumor Pathology, 3rd Series, Fascicle 20. Washington, DC: American Registry of Pathology; 1997.

48. Tanaka Y, Ijiri R, Yamanaka S, et al. Pancreatoblastoma: optically clear nuclei in squamoid corpuscles are rich in biotin. Mod Pathol 1998;11:945-9.

49. Tanaka Y, Kato K, Notohara K, et al. Significance of aberrant (cytoplasmic/nuclear) expression of beta-catenin in pancreatoblastoma. J Pathol 2003;199:185-90.

50. Vannier JP, Flamant F, Hemet J, et al. Pancreatoblastoma: response to chemotherapy. Med Pediatr Oncol 1991;19:187-91.

51. Vossen S, Goretzki PE, Goebel U, Willnow U. Therapeutic management of rare malignant pancreatic tumors in children. World J Surg 1998;22:879-82.

52. Wiley J, Posekany K, Riley R, et al. Cytogenetic and flow cytometric analysis of a pancreatoblastoma. Cancer Genet Cytogenet 1995;79: 115-8.

53. Yantiss RK, Chang HK, Farraye FA, Compton CC, Odze RD. Prevalence and prognostic significance of acinar cell differentiation in pancreatic endocrine tumors. Am J Surg Pathol 2002;26:893-901.

11 SOLID-PSEUDOPAPILLARY NEOPLASMS

DEFINITION

Solid-pseudopapillary neoplasm is a low-grade malignant epithelial neoplasm. It is composed of noncohesive polygonal cells that surround delicate blood vessels and form solid masses with frequent cystic degeneration and intracystic hemorrhage (24,31,61). The neoplastic cells have uniform nuclei, finely stippled chromatin, and nuclear grooves.

The name of this neoplasm and its definition are based on the gross and microscopic appearance of the tumor, because the direction of differentiation of solid-pseudopapillary neoplasms has not been defined. Synonyms include *solid-pseudopapillary tumor, papillary epithelial neoplasm, papillary cystic neoplasm, solid and papillary epithelial neoplasm, solid and cystic acinar cell tumor* (not advocated), *papillary and solid neoplasm, papillary-cystic epithelial neoplasm, papillary-cystic carcinoma, solid and papillary neoplasm, papillary cystic tumor, solid and cystic tumor, solid and papillary neoplasm, low-grade papillary neoplasm, Hamoudi's tumor,* and *Frantz's tumor.*

Solid-pseudopapillary neoplasms were called "tumors" and designated as "usually benign" or "borderline" neoplasms in the World Health Organization (WHO) classification and in the previous edition of this Fascicle (24,31,61). The current terminology reflects the recent literature that has established that these lesions harbor clonal mutations in cancer-associated genes and are therefore neoplastic, and that they have the ability to metastasize (1,2a,2b,66,67a).

GENERAL FEATURES

The distinctive features of solid-pseudopapillary neoplasms were first recognized by Frantz in 1959 (16). Since then, over 750 cases have been reported in the English literature. Despite these large numbers, solid-pseudopapillary neoplasms are, in fact, relatively rare, historically accounting for only 0.9 to 2.7 percent of all pancreatic malignancies (35,41,61). With the growing clinical and pathologic rec-

ognition of this entity, more recent estimates suggest that solid-pseudopapillary neoplasms may account for 6 percent of all exocrine pancreatic neoplasms and for as much as 24 percent of all surgically resected cystic lesions in the pancreas (30).

Solid-pseudopapillary neoplasms occur primarily in women in their twenties (7,41,57). The mean age at diagnosis of the over 750 cases reported to date is 28 years (range, 7 to 79 years), and 89 percent of the patients are female (40, 41). On average, men with solid-pseudopapillary neoplasms are 5 to 10 years older than women (35,64). Many of the reports of solid-pseudopapillary neoplasms come from Asia, and it has been suggested that these neoplasms are more common in Asians and African-Americans than they are in Caucasians (35,69).

Although a solid-pseudopapillary neoplasm has been reported in a patient with familial adenomatous polyposis (59), there is no established association with any recognized clinical or genetic syndrome. There has been a single case report of a patient with both a solid-pseudopapillary neoplasm and hairy cell leukemia, and a report of a patient with a solid-pseudopapillary neoplasm and a papillary carcinoma of the thyroid (2). A number of solid-pseudopapillary neoplasms have been reported in women who are pregnant or postpartum (7,14). This apparent association with pregnancy may simply reflect the propensity of these neoplasms to strike women of childbearing age; however, many solid-pseudopapillary neoplasms express progesterone receptors and a more rapid growth during pregnancy has been suggested.

CLINICAL FEATURES

Most patients present with relatively nonspecific symptoms related to an intraabdominal mass, including abdominal pain, dyspepsia, early satiety, and nausea and vomiting (7,41,42,71). An abdominal mass can often be palpated on physical examination (7). Up to a third of solid-

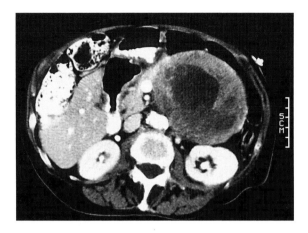

Figure 11-1

SOLID-PSEUDOPAPILLARY NEOPLASM

Computerized tomography (CT) shows a large expansile lesion in the tail of the pancreas. Mixed cystic and solid components include a large area of central cystic change. (Courtesy of Dr. S. S. Siegelman, Baltimore, MD.)

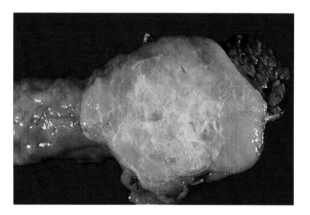

Figure 11-2

SOLID-PSEUDOPAPILLARY NEOPLASM

This neoplasm is mostly solid.

pseudopapillary neoplasms are discovered incidentally in asymptomatic patients by physical examination or imaging for another indication. Solid-pseudopapillary neoplasms can rupture and some patients (less than 10 percent) present acutely with hemoperitoneum (25,40, 54). Only rarely do patients develop jaundice.

The radiologic findings can be highly suggestive of a solid-pseudopapillary neoplasm. The radiologic findings reflect the variable gross findings, and imaging studies usually reveal a well-circumscribed neoplasm with solid and cystic components (13,70). Abdominal radiographs show calcifications in 30 percent (7,11, 57,70). Both ultrasound and computerized tomography (CT) examination show a well-demarcated heterogeneous mass (fig. 11-1) (7,58). The lesions often have variable echo texture on ultrasound and areas with differing attenuation ranging from that of soft tissue to water on CT scan (7,36,58). Fluid-debris levels are sometimes appreciated (7). The pancreatic and bile ducts are usually not dilated. Angiography typically shows a splaying and draping of the vessels, and mild vascularity in some areas (70). Other areas of the neoplasm can be relatively avascular. The solid areas have a signal intensity similar to liver on T1-weighted spin-echo magnetic resonance images (MRIs), while the areas of hemorrhage are hyperintense, and the areas with fluid

hypointense (8,52,58). Solid-pseudopapillary neoplasms often enhance during the arterial phase of gadolinium administration (8). Clinical laboratory data, including serum oncomarkers, are usually normal.

PATHOLOGIC FEATURES

Gross Findings

Solid-pseudopapillary neoplasms are relatively evenly distributed throughout the gland: approximately one third arise in the head, one third in the body, and one third in the tail (35,40,41,62, 71). An extrapancreatic solid-pseudopapillary neoplasm arising in the retroperitoneum behind the head of the pancreas has been reported, and one was reported arising in ectopic pancreas in the mesocolon (23). Most are solitary, although there have been multicentric neoplasms (33,53). Solid-pseudopapillary neoplasms are often large, with a mean diameter of 9 to 10 cm (range, 0.5 to 25.0 cm) (30,38). Most are well demarcated and some appear grossly encapsulated. Calcifications may be present within the capsule.

Cut section reveals soft, white-gray to yellow solid areas; irregularly shaped, often central, cavities containing friable necrotic material; and areas of recent or remote hemorrhage (figs. 11-2–11-7) (30,40). The contribution of each component varies from neoplasm to neoplasm. The vast majority (90 percent) are solid and cystic, however, some solid-pseudopapillary neoplasms are almost completely solid (especially the smaller ones) (fig. 11-2), while others are almost completely cystic, with only a thin peripheral rim of remaining neoplastic tissue (fig. 11-6) (40).

Microscopic Findings

Solid-pseudopapillary neoplasms have a distinctive microscopic appearance. The solid areas contain sheets of relatively uniform polygonal cells admixed with numerous, delicate capillary-sized blood vessels (fig. 11-8) (34,38,57,62). There is no gland formation. Other areas of the neoplasm show dramatic degenerative changes. Pseudopapillae are formed when the neoplastic cells drop away, leaving variable numbers of loosely cohesive cells surrounding delicate capillary-sized blood vessels (fig. 11-9). In these regions, the nuclei are sometimes oriented away from the vessels, resulting in a zone of cytoplasm that separates the capillaries from the nuclei (fig. 11-10). The cytoplasm of these cells is usually eosinophilic, but it can also be clear (fig. 11-11) or foamy (57). Cytoplasmic vacuoles are also common (fig. 11-12). The nuclei are round to oval and uniform, and have finely stippled chromatin and frequent longitudinal nuclear grooves (fig.

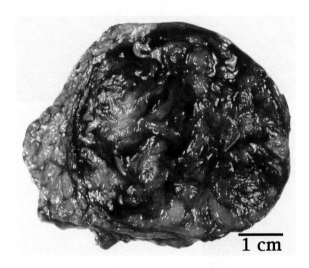

Figure 11-3

SOLID-PSEUDOPAPILLARY NEOPLASM

Focal hemorrhage and necrosis in a well-demarcated neoplasm.

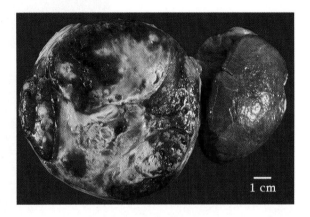

Figure 11-4

SOLID-PSEUDOPAPILLARY NEOPLASM

Partially hemorrhagic and necrotic large neoplasm in the tail of the pancreas.

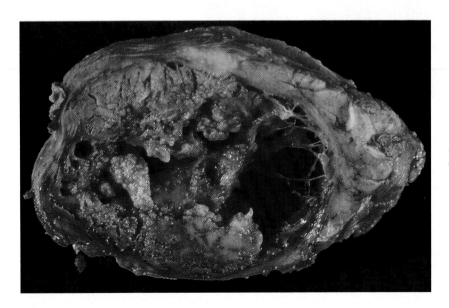

Figure 11-5

SOLID-PSEUDOPAPILLARY NEOPLASM

Prominent cystic degeneration with the formation of grossly visible pseudopapillae.

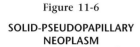

Figure 11-6

**SOLID-PSEUDOPAPILLARY
NEOPLASM**

An almost entirely cystic example in which only the capsule shows some solid areas. (Fig. 4-112 from Fascicle 20, Third Series.)

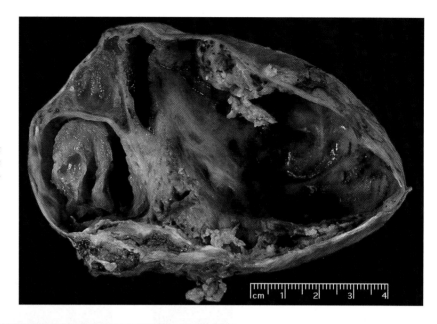

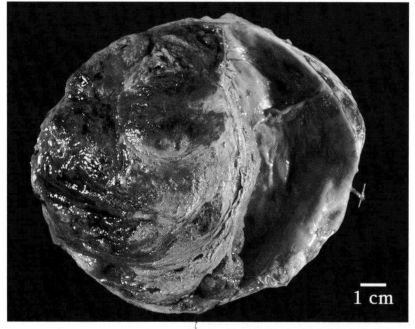

Figure 11-7

**SOLID-PSEUDOPAPILLARY
NEOPLASM**

A large hematoma fills the cavity of this mostly cystic example.

11-13). Mitoses are rare (range, 0 to 10 per 50 high-power fields), and pleomorphism is unusual but has been reported (57,66).

Some cells contain prominent intracytoplasmic eosinophilic hyaline globules that range in size from 1 to 20 µm, sometimes dwarfing the nuclei (figs. 11-13, 11-14). The globules are not uniformly distributed; they may be absent in much of the neoplasm only to be innumerable in isolated clusters of cells. These globules

stain with the periodic acid–Schiff (PAS) stain and are diastase resistant (fig. 11-15) (41). Other degenerative changes include foamy macrophages, cholesterol crystals, and hemorrhage (fig. 11-16). Rare solid-pseudopapillary neoplasms are pigmented, and this pigment may be either lipofuscin or melanin (9,12).

The stroma surrounding the delicate vessels is often imperceptible, but it can be hyalinized or myxoid. Some solid-pseudopapillary

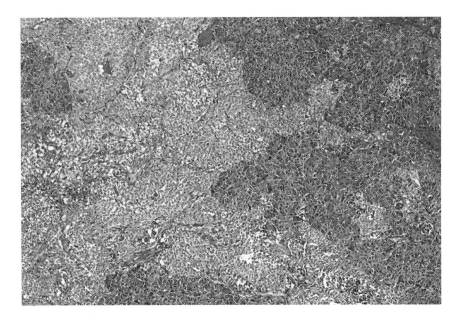

Figure 11-8

SOLID-PSEUDOPAPILLARY NEOPLASM

Neoplastic cells supported by delicate vessels (left) intimately interdigitate into the nonneoplastic pancreas (right).

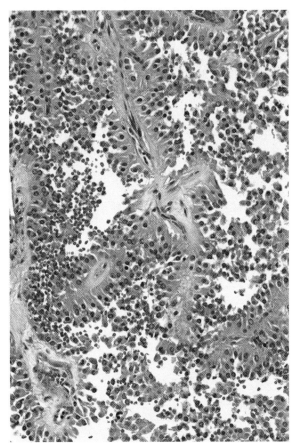

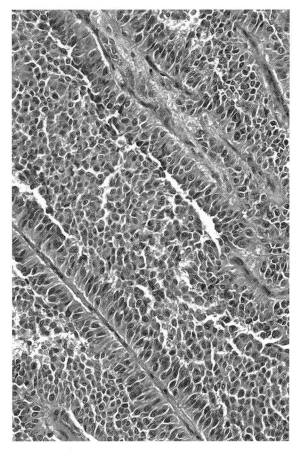

Figure 11-9

SOLID-PSEUDOPAPILLARY NEOPLASM

Prominent pseudopapillary growth pattern is present.

Figure 11-10

SOLID-PSEUDOPAPILLARY NEOPLASM

The slight polarization of the cells can create a "band" of cytoplasm around the vessels.

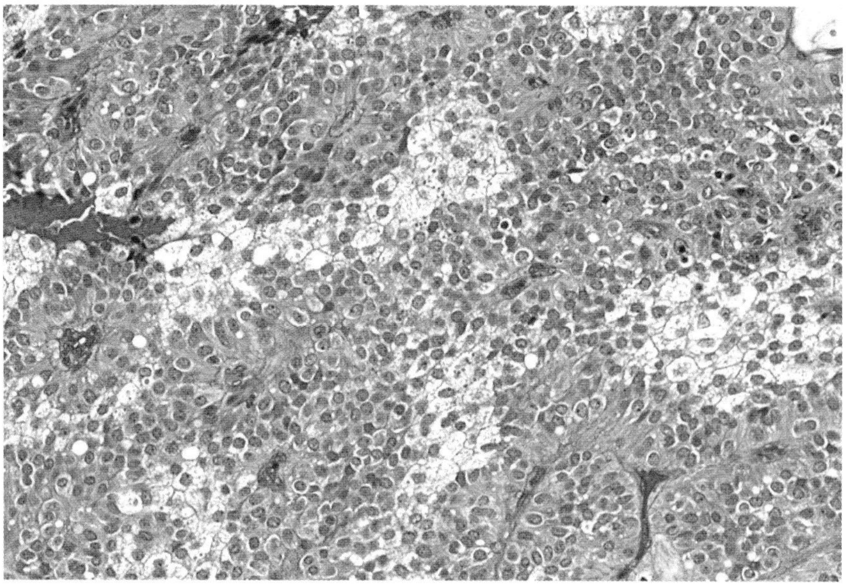

Figure 11-11

**SOLID-PSEUDOPAPILLARY
NEOPLASM**

Numerous foam cells are seen.

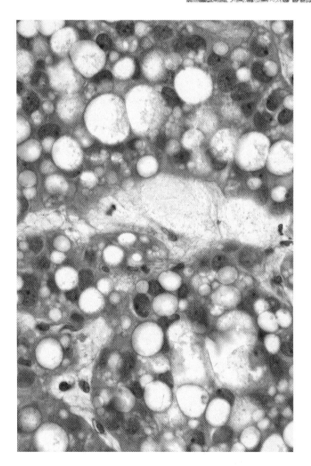

Figure 11-12

SOLID-PSEUDOPAPILLARY NEOPLASM

The neoplastic cells show cytoplasmic vacuolization.

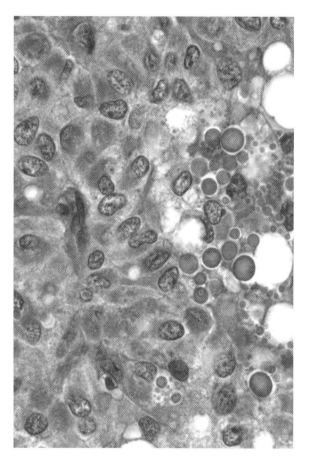

Figure 11-13

SOLID-PSEUDOPAPILLARY NEOPLASM

The neoplastic cells have prominent nuclear grooves. Multiple eosinophilic globules are also present.

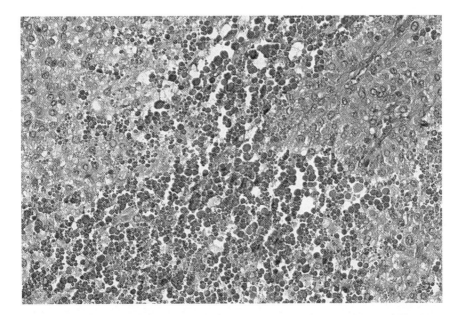

Figure 11-14

SOLID-PSEUDOPAPILLARY NEOPLASM

Numerous eosinophilic globules are seen.

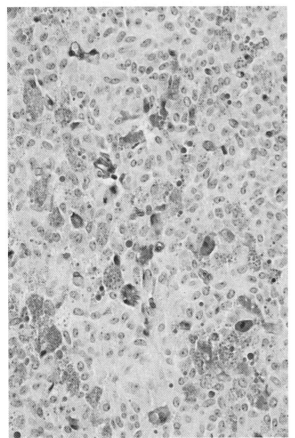

Figure 11-15

SOLID-PSEUDOPAPILLARY NEOPLASM

The hyaline globules stain with periodic acid–Schiff (PAS) stain.

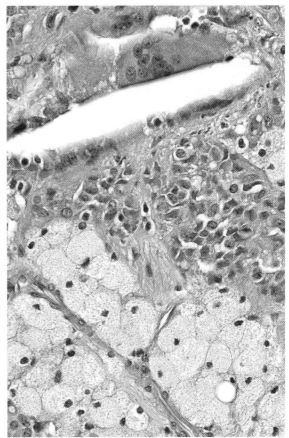

Figure 11-16

SOLID-PSEUDOPAPILLARY NEOPLASM

Degenerative changes here include foam cells, a cholesterol crystal, and an associated giant cell reaction.

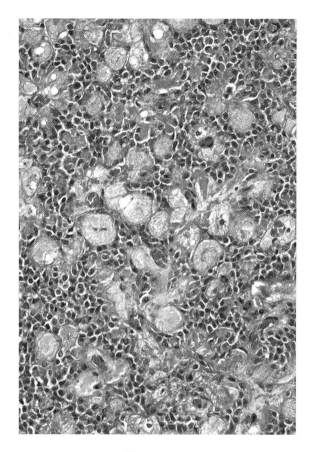

Figure 11-17

SOLID-PSEUDOPAPILLARY NEOPLASM

Delicate vessels surrounded by a myxoid stroma give the appearance of cylinders cut on end.

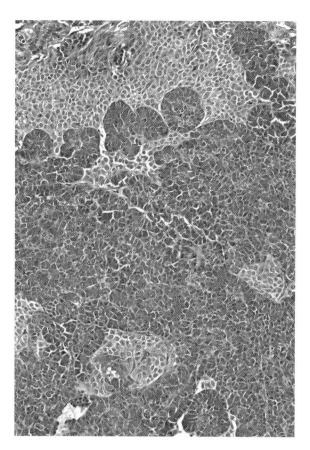

Figure 11-18

SOLID-PSEUDOPAPILLARY NEOPLASM

Neoplastic cells intimately intermingle with the non-neoplastic pancreatic parenchyma.

neoplasms have balls of myxoid stroma within the solid regions, resulting in a cylindromatous pattern (fig. 11-17). Rarely, there is extensive stromal hyalinization, leaving only scanty strands and nests of neoplastic cells surrounded by abundant collagen. Calcifications can be seen in the capsule, and focal ossification, although rare, has been reported (43,48).

Despite the well-circumscribed gross appearance, the neoplastic cells often infiltrate the adjacent non-neoplastic pancreas, intimately intermingling with the non-neoplastic cells without a desmoplastic reaction (figs. 11-8, 11-18) (57). In fact, the adjacent acini often appear separated from the neoplastic cells by only a basement membrane. Islands of entrapped non-neoplastic pancreatic tissue may likewise be found. Another characteristic finding is the presence of "blood lakes" at the periphery of the

neoplasm (fig. 11-19). Pools of red blood cells are admixed with nests of neoplastic cells, giving the appearance of vascular involvement, although true penetration of capsular vessels is hard to document in these regions. Perineural and true vascular invasion are seen in rare cases (fig. 11-20) (71).

Despite the presence of degenerative changes, true tumor necrosis is uncommon in solid-pseudopapillary neoplasms. Areas of infarction do occur, however, and we have seen almost completely infarcted lesions (fig. 11-21).

While metastases usually have the same morphologic appearance as the primary neoplasm, some metastases demonstrate increased nuclear pleomorphism and a higher mitotic rate than the primary (fig. 11-22) (41,42). The Grimelius/Cherukian-Schenk (argyrophilic) and Alcian blue stains are negative.

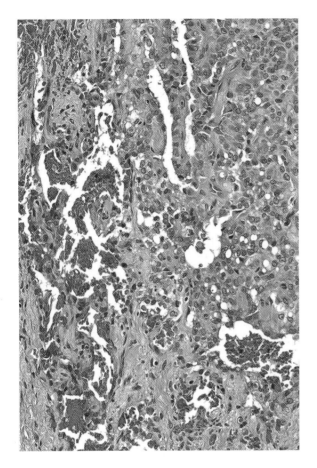

Figure 11-19

SOLID-PSEUDOPAPILLARY NEOPLASM

"Blood lakes" are at the leading edge of the neoplasm.

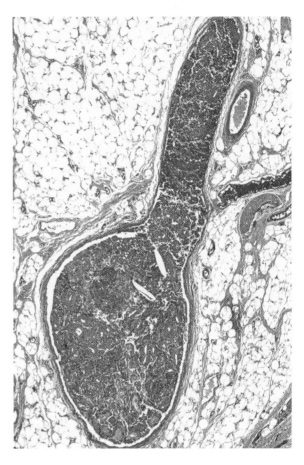

Figure 11-20

SOLID-PSEUDOPAPILLARY NEOPLASM

Invasion into a vessel.

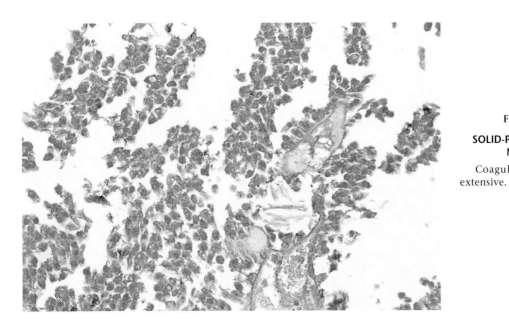

Figure 11-21

SOLID-PSEUDOPAPILLARY NEOPLASM

Coagulative necrosis is extensive.

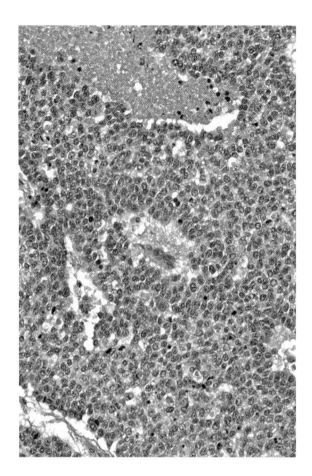

Figure 11-22

SOLID-PSEUDOPAPILLARY NEOPLASM

High-grade area with necrosis, pleomorphism, and an increased mitotic rate.

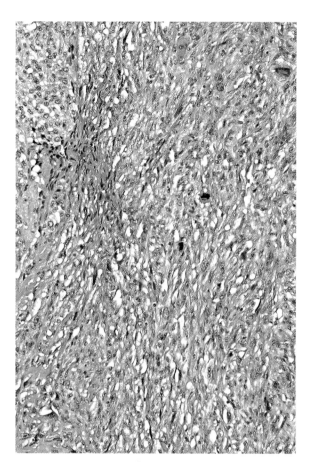

Figure 11-23

SOLID-PSEUDOPAPILLARY NEOPLASM

High-grade sarcomatoid focus with spindle-shaped cells.

Histologic Types

Solid nonencapsulated variants have been reported, but these may simply represent small solid-pseudopapillary neoplasms that haven't grown large enough to undergo cystic degeneration. A diffusely infiltrative variant has been described in which the entire neoplasm contained intimately associated islands of non-neoplastic pancreatic parenchyma.

Two cases of apparent high-grade malignant transformation in solid-pseudopapillary neoplasms have been reported (66). These cases showed residual areas of a conventional solid-pseudopapillary neoplasm but also demonstrated diffuse sheets of cells with marked nuclear pleomorphism, true tumor necrosis, and a relatively high mitotic rate (35 and 69 mito-ses per 50 high-power fields). One of these neoplasms contained a focus of sarcomatoid carcinoma as well (fig. 11-23). These two cases were regarded as undifferentiated carcinomas arising in solid-pseudopapillary neoplasms, and both patients experienced rapid disease progression.

Frozen Section

Solid-pseudopapillary neoplasms should be thought of at the time of frozen section diagnosis on all cystic masses in young women. The diagnosis should also be considered in males, as 10 percent of solid-pseudopapillary neoplasms occur in men. Uniform cells with a delicate vasculature should suggest the diagnosis, as should the presence of pseudopapillae, foam cells, eosinophilic globules, and cholesterol crystals. These features, particularly the pseudopapillae,

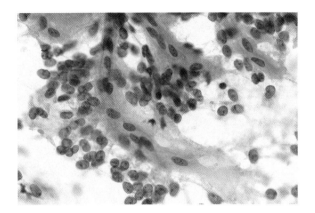

Figure 11-24

SOLID-PSEUDOPAPILLARY NEOPLASM

Papillary growth in an intraoperative touch preparation.

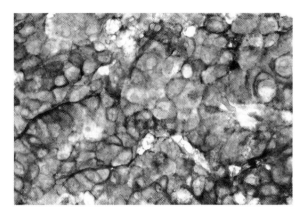

Figure 11-25

SOLID-PSEUDOPAPILLARY NEOPLASM

Immunohistochemical labeling for CD10.

eosinophilic globules, and foam cells, are often best appreciated in touch preparations, which can be an invaluable supplement to frozen-section diagnosis (fig. 11-24).

Immunohistochemical Findings

Almost all solid-pseudopapillary neoplasms strongly and diffusely express vimentin, alpha-1-antitrypsin, CD10, neuron-specific enolase, CD56, and progesterone receptors (fig. 11-25) (3,34,37,41,44,51,62,74). CD10, also known as neutral endopeptidase 24.11 or neprilysin, is a zinc metalloproteinase that functions as part of a regulatory loop to control concentrations of certain peptide substrates and associated peptide-mediated signal transduction (51). The role of CD10 differs from tissue to tissue depending on the substrate available (51). Progesterone receptors are expressed in solid-pseudopapillary neoplasms arising in both women and men (67). Solid-pseudopapillary neoplasms variably express synaptophysin and cytokeratin (AE1/AE3, CAM5.2). Labeling for cytokeratins (CKs) 7 and 19 is usually not seen (51,62).

Abnormal cytoplasmic and nuclear labeling for beta-catenin occurs in over 90 percent of solid-pseudopapillary neoplasms (fig. 11-26) (1,34,65); 75 percent also express cyclin D1 (1,47). The intracytoplasmic hyaline globules label with antibodies to alpha-1 antitrypsin (fig. 11-27) (46). Immunolabeling for chromogranin, insulin, glucagon, somatostatin, lipase, calretinin, alpha-inhibin, CD34, placental alkaline phos-

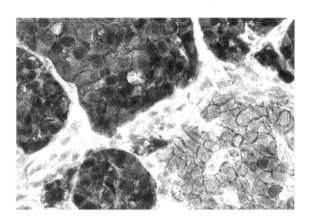

Figure 11-26

SOLID-PSEUDOPAPILLARY NEOPLASM

Immunohistochemical labeling for beta-catenin. The non-neoplastic pancreas shows a membranous pattern of labeling (lower right), while the neoplastic cells show abnormal nuclear labeling.

phatase, epithelial membrane antigen, carcinoembryonic antigen, S-100 protein, and estrogen receptors is usually negative, or at most focally positive (3,41,44,46). This pattern of immunolabeling does not correspond to any known normal cell type in the pancreas.

Ultrastructural Findings

Solid-pseudopapillary neoplasms show evidence of epithelial differentiation, including an incomplete basal lamina, rudimentary lumens, and poorly defined intercellular junctions (fig. 11-28) (3,21,42,49,62,68). The neoplastic cells usually contain numerous mitochondria,

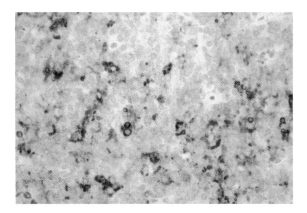

Figure 11-27

SOLID-PSEUDOPAPILLARY NEOPLASM

Alpha-1-antitrypsin labels the hyaline globules.

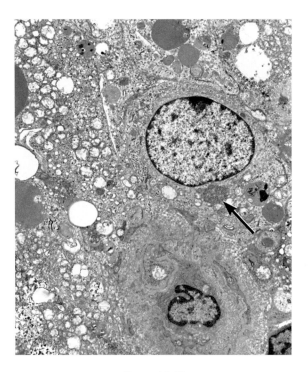

Figure 11-28

SOLID-PSEUDOPAPILLARY NEOPLASM

The neoplastic cells have intercellular junctions, numerous mitochondria, abundant rough endoplasmic reticulum, and annulate lamellae (arrow).

abundant rough endoplasmic reticulum, and some annulate lamellae (3,26,42,49). The mitochondria can be so numerous as to produce an oncocytic appearance by light microscopy (17). In most instances, large membrane-bound elec-

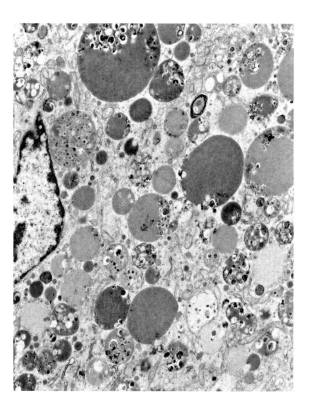

Figure 11-29

SOLID-PSEUDOPAPILLARY NEOPLASM

Numerous membrane-bound electron-dense vesicles (500 to 3,000 nm) resemble secondary lysosomes.

tron-dense granules (500 to 3,000 nm), suggestive of complex secondary lysosomes, are seen (fig. 11-29). These granules vary in morphology: some are homogeneous, resembling zymogen granules, whereas others contain abundant granular and membranous inclusions. Immunoelectron microscopic studies have demonstrated the presence of alpha-1-antitrypsin within these granules, confirming that they correspond to the eosinophilic hyaline globules identified by light microscopy (29). A minority of solid-pseudopapillary neoplasms contain smaller dense core granules that resemble neurosecretory granules (120 to 210 nm) (3,26,32,38,42,68).

Cytologic Findings

A preoperative diagnosis of solid-pseudopapillary neoplasm can typically be made by fine needle aspiration biopsy (4,55,56). One reported case was diagnosed by pancreatic duct brushing. Cell block preparation is optimal, not only to assess the cytologic and architectural features,

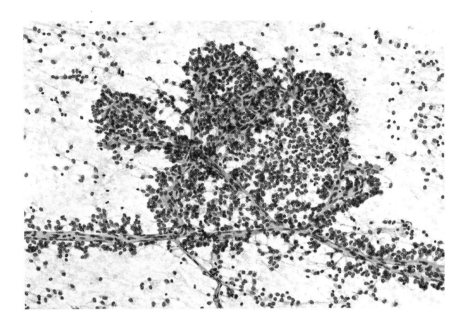

Figure 11-30

SOLID-PSEUDOPAPILLARY NEOPLASM

Cytology smear pattern on low-power microscopy reveals a cellular specimen with papillary groups and many single cells (direct smear; Papanicolaou stain).

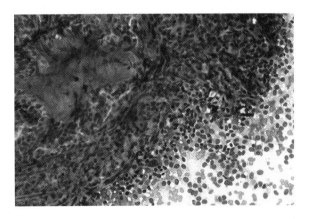

Figure 11-31

SOLID-PSEUDOPAPILLARY NEOPLASM

The myxoid stroma surrounding the vessels within the fibrovascular cores stains a bright magenta color on air-dried Romanowsky-stained smears (direct smear).

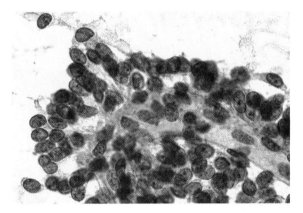

Figure 11-32

SOLID-PSEUDOPAPILLARY NEOPLASM

A zone of cytoplasm often separates the nuclei of the neoplastic cells from the vessels (direct smear; Papanicolaou stain).

but to provide tissue for ancillary studies in the often difficult differential diagnosis with pancreatic endocrine neoplasm (see below).

Aspirate smears of the viable solid areas of the neoplasm are often richly cellular and produce a smear pattern composed of a population of small, uniform cells in cohesive, often branching and papillary cell clusters (fig. 11-30). Small clusters and single neoplastic cells fill the background, which may be clean or filled with hemorrhagic cyst debris laden with foamy histiocytes and multinucleated giant cells. Iden-

tification of the usually delicate fibrovascular cores with myxoid stroma, a consistent finding in all reported cases, is a helpful diagnostic feature. This myxoid stroma is highlighted with a Romanowsky stain as magenta colored, metachromatic material (fig. 11-31). It is also PAS positive, diastase resistant. A zone of cytoplasm often separates the nuclei of the neoplastic cells from the fibrovascular cores to which they adhere (fig. 11-32).

Individual neoplastic cells are homogeneous in appearance, with little anisonucleosis and

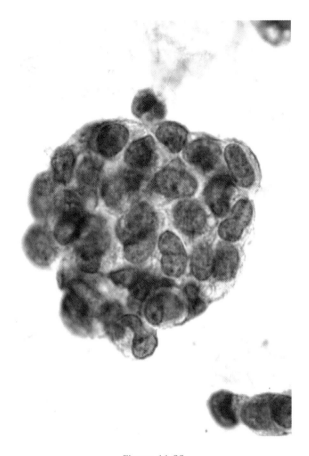

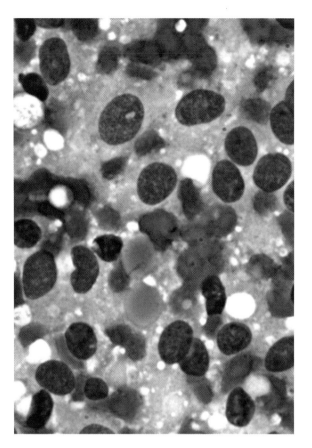

Figure 11-33

SOLID-PSEUDOPAPILLARY NEOPLASM

The individual small, uniform, monotonous-appearing cells have characteristic nuclear features: a bland even chromatin pattern, slightly indented and often grooved nuclear envelope, and inconspicuous nucleoli (ThinPrep®; Papanicolaou stain).

Figure 11-34

SOLID-PSEUDOPAPILLARY NEOPLASM

As with histology, the cells on cytology smears often display a clear perinuclear vacuole or, occasionally, a hyaline globule in the cytoplasm (Romanowsky stain).

no mitotic activity. The nuclei are round to oval, with smooth to slightly indented or grooved nuclear membranes, even and finely granular chromatin, and inconspicuous nucleoli (fig. 11-33). Many stripped nuclei are found. The cytoplasm is scant to moderate, nongranular to finely granular, and often contains a small perinuclear vacuole or intracytoplasmic hyaline globule (fig. 11-34).

Molecular and Other Special Techniques

Almost all (90 to 100 percent) solid-pseudo-papillary neoplasms harbor somatic point mutations in exon 3 of the *beta-catenin* gene (1,65). These mutations inactivate a glycogen synthase kinase-3 beta (GSK-3β) phosphorylation site,

and thereby interfere with the normal ubiquitin-mediated degradation of the β-catenin protein. The beta-catenin protein then abnormally accumulates in the cytoplasm of these cells and is translocated to the nucleus, where it can stimulate transcription of a variety of genes including *c-myc* and *cyclin D1*. As a result, over 90 percent of solid-pseudopapillary neoplasms show an abnormal pattern of immunolabeling for the beta-catenin protein (see fig. 11-26) (1,65). Normal cells in the pancreas show intense membranous labeling, while nuclear and cytoplasmic labeling is seen in the neoplastic cells. As one would expect in a neoplasm with β-catenin activation, cyclin D1 overexpression has also been reported in the majority of solid-pseudopapillary neoplasms (1).

In contrast to infiltrating ductal adenocarcinomas of the pancreas, alterations in the *KRAS*, *p16/CDKN2A*, and *SMAD4/DPC4* genes have not been reported in solid-pseudopapillary neoplasms, and less than 5 percent immunolabel for the *TP53* gene product (1,5,15,37,45,47,72).

A handful of solid-pseudopapillary neoplasms have been karyotyped (19,39). No distinct patterns have emerged; however, Grant et al. (19) reported unbalanced translocations resulting in a loss of 13q14-qter and 17p11-pter.

Most solid-pseudopapillary neoplasms are diploid, with a low S-phase by flow cytometry (20,37, 57). A minority of invasive/metastatic solid-pseudopapillary neoplasms are aneuploid (10,15,49).

DIFFERENTIAL DIAGNOSIS

Pseudocysts and solid-pseudopapillary neoplasms both produce well-defined cystic lesions containing necrotic and hemorrhagic material. A solid-pseudopapillary neoplasm with significant macrocystic degeneration may be grossly and radiologically mistaken for a pseudocyst and, hence, inadequately sampled for histologic analysis. When this happens, a solid-pseudopapillary neoplasm may be misdiagnosed as a pseudocyst, and the consequences of such an error are significant. Several case reports have documented the recurrence and even the metastasis of solid-pseudopapillary neoplasms that were incompletely resected because they were mistakenly diagnosed as pseudocysts (18,49). Pseudocysts, therefore, should be at the top of the list of entities in the differential diagnosis of solid-pseudopapillary neoplasms. These two entities can be distinguished from each other by the clinical and microscopic findings. Pseudocysts are more common in men than women, and patients with a pseudocyst typically have a history of pancreatitis and elevated serum amylase levels. In addition, chemical analysis of cyst fluid from a pseudocyst demonstrates high levels of amylase (6). By contrast, solid-pseudopapillary neoplasms are much more common in women than men, most of the patients do not develop pancreatitis, and patients usually have normal serum and low cyst fluid amylase levels (6). Microscopically, pseudocysts lack an epithelial lining, while solid-pseudopapillary neoplasms contain eosinophilic or clear neoplastic cells.

Infarct-like necrosis can be very extensive in solid-pseudopapillary neoplasms. In these cases, the presence of necrotic papillae (see fig. 11-21) should prompt an extensive search for viable tumor. Foamy macrophages, cholesterol crystals, and eosinophilic hyaline globules also suggest the diagnosis of solid-pseudopapillary neoplasm.

Well-differentiated pancreatic endocrine neoplasms should also be considered in the differential diagnosis. Both neoplasms are composed of homogeneous round to oval cells with uniform nuclei. The presence of solid areas admixed with pseudopapillae, foamy macrophages, cholesterol crystals, and eosinophilic hyaline globules should suggest the diagnosis of solid-pseudopapillary neoplasm, while a speckled chromatin pattern favors a pancreatic endocrine neoplasm. Immunohistochemical labeling is often needed to distinguish these two entities. Well-differentiated pancreatic endocrine neoplasms strongly and diffusely express the endocrine markers chromogranin and synaptophysin, and often express a pancreatic hormone (insulin, glucagon, somatostatin). Although both neoplasms express neuron-specific enolase and CD56, most solid-pseudopapillary neoplasms only focally and weakly express synaptophysin and never chromogranin. Instead, solid-pseudopapillary neoplasms strongly express CD10, alpha-1-antitrypsin, and vimentin; and show abnormal nuclear labeling for beta-catenin.

Acinar cell carcinomas should also be included in the differential diagnosis. The distinction between these two entities is usually straightforward. Acinar cell carcinomas are almost always solid, the cells are more cohesive and pleomorphic, mitoses are common, at least focal lumen formation is present, and the cells have a single prominent nucleolus and granular cytoplasm. In contrast, solid-pseudopapillary neoplasms are usually cystic, the cells are very uniform, lumen formation is never encountered at the light microscopic level, they lack mitoses, nuclei are grooved, the nucleoli are not prominent, and the neoplastic cells aggregate around delicate vessels rather than lumens. Immunolabeling for trypsin or chymotrypsin confirms a diagnosis of acinar cell carcinoma; staining for alpha-1-antitrypsin is not helpful, however, since both neoplasms can be positive.

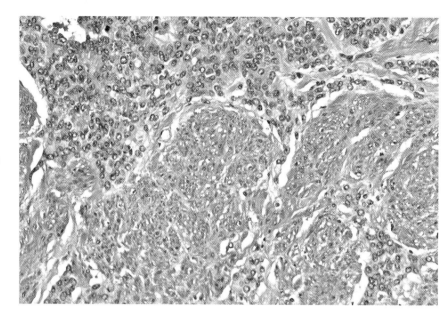

Figure 11-35

SOLID-PSEUDOPAPILLARY NEOPLASM

Invasion into the muscularis propria of the duodenum.

The entities in the differential diagnosis based on fine needle aspiration biopsy results parallels the histology-based entities. Most cystic lesions are readily distinguished from solid-pseudopapillary neoplasms cytologically on low power due to the typically hypercellular smears. Mucinous neoplasms produce frequently thick, viscous background mucin and columnar mucinous epithelial cells; pseudocysts, by definition, do not contain epithelial cells; and serous cystadenomas are, almost without exception, very scantily cellular. Solid-pseudopapillary neoplasms are most commonly mistaken for well-differentiated pancreatic endocrine neoplasms since both produce a similarly uniform, noncohesive smear pattern. The absence of coarse, speckled, "salt-and-pepper" chromatin helps to differentiate solid-pseudopapillary neoplasm from well-differentiated pancreatic endocrine neoplasm, as does the papillary architecture and myxoid stroma. As on histology, immunocytochemistry may be helpful for definitive classification. A full endocrine and exocrine panel, however, is not necessary; the most helpful label is chromogranin, with positive labeling supporting an endocrine neoplasm. Conversely, the expression of CD10 and nuclear labeling for beta-catenin support the diagnosis of solid-pseudopapillary neoplasm.

Injured acinar cells in the setting of pancreatitis may produce a cellular smear pattern mimicking a neoplasm.

For completeness, the other cystic neoplasms of the pancreas (serous cystic neoplasms, mucinous cystic neoplasms, and intraductal papillary mucinous neoplasms) should be included in the differential diagnosis. Beyond being cystic, however, these neoplasms are usually easily distinguished from solid-pseudopapillary neoplasms.

SPREAD AND METASTASES

Although they appear grossly well-demarcated, solid-pseudopapillary neoplasms often delicately infiltrate through the tumor capsule and into the adjacent pancreatic parenchyma (see figs. 11-8, 11-18). This subtle infiltration should not be taken as a sign of aggressiveness as it is a common finding. Direct extension into the stomach, duodenum, and spleen have been seen (fig. 11-35), and metastases to the liver or peritoneum occur in 10 to 15 percent of cases (figs. 11-36, 11-37) (22,29,35,40,41,49,67a). Lymph nodes and skin are exceptionally rare sites of metastatic disease (2a,2b). Peritoneal metastases appear to be more common in patients with a history of trauma and tumor rupture, and in patients whose neoplasms were drained instead of surgically resected (18,49). Serial CT scans of patients with unresected solid-pseudopapillary neoplasms have suggested that these neoplasms grow slowly, with a doubling time of 765 days (28). This slow growth is also reflected in a low Ki-67 labeling

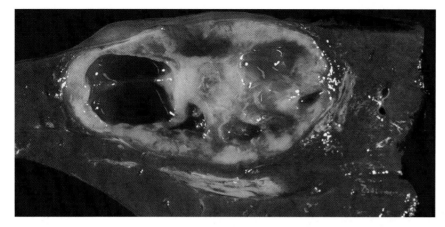

Figure 11-36

SOLID-PSEUDOPAPILLARY NEOPLASM

Metastasis to the liver.

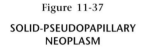

Figure 11-37

SOLID-PSEUDOPAPILLARY NEOPLASM

Metastasis to the liver.

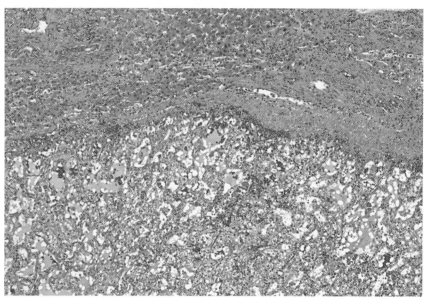

index, and by the calcification and even ossification of some of these neoplasms (48).

STAGING, TREATMENT, AND PROGNOSIS

The staging follows the staging for other carcinomas of the exocrine pancreas (see chapter 3).

Surgical resection is the treatment of choice (54,75). Long-term survival has even been achieved following the surgical resection of multiple liver metastases (30,60,73). There have only been a few isolated reports of clinical response following radiation or chemotherapy (63).

The prognosis for patients with solid-pseudopapillary neoplasms is excellent. Survival following surgical resection of lymph node–negative disease with negative margins (N0, M0, R0) results in a cure in the majority of patients (41, 49). Only 10 to 15 percent of patients have

metastases or recurrences (2a,2b,41). Most of these lesions are also surgically resectable, and long-term survival can be achieved in many patients with metastases; only rarely do patients die of their disease (30,60,73). Incompletely resected neoplasms (R1 disease) are more likely to recur (57). It has been suggested that older patients do worse than younger patients, and that those with aneuploid neoplasms do worse than those with diploid tumors (22,27,57,64).

There are no proven morphologic predictors of outcome, although vascular invasion, pleomorphism, and necrosis have been associated with the presence of metastases, as have certain morphometric features including mean nuclear diameter, mean standard deviation of the nuclear diameter, mean nuclear area, and the nuclear/non-nuclear ratio (10,41,49,50). In the absence of proven morphologic predictors of outcome, all patients with a solid-pseudopapillary neoplasm should be carefully followed after surgical resection.

A clinically aggressive variant of solid-pseudopapillary neoplasm in which an undifferentiated component is present has been described (66). Both reported patients died of disease 6 and 16 months after presentation, including one who had no evidence of metastatic disease at presentation other than a peripancreatic lymph node metastasis.

REFERENCES

1. Abraham SC, Klimstra DS, Wilentz RE, et al. Solid-pseudopapillary tumors of the pancreas are genetically distinct from pancreatic ductal adenocarcinomas and almost always harbor beta-catenin mutations. Am J Pathol 2002;160: 1361-9.
2. Acebo E, Rodilla IG, Torio B, et al Papillary cystic tumor of the pancreas coexisting with hairy cell leukemia. Pathology 2000;32:216-9.
2a. Alexandrescu DT, O'Boyle K, Feliz A, Fueg A, Wiernik PH. Metastatic solid-pseudopapillary tumour of the pancreas: clinico-biological correlates and management. Clin Oncol (R Coll Radiol) 2005;17:358-63.
2b. Arias de la Vega F, Gomez Dorronsoro ML, Jimenez FJ. Subcutaneous metastasis as the first manifestation of a solid-pseudopapillary tumor of the pancreas. Clin Trans Oncol 2006;8:136-8.
3. Balercia G, Zamboni G, Bogina G, Mariuzzi GM. Solid-cystic tumor of the pancreas. An extensive ultrastructural study of fourteen cases. J Submicrosc Cytol Pathol 1995;27:331-40.
4. Bardales RH, Centeno B, Mallery JS, et al. Endoscopic ultrasound-guided fine-needle aspiration cytology diagnosis of solid-pseudopapillary tumor of the pancreas: a rare neoplasm of elusive origin but characteristic cytomorphologic features. Am J Clin Pathol 2004;121:654-62.
5. Bartsch D, Bastian D, Barth P, et al. K-ras oncogene mutations indicate malignancy in cystic tumors of the pancreas. Ann Surg 1998; 228:79-86.
6. Brugge WR, Lauwers GY, Sahani D, Fernandez-del Castillo C, Warshaw AL. Cystic neoplasms of the pancreas. N Engl J Med 2004;351:1218-26.
7. Buetow PC, Buck JL, Pantongrag-Brown L, Beck KG, Ros PR, Adair CF. Solid and papillary epithelial neoplasm of the pancreas: imaging-pathologic correlation on 56 cases. Radiology 1996;199:707-11.
8. Cantisani V, Mortele KJ, Levy A, et al. MR imaging features of solid pseudopapillary tumor of the pancreas in adult and pediatric patients. AJR Am J Roentgenol 2003;181:395-401.
9. Chen C, Jing W, Gulati P, Vargas H, French SW. Melanocytic differentiation in a solid pseudopapillary tumor of the pancreas. J Gastroenterol 2004;39:579-83.
10. Cho NH, Go JH, Jung SH, Jung WH, Lee KK. Correlation between proliferating index and prognostic factors in papillary cystic tumors of the pancreas. J Korean Med Sci 1995;10:342-51.
11. Choi BI, Kim KW, Han MC, Kim YI, Kim CW. Solid and papillary epithelial neoplasms of the pancreas: CT findings. Radiology 1988;166:413-6.
12. Daum O, Sima R, Mukensnabl P, et al. Pigmented solid-pseudopapillary neoplasm of the pancreas. Pathol Int 2005;55:280-4.
13. Dong PR, Lu DS, Degregario F, Fell SC, Au A, Kadell BM. Solid and papillary neoplasm of the pancreas: radiological-pathological study of five cases and review of the literature. Clin Radiol 1996;51:702-5.
14. Duff P, Greene VP. Pregnancy complicated by solid-papillary epithelial tumor of the pancreas, pulmonary embolism, and pulmonary embolectomy. Am J Obstet Gynecol 1985;152:80-1.
15. Flejou JF, Boulange B, Bernades P, Belghiti J, Henin D. p53 protein expression and DNA ploidy in cystic tumors of the pancreas. Pancreas 1996;13:247-52.
16. Frantz VK. Tumors of the pancreas. Atlas of Tumor Pathology, 1st Series, Fascicles 27 & 28. Washington, DC: Armed Forces Institute of Pathology; 1959.
17. Goldstein J, Benharroch D, Sion-Vardy N, Arish A, Levy I, Maor E. Solid cystic and papillary tumor of the pancreas with oncocytic differentiation. J Surg Oncol 1994;56:63-7.
18. Gonzalez-Campora R, Rios Martin JJ, Villar Rodriguez JL, et al. Papillary cystic neoplasm of the pancreas with liver metastasis coexisting with thyroid papillary carcinoma. Arch Pathol Lab Med 1995;119:268-73.
19. Grant LD, Lauwers GY, Meloni AM, et al. Unbalanced chromosomal translocation, der(17) t(13;17)(q14;p11) in a solid and cystic papillary epithelial neoplasm of the pancreas. Am J Surg Pathol 1996;20:339-45.
20. Greenberg ML, Rennie Y, Grierson JM, Quin JW, Boadle RA. Solid and papillary epithelial tumour of the pancreas: cytological case study with ultrastructural and flow cytometric evaluation. Diagn Cytopathol 1993;9:541-6.

21. Hamoudi AB, Misugi K, Grosfeld JL, Reiner CB. Papillary epithelial neoplasm of pancreas in a child. Report of a case with electron microscopy. Cancer 1970;26:1126-34.

22. Horisawa M, Niinomi N, Sato T, et al. Frantz's tumor (solid and cystic tumor of the pancreas) with liver metastasis: successful treatment and long-term follow-up. J Pediatr Surg 1995;30:724-6.

23. Ishikawa O, Ishiguro S, Ohhigashi H, et al. Solid and papillary neoplasm arising from an ectopic pancreas in the mesocolon. Am J Gastroenterol 1990;85:597-601.

24. Japanese Pancreas Society. Classification of pancreatic carcinoma, 2nd English ed. Tokyo: Kanehara & Co, Ltd; 2003.

25. Jeng LB, Chen MF, Tang RP. Solid and papillary neoplasm of the pancreas. Emphasis on surgical treatment. Arch Surg 1993;128:433-6.

26. Jorgensen LJ, Hansen AB, Burcharth F, Philipsen E, Horn T. Solid and papillary neoplasm of the pancreas. Ultrastruct Pathol 1992;16:659-66.

27. Kamei K, Funabiki T, Ochiai M, Amano H, Kasahara M, Sakamoto T. Three cases of solid and cystic tumor of the pancreas. Analysis comparing the histopathological findings and DNA histograms. Int J Pancreatol 1991;10:269-78.

28. Kato T, Egawa N, Kamisawa T, et al. A case of solid pseudopapillary neoplasm of the pancreas and tumor doubling time. Pancreatology 2002; 2:495-8.

29. Klimstra DS, Wenig BM, Heffess CS. Solid-pseudopapillary tumor of the pancreas: a typically cystic carcinoma of low malignant potential. Semin Diagn Pathol 2000;17:66-80.

30. Klöppel G, Kosmahl M. Cystic lesions and neoplasms of the pancreas. The features are becoming clearer. Pancreatology 2001;1:648-55.

31. Klöppel G, Lüttges J, Klimstra DS, Hruban RH, Kern SE, Adler G. Solid-pseudopapillary neoplasm. In: Hamilton SR, Aaltonen LA, eds. World Health Organization classification of tumours. Pathology and genetics of tumours of the digestive system. Lyon: IARC Press; 2000:246-8.

32. Klöppel G, Morohoshi T, John HD, et al. Solid and cystic acinar cell tumour of the pancreas. A tumor in young women with favorable prognosis. Virchows Arch A Pathol Anat Histopathol 1981;392:171-83.

33. Kobayashi T, Kimura T, Takabayashi N, Sugimura H. Two synchronous solid and cystic tumors of the pancreas. J Gastroenterol 1998; 33:439-42.

34. Kosmahl M, Seada LS, Janig U, Harms D, Klöppel G. Solid-pseudopapillary tumor of the pancreas: its origin revisited. Virchows Arch 2000;436: 473-80.

35. Lam KY, Lo CY, Fan ST. Pancreatic solid-cystic-papillary tumor: clinicopathologic features in eight patients from Hong Kong and review of the literature. World J Surg 1999;23:1045-50.

36. Lee DH, Yi BH, Lim JW, Ko YT. Sonographic findings of solid and papillary epithelial neoplasm of the pancreas. J Ultrasound Med 2001;20: 1229-32.

37. Lee WY, Tzeng CC, Chen RM, Tsao CJ, Jin YT. Papillary cystic tumors of the pancreas: assessment of malignant potential by analysis of progesterone receptor, flow cytometry, and ras oncogene mutation. Anticancer Res 1997;17: 2587-97.

38. Lieber MR, Lack EE, Roberts JR Jr, et al. Solid and papillary epithelial neoplasm of the pancreas. An ultrastructural and immunocytochemical study of six cases. Am J Surg Pathol 1987;11:85-93.

39. Maitra A, Weinberg AG, Schneider N, Patterson K. Detection of t(11;22)(q24;q12) translocation and EWS-FLI-1 fusion transcript in a case of solid pseudopapillary tumor of the pancreas. Pediatr Dev Pathol 2000;3:603-5.

40. Mao C, Guvendi M, Domenico DR, Kim K, Thomford NR, Howard JM. Papillary cystic and solid tumors of the pancreas: a pancreatic embryonic tumor? Studies of three cases and cumulative review of the world's literature. Surgery 1995;118:821-8.

41. Martin RC, Klimstra DS, Brennan MF, Conlon KC. Solid-pseudopapillary tumor of the pancreas: a surgical enigma? Ann Surg Oncol 2002; 9:35-40.

42. Matsunou H, Konishi F. Papillary-cystic neoplasm of the pancreas. A clinicopathologic study concerning the tumor aging and malignancy of nine cases. Cancer 1990;65:283-91.

43. Matsunou H, Konishi F, Yamamichi N, Takayanagi N, Mukai M. Solid, infiltrating variety of papillary cystic neoplasm of the pancreas. Cancer 1990;65:2747-57.

44. Miettinen M, Partanen S, Fräki O, Kivilaakso E. Papillary cystic tumor of the pancreas. An analysis of cellular differentiation by electron microscopy and immunohistochemistry. Am J Surg Pathol 1987;11:855-65.

45. Moore PS, Orlandini S, Zamboni G, et al. Pancreatic tumours: molecular pathways implicated in ductal cancer are involved in ampullary but not in exocrine nonductal or endocrine tumorigenesis. Br J Cancer 2001;84:253-62.

46. Morohoshi T, Kanda M, Horie A, et al. Immunocytochemical markers of uncommon pancreatic tumors. Acinar cell carcinoma, pancreatoblastoma, and solid cystic (papillary-cystic) tumor. Cancer 1987;59:739-47.

47. Muller-Hocker J, Zietz CH, Sendelhofert A. Deregulated expression of cell cycle-associated proteins in solid pseudopapillary tumor of the pancreas. Mod Pathol 2001;14:47-53.

48. Nakamura S, Okayama Y, Imai H, et al. A solid cystic tumor of the pancreas with ossification and possible malignancy, coexisting nonfusion of the pancreatic ducts. J Clin Gastroenterol 2001;33:333-6.

49. Nishihara K, Nagoshi M, Tsuneyoshi M, Yamaguchi K, Hayashi I. Papillary cystic tumors of the pancreas. Assessment of their malignant potential. Cancer 1993;71:82-92.

50. Nishihara K, Tsuneyoshi M. Papillary cystic tumours of the pancreas: an analysis by nuclear morphometry. Virchows Arch A Pathol Anat Histopathol 1993;422:211-7.

51. Notohara K, Hamazaki S, Tsukayama C, et al. Solid-pseudopapillary tumor of the pancreas: immunohistochemical localization of neuroendocrine markers and CD10. Am J Surg Pathol 2000;24:1361-71.

52. Ohtomo K, Furui S, Onoue M, et al. Solid and papillary epithelial neoplasm of the pancreas: MR imaging and pathologic correlation. Radiology 1992;184:567-70.

53. Orlando CA, Bowman RL, Loose JH. Multicentric papillary-cystic neoplasm of the pancreas. Arch Pathol Lab Med 1991;115:958-60.

54. Panieri E, Krige JE, Bornman PC, Graham SM, Terblanche J, Cruse JP. Operative management of papillary cystic neoplasms of the pancreas. J Am Coll Surg 1998;186:319-24.

55. Pelosi G, Iannucci A, Zamboni G, Bresaola E, Iacono C, Serio G. Solid and cystic papillary neoplasm of the pancreas: a clinico-cyto-pathologic and immunocytochemical study of five new cases diagnosed by fine-needle aspiration cytology and a review of the literature. Diagn Cytopathol 1995;13:233-46.

56. Pettinato G, Di Vizio D, Manivel JC, Pambuccian SE, Somma P, Insabato L. Solid-pseudopapillary tumor of the pancreas: a neoplasm with distinct and highly characteristic cytological features. Diagn Cytopathol 2002;27:325-34.

57. Pettinato G, Manivel JC, Ravetto C, et al. Papillary cystic tumor of the pancreas. A clinico-pathologic study of 20 cases with cytologic, immunohistochemical, ultrastructural, and flow cytometric observations, and a review of the literature. Am J Clin Pathol 1992;98:478-88.

58. Procacci C, Graziani R, Bicego E, et al. Papillary cystic neoplasm of the pancreas: radiological findings. Abdom Imaging 1996;21:554-8.

59. Ruo L, Coit DG, Brennan MF, Guillem JG. Long-term follow-up of patients with familial adenomatous polyposis undergoing pancreaticoduodenal surgery. J Gastrointest Surg 2002; 6:671-5.

60. Saiura A, Umekita N, Matsui Y, et al. Successful surgical resection of solid cystic tumor of the pancreas with multiple liver metastases and a tumor thrombus in the portal vein. Hepatogastroenterology 2000;47:887-9.

61. Solcia E, Capella C, Klöppel G. Tumors of the pancreas. AFIP Atlas of Tumor Pathology, 3rd Series, Fascicle 20. Washington, DC: American Registry of Pathology; 1997.

62. Stömmer P, Kraus J, Stolte M, Giedl J. Solid and cystic pancreatic tumors. Clinical, histochemi-cal, and electron microscopic features in ten cases. Cancer 1991;67:1635-41.

63. Strauss JF, Hirsch VJ, Rubey CN, Pollock M. Resection of a solid and papillary epithelial neoplasm of the pancreas following treatment with cis-platinum and 5-fluorouracil: a case report. Med Pediatr Oncol 1993;21:365-7.

64. Takahashi H, Hashimoto K, Hayakawa H, et al. Solid cystic tumor of the pancreas in elderly men: report of a case. Surg Today 1999;29:1264-7.

65. Tanaka Y, Kato K, Notohara K, et al. Frequent beta-catenin mutation and cytoplasmic/nuclear accumulation in pancreatic solid-pseudopapillary neoplasm. Cancer Res 2001;61:8401-4.

66. Tang LH, Aydin H, Brennan MF, Klimstra DS. Clinically aggressive solid-pseudopapillary tumors of the pancreas. Am J Surg Pathol 2005;29: 512-9.

67. Tien YW, Ser KH, Hu RH, Lee CY, Jeng YM, Lee PH. Solid pseudopapillary neoplasms of the pancreas: Is there a pathologic basis for the observed gender differences in incidence? Surgery 2005;137:591-6.

67a. Tipton SG, Smyrk TC, Sarr MG, Thompson GB. Malignant potential of solid pseudopapillary neoplasm of the pancreas. Br J Surg 2006;93:733-7.

68. Ueda N, Nagakawa T, Ohta T, et al. Clinicopathological studies on solid and cystic tumors of the pancreas. Gastroenterol Jpn 1991;26:497-502.

69. Wang KS, Albanese C, Dada F, Skarsgard ED. Papillary cystic neoplasm of the pancreas: a report of three pediatric cases and literature review. J Pediatr Surg 1998;33:842-5.

70. Yamaguchi K, Hirakata R, Kitamura K. Papillary cystic neoplasm of the pancreas: radiological and pathological characteristics in 11 cases. Br J Surg 1990;77:1000-3.

71. Yamaguchi K, Miyagahara T, Tsuneyoshi M, et al. Papillary cystic tumor of the pancreas: an immunohistochemical and ultrastructural study of 14 patients. Jpn J Clin Oncol 1989;19:102-11.

72. Yamaue H, Tanimura H, Shono Y, et al Solid and cystic tumor of the pancreas: clinicopathologic and genetic studies of four cases. Int J Pancreatol 2000;27:69-76.

73. Yoon DY, Hines OJ, Bilchik AJ, Lewin K, Cortina G, Reber HA. Solid and papillary epithelial neoplasms of the pancreas: aggressive resection for cure. Am Surg 2001;67:1195-9.

74. Zamboni G, Bonetti F, Scarpa A, et al. Expression of progesterone receptors in solid-cystic tumour of the pancreas: a clinicopathological and immunohistochemical study of ten cases. Virchows Arch A Pathol Anat Histopathol 1993;423:425-31.

75. Zinner MJ, Shurbaji MS, Cameron JL. Solid and papillary epithelial neoplasms of the pancreas. Surgery 1990;108:475-80.

12 ENDOCRINE NEOPLASMS

Endocrine neoplasms of the pancreas constitute one of the more interesting families of pancreatic neoplasms. Most are well-differentiated, relatively low-grade neoplasms. The association with characteristic paraneoplastic syndromes has drawn attention to pancreatic endocrine neoplasms (PENs) out of proportion to their prevalence. Some PENs arise in patients with hereditary syndromes such as the multiple endocrine neoplasia, type 1 (MEN1) and von Hippel-Lindau syndromes, but most occur sporadically.

In 1902 Nicholls (174) reported the first well-documented case of an adenoma arising from an islet of Langerhans. Recognition that PENs can be functional came in 1927, when Wilder et al. (257) described a "carcinoma of the islands of the pancreas" that produced hyperinsulinism and hypoglycemia. Since then, nearly a dozen different functional types of PENs have been described.

PENs are classified in several ways: by grade, by size, and by functional status (Table 12-1). Most fall into the well-differentiated category, and it is generally assumed that a lesion designated "pancreatic endocrine neoplasm" is well-differentiated. Only rarely do PENs have sufficiently aggressive histologic features to be placed in the poorly differentiated endocrine carcinoma category (e.g., small cell carcinoma or large cell endocrine carcinoma). Within the predominant well-differentiated category, most PENs are malignant, and only the group measuring less than 0.5 cm, endocrine microadenoma, is designated with terminology suggesting a completely benign entity (91,118).

The well-differentiated PEN category is subclassified based on the presence or absence of an associated clinical endocrine paraneoplastic syndrome into functional and nonfunctional groups. Functional PENs include insulinomas, glucagonomas, somatostatinomas, gastrinomas, VIPomas (vasoactive intestinal polypeptide-omas), serotonin-secreting tumors, and other rare ectopic hormone-producing and mixed

hormone-producing entities (Table 12-2). A PEN not associated with a clinical syndrome is designated a *nonfunctional PEN*. It is important to recognize that the designation *functional PEN* only applies to those neoplasms associated with a corresponding clinical syndrome (91). Many other PENs can be shown to "function," in the sense that peptide hormone elevations are detected in the serum or in the neoplastic cells by immunohistochemistry (98,170); however, these "nonsyndromic" PENs are still categorized with the nonfunctional group. An exception to this rule, for historical reasons, is the pancreatic polypeptide cell PEN, or PPoma (142,243), a PEN that is demonstrated to produce predominantly pancreatic polypeptide (PP) by immunohistochemistry. Most such PENs also have serum elevations of PP, but patients are not generally symptomatic, so

---

Table 12-1

CLASSIFICATION OF ENDOCRINE NEOPLASMS OF THE PANCREAS

Endocrine microadenoma

Well-differentiated pancreatic endocrine neoplasm
  Functional pancreatic endocrine neoplasms
    Insulinoma
    Glucagonoma
    Somatostatinoma
    Gastrinoma
    VIPoma[a]
    PP-cell pancreatic endocrine neoplasm
    Other ectopic and mixed hormone–producing neoplasms
  Nonfunctional pancreatic endocrine neoplasms

Poorly differentiated endocrine carcinoma
  Small cell carcinoma
  Large cell poorly differentiated endocrine carcinoma

Mixed endocrine carcinomas
  Mixed ductal-endocrine carcinoma
  Mixed acinar-endocrine carcinoma[b]
  Mixed acinar-endocrine-ductal carcinoma[b]

[a]VIP = vasoactive intestinal polypeptide; PP = pancreatic polypeptide.
[b]See chapter 9.

Table 12-2

TYPES OF FUNCTIONAL PANCREATIC ENDOCRINE NEOPLASMS

	Cell Type	Syndrome	Clinical Findings
Insulinoma	β cell	Insulinoma syndrome	Hypoglycemia
Glucagonoma	α cell	Glucagonoma syndrome	Rash, stomatitis, diabetes, weight loss
Somatostatinoma	δ cell	Somatostatinoma syndrome	Diabetes, hypochlorhydria, cholelithiasis
Gastrinoma	G cell	Zollinger-Ellison syndrome	Peptic ulcers, diarrhea
VIPoma[a]	Unknown	Verner-Morrison syndrome	Watery diarrhea, hypokalemia, achlorhydria
PP-cell PEN[b]	PP cell	None	None

[a]VIP = vasoactive intestinal polypeptide; PP = pancreatic polypeptide.
[b]Usually not syndromic; included with functional neoplasms for historical purposes.

PPomas are technically nonsyndromic PENs, despite being traditionally classified with the functional group.

The sections that follow detail the clinical and pathologic features of endocrine neoplasms of the pancreas, including microadenomas, well-differentiated PENs, poorly differentiated endocrine carcinomas, and rare neoplasms with both endocrine and ductal elements (mixed ductal-endocrine carcinomas). Neoplasms with mixed acinar and endocrine differentiation are discussed in the chapter on acinar neoplasms (see chapter 9). Following the general section on well-differentiated PENs, there are individual sections discussing the distinctive features of each of the functional PENs.

ENDOCRINE MICROADENOMAS

Endocrine microadenomas are small and nonfunctional, and therefore they rarely come to clinical attention. Since they share many of the histologic features of larger PENs, it is tempting to assume that microadenomas represent an earlier phase in the development of clinically relevant PENs. Certainly, patients with MEN1 have numerous microadenomas in addition to clinically relevant PENs, and all PENs must pass through a microadenoma stage as they grow to sizes greater than 0.5 cm. There are a number of findings, however, including their prevalence, their peptide cell constitution, and their molecular profile that suggest that most microadenomas are not simply smaller versions of PENs. Importantly, it appears unlikely that most microadenomas progress beyond the stage of a small, biologically benign endocrine neoplasm.

Definition. *Pancreatic endocrine microadenoma* is a well-differentiated epithelial neoplasm characterized by organoid growth of cells cytologically resembling islet cells or other hormone-producing cells that measures less than 0.5 cm in greatest dimension and is not associated with a clinical syndrome due to hormone secretion. It is also known as *islet cell tumorlet*.

Clinical Features. The prevalence of endocrine microadenomas is estimated to be as high as 10 percent of the adult population based on autopsy studies in which numerous sections of the pancreas were examined; lower rates (1 percent) are found when fewer sections are reviewed (114,226). Endocrine microadenomas occur at any age, but since their detection usually depends upon resection of a portion of the pancreas for some other reason, most are detected in adults. Microadenomas are detected at a younger age in patients with MEN1 than are sporadic microadenomas (126).

Solitary microadenomas are almost always found incidentally, and they are generally asymptomatic, since they are, by definition, small and hormonally nonfunctional. Most microadenomas are only identified microscopically, either adjacent to other pancreatic neoplasms, in pancreata resected for pancreatitis or trauma, or at autopsy. In rare instances, an endocrine microadenoma situated near the surface of the pancreas may be recognized intraoperatively. In patients with MEN1, numerous microadenomas (microadenomatosis) are commonly present (5a) and may be identified by high-resolution cross-sectional imaging techniques, by nuclear medicine (octreotide) scanning, or during surgical

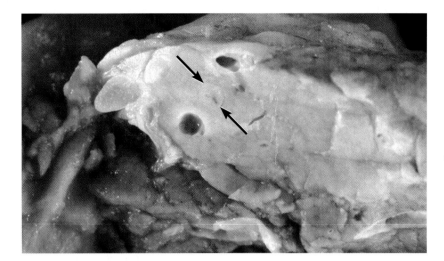

Figure 12-1

ENDOCRINE
MICROADENOMA

The 0.2-mm neoplasm (arrows) is
unencapsulated.

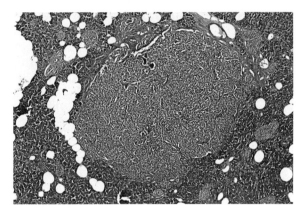

Figure 12-2

ENDOCRINE MICROADENOMA

The small endocrine neoplasm is circumscribed but lacks
a capsule.

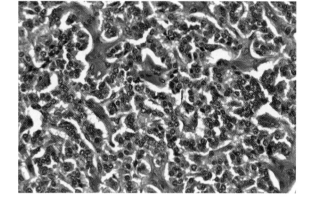

Figure 12-3

ENDOCRINE MICROADENOMA

Trabecular architecture.

exploration for other functional PENs. Rarely, microadenomatosis occurs in patients lacking MEN1, some of whom have hyperinsulinism in the absence of a solitary insulinoma (5a).

Gross Findings. Microadenomas are often overlooked on gross examination, especially since they usually are not the reason for surgical resection and attention is focused on the more substantial pathologic findings elsewhere in the gland. Microadenomas are usually sharply circumscribed but unencapsulated, soft tan nodules (fig. 12-1). By definition, they measure less than 0.5 cm, and the average size is 1 to 2 mm. Most arise in the tail of the gland, but some arise in the head. The surrounding pancreas is usually normal. Microadenomas occur in the presence of chronic pancreatitis, but there is no evidence that

they are more common in this setting or that pancreatitis plays a role in their pathogenesis.

Microscopic Findings. Endocrine microadenomas are microscopically circumscribed and usually separated from the surrounding pancreatic parenchyma by minimal fibrous tissue, if any (fig. 12-2). They do not invade into adjacent tissues or vessels. Microadenomas usually have a nesting or trabecular architecture, with minimal fibrous stroma between the neoplastic lobules, although hyalinized amyloid-like material may be found. The cells closely resemble normal islet cells and have moderate amounts of amphophilic cytoplasm and centrally located, cytologically bland nuclei (fig. 12-3). The chromatin is coarsely clumped. Mitotic figures are not identifiable in most instances.

Histochemical and Immunohistochemical Findings. Endocrine microadenomas demonstrate the same staining characteristics as non-neoplastic islet cells by silver impregnation techniques. Both the argyrophil and argentaffin stains may be positive. By immunohistochemistry, they express general endocrine markers including chromogranin, synaptophysin, and CD56. Most solitary microadenomas label for only one or two of the four islet peptides, and it is common to find either glucagon or PP labeling in the majority of the cells (226). In MEN1 patients with multiple microadenomas, the neoplasms are generally multihormonal (5a). The rare patients with microadenomatosis who lack MEN1 syndrome usually have microadenomas that express solely insulin (in those with hyperinsulinism) or glucagon (in those who are asymptomatic) (5a). Labeling for ectopic peptides such as vasoactive intestinal polypeptide (VIP) or gastrin is uncommon.

Differential Diagnosis. The differential diagnosis includes acinar cell nodules as well as non-neoplastic islets of Langerhans that are either enlarged (islet hyperplasia) or distorted due to chronic pancreatitis (islet aggregation).

Acinar cell nodules are also incidental pathologic findings (232,239). Acinar cell nodules are small, circumscribed collections of cytologically altered acinar cells that may be of either the eosinophilic or basophilic type (see chapter 1). Eosinophilic acinar cell nodules are common and demonstrate more abundant cytoplasm than normal acinar cells, with less basal basophilia due to dilatation of the rough endoplasmic reticulum. Since the apical eosinophilic zymogen granules are retained, acinar cell nodules have a more eosinophilic appearance than the surrounding acini. Careful examination reveals the basal polarization of the nuclei and the presence of large zymogen granules, distinguishing eosinophilic acinar cell nodules from endocrine microadenomas. Basophilic acinar cell nodules have markedly decreased zymogen granule content, and the nuclei are enlarged and have prominent nucleoli. These nodules are uncommon and may easily be confused for endocrine microadenomas, although they lack the characteristic chromatin pattern of the endocrine cells. In questionable cases, immunohistochemical labeling can be used to distinguish basophilic acinar cell nodules (which label for trypsin and chymotrypsin) from endocrine microadenomas (which label for chromogranin and synaptophysin).

Since normal non-neoplastic islets vary considerably in size, occasional islets may measure 1 to 2 mm in diameter, overlapping with the size of microadenomas. Furthermore, in chronic pancreatitis there is aggregation of islets as the exocrine elements atrophy, simulating a neoplasm (12). In some instances, the distortion of the islets by fibrosis, possibly accompanied by islet proliferation (see chapter 15), results in a pseudoinfiltrative appearance reminiscent of a neoplastic process. In general, microadenomas measure more than 0.5 mm. Furthermore, non-neoplastic islet cells retain their heterogeneous population of different peptide cell types, and immunohistochemical labeling of non-neoplastic islets for the major islet peptides (insulin, glucagon, somatostatin, and PP) reveals the presence of all cell types, in roughly normal numbers and distribution. By contrast, cells expressing one peptide typically predominate in endocrine microadenomas.

In patients with MEN1, dysplastic islets (126) are to be distinguished from endocrine microadenomas. Both have altered peptide cell type proportions and topography, but dysplastic islets measure less than 0.5 mm.

Treatment. Since patients are almost always asymptomatic, and most microadenomas are not detected until after they have been removed and therefore cured, there is no specific treatment for them. In patients with MEN1, it is impractical to attempt to remove the numerous microadenomas that are usually present, and since it is unclear that an individual microadenoma has a significant risk to progress to a clinically relevant PEN, only close follow-up is suggested. A similar argument applies if an incidental microadenoma is detected in a section of the surgical margin from a pancreatectomy performed for other reasons.

WELL-DIFFERENTIATED PANCREATIC ENDOCRINE NEOPLASMS

General Features and Nonfunctional Pancreatic Endocrine Neoplasms

The majority of clinically relevant PENs are nonfunctional and well differentiated. Since many of the clinical and pathologic features of nonfunctional PENs also apply to the functional examples, the general features of both nonfunctional and functional well-differentiated PENs are discussed together below.

Definition. *Well-differentiated pancreatic endocrine neoplasm* (PEN) is an epithelial neoplasm characterized by the organoid growth of cells cytologically resembling normal islet cells or other hormone-producing cells, with a relatively low mitotic rate (up to 10 mitoses per 10 high-power microscopic fields), that measures 0.5 cm or greater in largest dimension. PENs may be associated with clinical evidence of inappropriate hormone secretion in the form of several characteristic paraneoplastic syndromes (functional PENs, Tables 12-1, 12-2) or they may be nonfunctional. Synonyms include *pancreatic endocrine tumor, well-differentiated endocrine carcinoma of the pancreas,* and *islet cell tumor.* The last term remains popular despite falling into disfavor because all PENs are neoplastic and some PENs show differentiation towards endocrine cells not found in normal pancreatic islets (e.g., gastrinomas, VIPomas).

General Features. PENs are uncommon; they constitute 1 to 2 percent of pancreatic neoplasms (91). The prevalence of PENs in the general population is estimated to be 1/100,000 (164). Previously, functional PENs were considered more common than the nonfunctional type, the latter representing 15 to 35 percent of PENs in surgical series (25,90,112,123). In the past decade, the detection of PENs (especially nonfunctional PENs) has improved due to the increased use of sensitive imaging techniques, and in some institutions, nonfunctional PENs now comprise more than half of the surgically resected cases (98). Furthermore, since a significant number of nonfunctional PENs are detected only after they have metastasized, they often are not included in surgical studies. Among the functional variants (91), insulinomas are the most common, comprising 42 percent of functional PENs. Gastrinomas are also relatively common, reportedly making up 24 percent; however, many gastrinomas arise primarily within the duodenum, and this distinction is not always considered. Glucagonomas make up 14 percent of functional PENs; VIPomas, 10 percent; somatostatinomas, 6 percent; and the remaining ectopic and multiple hormone-producing neoplasms are rare (37,60,76).

There has been considerable debate about the histogenesis or cell of origin of PENs. The observation that the islet cells are derived from the embryonic ducts (40), along with the apparent neoformation of islet cells from ducts in persistent hyperinsulinemic hypoglycemia of infancy ("nesidioblastosis") (75,197,208,236) and the appearance in chronic pancreatitis of "ductuloinsular complexes" (intimately associated aggregates of ductules and islet cells) (12), have suggested that PENs may originate from cells within the ducts rather than from preexisting islet cells. Whether these intraductal cells are mature ductal epithelial cells, intraductal endocrine cells (which are documented), or undifferentiated intraductal stem cells (99) has never been clarified. In fact, observations of the histologic features of the islets in patients with MEN1 (126) suggest neoplastic transformation within the islets themselves. Also, mouse transgenic models of insulinomas have generated atypical proliferative lesions of the islet cells in addition to β-cell neoplasms (42,154, 240). In fact, there are no recognized precursor lesions for most PENs, making the identification of the elusive cell of origin difficult.

Clinical Features. PENs occur at any age but are most common between the ages of 40 and 60, with a mean of 58 years (90,226). Children are rarely affected, and examples presenting in the first decade are exceptional (85,105,219). Both men and women develop PENs with an equal frequency, although there are some differences in the male to female ratio among the different functional types.

The presenting clinical features are highly variable depending upon the presence and type of endocrine paraneoplastic syndrome. The specific presenting features of the functional PENs are detailed below (see Clinicopathologic Features of Functional PENs). Patients with nonfunctional PENs usually present with nonspecific symptoms including abdominal pain or nausea. In rare instances, PENs in the head of the pancreas compress the bile duct and cause jaundice, but invasion into the bile duct (as commonly seen in patients with ductal adenocarcinomas) rarely occurs. In 15 percent of patients, asymptomatic nonfunctional PENs are identified on abdominal imaging studies performed for other reasons (112); these incidental presentations are becoming increasingly frequent. Finally, a sizeable group of patients with PENs are asymptomatic until they develop metastases. Even in this circumstance, the symptoms may be relatively mild, and it is not uncommon for a patient with numerous hepatic metastases to appear relatively healthy and have only mild abdominal pain.

The production of specific hormones is common in both functional and nonfunctional PENs. Most functional PENs have associated serum elevations of the corresponding functional hormone (see below). Many nonfunctional PENs have serum elevations of one or more different peptide hormones, even in the absence of endocrinologic symptoms. Increased serum insulin, proinsulin, PP, glucagon, and gastrin levels can be used to predict the presence of PENs in patients with MEN1 syndrome. Elevated serum chromogranin A levels have a sensitivity of 70 percent for predicting the presence of a PEN (13). Interestingly, serum hormone types and levels do not correlate well with the patterns of hormone expression detected in the neoplasms by immunohistochemistry.

Familial Pancreatic Endocrine Neoplasms. PENs represent a major component of the hereditary multiple endocrine neoplasia syndrome, type 1 (MEN1) and are also more prevalent in patients with von Hippel-Lindau syndrome. There are a few reports of PENs in children with tuberous sclerosis (69,247). Somatostatinomas associated with neurofibromatosis (83,84) usually arise in the duodenum, but somatostatinomas in the pancreas also have been reported (34).

MEN1 syndrome is characterized by the development of endocrine lesions involving the parathyroid glands, pancreas, pituitary gland, and upper gastrointestinal tract (26); other less common sites of involvement include the lung, thymus, thyroid gland, and adrenal gland. The disease has an autosomal dominant pattern of inheritance with a very high degree of penetrance (95 percent), although the pancreas is involved in only 60 to 70 percent of cases. MEN1 syndrome is rare, but some autopsy studies have suggested up to 0.25 percent of the population has some features of the syndrome (149).

MEN1 syndrome is caused by a germline mutation in the *MEN1* tumor suppressor gene, located on chromosome 11q13. The *MEN1* gene codes for a 610 amino acid protein (menin) that suppresses cell proliferation (33). Affected patients have a germline inactivating mutation of one allele of this gene, accompanied in the endocrine neoplasms by an acquired somatic mutation of the remaining wild-type allele.

Most patients with MEN1 develop symptoms of endocrine neoplasia by age 25 to 30 years, and many of the endocrine lesions are hyperfunctional. Hyperplasia of the parathyroid glands is most common, affecting essentially all patients, and it is usually the first manifestation of the syndrome. PENs are found in over half of patients with MEN1 (126,129,144), and others likely have microadenomas that are nonfunctional (nearly all based on autopsy studies [157]). Pituitary abnormalities are less common (15 to 50 percent). Upper gastrointestinal manifestations include carcinoid tumors of the duodenum and stomach. The duodenal carcinoids may be functional, mostly by producing gastrin. The gastric carcinoid tumors arise in the fundus in a background of diffuse endocrine cell hyperplasia involving the enterochromaffin-like (ECL) cells (19). These proliferative lesions are due in part to the trophic action of gastrin on ECL cells, so MEN1 patients with gastrinomas in the duodenum or pancreas are particularly prone to develop gastric carcinoid tumors. It is likely, however, that the underlying genetic abnormality of the MEN1 syndrome also contributes to the progression of ECL cell hyperplasia to neoplasia, since patients with elevated gastrin levels of other etiologies (e.g., pernicious anemia or sporadic gastrinomas) develop fewer overt gastric carcinoids despite having a similar degree of ECL cell hyperplasia. The MEN1 syndrome can have different manifestations in different kindreds; in fact, even related individuals within an affected kindred can have different endocrine lesions (23,51).

Patients with MEN1 typically have multiple endocrine neoplasms in the pancreas, including both microadenomas and PENs (fig. 12-4) (126,144). These neoplasms occur throughout the pancreas but are concentrated in the tail. Although the majority are nonfunctional, most patients have at least one functional PEN (86, 126,144). Gastrinoma is the most common functional PEN in this population, followed by insulinoma, VIPoma, glucagonoma, and PENs

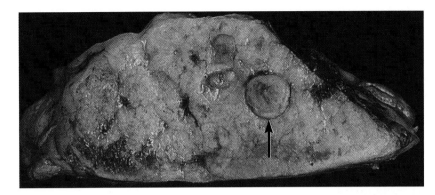

Figure 12-4

**PANCREATIC ENDOCRINE
NEOPLASMS IN PATIENT
WITH MULTIPLE
ENDOCRINE NEOPLASIA,
TYPE 1 (MEN1)**

Gross appearance. (Fig. 5-47A
from Fascicle 20, Third Series.)

producing growth hormone-releasing factor and
inducing acromegaly. Surgical enucleation of a
single functional PEN may be sufficient to control the symptoms, since total pancreatectomy
would be needed to remove all of the neoplasms.
Recurrence of symptoms is common, however,
either because of recurrence of the resected PEN
or the development of additional functional
PENs elsewhere in the pancreas.

Patients with von Hippel-Lindau syndrome develop a variety of neoplasms due to a dominantly
inherited germline mutation in the *VHL* tumor
suppressor gene on chromosome 3p25 (143).
Somatic inactivation of the second allele of the
VHL gene is found in the neoplasms. The most
common neoplasms in patients with von Hippel-
Lindau syndrome include hemangioblastomas of
the central nervous system and retina, renal cell
carcinoma, pheochromocytoma, cystadenomas
of the epididymis and pancreas, clear cell
carcinoids of the biliary tree, and PENs (40a,
51b,88,101,155). The presence of two of these
neoplasms establishes the diagnosis; for patients
with an affected family member, only one neoplasm is required. The type of neoplasm affecting a given patient depends upon the specific
mutation in the *VHL* gene. Von Hippel-Lindau
syndrome has a prevalence of 1/36,000 to 1/39,000.

PENs occur in about 5 to 10 percent of patients with von Hippel-Lindau syndrome and
may be multiple. The majority are nonfunctional.
Most are 0.4 to 8.0 cm and are confined to the
pancreas, although metastases occur (51b,147).
Grossly, they resemble other PENs but more often are yellow, reflecting a high fat content. The
fat may result in a foamy clear cell appearance,
and clear cell change is reported in 60 percent of
PENs in patients with the syndrome (96). Otherwise, the pathologic features of these PENs re-

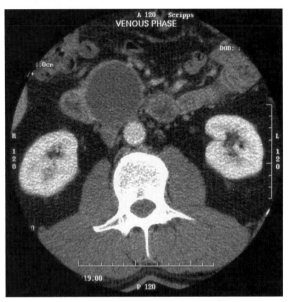

Figure 12-5

CYSTIC PANCREATIC ENDOCRINE NEOPLASM

Appearance on computerized tomography (CT) scan.

semble those of other nonfunctional PENs. Similar types of peptide are also expressed, although
two thirds of the cases show no peptide immunolabeling (155). Combined PEN/serous cystic neoplasms also occur in patients with von Hippel-
Lindau syndrome.

Radiologic Findings. Most PENs appear on
abdominal computerized tomography (CT) scans
as solid, circumscribed masses that enhance due
to their rich vascularity. PENs located in the head
of the pancreas generally do not dilate the pancreatic or biliary ducts. Even large PENs that
extend outside the pancreas usually displace
rather than invade adjacent structures such as
major blood vessels. Some PENs have calcifications, and cystic change may occur either

focally or extensively (see below) (fig. 12-5) (148). Octreotide scintigraphy takes advantage of the fact that most well-differentiated PENs possess somatostatin receptors. In this procedure, octreotide, a somatostatin analog, is labeled for nuclear imaging to identify PENs. Octreotide scanning is helpful in distinguishing PENs from other solid pancreatic masses; it may also be used to search for evidence of distant metastases or to look for an occult primary in patients who present with small, hormonally active PENs or metastatic disease with no obvious pancreatic primary.

Gross Findings. PENs occur throughout the pancreas. Functional types are more common in the head or the tail, and nonfunctional PENs are more common in the head, but taken all together, about 60 percent of PENs arise in the pancreatic tail (226). Smaller PENs are usually sharply circumscribed or even encapsulated, and are composed of uniform, red-tan to yellow parenchyma (figs. 12-6, 12-7). Larger PENs are multinodular and grossly demonstrate evidence of invasive growth (fig. 12-8). They may extend into peripancreatic tissues or adjacent structures (e.g., spleen, duodenum) (fig. 12-9). Occasionally, there is gross vascular invasion as well.

The consistency of PENs varies considerably: some are very soft whereas others have more fibrotic stroma, imparting a firm or even sclerotic consistency. Areas of hemorrhage may be found. Less commonly, there is necrosis that is usually infarct-like. Black PENs have been reported (220); the color appears to be caused by the accumulation of lipofuscin.

A minority of PENs have a grossly cystic appearance (148). Degenerative cystic changes are relatively common in larger PENs, but the cysts are generally a minor attribute of the predominantly solid neoplasm, and radiographic or gross confusion with a primarily cystic pancreatic neoplasm is unlikely. On rare occasion,

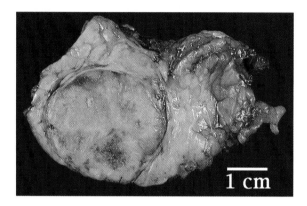

Figure 12-6

PANCREATIC ENDOCRINE NEOPLASM

Small, sharply circumscribed PEN without lobulation.

Figure 12-7

PANCREATIC ENDOCRINE NEOPLASM

Circumscribed PEN with a variegated appearance is surrounded by a fibrous pseudocapsule.

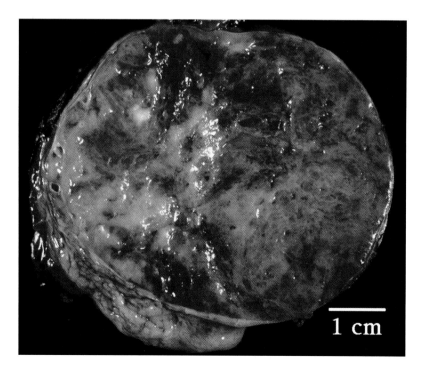

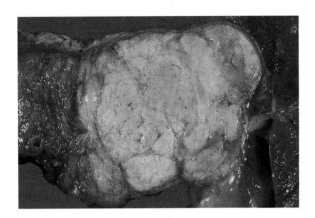

Figure 12-8

PANCREATIC ENDOCRINE NEOPLASM
Multilobulated PEN without encapsulation.

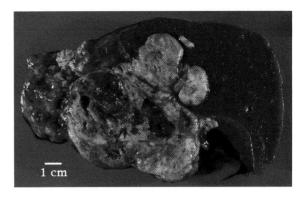

Figure 12-9

PANCREATIC ENDOCRINE NEOPLASM
Multinodular PEN with hemorrhage and gross invasion of the spleen.

however, extensive cystic change is found (148). In most of the reported cases, cystic PENs have a single central locule surrounded by a thin rim of neoplastic parenchyma; the parenchyma is often separated from the adjacent pancreas by a fibrous pseudocapsule (fig. 12-10).

Microscopic Findings. PENs usually have one or more of the characteristic organoid patterns of well-differentiated endocrine neoplasms of other organs, but there are many variations in the architecture of these neoplasms that, coupled with a wide array of cytologic appearances, produce a vast assortment of different histologic patterns, perhaps more so than any other family of endocrine neoplasms. In fact, a variegated appearance within an individual neoplasm is common (fig. 12-11).

Most PENs have a "pushing" periphery, which corresponds to their grossly expansile growth pattern (fig. 12-12). A fibrotic pseudocapsule sometimes surrounds the nests of neoplastic cells partially or entirely, although local invasion through the capsule into adjacent pancreatic parenchyma or into peripancreatic soft tissue is often found. Perineural and vascular invasion also occur and are most easily recognized in the peritumoral nerves and vessels within the pseudocapsule, or within the adjacent pancreas (fig. 12-13). Invasion of adjacent organs such as spleen, duodenum, or stomach may occur. Polypoid extension into the pancreatic ducts is uncommon but documented (115).

Most PENs have a nested, trabecular, or gyriform architectural pattern, although regions

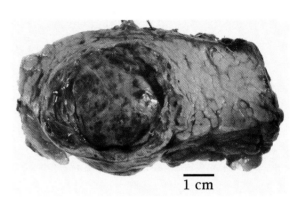

Figure 12-10

CYSTIC PANCREATIC ENDOCRINE NEOPLASM
Central unilocular cyst with a thin rim of neoplastic parenchyma at the periphery.

with a more diffuse arrangement can be found (fig. 12-14). Numerous small vessels, each accompanied by a variable amount of fibrotic stroma, surround the clusters of neoplastic cells. In some cases, there is little collagen adjacent to the vasculature, but in others, the stroma between the nests is densely hyalinized. Amyloid deposition may occur (124,254), especially in insulinomas (fig. 12-15), but usually the stroma is composed of acellular collagen. The cellular desmoplastic stroma of ductal adenocarcinomas is not typically found in PENs. Calcifications may occur in the stroma or within nests of neoplastic cells. Sometimes these are psammomatous. Psammoma bodies have been linked to insulinomas (and even more closely

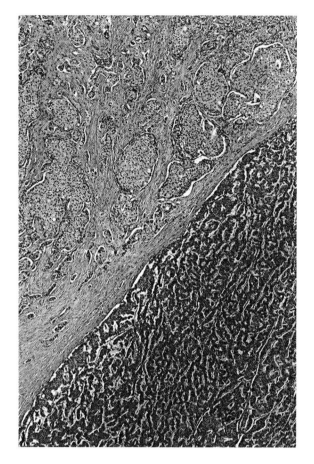

Figure 12-11

PANCREATIC ENDOCRINE NEOPLASM

Multiple histologic patterns are present.

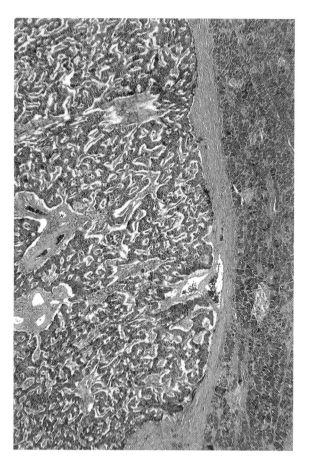

Figure 12-12

PANCREATIC ENDOCRINE NEOPLASM

Circumscribed neoplasm with a pushing border.

Figure 12-13

PANCREATIC ENDOCRINE NEOPLASM

Vascular invasion.

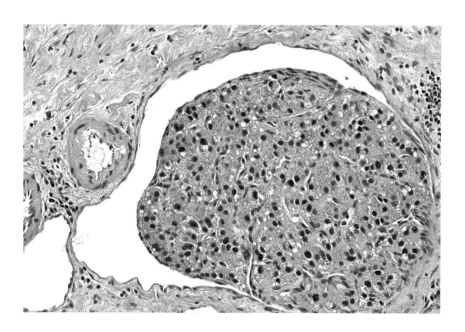

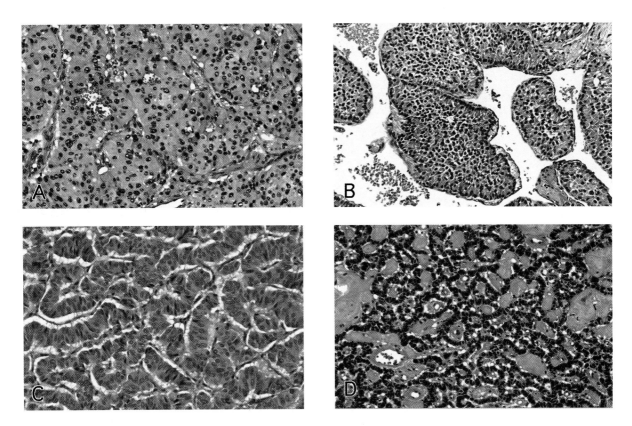

Figure 12-14

PANCREATIC ENDOCRINE NEOPLASM

Architectural patterns include nesting (A), macrotrabecular (B), microtrabecular (C), and gyriform (D).

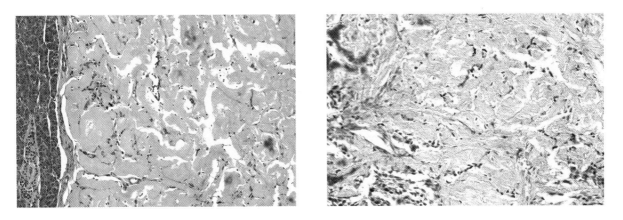

Figure 12-15

PANCREATIC ENDOCRINE NEOPLASM

Stromal amyloid deposition (left) stains with Congo red (right).

with the somatostatinomas that occur primarily within the periampullary duodenum [49]), although occasionally they are found associated with other types of PEN (22).

The nuclear features are characteristic. The round to oval nuclei are usually uniform in size and shape, and classically have the coarsely stippled "salt and pepper" appearance common

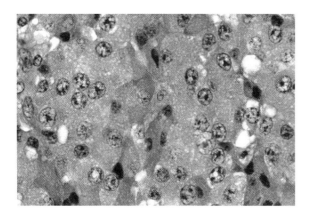

Figure 12-16

PANCREATIC ENDOCRINE NEOPLASM

Nuclear features show the coarsely clumped, "salt and pepper" chromatin pattern.

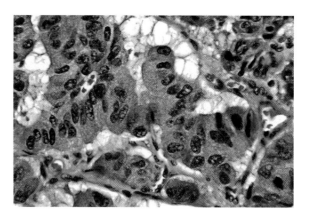

Figure 12-17

PANCREATIC ENDOCRINE NEOPLASM

The cytoplasm is amphophilic and nuclei are eccentrically located.

to well-differentiated endocrine neoplasms of other organs (fig. 12-16). There are many exceptions, however. Variable nuclear shape is common, and some PENs have scattered large nuclei, similar to the polyploid nuclei that are found in non-neoplastic islet cells (specifically, the β cells). Nucleoli are usually inconspicuous, but some PENs have prominent nucleoli. In general, the nuclei are centrally located within the cells, but basal polarization, with alignment of nuclei along the stroma-facing aspect of the cell, may occur.

The cells vary in size but are usually polygonal. The cytoplasm may be eosinophilic or amphophilic and is usually moderately abundant (fig. 12-17). Rare PENs with minimal cytoplasm may be confused with higher-grade neoplasms. Often the nucleus is peripherally located, resulting in a plasmacytoid appearance to the cytoplasm. Cytoplasmic hyaline globules may be found and resemble those of solid-pseudopapillary neoplasm.

Lumen formation may occur, usually within a large nest of cells, imparting a cribriform pattern (fig. 12-18). Less commonly, individual neoplastic glands are surrounded by stroma. In both of these circumstances, the cells lining the lumens are cytologically indistinguishable from the remainder of the endocrine cells in the solid regions; this is to be distinguished from PENs with a separate nonendocrine glandular component (see below).

The mitotic rate varies from undetectable (less than 1 mitosis per 50 high-power fields)

to 10 mitoses per 10 high-power fields; endocrine neoplasms with more than 10 mitoses per 10 high-power fields are poorly differentiated endocrine carcinomas by definition. Necrosis is not typically found in smaller PENs (less than 3 cm). When present, foci of necrosis may be large and confluent ("infarct-like") or they may appear as more punctate foci of true tumor necrosis in the center of the neoplastic nests.

Uncommon Histologic Findings. There are many morphologic variants in addition to the classic patterns of PEN described above. *Oncocytic PENs* are architecturally similar to conventional PENs but are composed of cells with abundant granular eosinophilic cytoplasm (fig. 12-19) (30,78,102,189). Oncocytic change may be focal, and it must occur in at least 25 percent of the neoplasm to qualify as an oncocytic PEN (102). Approximately 7 percent of PENs have oncocytic cytoplasm (102).

Clear cell change also occurs in PENs and is more common in patients with von Hippel-Lindau syndrome (96,219a). In these cases, the cells have abundant cytoplasm filled with numerous clear vesicles, some of which may scallop the nucleus (fig. 12-20). The resulting foamy cytoplasm resembles that of sebaceous cells, and intracellular fat can be demonstrated, leading some investigators to suggest the term *lipid-rich PEN* for this variant (219a). Since clear cell PENs are more common in patients with the von Hippel-Lindau syndrome, these primary pancreatic neoplasms need to be distinguished

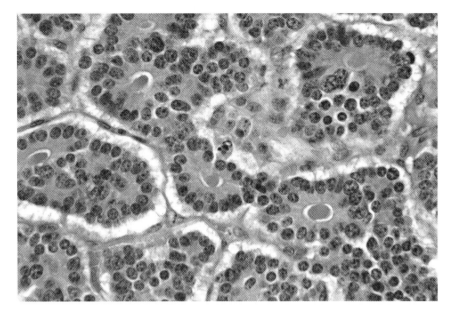

Figure 12-18

PANCREATIC ENDOCRINE NEOPLASM

Gland formation by the neoplastic cells.

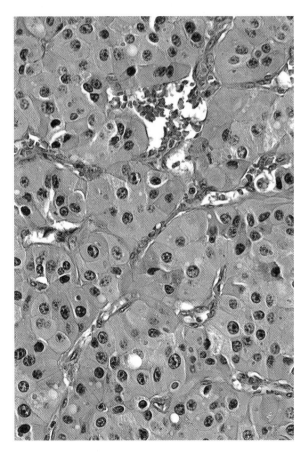

Figure 12-19

PANCREATIC ENDOCRINE NEOPLASM

Oncocytic variant, with abundant granular eosinophilic cytoplasm.

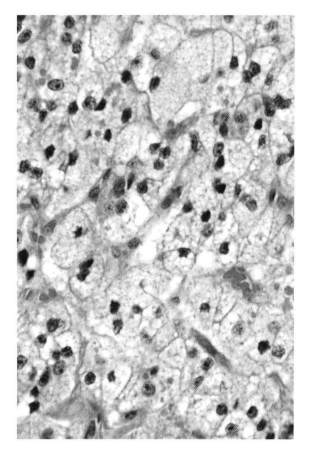

Figure 12-20

PANCREATIC ENDOCRINE NEOPLASM

Clear cell variant, with a foamy appearance caused by numerous lipid droplets.

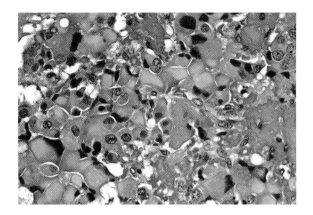

Figure 12-21

PANCREATIC ENDOCRINE NEOPLASM

Pleomorphic variant, with marked nuclear atypia and cytomegaly.

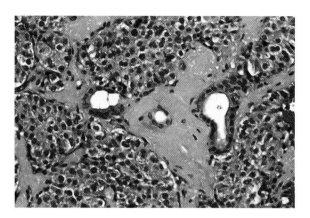

Figure 12-22

PANCREATIC ENDOCRINE NEOPLASM

Entrapped non-neoplastic ductules.

from renal cell carcinoma metastatic to the pancreas and the rare ectopic adrenal cortical nodule in the pancreas.

Some PENs have marked nuclear atypia throughout the neoplasm (fig. 12-21). These are called *pleomorphic PENs,* and many of the reported cases had been initially misdiagnosed as high-grade neoplasms such as ductal carcinomas or undifferentiated carcinomas (263). In fact, most pleomorphic PENs do not demonstrate an elevated mitotic rate or necrosis, and the enlarged nuclei are accompanied by abundant cytoplasm (cytomegaly). Despite their worrisome appearance, no studies have demonstrated that pleomorphic PENs have a more aggressive biology than PENs with uniform nuclear morphology.

Although it is common to find focal glandular differentiation in the form of lumen formation in PENs, some also contain a population of glands that are distinct from the surrounding endocrine elements. Most commonly, small exocrine ductules are scattered within the PEN, each closely surrounded by nests of endocrine cells (fig. 12-22). The endocrine and exocrine cells may be so intimately associated, that it often appears that they share the same basement membrane. These formations resemble the so-called ductuloinsular complexes seen in regions of chronic pancreatitis. The glands have features of non-neoplastic small intralobular ducts, although sometimes with somewhat more eosinophilic cytoplasm. Although PENs with sig-

nificant numbers of small glands have been designated *ductuloinsular tumors of the pancreas* (suggesting that the glands are an inherent, neoplastic component of the tumor) (53,199), recent studies have demonstrated that the ductules are not monoclonal and therefore represent a population of entrapped, non-neoplastic glands (245). It is not clear whether the reportedly higher frequency of entrapped ductules in insulinomas relative to other PEN types is merely a reflection of the small size of most insulinomas; it has been proposed that smaller PENs may be more likely to retain a noticeable component of entrapped non-neoplastic elements than larger PENs that have presumably displaced most of the remaining pancreatic tissue (34,245). True mixed ductal-endocrine carcinomas, in which there is a separate neoplastic (and malignant) component of ductal adenocarcinoma, although rare, do occur; these are discussed below.

Grossly cystic PENs generally do not have a distinctive microscopic appearance (148). The cysts are usually lined by a layer of fibrin adherent to the neoplastic cells, which are arranged in nests or trabeculae (fig. 12-23). Although the fibrin may suggest that the cyst arose by degeneration, there is usually no necrosis. In rare instances, the endocrine cells are separated from the cyst by a layer of ductal epithelium. In these cystic PENs, small ductules are also found within the remainder of the endocrine neoplasm, so the entire cyst has the appearance of a preexisting duct with surrounding ductules that has been

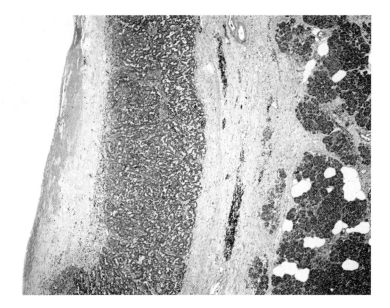

Figure 12-23

CYSTIC PANCREATIC ENDOCRINE NEOPLASM

A layer of fibrin separates the neoplastic cells from the cyst lumen.

colonized by the endocrine neoplasm and cystically dilated.

Also reported is a variant of PEN with rhabdoid morphology. These neoplasms have eccentrically located nuclei and inclusion-like, glassy cytoplasm. The resemblance of the cells to signet ring cells may cause confusion with adenocarcinoma. The inclusions, however, do not contain mucin but instead consist ultrastructurally of whorls of intermediate filaments, sometimes entrapping numerous neurosecretory granules (see below) (34,193,218). A spindle cell pattern is an unusual and generally focal feature in PENs. Also, PENs sometimes have widespread vacuolization of the cytoplasm. Rarely, squamoid nests resembling those of pancreatoblastoma are present. These neoplasms, however, lack the acinar differentiation seen in pancreatoblastomas.

A rhabdomyosarcoma component has been described (67,126,226). This may represent a mixed ductal-endocrine carcinoma in which the ductal component consists exclusively of sarcomatoid carcinoma.

Precursor Lesions. There are no well-accepted precursors of PENs, although presumably at some point in their evolution, PENs are small enough to qualify as microadenomas. Examination of the pancreas in patients with MEN1 syndrome demonstrates enlarged islets with irregular contours, nuclear abnormalities, and abnormal distribution of peptide cell types (fig.

12-24); these islets have been described as dysplastic (126,226), perhaps representing the earliest neoplastic change in MEN1. There is, however, considerable variation in the size and shape of normal islets, so the principal abnormal feature is the aberrant peptide immunolabeling pattern. Although small clusters of endocrine cells may be seen adjacent to ductules in MEN1, resembling nesidioblastosis, chronic pancreatitis secondary to ductal obstruction by mass-forming PENs may account for these changes, and they are not generally regarded as neoplastic precursors (136).

Frozen Section. Intraoperative frozen section evaluation may be performed to confirm the diagnosis of PEN, especially when a small functional PEN is suspected. However, it is not possible by frozen section analysis to determine whether a given PEN is the functional PEN in a patient with MEN1 who may have more than one lesion. If the diagnosis of PEN is expected due to clinical findings (e.g., an endocrinologic syndrome), the typical architectural and cytologic features are generally sufficient to confirm the diagnosis made on frozen section. Several other primary pancreatic neoplasms share the solid, hypercellular appearance of most PENs (see differential diagnosis, below), however, and are sometimes difficult to distinguish from a PEN by frozen section. Imprint cytology is useful for demonstrating the characteristic chromatin pattern and plasmacytoid cell shape of PENs.

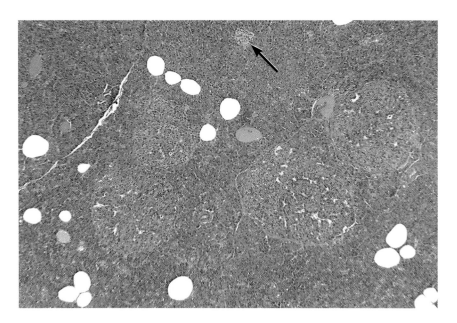

Figure 12-24

ISLETS FROM PATIENT WITH MEN1

The islets are enlarged and irregularly shaped. A normal islet (arrow) is shown for comparison.

Grading. Several different grading schemes have been proposed for PENs. In contrast to adenocarcinomas, the degree of nuclear pleomorphism and the architectural pattern do not correlate well with prognosis (263). Attempts to develop an effective grading system have analyzed the differences in histologic features between groups of patients with varying clinical outcomes. Based in part on the Capella classification of endocrine neoplasms (27), the most recent World Health Organization (WHO) classification (91) separates PENs into two general groups: well-differentiated endocrine tumors and well-differentiated endocrine carcinomas. Well-differentiated endocrine tumors are confined to the pancreas (or only extend locally into peripancreatic tissues) whereas well-differentiated endocrine carcinomas have either gross local invasion or metastases. Within the well-differentiated endocrine tumor category, those PENs that measure less than 2 cm in diameter, have less than 2 mitoses per 10 high-power fields (or have a Ki-67 labeling index less than 2 percent), and demonstrate no perineural or vascular invasion are predicted to have "benign behavior"; those that either are greater than 2 cm in diameter, have 2 to 10 mitoses per 10 high-power fields (or have a Ki-67 index greater than 2 percent), or have perineural or vascular invasion are considered to have "uncertain behavior" (91). In this scheme, no PEN other than microadenomas is designated as a benign neoplasm; the subcategories are intended to provide an indication of the likely clinical behavior based on relatively well-characterized prognostic factors.

It can be argued that by including size and the presence of metastases in the grading criteria, the WHO system includes factors that are generally regarded as staging parameters for other neoplasms. Certainly, a subset of PENs in the well-differentiated endocrine tumor group (mostly those in the uncertain behavior subgroup) will recur and metastasize (98), at which time they would be reclassified as well-differentiated endocrine carcinomas. So the "grade" in this system is not necessarily an inherent biologic feature of an individual PEN; for instance, this system would not allow for prognostic stratification of PENs that had already metastasized.

Another recently proposed grading system for PENs utilizes the strong prognostic correlation of proliferative rate and necrosis to separate PENs into low-grade and intermediate-grade categories (98). In this classification, low-grade PENs have no necrosis and less than 2 mitoses per 50 high-power fields whereas intermediate-grade PENs have either necrosis or a mitotic rate of 2 to 50 per 50 high-power fields. (Note that in this system, the mitotic rate separating PENs from poorly differentiated endocrine carcinomas is 50 per 50 high-power fields.) Again, no group of PENs is classified as benign, but in this system the prognostic significance applies

Table 12-3

GRADING OF PANCREATIC ENDOCRINE NEOPLASMS

World Health Organization (WHO) System	Mitotic Count System

Well-differentiated pancreatic endocrine tumor
  "Benign" behavior (confined to the pancreas; no vascular or
    perineural invasion, <2 cm, and <2 mitoses/10 hpf[a])
  Uncertain behavior (confined to the pancreas; vascular invasion,
    perineural invasion, ≥2 cm or 2 to 10 mitoses/10 hpf)
Well-differentiated pancreatic endocrine carcinoma (gross local
  invasion or metastases)
	Low-grade pancreatic endocrine neoplasm (no
	  necrosis and <2 mitoses/50 hpf)
	
	Intermediate-grade pancreatic endocrine neoplasm
	  (necrosis present or 2 to 50 mitoses/50 hpf)

[a]hpf = high-power microscopic fields.

independent of the stage of the neoplasm (98). Some PENs in the low-grade group may still recur or metastasize. Interestingly, some of the PENs in the WHO benign behavior subgroup fall into the intermediate-grade group (i.e., those with 2 to 9 mitoses per 50 high-power fields). A comparison of these two grading schemes is shown in Table 12-3.

We recommend histologically grading PENs based on their mitotic rate and the presence of necrosis into low- and intermediate-grade categories (98). Other prognostic features (see below), including tumor size, the presence of extrapancreatic or vascular invasion, and lymph node metastases, should also be noted.

Histochemical and Immunohistochemical Findings. Classic silver staining techniques have been used to identify neurosecretory granules in PENs. Either argyrophil (such as the Grimelius stain) or argentaffin (such as the Fontana-Masson stain) reactions may be positive. Currently, these stains have been supplanted by immunohistochemistry, a much more specific method to document endocrine differentiation and to determine the type of hormones produced by a PEN. The periodic acid–Schiff (PAS) stain is typically negative in PENs. Mucin stains such as mucicarmine are also usually negative, although luminal positivity can be detected in PENs with gland formation. Substantial intracellular mucin staining suggests the diagnosis of a mixed ductal-endocrine neoplasm.

By immunohistochemistry, more than 95 percent of PENs label for at least one of the general markers of endocrine differentiation, such as chromogranin, synaptophysin, CD57 (leu-7), or CD56 (neural cell adhesion molecule) (152).

Neuron-specific enolase is also typically expressed, but the poor specificity of this marker has limited its diagnostic utility. Among the two most specific markers, synaptophysin is more consistently expressed than chromogranin, and labeling for synaptophysin is generally diffuse (fig. 12-25, left). Chromogranin labeling is patchy and variable in intensity (fig. 12-25, right), with up to 20 percent of PENs showing only focal positivity. There is some correlation of the peptide cell type of a PEN and chromogranin labeling: PENs with β-cell differentiation often label less intensely, as do non-neoplastic β cells (116).

PENs show a wide range of positivity for specific peptides. Many different peptides have been detected (170), including the normal islet peptides (insulin, glucagon, somatostatin, and pancreatic polypeptide) as well as many ectopic peptides (gastrin, vasoactive intestinal polypeptide, cholecystokinin, adrenocorticotrophic hormone) (226). The neoplastic cells may also express bioamines such as serotonin. The pattern of labeling for these hormones varies widely; some PENs are diffusely positive for one peptide, others show only focal labeling for one or more peptides (90,140,150). It is common to demonstrate the production of more than one hormone in a single PEN. Even examples with widespread immunolabeling for a single hormone may show additional labeling of scattered cells for other peptides.

Often, but not always, there is a good correlation between the specific functional syndrome associated with a PEN and the peptide identified by immunohistochemistry (see sections on specific tumor types, below, for the rates of peptide detection for each type of functional PEN). Some clinically nonfunctional PENs fail

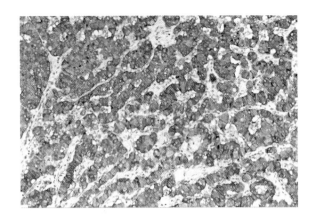
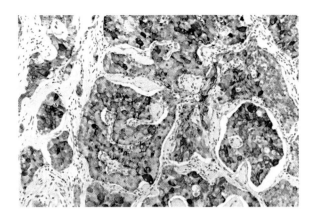

Figure 12-25

PANCREATIC ENDOCRINE NEOPLASM

Immunolabeling is diffuse for synaptophysin (left) but more heterogeneous for chromogranin (right).

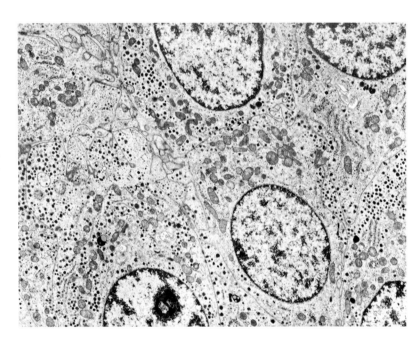

Figure 12-26

PANCREATIC ENDOCRINE NEOPLASM

Ultrastructurally, numerous randomly oriented, 100-nm neurosecretory granules are present.

to demonstrate immunolabeling for any of the hormones, but this does not preclude the possibility of hormone production. These apparent discrepancies between immunolabeling for hormones and clinical function (or serum hormone elevations) can be explained in several ways. For functional PENs that do not label for the corresponding hormone, it has been proposed that the neoplastic cells are secreting the hormone as fast as they are making it, preventing the hormone from accumulating to levels needed for immunodetection. Also, the neoplastic cells may produce antigenically altered peptides that

may not be detected by immunohistochemistry, while retaining functional activity. Of course, there is always a possibility that some nonfunctional PENs produce other hormones not examined by immunohistochemical labeling.

PENs also commonly focally express markers of acinar or ductal differentiation. Scattered cells that immunolabel for trypsin or chymotrypsin can be found in PENs, where they generally constitute less than 5 percent of the neoplastic cells (98,108,261). The reported frequency of focal acinar differentiation has varied widely, from 5 percent in one study (98) to 66 percent in another (261). If more than 25 percent of the neoplastic cells in a predominantly endocrine neoplasm express markers of acinar differentiation, the neoplasm should be classified as a mixed acinar-endocrine carcinoma (119). Immunolabeling for alpha-1-antitrypsin is found in 36 percent of PENs, but this is not a specific marker of acinar differentation and should not be taken as evidence of a mixed acinar-endocrine carcinoma (185a).

PENs also label for glycoprotein markers of ductal differentiation. Focal expression of DUPAN-2 or carbohydrate antigen (CA) 19-9 is found in 22 and 13 percent of PENs, respectively (7,98,108). Carcinoembryonic antigen (CEA) is much less commonly expressed. In those cases with histologic evidence of glandular differentiation, the labeling for these glycoproteins is often most intense in the glandular regions. Oncocytic PENs more frequently label for CEA; in addition, polyclonal antibodies to CEA may label the cell surface, resulting in a branching linear pattern similar to the canalicular pattern of labeling in hepatocellular carcinomas (102). Some oncocytic PENs also label with hepatocyte paraffin-1, which, along with the granular eosinophilic cytoplasm of these neoplasms, furthers the similarity to hepatocellular carcinoma (102). Immunohistochemical labeling for glycoproteins in a PEN is not sufficient evidence for a diagnosis of mixed ductal-endocrine carcinoma unless a morphologically separate component of ductal adenocarcinoma is recognized.

Cytokeratins (CKs) 8 and 18 are generally expressed in PENs, and antibodies such as CAM5.2 and AE1/AE3 are usually positive. Little work has been done regarding the expression of specific keratin types in PENs. Some label for CK19, which is usually regarded as a marker of ductal epithelium and may have prognostic significance (52).

Normal islet cells express progesterone receptors and CD99, but only some PENs retain expression of these markers (44 and 48 percent, respectively) (79,98,250). Some clear cell PENs label for inhibin, potentially causing confusion with adrenal cortical neoplasms (96), but preliminary studies suggest that the majority of clear cell PENs do not express inhibin (219a).

Proliferation markers such as Ki-67 and proliferating cell nuclear antigen (PCNA) are expressed at relatively low levels in PENs. In general, less than 10 percent of the neoplastic cells are positive, and in most cases the rate is between 5 percent and less than 1 percent (38,91,192,226).

Ultrastructural Findings. Prior to the availability of immunohistochemistry, electron microscopy was widely used to characterize PENs (68,81). In addition to demonstrating well-developed features of endocrine differentiation, some PENs also contain neurosecretory granules that resemble those of non-neoplastic islet cells, and in some cases, the granule morphology correlates with the specific clinical syndrome of the neoplasm (see sections on functional PEN types, below).

Neurosecretory granules are common to all PENs (64,68). In most examples, the granules are numerous and are randomly distributed in the cytoplasm (fig. 12-26). In PENs with well-developed cellular polarity, the granules may be concentrated in the basal region of the cytoplasm, adjacent to the vasculature of the stroma. The individual granules range from 50 to 300 nm in diameter and most have a lucent halo separating the limiting membrane from the dense granule content (dense core granules). Some of the morphologic variants of PENs have distinctive ultrastructural findings, including abundant mitochondria in oncocytic PENs, lipid vacuoles in clear cell PENs (219a), and paranuclear aggregates of intermediate filaments in PENs with a rhabdoid morphology (218).

Cytologic Findings. Cytologic sampling of PENs is largely by fine needle aspiration biopsy. The parenchymal location and lack of continuity with the pancreatic ductal system renders duct brushing cytology of no diagnostic use. CT and endoscopic ultrasound (EUS) fine needle aspiration biopsy have equal sensitivity (94 to 95 percent) and specificity (100 percent) for the diagnosis of PEN (237).

Aspirate smears are hypercellular and composed of a monotonous population of small to medium-sized polygonal cells. The rich vascular network of these neoplasms typically produces a bloody background on cytology smears. The cells are mostly noncohesive and arranged singly or in small to medium-sized groups (fig. 12-27, left) which occasionally form acinar arrangements (fig. 12-27, right). Stripped naked nuclei are uncommon. The cells have round nuclei and generally visibly coarse, stippled, evenly distributed

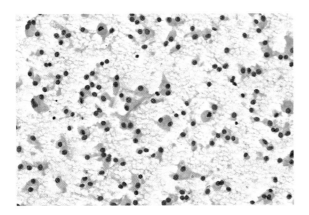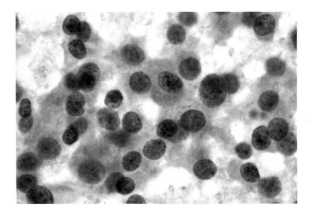

Figure 12-27

PANCREATIC ENDOCRINE NEOPLASM

Left: The typical aspirate cytologic smear pattern demonstrates a noncohesive single cell pattern.

Right: Acinar arrangements of neoplastic cells are occasionally seen on aspiration cytology (direct smear; Papanicolaou stain).

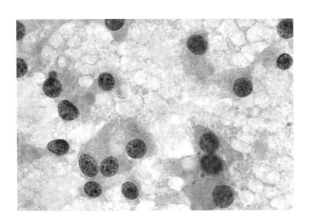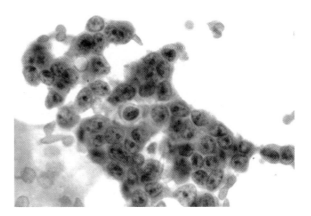

Figure 12-28

PANCREATIC ENDOCRINE NEOPLASM

Left: The characteristic coarse, stippled salt and pepper chromatin pattern characterizes the cells as endocrine in origin (direct smear; Papanicolaou stain).

Right: Nucleoli are occasionally quite prominent, creating difficulty in distinguishing a pancreatic endocrine neoplasm from acinar cell carcinoma and adenocarcinoma (cytospin; Papanicolaou stain).

chromatin (salt and pepper chromatin pattern) (fig. 12-28, left). Nucleoli are usually inconspicuous but may be quite prominent (fig. 12-28, right). Nuclear atypia is variable, and although the nuclei are usually bland and uniform, they may display significant pleomorphism. The cytoplasm is relatively scant and usually dense and eccentric, yielding a plasmacytoid appearance; this feature best appreciated in single cells (3,14,39, 107,206,216,221). Rare variants of PEN, such as clear cell (fig. 12-29) and oncocytic (fig. 12-30), are recognized by their distinctive cytoplasmic features. Mitotic figures and necrosis are uncommon but

may be seen. The cytologic features of cystic PEN are similar to those of solid PEN (31,32).

As with histology, the degree of nuclear atypia cannot be used to predict the outcome of a patient with PEN. As such, the cytologic diagnosis should specify simply a "well-differentiated pancreatic endocrine neoplasm" with a note documenting any unfavorable features such as necrosis or mitotic activity.

Given the characteristic cytologic features of most aspirates, immunocytochemical confirmation of the diagnosis is not always necessary. In difficult cases, confirmatory immunolabeling

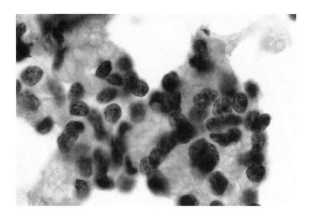

Figure 12-29

PANCREATIC ENDOCRINE NEOPLASM

The clear, vacuolated cytoplasm and the characteristic chromatin pattern help to define this neoplasm cytologically as a clear cell variant (direct smear; Papanicolaou stain).

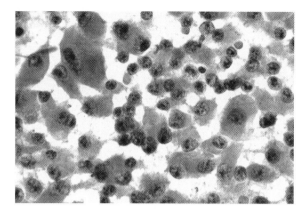

Figure 12-30

PANCREATIC ENDOCRINE NEOPLASM

The abundant, oncocytic cytoplasm and the characteristic chromatin pattern help to define this neoplasm cytologically as an oncocytic variant (direct smear; Papanicolaou stain).

with chromogranin and/or synaptophysin can be performed either on destained smears or on formalin-fixed cell block preparations. The cells on cytology smears can be labeled with specific endocrine hormones but this is not necessary to establish the diagnosis of PEN.

Molecular and Other Special Techniques. Cytogenetic and molecular genetic studies have identified many chromosomal alterations in PENs; however, activation of oncogenes does not appear to play a major role in their development. Chromosomal losses are more common than gains (228,234,264). The most consistent chromosomal alterations described in sporadic PENs include gains at 4p, 4q, 5q, 7p, 7q, 9q, 12q, 14q, 17p, 17q, and 20q, and losses at 1p, 3p, 6q, 9p, 10p, 10q, 11q, 18q, 22q, Y, and X (10,11,62,93, 163,201,228,234,256,264). Some of these losses are associated with more aggressive clinical behavior (see below). The specific genes involved at most of these loci have yet to be identified.

Neoplasms arising in patients with the MEN1 syndrome have germline mutations in the *MEN1* gene on chromosome 11q13 coupled with a somatic (acquired) loss of the second allele of this gene. Losses at 11q13 or elsewhere on the short arm of chromosome 11 are also present in 70 percent of sporadic PENs, but specific intragenic *MEN1* gene mutations are only present in approximately 20 percent of sporadic PENs, suggesting involvement of another tumor suppressor gene on this chromosome (9,47,77,

93,129,165,166,214,252,265). Insulinomas have a much lower frequency of mutations in the *MEN1* gene than most other PENs. PENs arising in patients with the von Hippel-Lindau syndrome usually show biallelic inactivation of the *VHL* gene (155), but this gene is usually not targeted in sporadic PENs (165).

Many of the genes targeted in the development of ductal adenocarcinoma of the pancreas are not targeted in PENs (36,77,166,190). In particular, *KRAS, TP53, p16/CDKN2A*, and *SMAD4/DPC4* are not mutated in most PENs, although the *p16/CDKN2A* gene is inactivated by hypermethylation of the *p16/CDKN2A* promotor in 40 percent of PENs (100,171,209). It appears that promotor methylation, rather than mutation, may be a relatively common mechanism of tumor suppressor gene inactivation in PENs (100). PENs also usually lack *HER2/neu* amplification (74). Some PENs have loss of nuclear expression of p27 (198).

Recent global gene expression analyses have determined which genes are significantly overexpressed or underexpressed in PENs relative to normal islet cells (29a,156). Overexpressed genes include putative oncogenes, growth factors, and cell adhesion and migration molecules, whereas the cell cycle regulator p21, the cell surface glycoprotein MIC2 (CD99), and putative metastasis suppressor genes are among those underexpressed (156).

Table 12-4

DIFFERENTIAL DIAGNOSIS OF PANCREATIC ENDOCRINE NEOPLASM

	Pancreatic Endocrine Neoplasm	Acinar Cell Carcinoma	Pancreato-blastoma	Solid-Pseudo-papillary Neoplasm	Ductal Adeno-carcinoma
Solid, cellular low-power appearance	++[a]	++	++	++	–
Nesting pattern	++	++	++	++	+
Trabecular or gyriform pattern	+	–	–	–	–
Pseudopapillae	–	–	–	++	–
Squamoid nests	–	–	++	–	–
Abundant stroma	+	–	+[b]	+	++[b]
Intracellular mucin	–	–	–	–	++
Hyaline globules	–	–	–	++	–
"Salt and pepper" chromatin	++	–	–	–	–
Nuclear grooves	–	–	–	++	–
Nucleoli	+	++	++	–	+

[a]++ = usually present; + = may be present; – = usually absent.
[b]Often hypercellular.

In general, PENs that are larger or of more advanced stage have more genetic alterations than smaller PENs limited to the pancreas. Thus, there appears to be continuing genetic progression in PENs that parallels clinical progression. Fewer gains and losses of genetic material are found in PENs less than 2 cm, although losses at 1p and 11q and gains at 9q are usually already present (264). In fact, some data suggest that small PENs may represent polyclonal or oligoclonal proliferations from which more aggressive monoclonal neoplasms may arise (194). However, gene expression profiles comparing primary neoplasms with their metastases have not identified significantly differentially expressed genes (29a).

Differential Diagnosis. Because PENs have a wide variety of histologic appearances, the histologic differential diagnosis includes many of the other noncystic primary neoplasms of the pancreas (Table 12-4). In most instances, it is the distinction of PENs from other solid, cellular pancreatic neoplasms that is most problematic; these include acinar cell carcinoma, pancreatoblastoma, mixed acinar-endocrine carcinoma, and solid-pseudopapillary neoplasm. Since PENs are relatively more common than any of these entities, and since all may show some immunolabeling for endocrine markers, it may

be tempting to render a diagnosis of PEN based on the general architectural pattern, with the support of immunohistochemical results, if other considerations are not properly excluded.

Acinar cell carcinoma, pancreatoblastoma, and mixed acinar-endocrine carcinoma are all predominantly acinar neoplasms (117,119,120,184). Recognition of acinar formations is therefore helpful in the diagnosis. All three, however, may have extensive solid areas, and gland formation does occur in PENs. Acinar neoplasms often have single prominent nucleoli and may have an elevated mitotic rate. Pancreatoblastomas generally affect young children and have distinctive squamoid corpuscles usually not encountered in PENs (195). If any of these acinar neoplasms is considered, immunohistochemical labeling for pancreatic enzymes (trypsin, chymotrypsin, and lipase) will demonstrate the acinar differentiation in the majority of cases (117,119,120).

Solid-pseudopapillary neoplasm shares some architectural features with PENs but the former has the characteristic degenerative pseudopapillae in addition to aggregates of foamy histiocytes, large cytoplasmic hyaline globules, and longitudinal nuclear grooves (121). Although PENs and solid-pseudopapillary neoplasms both express synaptophysin and CD56, solid-pseudopapillary neoplasms are never chromogranin positive and, in contrast to PENs, express CD10, and show an abnormal nuclear pattern of labeling for beta-catenin (1).

When PENs display variations in nuclear morphology and gland formation, they may be mistaken for ductal adenocarcinomas. Of the reported pleomorphic PENs (263), 75 percent of the cases were initially diagnosed as adenocarcinomas, and some were felt to be poorly differentiated based on the predominantly solid growth pattern. In contrast to ductal adenocarcinomas, PENs generally maintain some degree of a pushing growth pattern (at least grossly), and they usually lack significant mitotic activity and necrosis. Careful attention to the cytologic appearance as well as recognition of the wide array of patterns encountered in PENs aid in proper diagnosis. Immunolabeling for chromogranin and synaptophysin helps in difficult cases.

When foci of metastatic disease are sampled (often in the liver), the distinction of PENs from neoplasms of other sites becomes important, especially since some small PENs may give rise to metastases while still occult in the primary site. PENs with oncocytic cytoplasm may resemble hepatocellular and adrenal cortical carcinomas, clear cell PENs may be confused with renal cell carcinoma, and PENs with nuclear pleomorphism may resemble carcinomas of many different sites. The features of PENs that are prone to cause confusion include moderate variation in nuclear size, the occasional abundance of fibrotic stroma, eosinophilic cytoplasm, and foci of gland formation. The absence of necrosis and a low mitotic rate suggest a low-grade neoplasm.

The most important factor in achieving the correct diagnosis is to consider the possibility of a PEN based on the routine microscopy; the immunohistochemical evaluation of these cases is generally straightforward. Once such a lesion is recognized as a well-differentiated endocrine neoplasm, distinguishing a carcinoid tumor or other endocrine neoplasm from a PEN may not be possible. Since ectopic hormone production is well-recognized among endocrine neoplasms of diverse sites, immunohistochemical labeling for peptide hormones is not usually helpful. A proportion of pulmonary carcinoid tumors labels for thyroid transcription factor-1 (TTF1) (61), but there are no specific markers for pancreatic origin. In our experience, the less "carcinoid-like"

(i.e., insular and cytologically monotonous) a well-differentiated endocrine neoplasm appears, the more likely it is to have arisen in the pancreas.

Another diagnostic problem results from the dissociation of the neoplastic cells from the bands of fibrotic stroma, as may occur during a needle biopsy procedure, resulting in fragments of naked stromal latticework, and simulating a cavernous hemangioma (see chapter 17). Even when no residual epithelial cells are recognized, immunohistochemical labeling for synaptophysin or chromogranin generally reveals labeling at the edges of the stroma.

The cytologic differential diagnosis of PEN parallels that on histology and is dependent on the degree of cellular atypia. It includes acinar cell carcinoma, solid-pseudopapillary neoplasm, non-Hodgkin's lymphoma, and pancreatoblastoma. Islet cell hyperplasia or aggregation and extramedullary plasmacytoma can also be confused with PENs. Clear cell and oncocytic PEN variants can be confused with primary and metastatic neoplasms with similar cytoplasmic features. Smear artifact of normal acinar cells may also be mistaken for a PEN.

The cytologic distinction between PEN and acinar cell carcinoma rests with the smear pattern, the nuclear chromatin pattern, and the quality of the cytoplasm; there is often significant overlap in these features (138,233a). Endocrine neoplasms tend to produce a richly cellular smear with mostly single cells and some cell clusters in contrast to acinar cell carcinoma where cell clusters predominate over single cells. The stippled salt and pepper chromatin pattern so characteristic of a PEN is absent in acinar cell carcinoma, but this nuclear feature is not always fully defined in a PEN. Nucleoli are typically much more prominent in acinar cell carcinoma than in a PEN, but as noted above and seen in figure 12-28, right, a PEN can, rarely, demonstrate very prominent nucleoli. Granular cytoplasm, when present and visible on smears, helps to define an acinar cell carcinoma in contrast to the dense, not visibly granular, eccentric cytoplasm of PENs. PENs label with antibodies to chromogranin and synaptophysin, while acinar cell carcinomas label with exocrine markers such as trypsin and chymotrypsin (138).

In cytologic preparations, solid-pseudopapillary neoplasms are distinguished by papillary groups with vascular cores and myxoid stroma, but this pattern may not be well demonstrated. When these features are absent, the small uniform cells with bland nuclei and scant cytoplasm of a solid-pseudopapillary neoplasm can be confused with a PEN. The former has a chromatin pattern that is fine and evenly distributed rather than stippled as in PEN. Also, the nuclei tend to have a delicate nuclear groove and the cytoplasm of intact cells is scant and wispy rather than dense and eccentric as in PEN. When present, PAS-positive globules support the diagnosis of solid-pseudopapillary neoplasm.

Non-Hodgkin's lymphoma enters the cytologic differential diagnosis owing to the single cell smear pattern common to both neoplasms. The chromatin pattern is most helpful in distinguishing lymphoma cells, which demonstrate peripherally clumped chromatin, from PEN cells, which have coarse, stippled chromatin. Nucleoli can be prominent in both (immunoblastic lymphoma in particular) and the cytoplasm of both neoplasms can be eccentric, yielding a plasmacytoid appearance (lymphoplasmacytic lymphoma especially). The distinction of lymphoma is aided by the identification in the smear background of globules of the stripped delicate cytoplasm of lymphoma cells (lymphoglandular bodies), a finding that helps to identify the neoplasm as lymphoid rather than epithelial.

Although uncommon in the pancreas, extramedullary plasmacytoma shares the features of eccentric cytoplasm and stippled chromatin (55). In most cases, the diagnosis of extrapancreatic hematologic malignancy is established, prompting ancillary studies for diagnostic confirmation. Because light chain analysis is best performed on fresh tissue, it may be prudent to save unfixed tissue from the fine needle aspiration biopsy. This can be accomplished by rinsing the needle after puncture; however, an aspirate dedicated to flow cytometric analyses may be needed.

In cytologic material, clear cell PENs can be confused with primary clear cell neoplasms of the pancreas (foamy gland adenocarcinoma, PEComa [clear cell "sugar tumor"]) and especially, metastases with clear cytoplasm, most notably metastatic renal cell carcinoma. The distinction between clear cell PEN and metastatic renal cell carcinoma can be impossible on cytology alone, as both neoplasms have a polygonal cell shape, round nuclei, prominent nucleoli, and clear, vacuolated cytoplasm. Renal cell carcinoma, however, normally does not demonstrate the stippled chromatin pattern that is at least focally noted in a clear cell PEN. Immunocytochemical markers are helpful in this differential diagnosis.

Polygonal cells with abundant oncocytic cytoplasm are extremely unusual in smears of pancreatic neoplasms, but when present, oncocytic PEN needs to be differentiated from intraductal oncocytic papillary neoplasm. Both are rare, but clinical, radiologic, and nuclear features aid in their distinction.

A smear containing non-neoplastic acinar or endocrine cells from either normal pancreatic acinar tissue or islet hyperplasia (173) or aggregation can be mistaken for a PEN, particularly when there is radiologic evidence of a mass lesion. The absence of high overall cellularity and well-preserved cells with the clear nuclear features of endocrine cells help avoid this pitfall.

Spread and Metastases. PENs in the head of the gland may encase the superior mesenteric and portal vessels, but this is much less common than in ductal adenocarcinomas. PENs generally metastasize to the regional lymph nodes and the liver. The direct invasion of veins around the neoplasm may result in hepatic metastases in the absence of lymph node spread. Late in the course of the disease, widespread distant metastases may develop, although some patients die of PENs with the metastases largely restricted to the liver. Other typical metastatic sites include lung and bone.

Staging. PENs are not staged.

Treatment. The treatment for primary solitary PEN is surgical resection. The situation is more complicated in the setting of MEN1. These patients generally have multiple PENs, including some that are functional and many that fall into the size range of microadenomas. In some cases, it would be necessary to remove the entire pancreas to ensure complete excision of all neoplasms, but the morbidity of this procedure probably does not justify the benefit of removing microadenomas. Functional PENs can be selectively removed, and elaborate intraoperative techniques (e.g., selected venous blood sampling for hormone levels) have been developed to help identify and localize functional PENs. Otherwise, conservative surgical resection of the larger neoplasms is recommended.

The treatment of metastatic PEN is controversial. There is no proven benefit of adjuvant chemotherapy or radiation after surgical resection of a primary PEN, and patients with regional lymph node metastases are generally observed, despite the relatively high risk of recurrence. If hepatic or other distant metastases are present, some oncologists believe that the timing and type of chemotherapy should depend upon the presence of symptoms (24). If a patient suffers from endocrinologic symptoms, a variety of options are available, including treatment of the primary symptom (e.g., proton pump inhibitors for gastrinomas) or ablation of the largest foci of metastatic disease using hepatic artery embolization, alcohol injection, or surgical resection. Treatment with the somatostatin analog octreotide can provide symptomatic relief. Some partial responses are achieved with chemotherapy such as 5-fluorouracil and streptozotocin (24). In highly selected patients, primary surgical resection of hepatic metastases may be associated with long-term survival, but some patients with metastatic PENs survive for many years without treatment.

Prognosis. The natural history of PENs is often unpredictable, like that of other well-differentiated endocrine neoplasms, although taken as a group, PENs are more aggressive than well-differentiated endocrine neoplasms of the tubular gastrointestinal tract (189a). Small PENs lacking adverse prognostic features (see below) can be cured by surgical resection. Many insulinomas fit this category, since they are generally less than 2 cm when detected. Since insulinomas comprise nearly half of functional PENs, the overall prognosis of patients with functional PENs is better than that for those with nonfunctional PENs. Most PENs other than insulinomas are larger at diagnosis, and the prognosis for these patients is less favorable (24). Approximately 50 to 80 percent of these neoplasms recur or metastasize (54,63,112,151,246), although sometimes only after many years. Thus, studies with short follow-up periods often underestimate the proportion of PENs that ultimately behave in a malignant fashion. The 5-year survival rate after surgical resection for nonfunctional PENs is 65 percent, and the 10-year rate is 45 percent (98). Up to 30 percent of patients with PENs already have metastases when first diagnosed, and the contribution of this group to the overall outcome of patients often is not considered in studies based on surgically resected cases. Functional PENs with mixed or "ectopic" syndromes are reportedly more aggressive (37,60).

Although PENs frequently recur or metastasize, many patients survive for several years or even decades following the appearance of metastases due to the slowly progressive nature of the neoplasm. PENs are not very sensitive to chemotherapy (24), and cure is generally not possible after the development of metastases.

Prognostic studies of PENs have attempted to identify absolute criteria for malignancy. Some PENs that behave aggressively have deceptively bland histologic features, so some authorities consider that only PENs with locally invasive growth, large vessel invasion, or distant metastases can be considered definitely malignant (226). PENs lacking these features are regarded as benign or having uncertain malignant potential, depending upon the size and mitotic rate of the neoplasm (27,226). However, some PENs lacking features of malignancy nonetheless metastasize and ultimately cause the death of the patient (98). The grading system advocated by Capella et al. (27) has been shown to have prognostic significance (94). Nonetheless, some PENs lacking features of malignancy metastasize and ultimately cause the death of the patient (98). The newest WHO grading system has avoided classifying PENs into benign and malignant categories, rather using a variety of prognostic factors to predict "benign behavior" or "malignant behavior" (91).

Although efforts to strictly classify PENs into prognostically distinct subgroups have had limited success, many studies agree on the features most predictive of recurrence or metastasis following surgical resection. Some authors now regard all clinically relevant PENs (i.e., those other than microadenomas) as malignant neoplasms (98), and this is the position we advocate. Features well recognized to have prognostic significance in PENs include tumor size, mitotic rate, presence of necrosis, extrapancreatic invasion,

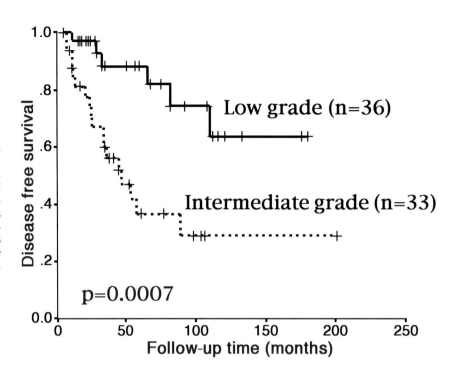

Figure 12-31

PATIENT SURVIVAL AFTER SURGICAL RESECTION

Disease-free survival is markedly different between patients with low-grade and intermediate-grade PENs, as defined by mitotic rate and necrosis. (Fig. 3 from Hochwald SN, Zee S, Conlon KC, et al. Prognostic factors in pancreatic endocrine neoplasms: an analysis of 136 cases with a proposal for low-grade and intermediate-grade groups. J Clin Oncol 2002;20:2638.)

and vascular invasion, in addition to the presence of nodal or distant metastases (91,98,118, 137,226). The grading of PENs based on the presence of necrosis or a mitotic rate of greater than or equal to 2 per 50 high-power fields (98) stratifies the neoplasms into low- and intermediate-grade categories that have highly significant differences in disease-free and disease-specific survival rates (fig. 12-31). Peptide production, as detected in the serum or by immunohistochemistry, is not a prognostic factor for nonfunctional PENs (98). Nuclear pleomorphism is also not a useful predictor (263), although some studies have demonstrated a correlation between overall nuclear grade and prognosis (98). Other factors reportedly predictive of more aggressive behavior include loss of progesterone receptor expression (192,250), aneuploidy (22,111), increased Ki-67 or PCNA labeling index (38,192), loss of heterozygosity (LOH) of chromosome 17p13 (86), LOH of chromosome 22q (256), increased fractional allelic loss (201), upregulated CD44 isoform expression (104,132), and immunohistochemical expression of CK19 (52).

Clinicopathologic Features of Functional Pancreatic Endocrine Neoplasms

As discussed previously, functional PENs are defined based primarily on their clinical features, with the associated hormonal syndromes serving to separate these neoplasms from nonfunctional PENs. Although some of the functional PENs have histologic features that are characteristic, none of the routine pathologic findings are sufficiently specific to recognize each functional PEN without knowledge of the clinical findings. Elevated serum peptide levels and immunohistochemical labeling for the specific peptides usually correlate well with the clinical syndromes in functional PENs, but identification of a predominant peptide cell type by immunohistochemistry does not necessarily imply that the PEN is functional (with the exception of pancreatic polypeptide in a PPoma). In the sections that follow, the clinical features of each type of functional PEN are described along with any specific pathologic and molecular findings that are characteristic of that type of neoplasm (Tables 12-2, 12-5).

Insulinoma

Definition. *Insulinoma* is a functionally active, well-differentiated PEN that produces clinical symptoms of hypoglycemia due to inappropriate secretion of insulin. PENs that demonstrate β-cell differentiation based on immunohistochemistry but are not associated with the clinical syndrome may be designated *β-cell neoplasms* but they are not considered insulinomas.

Table 12-5
FUNCTIONAL PANCREATIC ENDOCRINE NEOPLASMS

	M:F	Age Mean (Range)	Head (%)	Body (%)	Tail (%)
Insulinoma	1:1.4	46.7 (1-88)	30	29	41
Glucagonoma	1:1.4	52.5 (11-88)	26	22	52
Somatostatinoma	1:2	52.2 (25-84)	63	10	27
Gastrinoma	1.3:1	46.7 (7-85)	55	18	27
VIPoma[a]	1.1:1	49.2 (12-79)	23	19	47
PP-cell PEN[a]	1:1.4	51.3 (20-84)	37	15	48

[a]VIP = vasoactive intestinal polypeptide; PP = pancreatic polypeptide; PEN = pancreatic endocrine neoplasm.

Synonyms for insulinoma include *functional β-cell tumor* and *insulin-producing islet cell tumor*.

General Features. Insulinomas were among the first PENs recognized to cause a clinical syndrome due to excessive hormone secretion (89, 257). They are the most common functional PEN at 42 percent (130) and have an incidence of 2 to 4/million population/year, which becomes higher in patients with MEN1 (139,212). Approximately 4 to 6 percent of insulinomas arise in patients with MEN1 syndrome, and 10 to 30 percent of functional PENs in MEN1 patients are insulinomas (71,73,145,211,215). Insulinomas have also been reported in patients with neurofibromatosis. The majority of insulinomas, however, are sporadic. Almost all functioning insulinomas are primary in the pancreas, although some have been reported in the duodenum, ileum, jejunum, stomach, and elsewhere (2,113,127,191,213,217,262).

Clinical Features. Insulinomas occur at all ages but are most common between the ages of 40 and 60 years; 80 percent occur between the ages of 20 and 60 years (mean, 46.7 years) (71, 73,145,150,211,233). The majority arise in women (female to male ratio, 1.4 to 1). Insulinomas arise anywhere in the pancreas. Most are solitary, but multiple examples have been reported both in patients with or without MEN1.

The hyperinsulinemic hypoglycemia seen in patients with insulinomas is generally the first manifestation of the neoplasm, rather than the local effects of the pancreatic mass (130). Affected patients most commonly experience the central nervous system effects of hypoglycemia and the resulting catecholamine response. Visual changes (diplopia, blurred vision), confusion, amnesia,

and behavioral changes may occur, and some patients lose consciousness or have seizures. The secondary effects of catecholamine release include hunger, weakness, perspiration, nausea, palpitations, and anxiety; these symptoms, associated with a low blood glucose level, strongly suggest hypoglycemia. The classically described "Whipple triad" of insulinoma includes symptoms of hypoglycemia, low blood glucose levels (below 3.0 mmol/L), and relief of symptoms with administration of glucose (179,210,215,266).

Because of the early symptomatology, most insulinomas are detected while relatively small, and in fact, some are so small they are difficult to detect with conventional imaging. The size of the neoplasm has no relationship to the severity of the symptoms (130,133). Both endoscopic ultrasonography and CT scanning identify only about two thirds of cases; angiography finds up to three quarters. More recently, octreotide scintigraphy and positron emission tomography (PET) scanning have improved preoperative detection.

The serologic tests for insulinoma are highly sensitive in the face of suggestive clinical symptoms. Plasma insulin and proinsulin levels are elevated in relation to the blood glucose levels (130). A high insulin level following a period of fasting is also indicative of an insulinoma. In some cases, surgical exploration is justified based on the laboratory data, even if the location of the insulinoma cannot be determined preoperatively. Intraoperative ultrasonography is almost always successful in localizing the neoplasm if direct visualization and palpation fail (130).

Pathologic Findings. Most insulinomas are less than 2 cm in diameter, and many measure

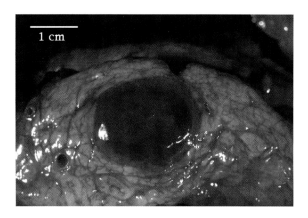

1 cm

Figure 12-32

INSULINOMA

The neoplasm is small, circumscribed, and homogeneous.

between 0.5 and 1.0 cm (133); only 25 percent are larger than 2 cm, although cases in excess of 10 cm have been documented (225). It is also unusual for insulin-producing PENs smaller than 0.5 cm (microadenomas) to be clinically functional even in patients with MEN1. On cut section, insulinomas are usually red to brown, well circumscribed, and soft (fig. 12-32). Necrosis is uncommon.

Histologically, most insulinomas resemble other small PENs. They are circumscribed but not encapsulated; large insulinomas may have a fibrotic pseudocapsule. Extension of nests of neoplastic cells into the adjacent pancreatic parenchyma should not be taken as evidence of aggressive behavior. The most common architectural patterns are solid (nested), trabecular, and acinar (fig. 12-33, left); some insulinomas have a pronounced microglandular pattern. Larger insulinomas are more likely to display multiple patterns. Stromal hyalinization may occur, as may amyloid deposition, a characteristic if uncommon feature. Stromal amyloid consists of islet amyloid polypeptide (IAPP) or amylin (258).

The cytologic features of insulinomas are not distinctive, although they are less likely than other PENs to show nuclear pleomorphism. Sometimes calcifications, including psammoma bodies, are present.

Most insulinomas label intensely for insulin and proinsulin (fig. 12-33, right) (133,203,204). The intensity of immunolabeling does not, however, correlate with the severity of the clini-

cal syndrome. Interestingly, some insulinomas display only focal positivity for chromogranin (despite uniform immunolabeling for synaptophysin), perhaps reflecting the fact that non-neoplastic β cells also label less intensely for chromogranin than the other islet cell types.

Classic ultrastructural studies defined several different types of neurosecretory granules in insulinomas, some of which resemble the granules in non-neoplastic β cells (fig. 12-34) (15,43, 46,133,203,204,238). Many cases have multiple different types of granules in the same neoplasm, and electron microscopy is no longer used to subclassify insulinomas.

Treatment and Prognosis. The treatment of choice for symptomatic patients is surgical resection. Because of their generally small size and lack of mitotic activity and necrosis, most insulinomas are extremely indolent and can be cured by simple enucleation. Malignant behavior only occurs in approximately 10 percent of insulinomas (130,225,226), usually in those uncommon examples measuring more than 2 cm. In addition to size, the presence of gross local invasion or vascular invasion, an elevated proliferative rate (more than 2 to 10 mitoses per 50 high-power fields), and necrosis are considered adverse prognostic factors (98). Of course, lymph node or distant metastases portend a poor outcome. Like other PENs, relatively long-term survival in the presence of distant metastases may occur if the endocrinologic syndrome can be controlled. Chromosomal losses at 3p, 3q, and 6q and gains at 17p, 17q, and 20q are more commonly detected in insulinomas with malignant behavior (229).

It may be reasonable to perform a more extended resection for large insulinomas, despite the overall favorable prognosis associated with the group as a whole. In MEN1 patients with insulinomas, there may be several macroscopically visible endocrine neoplasms at surgery, and it is often impossible to determine intraoperatively which lesion is the functional PEN. Since it is rare for insulinomas to be less than 0.5 cm, enucleation of the larger neoplasms is likely to include the functional insulinoma.

Discussion. It has long been held that most insulinomas are benign. It is true that most are small and can be cured by relatively conservative surgery. It is also true that smaller PENs have

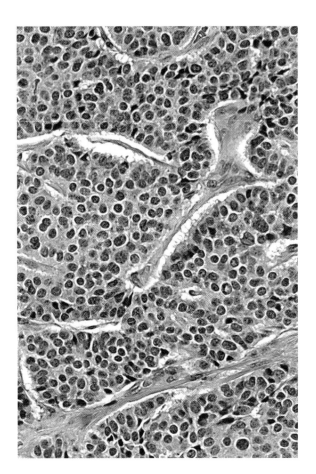
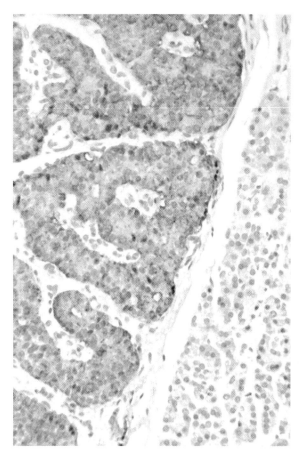

Figure 12-33

INSULINOMA

Uniform cells are arranged in nests (left), and immunolabeling for insulin shows diffuse positivity (right).

fewer genetic abnormalities and probably therefore represent "less malignant" neoplasms than large PENs with more accumulated genetic alterations (264). Nevertheless, it remains to be proven that, independent of tumor size, patients with insulinomas have a better prognosis than those with other PENs. In addition to their small size, most insulinomas have few mitoses and no necrosis and fall into the low-grade category (98). Whether an insulinoma, left untreated, would evolve into a larger and more aggressive PEN is a matter for speculation. We prefer not to designate them as benign neoplasms but rather recommend enumerating their prognostic features in the same manner as other PENs; in most cases, this will place the insulinoma into a very low-risk category.

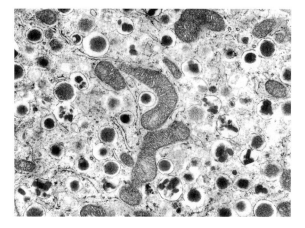

Figure 12-34

INSULINOMA

Some of the neurosecretory granules have a crystalline core, similar to the granules of normal β cells.

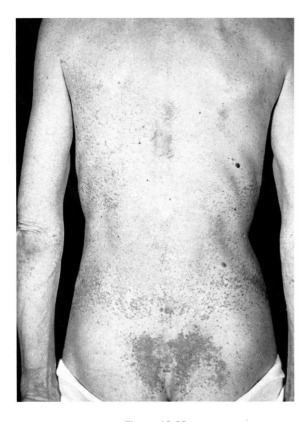

Figure 12-35

GLUCAGONOMA

Necrolytic migratory erythema. (Fig. 5-23 from Fascicle 20, Third Series.)

Glucagonoma

Definition. *Glucagonoma* is a functionally active, well-differentiated PEN that is associated with the clinical manifestations of inappropriate secretion of glucagon, i.e., rash, stomatitis, diabetes, and weight loss (*glucagonoma syndrome*). PENs that demonstrate α-cell differentiation based on immunohistochemical labeling but are not associated with the clinical syndrome are designated α-cell neoplasms but they are not considered glucagonomas.

Clinical Features. Glucagonomas make up 8 to 13 percent of functional PENs and 5 percent of all PENs (excluding microadenomas) (226). The incidence of the glucagonoma syndrome is roughly 1/20 million/year (196). Most patients are adults between the ages of 40 and 70 years; females are more commonly affected. Only rarely are glucagonomas associated with the MEN1 syndrome. Most glucagonomas oc-

cur sporadically, and almost all arise in the pancreas (202,205).

The characteristic rash, necrolytic migratory erythema, begins centrally, often in the groin, and progresses to involve the trunk and extremities (fig. 12-35) (95,158,196). About two thirds of patients present with this rash, along with symptoms of stomatitis, cheilitis, alopecia, vulvovaginitis, and urethritis. The cause of the rash is poorly understood. Possible etiologies include the direct effect of glucagon on the skin, prostaglandin release, and deficiency of amino acids, free fatty acids, or zinc (125). Other findings of the glucagonoma syndrome include glucose intolerance; diabetes mellitus (50 percent); weight loss (65 percent), which may be marked; normochromic, normocytic anemia (33 percent); diarrhea (20 percent); and psychiatric disturbances (5,18,196). Patients also appear to have an increased risk of deep vein thrombosis.

If symptoms of the glucagonoma syndrome are suspected, the diagnosis is supported by an elevated fasting serum glucagon level and a pancreatic mass (125). In most patients, a marked elevation of the level of serum glucagon (10 to 20 times normal) is found; in patients with a borderline elevation, tolbutamide or arginine stimulation tests can be used (125). Gastrin levels may also be elevated in 20 percent of patients. Since most glucagonomas are large, imaging tests, such as CT scans, are usually effective in confirming the presence of a pancreatic mass. Octreotide scans are helpful as well.

Pathologic Findings. Most glucagonomas occur in the tail of the pancreas. On average, these neoplasms are large (7 to 8 cm), and one example measured 35 cm (205,226). They are usually red to brown and soft in consistency; cystic changes or hemorrhage may occur.

The microscopic patterns are not specific to this functional type, with solid, nesting, and trabecular architectural patterns predominating (fig. 12-36) (21). As with other large PENs, a heterogeneous appearance often results from regions with varying architecture. Some reports suggest that glucagonomas have more abundant cytoplasm. Foci of necrosis may be found, and the mitotic rate is variable, usually 2 to 10 mitoses per 50 high-power fields, but sometimes more.

Glucagon may be immunohistochemically detectable, but less consistently and intensely than other hormones in their corresponding functional PEN types (21,87,205). Reactivity for proglucagon-derived peptide fragments (glycentin, glucagon-like peptides 1 and 2) has been reported, but antibodies against these proteins are not in general use. Electron microscopy sometimes reveals the characteristic neurosecretory granules of α cells, with their eccentrically dense cores, but most glucagonomas have rather nonspecific granules (21).

Treatment and Prognosis. The treatment of glucagonomas depends upon the stage of the neoplasm. For glucagonomas limited to the pancreas, surgical resection is indicated; however, more than half have already metastasized when detected. Endocrine symptoms can be controlled in some patients with somatostatin analogs. In the case of symptomatic hepatic metastases, surgical debulking has been employed to treat the hormonal symptoms, but this probably does not increase the disease-specific survival rate. Local therapies, such as embolization or cryotherapy, may prove equally effective. Up to 75 percent of glucagonomas are ultimately fatal (95,196,205), and cure is exceptional after metastases develop. As with other PENs, however, patients may survive for many years following the development of metastases if the hormonal symptoms are controlled.

Somatostatinoma

Definition. A pancreatic *somatostatinoma* is a functionally active, well-differentiated PEN associated with the clinical manifestations of inappropriate secretion of somatostatin, which include diabetes mellitus, hypochlorhydria, cholelithiasis, diarrhea or steatorrhea, anemia, and weight loss (*somatostatinoma syndrome*). PENs that demonstrate δ-cell differentiation based on immunohistochemical labeling but are not associated with the clinical syndrome may be designated δ-cell neoplasms but they are not considered somatostatinomas.

General Features. True pancreatic somatostatinomas are very rare, representing no more than 2 percent of PENs (48). In fact, much attention has been devoted in the literature to another somatostatinoma, the psammomatous somatostatinoma or, more appropriately, the "glandular duodenal carcinoid" of the periampullary duodenum (83). These histologically

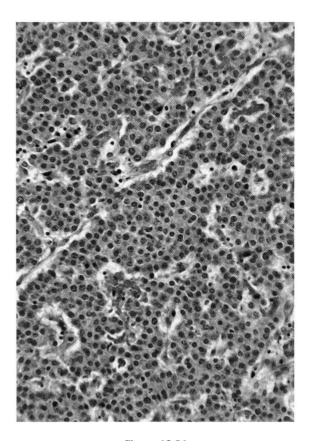

Figure 12-36

GLUCAGONOMA

Nesting and trabecular patterns are present.

distinctive gland-forming endocrine neoplasms with frequent psammoma body formation may express somatostatin immunohistochemically, but they almost never produce the somatostatinoma syndrome. Although duodenal somatostatinomas have some very interesting associations, such as with neurofibromatosis, they do not appear to be related to pancreatic somatostatinomas (other than that both are well-differentiated endocrine neoplasms).

Clinical Features. Pancreatic somatostatinomas occur more commonly in females and affect middle-aged to older individuals (35 to 60 years) (49,223,251). The clinical findings indicative of excess somatostatin secretion are not as dramatic or distinctive as the features of other functional PENs, and most patients are not symptomatic unless the serum levels of somatostatin are markedly elevated. Somatostatinomas are accompanied by diabetes mellitus of

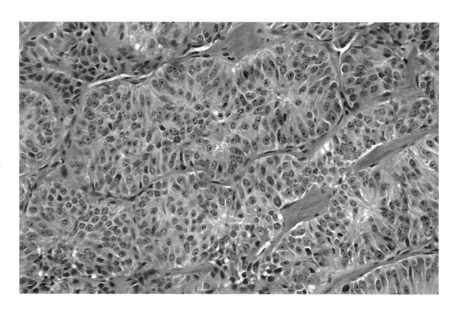

Figure 12-37

PANCREATIC SOMATOSTATINOMA

The nesting architecture is not specific for pancreatic somatostatinomas, in contrast to the glandular pattern typical of somatostatinomas of the duodenum.

new onset, hypochlorhydria, gallbladder dysmotility and cholelithiasis, diarrhea with steatorrhea, anemia, and weight loss (135). Often, only some of these manifestations occur, and their nonspecific nature may cause a delay in diagnosis by suggesting other primary disorders of the intestines, gallbladder, or endocrine pancreas. The common etiology of the symptoms is related to the inhibitory effects of somatostatin on the other endocrine cells of the gastroenterohepatic axis (48). If a somatostatinoma is considered, the diagnosis can be confirmed by documenting the marked serum elevations of somatostatin that accompany the symptoms.

Pathologic Findings. Somatostatinomas appear to be more common in the head of the pancreas. Most measure 5 to 6 cm. They are not grossly distinguishable from other PENs.

Although gland formation and psammomatous calcifications are typical of duodenal somatostatin-producing endocrine neoplasms, pancreatic somatostatinomas are not as histologically distinctive (fig. 12-37). Most have the typical patterns of other PENs, with a solid or nesting architecture, uniform nuclei, and moderate amounts of amphophilic cytoplasm.

By immunohistochemistry, synaptophysin and somatostatin are strongly expressed, although immunolabeling for chromogranin is inconsistent (48). Ultrastructurally, somatostatinomas may contain relatively large (250 to 450 nm), homogeneous neurosecretory granules that resemble the zymogen granules of acinar neo-

plasms. In addition, a population of smaller granules with denser cores is generally present.

Prognosis. Approximately half of the patients with somatostatinomas are dead 10 years after diagnosis (223). Extreme morbidity is usually not associated with the hormonal symptoms.

Gastrinoma

Definition. Pancreatic *gastrinoma* is a functionally active, well-differentiated PEN that produces the manifestations of inappropriate secretion of gastrin such as duodenal ulceration (Zollinger-Ellison syndrome). PENs that demonstrate G-cell differentiation based on immunohistochemical labeling but are not associated with the clinical syndrome may be designated G-cell neoplasms but they are not considered gastrinomas.

General Features. PENs were first associated with ulcer disease by Zollinger and Ellison in 1955 (268), and gastrin was isolated from a pancreatic gastrinoma by Gregory in 1960 (80). After insulinomas, gastrinomas are the most frequently encountered functional PEN, and gastrinomas are the most common type of functional pancreatoduodenal endocrine neoplasm in patients with the MEN1 syndrome (144). Approximately 20 percent of gastrinomas occur in patients with the MEN1 syndrome, and 20 to 60 percent of patients with MEN1 develop gastrinomas (58,59).

The gastrinomas are not always located within the pancreas, however, and a significant proportion are primary in the duodenum (179). Other possible sites include the stomach, jejunum, and bile ducts, as well as exotic sites like the liver, kidney, and heart (6,72,141,159,176,230, 242). Early data suggested that 53 percent of gastrinomas were pancreatic, but with advances in imaging and diagnosis, only 24 percent are now felt to be pancreatic, or even less (14 percent) in the case of sporadic gastrinomas (178). The duodenum is now regarded to be the most common site (178). Some gastrinomas are found only in the lymph nodes around the head of the pancreas or common bile duct (16,50,259). The concept of a primary nodal endocrine neoplasm has been suggested, supported by the finding of rare endocrine cells in normal lymph nodes from the region (92) as well as the apparent cure of patients with nodal gastrinomas by simple lymphadenectomy (4, 177); however, the alternative possibility of nodal metastases from an occult duodenal primary may account for some of these cases. Duodenal gastrinomas are often smaller (62 percent measure less than 1 cm [267]), than those in the pancreas, which are usually over 2 cm. Since small gastrinomas may still be highly functional, the search for the primary neoplasm is often difficult. Almost all gastrinomas arise within the region encompassed by the head of the pancreas, duodenum, and regional lymph nodes (the so-called gastrinoma triangle), so blind pancreatoduodenectomy has been performed to treat occult gastrinomas.

Clinical Features. Gastrinomas occur at all ages but are most common between the ages of 40 and 50 years (224). Males are more often affected (male to female ratio, 1.3 to 1). Gastrinomas may arise anywhere in the pancreas but are most common in the head of the gland (58,230). Most are solitary; multiple PENs may occur in patients with MEN1, but generally only one is the functional gastrinoma.

Most patients with gastrinomas present with duodenal ulcers and symptoms thereof, usually severe abdominal pain (131,174a). Gastroesophageal reflux also occurs. Approximately 20 percent have no ulcer disease and present with diarrhea due to malabsorption secondary to the inactivation of pancreatic enzymes by the high duodenal acid content (131). Rarely, patients present with symptoms related to the location of the neoplasm, such as jaundice or an enlarg-

ing abdominal mass. Earlier diagnosis and more effective acid inhibition therapy have reduced the once common complications of severe ulcer disease such as perforation or hemorrhage.

A diagnosis of gastrinoma can be made by demonstrating a serum gastrin level over 1,000 pg/mL (normal, less than 100 pg/mL) in the face of a gastric pH of less than 2.5 (131). Nearly half of gastrinoma patients, however, have gastrin levels of less than 500 pg/mL. Thus, the secretin stimulation test is used as a further diagnostic aid. Gastrinomas can be localized using CT and MRI scans, but the small size of many duodenal primaries renders these tests insensitive. Endoscopic ultrasound, octreotide scintigraphy, and PET scanning are the most sensitive diagnostic tests.

An interesting endocrine proliferative syndrome occurs in the stomach of patients with gastrinomas, especially in the setting of MEN1 (19). Chronically elevated serum gastrin levels cause hyperplasia and then neoplasia of the enterochromaffin-like (ECL) cells in the gastric fundus. Thus, carcinoid tumors of the stomach may develop (so-called type 2 gastric carcinoids). Removal of the gastrinoma can induce regression of the hyperplasia and some of the early carcinoid tumors in the stomach. Gastric endocrine proliferations and neoplasms are the result of hypergastrinemia from any source (e.g., pernicious anemia or advanced chronic atrophic gastritis), so their presence does not always signify a gastrinoma.

Pathologic Findings. Pancreatic gastrinomas resemble other types of PENs, both grossly and microscopically. They are usually over 2 cm, are circumscribed and tan to red, and have a variable consistency. Microscopic patterns include solid and trabecular formations (fig. 12-38), and a prevalent glandular architecture also has been described (82). The nuclear features are bland and mitoses are infrequent.

By immunohistochemistry, general endocrine markers are expressed consistently. Gastrin immunolabeling is usually present but may not be diffuse. Some cases fail to label with antibodies to gastrin, presumably due to modification of the antigenic site on the gastrin molecules or because of rapid secretion (131). Gastrin mRNA has been detected by in situ hybridization in such cases. Electron microscopy

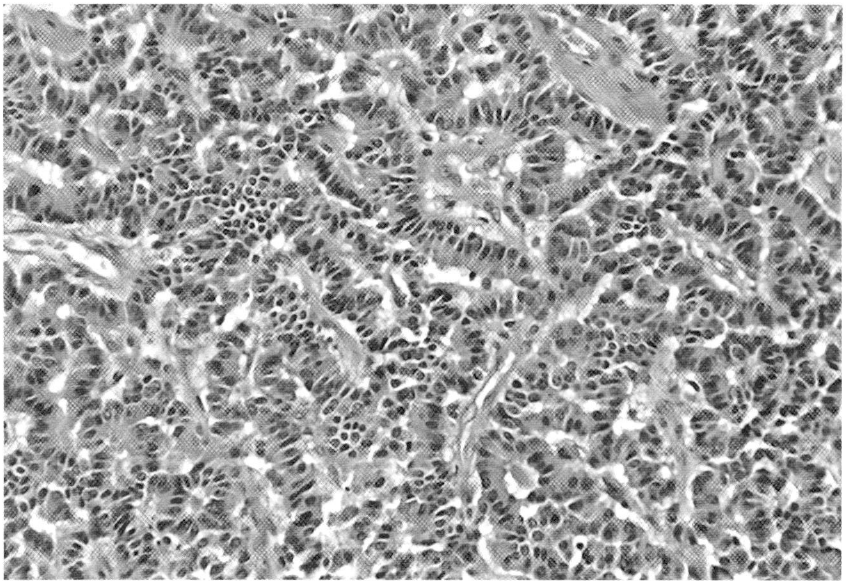

Figure 12-38

PANCREATIC GASTRINOMA

The trabecular architecture is a common, if nonspecific, finding.

reveals neurosecretory granules without specific distinguishing features (44).

Treatment and Prognosis. Gastrinomas are treated by resection when limited to the pancreas and regional lymph nodes. Surgical debulking of metastatic disease to control the ulcerogenic syndrome is generally no longer necessary due to improvements in the medical suppression of acid secretion.

The majority of pancreatic gastrinomas (60 to 70 percent) display malignant behavior, with metastases to regional lymph nodes and liver (131,162). In contrast, duodenal gastrinomas have a lower rate of malignant behavior (38 percent) (50,231). Gastrinomas in patients with MEN1 are clinically less aggressive, perhaps due to earlier detection (72).

Patients with metastases limited to regional lymph nodes have a relatively favorable long-term survival rate, and it has been suggested that nodal involvement may not be an adverse prognostic factor (50). Those with hepatic metastases have a significantly worse prognosis. Some authorities have divided gastrinomas into aggressive and nonaggressive varieties based on the growth rate of their hepatic metastases (72), although no histologic correlations have been made with these subsets. The overall 5-year survival rate for patients with pancreatic gastrinomas is approximately 65 percent and the 10-year rate is 51 percent, so slow progression is typical (106).

VIPoma

Definition. A pancreatic *VIPoma* is a functionally active, well-differentiated PEN that produces the clinical symptoms associated with inappropriate secretion of vasoactive intestinal polypeptide (VIP), i.e., watery diarrhea associated with hypokalemia and achlorhydria (*WDHA, pancreatic cholera,* or *Verner-Morrison syndrome*). Symptomatic VIP production occurs in two different families of neoplasms: epithelial neoplasms like PENs and neurogenic neoplasms (128,174b,226); both types of VIPomas can produce the WDHA syndrome, although the pathologic and biologic features of these different families of neoplasms are quite different. PENs that produce VIP, as assessed by immunohistochemistry, but are not associated with the clinical syndrome, are not considered to be VIPomas. Synonyms include *diarrheagenic tumor of the pancreas* and *islet cell tumor with watery diarrhea*.

General Features. Verner and Morrison first described the association of watery diarrhea and hypokalemia with a PEN in 1958 (249). VIPomas constitute 3 to 8 percent of all PENs and about 10 percent of functional PENs (123). Rarely, VIPomas occur in patients with the MEN1 syndrome (103,183). There is no association with von Hippel-Lindau syndrome or neurofibromatosis. VIP-producing neurogenic neoplasms have also been designated VIPomas;

these include ganglioneuromas, ganglioneuro-blastomas, neuroblastomas, and paragangliomas that usually arise in the retroperitoneum or mediastinum (128,226), especially in children (109,153). Rarely, extrapancreatic well-differentiated endocrine (i.e., epithelial) neoplasms produce VIP, and these extrapancreatic VIPomas may be found in the esophagus (253), small bowel (29), kidney, and other sites. Pancreatic VIPomas constitute 80 percent of the functional VIP-producing neoplasms; most of the remainder are neurogenic neoplasms.

Although VIP can be detected in neurons within the pancreas, it is not normally expressed in islet cells. Thus, it is unclear why the pancreas should be the predominant site for epithelial VIPomas. It is also interesting that neurogenic neoplasms producing VIP do not arise within the pancreas.

Clinical Features. Pancreatic VIPomas occur at all ages but are most common between the ages of 40 and 50 years (mean, 49.2 years) (29, 168,174b,224). More VIPomas occur in the tail of the pancreas (47 percent) than in the head (23 percent) or body (19 percent) (29,123,183,224).

The WDHA syndrome is the defining feature of VIPomas and includes watery diarrhea, hypokalemia, and achlorhydria (or hypochlorhydria) (167,248). Other substances produced by the neoplasm, such as peptide histidine methionine, PP, and neurotensin, may also contribute to the symptoms (146). Most patients present with profuse secretory diarrhea in amounts ranging from 0.5 to 6.0 L per day. The resulting loss of potassium and bicarbonate leads to dehydration and metabolic acidosis. Some patients also have hypercalcemia, hyperglycemia, and flushing. Loss of magnesium leads to tetany on rare occasion (103,134).

In patients with suggestive symptomatology, a diagnosis of VIPoma is established by demonstrating a serum VIP level over 60 pmol/L (146). VIP is sensitive to proteolysis, however, and false negative blood tests occur. An elevated serum peptide histidine methionine level supports the diagnosis. Pancreatic VIPomas can be localized using CT and MRI scans, octreotide scintigraphy, and PET scans (174b).

Pathologic Findings. Pancreatic VIPomas resemble other types of PENs grossly and microscopically. They are usually solitary and are

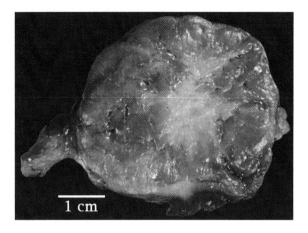

Figure 12-39

VIPOMA

The 4.5-cm neoplasm is tan and lobulated, with a central scar.

larger than 2 cm (mean, 4.5 cm). VIPomas are circumscribed and red-tan or yellow, and may have fibrous septa, cystic changes, or calcifications (fig. 12-39). The histologic patterns include solid, acinar, gyriform, and trabecular, the most common (fig. 12-40, left). The cells have modest amounts of cytoplasm and bland nuclei without prominent nucleoli, and most examples have few mitoses.

By immunohistochemistry, general endocrine markers are expressed. Immunolabeling for VIP is present in nearly 90 percent of neoplasms (fig. 12-40, right). Many VIPomas (53 percent) also express PP, and studies have also identified peptide histidine methionine, growth hormone-releasing hormone, and human chorionic gonadotrophin (29,183,226,227); these peptides are not generally useful diagnostically. Electron microscopy reveals neurosecretory granules without specific distinguishing features.

Treatment and Prognosis. Most pancreatic VIPomas demonstrate malignant behavior, and more than half of patients have liver metastases at presentation (174b,226). Lymph node metastases are less common. Like other PENs, VIPomas with metastases progress slowly but inexorably, and despite a reported 60 percent 5-year survival rate (226), most patients ultimately die of their disease. Some VIPomas that are resected prior to the development of metastases can be cured surgically. The WDHA syndrome causes morbidity and mortality in patients with VIPomas.

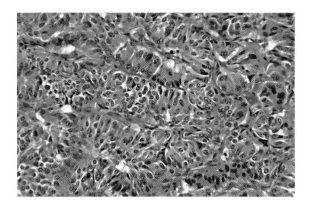 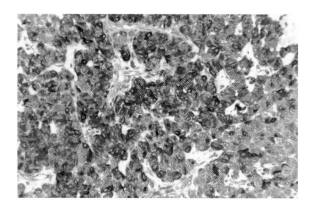

Figure 12-40

VIPOMA

Left: Trabecular architecture with variably sized nuclei.
Right: Immunolabeling for vasoactive intestinal polypeptide (VIP).

Pancreatic Polypeptide-Cell Pancreatic Endocrine Neoplasm

Definition. The *PP-cell PEN*, or *PPoma*, is a well-differentiated PEN measuring at least 0.5 cm that produces predominantly PP, as assessed by immunohistochemistry or by measurement of elevated levels in the serum.

General Features. In contrast to all other hormonally designated types of PENs, PP-cell neoplasms are not associated with specific endocrinologic symptoms. Thus, PP-cell neoplasms are technically nonfunctional PENs and some classification systems do not recognize them separately (91). It is possible that some of the symptoms experienced by patients with PP-producing PENs (see below) may be referable to elevated levels of PP. It is relatively common to detect focal immunoreactivity for PP (in addition to other hormones) in nonfunctional PENs; in order for such a neoplasm to qualify as a PP-cell PEN, there should be predominant PP immunolabeling (i.e., in more than half of the neoplastic cells) and, ideally, there should be an associated elevation in the serum PP levels. Diffuse PP positivity is not uncommon in endocrine microadenomas; thus, the definition of PP-cell PEN is specifically restricted to larger PENs. MEN1 syndrome is present in 18 to 44 percent of patients with PP-cell PENs (243).

Clinical Features. PP-cell PENs occur at all ages but are most common between the ages of 50 and 60 years (mean, 51.3 years). There is a slight female predominance (222).

Patients generally do not have symptoms referable to the elevated levels of PP in the serum (243). Thus, the presenting symptoms are those of other nonfunctional PENs, such as abdominal pain and nausea. Some patients have the watery diarrhea, hypokalemia, and achlorhydria (WDHA) syndrome usually associated with VIPomas (142), but there is no specific evidence that the symptoms are caused by the secretion of PP. Since some VIPomas secrete PP as well as other bioactive substances (such as prostaglandins), and VIP is relatively sensitive to proteolysis during serum assays, it is possible that something other than PP is responsible for the diarrhea in these patients. In fact, PP-cell PENs with massive serum levels of PP have been described in patients without any endocrinologic symptoms.

The clinical diagnosis of a PP-cell PEN is complicated by the fact that other types of PENs also secrete PP into the blood, so the finding of elevated PP levels does not preclude the possibility of another functional or nonfunctional PEN. In fact, plasma PP levels have been used in MEN1 syndrome patients to predict the presence of a PEN (70), most of which are not PP-cell neoplasms.

Pathologic Findings. The pathologic features of PP-cell PEN are not specific and resemble those of other nonfunctional PENs (fig. 12-41, left). PP-cell PENs vary in size from 0.7 to 15.0 cm (mean, 6.2 cm), and are more common in the tail of the pancreas. These neoplasms are generally defined immunohistochemically by the expression of PP in more than half of the

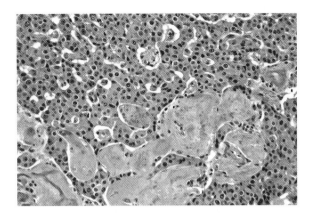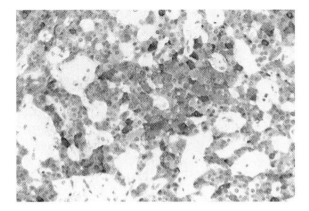

Figure 12-41

PANCREATIC POLYPEPTIDE–CELL PANCREATIC ENDOCRINE NEOPLASM

Left: The histologic appearance is nonspecific, with hyalinized stroma and a trabecular architecture.
Right: Immunolabeling for pancreatic polypeptide (PP) shows positivity in the majority of the neoplastic cells.

neoplastic cells (fig. 12-41, right). Other hormones may also be expressed in fewer cells.

Treatment and Prognosis. The biologic behavior of reported PP-cell PENs has been variable. Microadenomas producing PP are considered benign (and do not technically qualify as PP-cell PENs). PP-cell neoplasms less than 2 cm are generally curable surgically. Larger examples are more prone to metastasize, and the mean size of cases with metastases in a review by Tomita et al. (243) was 8.1 cm, compared with 4.3 cm for those without metastases. Overall metastases are reported in 44 percent of cases.

Serotonin-Secreting Pancreatic Endocrine Neoplasm

Definition. The *serotonin-secreting PEN* is a rare, well-differentiated PEN associated with significant serotonin production by the neoplastic cells and elevations in serum 5-hydroxytryptamine (5-HT) levels or urinary 5-hydroxyindole acetic acid (5-HIAA) levels (188,221a). Patients may develop the carcinoid syndrome of flushing, diarrhea, and bronchoconstriction, usually only after the neoplasm metastasizes to the liver. A synonym is *pancreatic carcinoid tumor*.

General Features. PENs associated with the carcinoid syndrome are rare (57,161,186,255). Like other functional PENs, serotonin-secreting PENs should produce symptoms of the carcinoid syndrome to be so designated. As in carcinoids of the tubular gastrointestinal tract, however, the 5-HT produced by pancreatic se-

rotonin-secreting neoplasms is usually neutralized as the portal blood passes through the liver, and patients do not develop the classic symptoms of the carcinoid syndrome until liver metastases develop. It is possible that if the tumors are resected before the development of liver metastases, some serotonin-secreting PENs are unrecognized and classified as nonfunctional PENs, and thus, the prevalence of these neoplasms is unknown. Serotonin-secreting PENs have not been described in patients with MEN1 or von Hippel-Lindau syndrome.

Clinical Features. The carcinoid syndrome associated with serotonin-secreting PENs is the same as that associated with carcinoid tumors of other organs, characterized by flushing, bronchoconstriction, and diarrhea (188). The diagnosis is further supported by demonstration of elevations in serum 5-HT and urinary 5-HIAA levels. The symptoms are also related to the liberation of other substances, such as kallikreins, substance P, prostaglandins, and other tachykinins (188). Confirmation that the carcinoid syndrome is due to a pancreatic neoplasm can be achieved by demonstrating an endocrine neoplasm in the pancreas in the absence of involvement of organs more commonly associated with carcinoid tumors, such as the lung and intestines. Octreotide scintigraphy is particularly helpful for identifying occult foci of disease not detected by CT or MRI.

Pathologic Findings. The gross and histologic features of serotonin-secreting PENs resemble those of other PENs; the typical features of classic small intestinal carcinoid tumors are not usually noted. Immunolabeling for serotonin is found in most cases (188); other hormones may also be detected. Since serotonin may be detected in some cells in PENs unassociated with the carcinoid syndrome (66), and because it is not commonly assayed for, the true frequency of this neoplasm may be higher than reports would suggest.

Differential Diagnosis. Most endocrine neoplasms associated with the carcinoid syndrome are carcinoid tumors of the midgut or lung, so the determination that an endocrine neoplasm metastatic in the liver is a serotonin-secreting PEN requires excluding a small bowel or lung primary. Most pathologic specimens from liver metastases consist of core biopsies or fine needle aspiration cytology specimens, and detailed architectural features may be hard to demonstrate. Histologically, the presence of classic carcinoid features such as tight, sharply defined cell nests, abundant lumen formation, monotonous cytology with coarsely clumped chromatin, and basally polarized eosinophilic cytoplasmic microgranularity, suggest origin in the midgut, although all such features can occur in PENs as well. Correlation with imaging findings (octreotide scintigraphy in particular) is recommended to identify the primary site.

Treatment and Prognosis. Since serotonin-secreting PENs are only definable in patients with hepatic metastases, the prognosis is ultimately poor, although patients may survive for many years. Somatostatin analogs may help alleviate the symptoms of the carcinoid syndrome.

Pancreatic Endocrine Neoplasms Producing Other Ectopic Syndromes

Rare well-differentiated PENs occur that secrete other ectopic hormones and produce the related endocrinologic syndromes. Symptomatic secretion of adrenal corticotropic hormone (ACTH), parathyroid hormone (PTH), growth hormone (GH), calcitonin, and others has been described (51a,187,226). Of these, the most common is the *ACTH-secreting PEN*; pancreatic primaries account for 10 percent of ectopic (i.e., nonpituitary, nonadrenal) Cushing's syndrome cases (187). Affected patients develop some or all of the symptoms of Cushing's syndrome (37,60), such

as muscle wasting, truncal obesity, abdominal striae, and hypertension. Relatively rapid onset of symptoms has been described for pancreatic ACTH-producing neoplasms, compared with those of the pituitary. *Growth hormone–producing PENs* cause acromegaly (65,207), *calcitonin-producing PENs* cause diarrhea, and *parathyroid hormone–producing PENs* cause hypercalcemia (8). Some ectopic hormone-producing PENs occur in patients with MEN1 (56,235).

The gross and microscopic feature of these functional PENs are not distinctive. Immunolabeling for the associated hormones can generally be found in varying numbers of neoplastic cells, and other hormones may also be detected. The ultimate prognosis of patients with these PENs is poor.

Pancreatic Endocrine Neoplasms Producing Mixed Syndromes

Rare functional PENs produce symptoms related to the overproduction of more than one hormone. The different syndromes may appear synchronously or metachronously. Many of these multihormonal PENs are rare enough to be documented only in single case reports. Examples include insulinoma syndrome with glucagonoma syndrome (182), glucagonoma syndrome with Zollinger-Ellison syndrome (260), carcinoid syndrome with hypoglycemia (244), hypercalcemia with Zollinger-Ellison syndrome (45), and Cushing's syndrome with Zollinger-Ellison syndrome (37,160). Sometimes the second syndrome appears following chemotherapy; this phenomenon has been reported to occur in as many as 7 percent of functional PENs (260). The coexpression of Cushing's and Zollinger-Ellison syndromes occurs in 5 percent of patients with Zollinger-Ellison syndrome and 14 percent of patients with Cushing's syndrome due to pancreatic primaries (37,160).

Almost all PENs with mixed syndromes demonstrate malignant behavior. The mean survival period after the appearance of the second hormonal syndrome is only 5 to 7 months (226). Many PENs (both functional and nonfunctional) immunolabel for multiple hormones; the aggressive multihormonal PENs discussed here include only those associated with multiple clinical hormonal syndromes, independent of the immunohistochemical findings.

POORLY DIFFERENTIATED ENDOCRINE CARCINOMA

Definition. *Poorly differentiated endocrine carcinomas* of the pancreas are clinically aggressive, poorly differentiated carcinomas with morphologic features suggesting endocrine differentiation, a high proliferative rate (more than 10 mitoses per 10 high-power fields) or abundant necrosis, and, for those lacking the characteristic cytologic features of small cell carcinoma, immunohistochemical labeling for endocrine markers. The category of poorly differentiated endocrine carcinoma includes two well-defined entities: *small cell carcinoma* and *large cell endocrine carcinoma*. Alternative terminology includes *high-grade neuroendocrine carcinoma*.

General Features. Poorly differentiated endocrine carcinomas constitute a rare and rather poorly characterized group of neoplasms in the pancreas. At most, they constitute 2 to 3 percent of all PENs (226). Some examples have the typical pathologic features of small cell carcinomas (15a,35,180,200) and have been designated as such in the literature. Other poorly differentiated endocrine carcinomas are composed of larger cells with more abundant cytoplasm, and these resemble large cell neuroendocrine carcinomas of the lung and other sites. Due to the rarity of poorly differentiated endocrine carcinomas in the pancreas, the possibility of a metastasis from the lung or direct extension from a contiguous site (e.g., the ampulla of Vater, where poorly differentiated endocrine carcinomas are more common [172]) must always be considered. Although it is possible that with disease progression, conventional PENs may transform genetically into more aggressive neoplasms, there is no evidence that most poorly differentiated endocrine carcinomas of the pancreas arise from well-differentiated PENs. In fact, some poorly differentiated endocrine carcinomas arise in association with conventional ductal adenocarcinomas. The genetic features of pancreatic poorly differentiated endocrine carcinomas have not been studied, but by analogy with similar neoplasms of other organs, it is likely that they are more closely related to ductal adenocarcinomas than to well-differentiated PENs.

Clinical Features. Poorly differentiated endocrine carcinomas usually arise in adults, and the mean age is similar to that for ductal adeno-

carcinoma (20). There is a male predominance (200). Some patients have associated paraneoplastic syndromes including Cushing's syndrome (41), hypercalcemia (97), and carcinoid syndrome (76). Most patients present with symptoms similar to those of ductal adenocarcinomas, including back pain, cachexia, and jaundice. In contrast to well-differentiated PENs, poorly differentiated endocrine carcinomas are highly aggressive, with early dissemination and a rapidly fatal course (15a). All patients have died, usually within a few months of diagnosis, despite initial favorable response to chemotherapy. For patients presenting with metastatic disease, it is particularly difficult to confirm the pancreas as the site of origin of the carcinoma, since the lung is often involved and constitutes a much more common primary location.

Pathologic Findings. Grossly, poorly differentiated endocrine carcinomas are solid, white to tan tumors with a variable consistency, ill-defined borders, and areas of necrosis. They are divided into small cell and large cells types. The small cell type (small cell carcinoma) histologically resembles small cell carcinomas of other sites (35,180,200), with a diffuse, infiltrative growth pattern, small to medium-sized cells with minimal cytoplasm, and fusiform nuclei with a finely granular chromatin pattern, inconspicuous nucleoli, and nuclear molding against adjacent nuclei (fig. 12-42). Necrosis is abundant and the mitotic rate is typically more than 50 mitoses per 10 high-power fields. Widely invasive growth is common, and entrapment of pancreatic parenchyma within the neoplasm may occur.

The large cell type exhibits a more pronounced nesting pattern and may be less extensively infiltrative (fig. 12-43). The cells have a moderate amount of amphophilic cytoplasm and the nuclei are large and round to oval, with coarsely clumped chromatin and prominent nucleoli. Some gland formation may be present, but a separate component of conventional ductal adenocarcinoma with mucin-containing cytoplasm should suggest a diagnosis of mixed ductal-endocrine carcinoma (see below). The mitotic rate is not as high as in the small cell type of poorly differentiated endocrine carcinoma: 30 to 40 mitoses per 10 high-power fields.

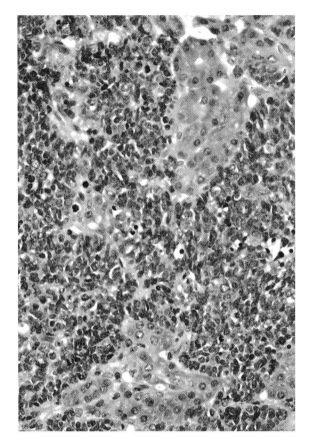

Figure 12-42

SMALL CELL CARCINOMA

This poorly differentiated endocrine carcinoma is composed of small cells with minimal cytoplasm and a high mitotic rate. There is diffuse infiltration into the pancreatic parenchyma, with a few residual acini.

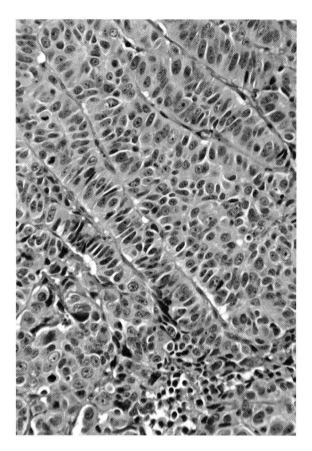

Figure 12-43

LARGE CELL ENDOCRINE CARCINOMA

The cells are large and have abundant cytoplasm. There is a small focus of necrosis (bottom) and numerous mitoses are present.

Immunohistochemical labeling reveals positivity for synaptophysin and chromogranin in most poorly differentiated endocrine carcinomas of the pancreas, although the labeling may be focal (especially for chromogranin). For histologically typical examples of small cell carcinoma, it is not necessary to document endocrine differentiation to establish the diagnosis, but for the large cell type, positivity for one of these markers should be found. Reflecting the high mitotic rate, Ki-67 labels 40 to 90 percent of the neoplastic cells. In contrast to well-differentiated PENs, some poorly differentiated endocrine carcinomas display abnormal labeling with antibodies to p53 (20). Expression of the cell adhesion molecule L1 (CD171) has been demonstrated in poorly differentiated endocrine carcinomas of the pancreas; this marker is not expressed in well-differentiated PENs or ductal adenocarcinomas (107a,107b).

In cytologic samples, small cell carcinoma of the pancreas resembles small cell carcinoma of the lung and is characterized by small blue cells with irregular nuclei, coarse chromatin, nuclear molding, and scant ill-defined cytoplasm (fig. 12-44). Large cell endocrine carcinoma is similar morphologically to conventional PEN but displays larger cells with more nuclear irregularity and pleomorphism. Although small cell carcinoma has characteristic features allowing a cytologic diagnosis, large cell endocrine carcinoma has cytologic features that overlap with well-differentiated PEN and, despite, the apparent cytologic atypia, a high-grade malignant diagnosis is not warranted based on cytology alone.

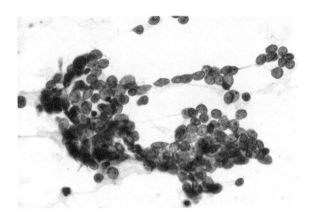

Figure 12-44

SMALL CELL CARCINOMA OF THE PANCREAS

The cytologic appearance resembles small cell carcinoma of the lung (direct smear; Papanicolaou stain).

Differential Diagnosis. The differential diagnosis of a poorly differentiated endocrine carcinoma includes metastases from an extrapancreatic primary, well-differentiated PENs, and poorly differentiated pancreatic adenocarcinomas lacking endocrine differentiation. Due to the rarity of a poorly differentiated endocrine carcinomas primary in the pancreas relative to the lung and other sites, the possibility of a metastasis to the pancreas must always be considered, and careful clinical and radiologic correlation is necessary before accepting such a neoplasm as primary in the pancreas. In the case of lung primaries, both small cell carcinomas and large cell neuroendocrine carcinomas commonly express thyroid transcription factor 1 (TTF1) by immunohistochemistry, a marker that suggests pulmonary origin, despite reports of expression in extrapulmonary small cell carcinomas (185).

PENs are distinguished from poorly differentiated endocrine carcinomas by their lower proliferative rate, which is defined as no more that 10 mitoses per 10 high-power fields (50 mitoses per 50 high-power fields). Pancreatic small cell carcinomas also have distinctive cytologic features not encountered in well-differentiated PENs. Immunohistochemical labeling for chromogranin and synaptophysin are typically more intense in PENs than in poorly differentiated endocrine carcinomas, but this finding is not sufficient to separate the two entities.

Poorly differentiated adenocarcinoma may share with poorly differentiated endocrine car-

cinomas a solid, nesting growth pattern. The nuclear morphology, however, does not suggest endocrine differentiation, and there is no significant immunolabeling for endocrine markers. Most such neoplasms also have foci of better-differentiated adenocarcinoma, but immunohistochemistry is still necessary to explore the possibility of a mixed ductal-endocrine carcinoma (see below).

Two other neoplasms that can resemble poorly differentiated endocrine carcinoma and occasionally involve the pancreas are primitive neuroectodermal tumors (PNETs) (169) and desmoplastic small round cell tumors (DSRCTs) (17). Both typically affect younger patients than do poorly differentiated endocrine carcinomas, but they share with the latter the presence of endocrine differentiation. The characteristic architecture of DSRCTs, the abundant desmoplastic stroma, and the immunohistochemical positivity for desmin and WT1, are helpful diagnostic features. PNETs may be less histologically distinctive but demonstrate intense diffuse immunolabeling for CD99 (79,98), which, although common in well-differentiated PENs, has not been reported in poorly differentiated endocrine carcinomas of the pancreas. Some reported pancreatic PNETs immunolabel for cytokeratin (169), another feature that may cause confusion with poorly differentiated endocrine carcinomas. For both PNETs and DSRCTs, molecular testing is now widely used for ultimate diagnostic confirmation.

MIXED DUCTAL-ENDOCRINE CARCINOMA

Definition. *Mixed ductal-endocrine carcinoma* of the pancreas is a malignant epithelial neoplasm with separate, morphologically recognizable ductal adenocarcinoma and endocrine elements, each constituting at least 25 percent of the neoplasm. Conventional PENs with focal gland formation, PENs with entrapped nonneoplastic ductules, and infiltrating ductal adenocarcinomas that contain endocrine cells only recognizable based on immunohistochemical labeling are not considered mixed ductal-endocrine carcinomas.

General Features. Since pancreatic ductal adenocarcinomas commonly contain scattered endocrine cells, it is not surprising that in some cases, a significant endocrine component may

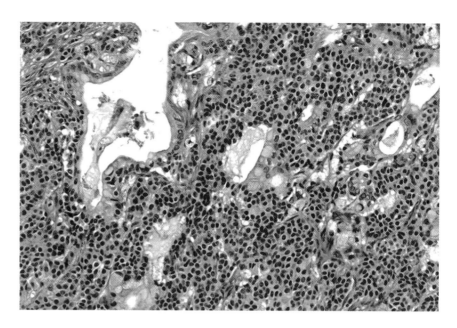

Figure 12-45

MIXED DUCTAL-ENDOCRINE CARCINOMA

Solid nests of the endocrine component are intimately mixed with the mucinous glands of the ductal component in this lymph node metastasis.

be present. Mixed ductal-endocrine carcinomas are among the least common pancreatic neoplasms (9a,110,122,175,181). Although the literature contains case reports and a number of small series of "ductuloinsular" neoplasms (53,199), many of the described cases appear to represent PENs with entrapped non-neoplastic ductules, a phenomenon that, while interesting, is not associated with biologic behavior different than other PENs. Furthermore, focal ductal differentiation in the form of lumen formation or immunohistochemical labeling for glycoproteins is relatively common in PENs and has no prognostic significance. Finally, the incidental coexistence of a PEN or endocrine microadenoma in a pancreas also harboring a conventional ductal adenocarcinoma has been documented, but these are regarded as separate independent neoplasms rather than mixed carcinomas. The above definition is intended to include only those neoplasms with obvious endocrine and ductal components, and using this restrictive definition, there are few well-documented cases. In most, the endocrine elements have the appearance of a poorly differentiated endocrine carcinoma rather than a well-differentiated PEN.

Clinical Features. Patients with mixed ductal-endocrine carcinomas are usually older adults, and there is a predominance in men (28, 122). The head of the gland is more commonly involved (122,181). Most patients present with nonspecific symptoms; a single reported hormon-

ally active neoplasm was associated with Zollinger-Ellison syndrome (241). Mixed ductal-endocrine carcinomas are highly aggressive neoplasms, similar to pure ductal adenocarcinomas.

Pathologic Findings. Mixed ductal-endocrine carcinoma appears grossly as a solid, tan to yellow, circumscribed mass with a variable degree of fibrosis.

Microscopically, the ductal adenocarcinoma component is intimately mixed with the endocrine component (fig. 12-45), and in some regions there appears to be a subtle transition between the two different elements. The ductal adenocarcinoma component is usually moderately to poorly differentiated and may be mucinous. The cytoarchitectural features are similar to those of conventional ductal adenocarcinomas, although the amount of desmoplastic stroma may be less. Intracellular and luminal mucin is usually obvious and can be highlighted with histochemical stains (mucicarmine or Alcian blue). The endocrine elements consist of uniform, small to medium-sized cells arranged in solid sheets and nests. The chromatin pattern is stippled and nucleoli are usually inconspicuous. The mitotic rate in the endocrine component is often significant, higher than the 10 mitoses per 10 high-power fields rate that separates well-differentiated PENs from poorly differentiated endocrine carcinomas. Foci of necrosis may be found. Rarely, a well-differentiated endocrine component is present.

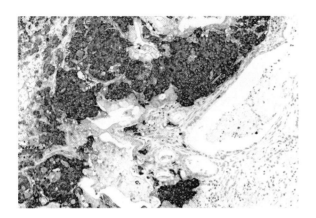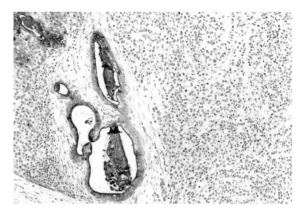

Figure 12-46

MIXED DUCTAL -ENDOCRINE CARCINOMA

Immunolabeling for chromogranin (left) highlights the endocrine component whereas that for CA19.9 (right) labels only the ductal elements.

By immunohistochemistry, the two components display distinct patterns (fig. 12-46). The ductal components label for CK19, CEA, and CA19-9 whereas the endocrine cells express synaptophysin and chromogranin. Focal expression of peptide hormones has also been documented, including gastrin in a reported patient with Zollinger-Ellison syndrome (241).

Differential Diagnosis. Since gland formation is not uncommon in conventional PENs, and other PENs entrap non-neoplastic ductules, the appearance of lumens in an endocrine neoplasm of the pancreas usually does not signify a mixed ductal-endocrine carcinoma. In the former circumstance, the lumens are lined by cells with the same cytoarchitectural features as the more solid portions of the neoplasm. Although immunolabeling for ductal markers such as CA19-9 may be found in these cells, there is also ex-

pression of endocrine markers (chromogranin or synaptophysin) and a dual cell population cannot be demonstrated. Entrapped non-neoplastic ductules in PENs indeed represent a second cell population (245), but they have no cytoarchitectural features of malignancy, in contrast to the glands of mixed ductal-endocrine carcinoma. In both of these cases, the endocrine components are usually well differentiated, and there is no adverse prognostic significance to the glandular differentiation or entrapment.

Conventional ductal adenocarcinoma may also contain scattered endocrine cells, detectable by immunolabeling for chromogranin. But these are much less than the 25 percent component required for a diagnosis of mixed ductal-endocrine carcinoma, and are usually not recognizable by routine microscopy (181).

REFERENCES

1. Abraham SC, Klimstra DS, Wilentz RE, et al. Solid-pseudopapillary tumors of the pancreas are genetically distinct from pancreatic ductal adenocarcinomas and almost always harbor beta-catenin mutations. Am J Pathol 2002;160:1361-9.
2. Adamson AR, Grahame-Smith DG, Bogomoletz V, Maw DS, Rothnie NG. Malignant argentaffinoma with carcinoid syndrome and hypoglycaemia. Br Med J 1971;3:93-4.
3. Al-Kaisi N, Weaver MG, Abdul-Karim FW, Siegler E. Fine needle aspiration cytology of neuroendocrine tumors of the pancreas. A cytologic, immunocytochemical and electron microscopic study. Acta Cytol 1992;36:655-60.
4. Andersen DK. Current diagnosis and management of Zollinger-Ellison syndrome. Ann Surg 1989;210:685-703.

5. Anderson MA, Carpenter S, Thompson NW, Nostrant TT, Elta GH, Scheiman JM. Endoscopic ultrasound is highly accurate and directs management in patients with neuroendocrine tumors of the pancreas. Am J Gastroenterol 2000; 95:2271-7.

5a. Anlauf M, Schlenger R, Bauersfeld J, et al. Microadenomatosis of the endocrine pancreas in patients with and without the multiple endocrine neoplasia type 1 syndrome. Am J Surg Pathol 2006;30:560-74.

6. Antonioli DA, Dayal Y, Dvorak AM, Banks PA. Zollinger-Ellison syndrome. Cure by surgical resection of a jejunal gastrinoma containing growth hormone releasing factor. Gastroenterology 1987;92:814-23.

7. Arihiro K, Inai K. Malignant islet cell tumor of the pancreas with multiple hormone production and expression of CEA and CA19-9. Report of an autopsy case. Acta Pathol Jpn 1991;41:150-7.

8. Arps H, Dietel M, Schulz A, Janzarik H, Klöppel G. Pancreatic endocrine carcinoma with ectopic PTH-production and paraneoplastic hypercalcaemia. Virchows Arch A Pathol Anat Histopathol 1986;408:497-503.

9. Asteria C, Anagni M, Fugazzola L, Faglia G, Vezzadini P, Beck-Peccoz P. MEN1 gene mutations are a rare event in patients with sporadic neuroendocrine tumors. Eur J Intern Med 2002; 13:319-23.

9a. Ballas KD, Rafailidis SF, Demertzidis C, Alatsakis MB, Pantzaki A, Sakadamis AK. Mixed exocrine-endocrine tumor of the pancreas. JOP 2005;6: 449-54.

10. Barghorn A, Komminoth P, Bachmann D, et al. Deletion at 3p25.3-p23 is frequently encountered in endocrine pancreatic tumours and is associated with metastatic progression. J Pathol 2001;194:451-8.

11. Barghorn A, Speel EJ, Farspour B, et al. Putative tumor suppressor loci at 6q22 and 6q23-q24 are involved in the malignant progression of sporadic endocrine pancreatic tumors. Am J Pathol 2001;158:1903-11.

12. Bartow SA, Mukai K, Rosai J. Pseudoneoplastic proliferation of endocrine cells in pancreatic fibrosis. Cancer 1981;47:2627-33.

13. Baudin E, Bidart JM, Bachelot A, et al. Impact of chromogranin A measurement in the workup of neuroendocrine tumors. Ann Oncol 2001; 12(suppl 2):S79-82.

14. Bell DA. Cytologic features of islet-cell tumors. Acta Cytol 1987;31:485-92.

15. Berger M, Bordi C, Cuppers HJ, et al. Functional and morphologic characterization of human insulinomas. Diabetes 1983;32:921-31.

15a. Berkel S, Hummel F, Gaa J, et al. Poorly differentiated small cell carcinoma of the pancreas. A case report and review of the literature. Pancreatology 2004;4:521-6.

16. Bhagavan BS, Slavin RE, Goldberg J, Rao RN. Ectopic gastrinoma and Zollinger-Ellison syndrome. Hum Pathol 1986;17:584-92.

17. Bismar TA, Basturk O, Gerald WL, Schwarz K, Adsay NV. Desmoplastic small cell tumor in the pancreas. Am J Surg Pathol 2004;28:808-12.

18. Bloom SR, Polak JM. Glucagonoma syndrome. Am J Med 1987;82:25-36.

19. Bordi C, Corleto VD, Azzoni C, et al. The antral mucosa as a new site for endocrine tumors in multiple endocrine neoplasia type 1 and Zollinger-Ellison syndromes. J Clin Endocrinol Metab 2001;86:2236-42.

20. Bordi C, Oberg K, Papotti M, Volante M, Capella C. Pancreatic endocrine tumours: poorly differentiated endocrine carcinoma. In: DeLellis RA, Lloyd RV, Heitz PU, Eng C, eds. World Health Organization Classification of Tumours. Pathology and genetics of tumours of endocrine organs. Lyon: IARC Press; 2004:207-8.

21. Bordi C, Ravazzola M, Baetens D, Gorden P, Unger RH, Orci L. A study of glucagonomas by light and electron microscopy and immunofluorescence. Diabetes 1979;28:925-36.

22. Bottger T, Seidl C, Seifert JK, Heintz A, Bretz B, Junginger T. Value of quantitative DNA analysis in endocrine tumors of the pancreas. Oncology 1997;54:318-23.

23. Brandi ML, Marx SJ, Aurbach GD, Fitzpatrick LA. Familial multiple endocrine neoplasia type I: a new look at pathophysiology. Endocr Rev 1987;8:391-405.

24. Brentjens R, Saltz L. Islet cell tumors of the pancreas: the medical oncologist's perspective. Surg Clin North Am 2001;81:527-42.

25. Broughan TA, Leslie JD, Soto JM, Hermann RE. Pancreatic islet cell tumors. Surgery 1986;99: 671-8.

26. Calender A, Giraud S, Porchet N, Gaudray P, Cadiot G, Mignon M. [Clinicogenetic study of MEN1: recent physiopathological data and clinical applications. Study Group of Multiple Endocrine Neoplasia (GENEM)]. Ann Endocrinol (Paris) 1998;59:444-51. [French.]

27. Capella C, Heitz PU, Hofler H, Solcia E, Klöppel G. Revised classification of neuroendocrine tumors of the lung, pancreas and gut. Digestion 1994;55(suppl 3):11-23.

28. Capella C, Oberg K, Papotti M, Volante M, Bordi C. Pancreatic endocrine tumours: mixed exocrine-endocrine carcinomas. In: DeLellis RA, Lloyd RV, Heitz PU, Eng C, eds. World Health Organization Classification of Tumours. Pathology and genetics of tumours of endocrine organs. Lyon: IARC Press; 2004:205-6.

29. Capella C, Polak JM, Buffa R, et al. Morphologic patterns and diagnostic criteria of VIP-producing endocrine tumors. A histologic, histochemical, ultrastructural, and biochemical study of 32 cases. Cancer 1983;52:1860-74.

29a. Capurso G, Lattimore S, Crnogorac-Jurcevic T, et al. Gene expression profiles of progressive pancreatic endocrine tumours and their liver metastases reveal potential novel markers and therapeutic targets. Endocr Relat Cancer 2006;13:541-58.

30. Carstens PH, Cressman FK. Malignant oncocytic carcinoid of the pancreas. Ultrastruct Pathol 1989;13:69-75.

31. Centeno BA, Lewandrowski KB, Warshaw AL, Compton CC, Southern JF. Cyst fluid cytologic analysis in the differential diagnosis of pancreatic cystic lesions. Am J Clin Pathol 1994;101:483-7.

32. Centeno BA, Warshaw AL, Mayo-Smith W, Southern JF, Lewandrowski KB. Cytologic diagnosis of pancreatic cystic lesions. A prospective study of 28 percutaneous aspirates. Acta Cytol 1997;41:972-80.

33. Chandrasekharappa SC, Guru SC, Manickam P, et al. Positional cloning of the gene for multiple endocrine neoplasia-type 1. Science 1997;276:404-7.

34. Chetty R, Asa SL. Pancreatic endocrine tumors: an update. Adv Anat Pathol 2004;11:202-10.

35. Chetty R, Clark SP, Pitson GA. Primary small cell carcinoma of the pancreas. Pathology 1993;25:240-2.

36. Chung DC, Smith AP, Louis DN, Graeme-Cook F, Warshaw AL, Arnold A. A novel pancreatic endocrine tumor suppressor gene locus on chromosome 3p with clinical prognostic implications. J Clin Invest 1997;100:404-10.

37. Clark ES, Carney JA. Pancreatic islet cell tumor associated with Cushing's syndrome. Am J Surg Pathol 1984;8:917-24.

38. Clarke MR, Baker EE, Weyant RJ, Hill L, Carty SE. Proliferative activity in pancreatic endocrine tumors: association with function, metastases, and survival. Endocr Pathol 1997;8:181-7.

39. Collins BT, Cramer HM. Fine-needle aspiration cytology of islet cell tumors. Diagn Cytopathol 1996;15:37-45.

40. Conklin JL. Cytogenesis of the human fetal pancreas. Am J Anat 1962;111:181-93.

40a. Corcos O, Couvelard A, Giraud S, et al. Endocrine pancreatic tumors in von Hippel-Lindau disease: clinical, morphological, histological and genetic features. Am J Gastroenterol (in press).

41. Corrin B, Gilby ED, Jones NF, Patrick J. Oat cell carcinoma of the pancreas with ectopic ACTH secretion. Cancer 1973;31:1523-7.

42. Crabtree JS, Scacheri PC, Ward JM, et al. Of mice and MEN1: insulinomas in a conditional mouse knockout. Mol Cell Biol 2003;23:6075-85.

43. Creutzfeldt W. Endocrine tumors of the pancreas. In: Volk BW, Arquilla ER, eds. The diabetic pancreas, 2nd ed. New York: Plenum; 1985:543-86.

44. Creutzfeldt W, Arnold R, Creutzfeldt C, Track NS. Pathomorphologic, biochemical, and diagnostic aspects of gastrinomas (Zollinger-Ellison syndrome). Hum Pathol 1975;6:47-76.

45. Cryer PE, Hill GJ. Pancreatic islet cell carcinoma with hypercalcemia and hypergastrinemia. Response to streptozotocin. Cancer 1976;38:2217-21.

46. Cubilla AL, Hajdu SI. Islet cell carcinoma of the pancreas. Arch Pathol 1975;99:204-7.

47. Cupisti K, Hoppner W, Dotzenrath C, et al. Lack of MEN1 gene mutations in 27 sporadic insulinomas. Eur J Clin Invest 2000;30:325-9.

48. Dayal Y, Oberg K, Perren A, Komminoth P. Pancreatic endocrine tumours: somatostatinoma. In: DeLellis RA, Lloyd RV, Heitz PU, Eng C, eds. World Health Organization Classification of Tumours. Pathology and genetics of tumours of endocrine organs. Lyon: IARC Press; 2004:189-90.

49. Dayal Y, Tallberg KA, Nunnemacher G, DeLellis RA, Wolfe HJ. Duodenal carcinoids in patients with and without neurofibromatosis. A comparative study. Am J Surg Pathol 1986;10:348-57.

50. Delcore R Jr, Cheung LY, Friesen SR. Outcome of lymph node involvement in patients with the Zollinger-Ellison syndrome. Ann Surg 1988;208:291-8.

51. DeLellis RA, Dayal Y, Tischler AS, Lee AK, Wolfe HJ. Multiple endocrine neoplasia (MEN) syndromes: cellular origins and interrelationships. Int Rev Exp Pathol 1986;28:163-215.

51a. Delis S, Bakoyiannis A, Giannakou N, Tsigka A, Avgerinos C, Dervenis C. Asymptomatic calcitonin-secreting tumor of the pancreas. A case report. JOP 2006;7:70-3.

51b. Delman KS, Shapiro SE, Jonasch EW, et al. Abdominal visceral lesions in von Hippel-Lindau disease: incidence and clinical behavior of pancreatic and adrenal lesions at a single center. World J Surg 2006;30:665-9.

52. Deshpande V, Fernandez-del Castillo C, Muzikansky A, et al. Cytokeratin 19 is a powerful predictor of survival in pancreatic endocrine tumors. Am J Surg Pathol 2004;28:1145-53.

53. Deshpande V, Selig MK, Nielsen GP, Fernandez-del Castillo C, Lauwers GY. Ductulo-insular pancreatic endocrine neoplasms: clinicopathologic analysis of a unique subtype of pancreatic endocrine neoplasms. Am J Surg Pathol 2003;27:461-8.

54. Dial PF, Braasch JW, Rossi RL, Lee AK, Jin G. Management of nonfunctioning islet cell tumors of the pancreas. Surg Clin North Am 1985;65:291-9.

55. Dodd LG, Evans DB, Symmans F, Katz RL. Fine-needle aspiration of pancreatic extramedullary plasmacytoma: possible confusion with islet cell tumor. Diagn Cytopathol 1994;10:371-4.

56. Doi M, Imai T, Shichiri M, et al. Octreotide-sensitive ectopic ACTH production by islet cell carcinoma with multiple liver metastases. Endocr J 2003;50:135-43.

57. Dollinger MR, Ratner LH, Shamoian CA, Blackbourne BD. Carcinoid syndrome associated with pancreatic tumors. Arch Intern Med 1967;120:575-80.

58. Donow C, Pipeleers-Marichal M, Schröder S, Stamm B, Heitz PU, Klöppel G. Surgical pathology of gastrinoma. Site, size, multicentricity, association with multiple endocrine neoplasia type 1, and malignancy. Cancer 1991;68:1329-34.

59. Donow C, Pipeleers-Marichal M, Stamm B, Heitz PU, Klöppel G. [The pathology of insulinoma and gastrinoma. The location, size, multicentricity, association with multiple endocrine type-I neoplasms and malignancy]. Dtsch Med Wochenschr 1990;115:1386-91. [German.]

60. Doppman JL, Nieman LK, Cutler GB Jr, et al. Adrenocorticotropic hormone—secreting islet cell tumors: are they always malignant? Radiology 1994;190:59-64.

61. Du EZ, Goldstraw P, Zacharias J, et al. TTF-1 expression is specific for lung primary in typical and atypical carcinoids: TTF-1-positive carcinoids are predominantly in peripheral location. Hum Pathol 2004;35:825-31.

62. Ebrahimi SA, Wang EH, Wu A, Schreck RR, Passaro E Jr, Sawicki MP. Deletion of chromosome 1 predicts prognosis in pancreatic endocrine tumors. Cancer Res 1999;59:311-5.

63. Eckhauser FE, Cheung PS, Vinik AI, Strodel WE, Lloyd RV, Thompson NW. Nonfunctioning malignant neuroendocrine tumors of the pancreas. Surgery 1986;100:978-88.

64. Erlandson RA. Diagnostic transmission electron microscopy of tumors. New York: Raven Press; 1994.

65. Ezzat S, Ezrin C, Yamashita S, Melmed S. Recurrent acromegaly resulting from ectopic growth hormone gene expression by a metastatic pancreatic tumor. Cancer 1993;71:66-70.

66. Feldman JM. Carcinoid tumors and syndrome. Semin Oncol 1987;14:237-46.

67. Ferreiro J, Lewin K, Herron RM, Bhuta S. Malignant islet cell tumor with rhabdomyosarcomatous differentiation. Am J Surg Pathol 1989;13:422-7.

68. Fitzpatrick B, Ordonez NG, Mackay B. Islet cell tumor. Ultrastruct Pathol 1991;15:579-84.

69. Francalanci P, Diomedi-Camassei F, Purificato C, et al. Malignant pancreatic endocrine tumor in a child with tuberous sclerosis. Am J Surg Pathol 2003;27:1386-9.

70. Friesen SR, Tomita T, Kimmel JR. Pancreatic polypeptide update: its role in detection of the trait for multiple endocrine adenopathy syndrome, type I and pancreatic polypeptide-secreting tumors. Surgery 1983;94:1028-37.

71. Galbut DL, Markowitz AM. Insulinoma: diagnosis, surgical management and long-term follow-up. Review of 41 cases. Am J Surg 1980;139:682-90.

72. Gibril F, Venzon DJ, Ojeaburu JV, Bashir S, Jensen RT. Prospective study of the natural history of gastrinoma in patients with MEN1: definition of an aggressive and a nonaggressive form. J Clin Endocrinol Metab 2001;86:5282-93.

73. Glickman MH, Hart MJ, White TT. Insulinoma in Seattle: 39 cases in 30 years. Am J Surg 1980;140:119-25.

74. Goebel SU, Iwamoto M, Raffeld M, et al. Her-2/neu expression and gene amplification in gastrinomas: correlations with tumor biology, growth, and aggressiveness. Cancer Res 2002;62:3702-10.

75. Goossens A, Gepts W, Saudubray JM, et al. Diffuse and focal nesidioblastosis. A clinicopathological study of 24 patients with persistent neonatal hyperinsulinemic hypoglycemia. Am J Surg Pathol 1989;13:766-75.

76. Gordon DL, Lo MC, Schwartz MA. Carcinoid of the pancreas. Am J Med 1971;51:412-5.

77. Gortz B, Roth J, Krahenmann A, et al. Mutations and allelic deletions of the MEN1 gene are associated with a subset of sporadic endocrine pancreatic and neuroendocrine tumors and not restricted to foregut neoplasms. Am J Pathol 1999;154:429-36.

78. Gotchall J, Traweek T, Stenzel P. Benign oncocytic endocrine tumor of the pancreas in a patient with polyarteritis nodosa. Hum Pathol 1987;18:967-9.

79. Goto A, Niki T, Terado Y, Fukushima J, Fukayama M. Prevalence of CD99 protein expression in pancreatic endocrine tumours (PETs). Histopathology 2004;45:384-92.

80. Gregory RA, Tracy HJ, French JM, Sircus W. Extraction of a gastrin-like substance from a pancreatic tumour in a case of Zollinger-Ellison syndrome. Lancet 1960;1:1045-8.

81. Greider MH, Elliott DW. Electron microscopy of human pancreatic tumors of islet cell origin. Am J Pathol 1964;44:663-78.

82. Greider MH, Rosai J, McGuigan JE. The human pancreatic islet cells and their tumors. II. Ulcerogenic and diarrheogenic tumors. Cancer 1974;33:1423-43.

83. Griffiths DF, Jasani B, Newman GR, Williams ED, Williams GT. Glandular duodenal carcinoid—a somatostatin rich tumour with neuroendocrine associations. J Clin Pathol 1984;37:163-9.

84. Griffiths DF, Williams GT, Williams ED. Duodenal carcinoid tumours, phaeochromocytoma and neurofibromatosis: islet cell tumour, phaeochromocytoma and the von Hippel-Lindau complex: two distinctive neuroendocrine syndromes. Q J Med 1987;64:769-82.

85. Grosfeld JL, Vane DW, Rescorla FJ, McGuire W, West KW. Pancreatic tumors in childhood: analysis of 13 cases. J Pediatr Surg 1990;25: 1057-62.

86. Gumbs AA, Moore PS, Falconi M, et al. Review of the clinical, histological, and molecular aspects of pancreatic endocrine neoplasms. J Surg Oncol 2002;81:45-53.

87. Hamid QA, Bishop AE, Sikri KL, Varndell IM, Bloom SR, Polak JM. Immunocytochemical characterization of 10 pancreatic tumours, associated with the glucagonoma syndrome, using antibodies to separate regions of the proglucagon molecule and other neuroendocrine markers. Histopathology 1986;10:119-33.

88. Hammel PR, Vilgrain V, Terris B, et al. Pancreatic involvement in von Hippel-Lindau disease. Gastroenterology 2000;119:1087-95.

89. Harris S. Hyperinsulinism and dysinsulinism. JAMA 1924;83:729-33.

90. Heitz PU, Kasper M, Polak JM, Klöppel G. Pancreatic endocrine tumors. Hum Pathol 1982;13: 263-71.

91. Heitz PU, Komminoth P, Perren A, et al. Pancreatic endocrine tumours: introduction. In: DeLellis RA, Lloyd RV, Heitz PU, Eng C, eds. World Health Organization Classification of Tumours. Pathology and genetics of tumours of endocrine organs. Lyon: IARC Press; 2004: 177-82.

92. Herrmann ME, Ciesla MC, Chejfec G, DeJong SA, Yong SL. Primary nodal gastrinomas. Arch Pathol Lab Med 2000;124:832-5.

93. Hessman O, Lindberg D, Einarsson A, et al. Genetic alterations on 3p, 11q13, and 18q in nonfamilial and MEN 1-associated pancreatic endocrine tumors. Genes Chromosomes Cancer 1999;26:258-64.

94. Heymann MF, Joubert M, Nemeth J, et al. Prognostic and immunohistochemical validation of the Capella classification of pancreatic neuroendocrine tumours: an analysis of 82 sporadic cases. Histopathology 2000;36:421-32.

95. Higgins GA, Recant L, Fischman AB. The glucagonoma syndrome: surgically curable diabetes. Am J Surg 1979;137:142-8.

96. Hoang MP, Hruban RH, Albores-Saavedra J. Clear cell endocrine pancreatic tumor mimicking renal cell carcinoma: a distinctive neoplasm of von Hippel-Lindau disease. Am J Surg Pathol 2001;25:602-9.

97. Hobbs RD, Stewart AF, Ravin ND, Carter D. Hypercalcemia in small cell carcinoma of the pancreas. Cancer 1984;53:1552-4.

98. Hochwald SN, Zee S, Conlon KC, et al. Prognostic factors in pancreatic endocrine neoplasms: an analysis of 136 cases with a proposal for low-grade and intermediate-grade groups. J Clin Oncol 2002;20:2633-42.

99. Holland AM, Gonez LJ, Harrison LC. Progenitor cells in the adult pancreas. Diabetes Metab Res Rev 2004;20:13-27.

100. House MG, Herman JG, Guo MZ, et al. Aberrant hypermethylation of tumor suppressor genes in pancreatic endocrine neoplasms. Ann Surg 2003;238:423-31.

101. Hull MT, Warfel KA, Muller J, Higgins JT. Familial islet cell tumors in Von Hippel-Lindau's disease. Cancer 1979;44:1523-6.

102. Hussain S, Arwini A, Chetty R, Klimstra DS. Oncocytic pancreatic endocrine neoplasms: a clinicopathologic and immunohistochemical analysis of 21 cases. Mod Pathol 2005;18:279A.

103. Hutcheon DF, Bayless TM, Cameron JL, Baylin SB. Hormone-mediated watery diarrhea in a family with multiple endocrine neoplasms. Ann Intern Med 1979;90:932-4.

104. Imam H, Eriksson B, Oberg K. Expression of CD44 variant isoforms and association to the benign form of endocrine pancreatic tumours. Ann Oncol 2000;11:295-300.

105. Jaksic T, Yaman M, Thorner P, Wesson DK, Filler RM, Shandling B. A 20-year review of pediatric pancreatic tumors. J Pediatr Surg 1992;27:1315-7.

106. Jensen RT, Doppman JL, Gardner JD. Gastrinoma. In: Go VL, Gardner JD, Brooks FP, Lebenthal E, DiMagno EP, Schleele GAeds. The pancreas: biology, pathobiology and disease. New York: Raven Press; 1993:727-4.

107. Jimenez-Heffernan JA, Vicandi B, Lopez-Ferrer P, Gonzalez-Peramato P, Perez-Campos A, Viguer JM. Fine needle aspiration cytology of endocrine neoplasms of the pancreas. Morphologic and immunocytochemical findings in 20 cases. Acta Cytol 2004;48:295-301.

107a. Kaifi JT, Heidtmann S, Schurr PG, et al. Absence of L1 in pancreatic masses distinguishes adenocarcinomas from poorly differentiated neuroendocrine carcinomas. Anticancer Res 2006;26: 1167-70.

107b. Kaifi JT, Zinnkann U, Yekebas EF, et al. L1 is a potential marker for poorly-differentiated pancreatic neuroendocrine carcinoma. World J Gastroenterol 2006;12:94-8.

108. Kamisawa T, Tu Y, Egawa N, et al. Ductal and acinar differentiation in pancreatic endocrine tumors. Dig Dis Sci 2002;47:2254-61.

109. Kaplan SJ, Holbrook CT, McDaniel HG, Buntain WL, Crist WM. Vasoactive intestinal peptide secreting tumors of childhood. Am J Dis Child 1980;134:21-4.

110. Kashiwabara K, Nakajima T, Shinkai H, et al. A case of malignant duct-islet cell tumor of the pancreas immunohistochemical and cytofluorometric study. Acta Pathol Jpn 1991;41:636-41.

111. Kenny BD, Sloan JM, Hamilton PW, Watt PC, Johnston CF, Buchanan KD. The role of morphometry in predicting prognosis in pancreatic islet cell tumors. Cancer 1989;64:460-5.

112. Kent RB, van Heerden JA, Weiland LH. Nonfunctioning islet cell tumors. Ann Surg 1981; 193:185-90.

113. Kiang DT, Bauer GE, Kennedy BJ. Immunoassayable insulin in carcinoma of the cervix associated with hypoglycemia. Cancer 1973;31: 801-5.

114. Kimura W, Kuroda A, Morioka Y. Clinical pathology of endocrine tumors of the pancreas. Analysis of autopsy cases. Dig Dis Sci 1991;36: 933-42.

115. Kitami CE, Shimizu T, Sato O, et al. Malignant islet cell tumor projecting into the main pancreatic duct. J Hepatobiliary Pancreat Surg 2000;7:529-33.

116. Klimstra DS. Pancreas. In: Sternberg SS, ed. Histology for pathologists. Philadelphia: Lippincott-Raven; 1997:613-47.

117. Klimstra DS, Heffess CS, Oertel JE, Rosai J. Acinar cell carcinoma of the pancreas: a clinicopathologic study of 28 cases. Am J Surg Pathol 1992;16:815-37.

118. Klimstra DS, Perren A, Oberg K, Komminoth P, Bordi C. Pancreatic endocrine tumours: nonfunctioning tumours and microadenomas. In: DeLellis RA, Lloyd RV, Heitz PU, Eng C, eds. World Health Organization Classification of Tumours. Pathology and genetics of tumours of endocrine organs. Lyon: IARC Press; 2004: 201-4.

119. Klimstra DS, Rosai J, Heffess CS. Mixed acinar-endocrine carcinomas of the pancreas. Am J Surg Pathol 1994;18:765-78.

120. Klimstra DS, Wenig BM, Adair CF, Heffess CS. Pancreatoblastoma. A clinicopathologic study and review of the literature. Am J Surg Pathol 1995;19:1371-89.

121. Klimstra DS, Wenig BM, Heffess CS. Solid-pseudopapillary tumor of the pancreas: a typically cystic carcinoma of low malignant potential. Semin Diagn Pathol 2000;17:66-80.

122. Klöppel G. Mixed exocrine-endocrine tumors of the pancreas. Semin Diagn Pathol 2000;17: 104-8.

123. Klöppel G, Heitz PU. Pancreatic endocrine tumors. Pathol Res Pract 1988;183:155-68.

124. Klöppel G, Heitz PU, Capella C, Solcia E. Endocrine tumours of the pancreas. In: Solcia E, Klöppel G, Sobin LH, eds. Histological typing of endocrine tumours, 2nd ed. Berlin: Springer-Verlag; 2000:56-60.

125. Klöppel G, Komminoth P, Perren A, Oberg K, Matias-Guiu X, Heitz PU. Pancreatic endocrine tumours: glucagonoma. In: DeLellis RA, Lloyd RV, Heitz PU, Eng C, eds. World Health Organization Classification of Tumours. Pathology and genetics of tumours of endocrine organs. Lyon: IARC Press; 2004:187-8.

126. Klöppel G, Willemer S, Stamm B, Hacki WH, Heitz PU. Pancreatic lesions and hormonal profile of pancreatic tumors in multiple endocrine neoplasia type I. An immunocytochemical study of nine patients. Cancer 1986;57:1824-32.

127. Koga A, Tabata M, Kido H, et al. [Successful treatment of ectopic insulinoma. Report of a case (author's transl)]. Nippon Shokakibyo Gakkai Zasshi 1979;76:279-84. [Japanese.]

128. Kogut MD, Kaplan SA. Systemic manifestations of neurogenic tumors. J Pediatr 1962;60:694-704.

129. Komminoth P. Review: multiple endocrine neoplasia type 1, sporadic neuroendocrine tumors, and MENIN. Diagn Mol Pathol 1999;8:107-12.

130. Komminoth P, Perren A, Oberg K, et al. Pancreatic endocrine tumours: insulinoma. In: DeLellis RA, Lloyd RV, Heitz PU, Eng C, eds. World Health Organization Classification of Tumours. Pathology and genetics of tumours of endocrine organs. Lyon: IARC Press; 2004.

131. Komminoth P, Perren A, Oberg K, et al. Pancreatic endocrine tumours: gastrinoma. In: DeLellis RA, Lloyd RV, Heitz PU, Eng C, eds. World Health Organization Classification of Tumours. Pathology and genetics of tumours of endocrine organs. Lyon: IARC Press; 2004:191-4.

132. Komminoth P, Seelentag WK, Saremaslani P, Heitz PU, Roth J. CD44 isoform expression in the diffuse neuroendocrine system. II. Benign and malignant tumors. Histochem Cell Biol 1996;106:551-62.

133. Kovacs K, Asa SL. Functional endocrine pathology, 2nd ed. Malden, Mass: Blackwell Science; 1998.

134. Krejs GJ. VIPoma syndrome. Am J Med 1987;82: 37-48.

135. Krejs GJ, Orci L, Conlon JM, et al. Somato-statinoma syndrome. Biochemical, morphologic and clinical features. N Engl J Med 1979; 301:285-92.

136. Kunz J, Amendt P, Hahn von Dorsche H, Gerl H, Knappe E, Lorenz D. [The endocrine pancreas in pluriglandular neoplasia type I. A report of two cases and review of the literature]. Zentralbl Allg Pathol 1983;127:375-83. [German.]

137. La Rosa S, Sessa F, Capella C, et al. Prognostic criteria in nonfunctioning pancreatic endocrine tumors. Virchows Arch 1996;429:323-33.

138. Labate AM, Klimstra DS, Zakowski MF. Comparative cytologic features of pancreatic acinar cell carcinoma and islet cell tumor. Diagn Cytopathol 1997;16:112-6.

139. Lam KY, Lo CY. Pancreatic endocrine tumour: a 22-year clinico-pathological experience with morphological, immunohistochemical observation and a review of the literature. Eur J Surg Oncol 1997;23:36-42.

140. Larsson LI, Grimelius L, Hakanson R, et al. Mixed endocrine pancreatic tumors producing several peptide hormones. Am J Pathol 1975;79:271-84.

141. Larsson LI, Ljungberg O, Sundler F, et al. Antropyloric gastrinoma associated with pancreatic nesidioblastosis and proliferation of islets. Virchows Arch A Pathol Pathol Anat 1973;360: 305-14.

142. Larsson LI, Schwartz T, Lundqvist G, et al. Occurrence of human pancreatic polypeptide in pancreatic endocrine tumors. Possible implication in the watery diarrhea syndrome. Am J Pathol 1976;85:675-84.

143. Latif F, Tory K, Gnarra J, et al. Identification of the von Hippel-Lindau disease tumor suppressor gene. Science 1993;260:1317-20.

144. Le Bodic MF, Heymann MF, Lecomte M, et al. Immunohistochemical study of 100 pancreatic tumors in 28 patients with multiple endocrine neoplasia, type I. Am J Surg Pathol 1996;20: 1378-84.

145. Le Quesne LP, Nabarro JD, Kurtz A, Zweig S. The management of insulin tumours of the pancreas. Br J Surg 1979;66:373-8.

146. Lechago J, Speel EJ, Perren A, Papotti M. Pancreatic endocrine tumours: VIPoma. In: DeLellis RA, Lloyd RV, Heitz PU, Eng C, eds. World Health Organization Classification of Tumours. Pathology and genetics of tumours of endocrine organs. Lyon: IARC Press; 2004:195-7.

147. Libutti SK, Choyke PL, Bartlett DL, et al. Pancreatic neuroendocrine tumors associated with von Hippel-Lindau disease: diagnostic and management recommendations. Surgery 1998; 124:1153-9.

148. Ligneau B, Lombard-Bohas C, Partensky C, et al. Cystic endocrine tumors of the pancreas: clinical, radiologic, and histopathologic features in 13 cases. Am J Surg Pathol 2001;25:752-60.

149. Lips CJ, Vasen HF, Lamers CB. Multiple endocrine neoplasia syndromes. Crit Rev Oncol Hematol 1984;2:117-84.

150. Liu TH, Tseng HC, Zhu Y, Zhong SX, Chen J, Cui QC. Insulinoma. An immunocytochemical and morphologic analysis of 95 cases. Cancer 1985;56:1420-9.

151. Liu TH, Zhu Y, Cui QC, et al. Nonfunctioning pancreatic endocrine tumors. An immunohistochemical and electron microscopic analysis of 26 cases. Pathol Res Pract 1992;188:191-8.

152. Lloyd RV, Mervak T, Schmidt K, Warner TF, Wilson BS. Immunohistochemical detection of chromogranin and neuron-specific enolase in pancreatic endocrine neoplasms. Am J Surg Pathol 1984;8:607-14.

153. Long RG. Vasoactive intestinal polypeptide-secreting tumours (vipomas) in childhood. J Pediatr Gastroenterol Nutr 1983;2:122-6.

154. Lopez T, Hanahan D. Elevated levels of IGF-1 receptor convey invasive and metastatic capability in a mouse model of pancreatic islet tumorigenesis. Cancer Cell 2002;1:339-53.

155. Lubensky IA, Pack S, Ault D, et al. Multiple neuroendocrine tumors of the pancreas in von Hippel-Lindau disease patients: histopathological and molecular genetic analysis. Am J Pathol 1998;153:223-31.

156. Maitra A, Hansel DE, Argani P, et al. Global expression analysis of well-differentiated pancreatic endocrine neoplasms using oligonucleotide microarrays. Clin Cancer Res 2003;9:5988-95.

157. Majewski JT, Wilson SD. The MEA-I syndrome: an all or none phenomenon? Surgery 1979;86: 475-84.

158. Mallinson CN, Bloom SR, Warin AP, Salmon PR, Cox B. A glucagonoma syndrome. Lancet 1974;2:1-5.

159. Martignoni ME, Friess H, Lubke D, et al. Study of a primary gastrinoma in the common hepatic duct—a case report. Digestion 1999;60: 187-90.

160. Maton PN, Gardner JD, Jensen RT. Cushing's syndrome in patients with the Zollinger-Ellison syndrome. N Engl J Med 1986;315:1-5.

161. Migliori M, Tomassetti P, Lalli S, et al. Carcinoid of the pancreas. Pancreatology 2002;2: 163-6.

162. Mignon M, Cadiot G. Gastrinomas (Zollinger-Ellison syndrome). In: Howard JM, Idezuki Y, Ihse I, Prinz RA, eds. Cancer. Surgical diseases of the pancreas. Philadelphia: Williams & Wilkins; 1998:733-44.

163. Missiaglia E, Moore PS, Williamson J, et al. Sex chromosome anomalies in pancreatic endocrine tumors. Int J Cancer 2002;98:532-8.

164. Moldow RE, Connelly RR. Epidemiology of pancreatic cancer in Connecticut. Gastroenterology 1968;55:677-86.

165. Moore PS, Missiaglia E, Antonello D, et al. Role of disease-causing genes in sporadic pancreatic endocrine tumors: MEN1 and VHL. Genes Chromosomes Cancer 2001;32:177-81.

166. Moore PS, Orlandini S, Zamboni G, et al. Pancreatic tumours: molecular pathways implicated in ductal cancer are involved in ampullary but not in exocrine nonductal or endocrine tumorigenesis. Br J Cancer 2001;84:253-62.

167. Morrison AB. Islet cell tumors and the diarrheogenic syndrome. Monogr Pathol 1980;21:185-207.

168. Morrison AB, Rawson AJ, Fitts WT. The syndrome of refractory watery diarrhea and hypokalemia in patients with a non-insulin-secreting islet cell tumor. A further case study and review of the literature. Am J Med 1962;32:119-27.

169. Movahedi-Lankarani S, Hruban RH, Westra WH, Klimstra DS. Primitive neuroectodermal tumors of the pancreas: a report of seven cases of a rare neoplasm. Am J Surg Pathol 2002;26:1040-7.

170. Mukai K, Grotting JC, Greider MH, Rosai J. Retrospective study of 77 pancreatic endocrine tumors using the immunoperoxidase method. Am J Surg Pathol 1982;6:387-99.

171. Muscarella P, Melvin WS, Fisher WE, et al. Genetic alterations in gastrinomas and nonfunctioning pancreatic neuroendocrine tumors: an analysis of p16/MTS1 tumor suppressor gene inactivation. Cancer Res 1998;58:237-40.

172. Nassar H. High grade neuroendocrine carcinoma of the ampulla of Vater: a clinicopathologic and immunohistochemical analysis of 14 cases. Am J Surg Pathol 2005;29:588-94.

173. Nguyen GK. Cytology of hyperplastic endocrine cells of the pancreas in fine needle aspiration biopsy. Acta Cytol 1984;28:499-502.

174. Nicholls AG. Simple adenoma of the pancreas arising from an island of Langerhans. J Med Res 1902;8:358-95.

174a. Nikou GC, Toubanakis C, Nikolaou P, et al. Gastrinomas associated with MEN-1 syndrome: new insights for the diagnosis and management in a series of 11 patients. Hepatogastroenterology 2005;52:1668-76.

174b. Nikou GC, Toubanakis C, Nikolaou P, et al. VIPomas: an update in diagnosis and management in a series of 11 patients. Hepatogastroenterology 2005;52:1259-65.

175. Nonomura A, Mizukami Y, Matsubara F, Kono N, Nakanuma Y. Duct-islet cell tumor of the pancreas. A case report with immunohistochemical and electron microscopic findings. Acta Pathol Jpn 1989;39:328-35.

176. Nord KS, Joshi V, Hanna M, et al. Zollinger-Ellison syndrome associated with a renal gastrinoma in a child. J Pediatr Gastroenterol Nutr 1986;5:980-6.

177. Norton JA, Doppman JL, Collen MJ, et al. Prospective study of gastrinoma localization and resection in patients with Zollinger-Ellison syndrome. Ann Surg 1986;204:468-79.

178. Norton JA, Fraker DL, Alexander HR, et al. Surgery to cure the Zollinger-Ellison syndrome. N Engl J Med 1999;341:635-44.

179. Norton JA, Shawker TH, Doppman JL, et al. Localization and surgical treatment of occult insulinomas. Ann Surg 1990;212:615-20.

180. O'Connor TP, Wade TP, Sunwoo YC, et al. Small cell undifferentiated carcinoma of the pancreas. Report of a patient with tumor marker studies. Cancer 1992;70:1514-9.

181. Ohike N, Kosmahl M, Klöppel G. Mixed acinar-endocrine carcinoma of the pancreas. A clinicopathological study and comparison with acinar-cell carcinoma. Virchows Arch 2004; 445:231-5.

181a. Ohike N, Morohoshi T. Pathological assessment of pancreatic endocrine tumors for metastatic potential and clinical prognosis. Endocr Pathol 2005;16:33-40.

182. Ohneda A, Otsuki M, Fujiya H, Yaginuma N, Kokubo T, Ohtani H. A malignant insulinoma transformed into a glucagonoma syndrome. Diabetes 1979;28:962-9.

183. Ooi A, Kameya T, Tsumuraya M, et al. Pancreatic endocrine tumours associated with WDHA syndrome. An immunohistochemical and electron microscopic study. Virchows Arch A Pathol Anat Histopathol 1985;405:311-23.

184. Ordonez NG. Pancreatic acinar cell carcinoma. Adv Anat Pathol 2001;8:144-59.

185. Ordonez NG. Value of thyroid transcription factor-1 immunostaining in distinguishing small cell lung carcinomas from other small cell carcinomas. Am J Surg Pathol 2000;24: 1217-23.

185a. Ordonez NG, Manning JT, Hanssen G. Alpha-1-antitrypsin in islet cell tumors of the pancreas. Am J Clin Pathol 1983;80:277-82.

186. Ordonez NG, Manning JT, Raymond AK. Argentaffin endocrine carcinoma (carcinoid) of the pancreas with concomitant breast metastasis: an immunohistochemical and electron microscopic study. Hum Pathol 1985;16:746-51.

187. Osamura RY, Oberg K, Perren A. Pancreatic endocrine tumours: ACTH and other ectopic hormone producing tumours. In: DeLellis RA, Lloyd RV, Heitz PU, Eng C, eds. World Health Organization Classification of Tumours. Pathology and genetics of tumours of endocrine organs. Lyon: IARC Press; 2004:199-200.

188. Osamura RY, Oberg K, Speel EJ, Volante M, Perren A. Pancreatic endocrine tumours: serotonin-secreting tumour. In: DeLellis RA, Lloyd RV, Heitz PU, Eng C, eds. World Health Organization Classification of Tumours. Pathology and genetics of tumours of endocrine organs. Lyon: IARC Press; 2004:198.

189. Pacchioni D, Papotti M, Macri L, Forte G, Bussolati G. Pancreatic oncocytic endocrine tumors. Cytologic features of two cases. Acta Cytol 1996;40:742-6.

189a. Panzuto F, Nasoni S, Falconi M, et al. Prognostic factors and survival in endocrine tumor patients: comparison between gastrointestinal and pancreatic localization. Endocr Relat Cancer 2005;12:1083-92.

190. Pellegata NS, Sessa F, Renault B, et al. K-ras and p53 gene mutations in pancreatic cancer: ductal and nonductal tumors progress through different genetic lesions. Cancer Res 1994;54:1556-60.

191. Pelletier G, Cortot A, Launay JM, et al. Serotonin-secreting and insulin-secreting ileal carcinoid tumor and the use of in vitro culture of tumoral cells. Cancer 1984;54:319-22.

192. Pelosi G, Bresaola E, Bogina G, et al. Endocrine tumors of the pancreas: Ki-67 immunoreactivity on paraffin sections is an independent predictor for malignancy: a comparative study with proliferating-cell nuclear antigen and progesterone receptor protein immunostaining, mitotic index, and other clinicopathologic variables. Hum Pathol 1996;27:1124-34.

193. Perez-Montiel MD, Frankel WL, Suster S. Neuroendocrine carcinomas of the pancreas with 'Rhabdoid' features. Am J Surg Pathol 2003;27:642-9.

194. Perren A, Roth J, Muletta-Feurer S, et al. Clonal analysis of sporadic pancreatic endocrine tumours. J Pathol 1998;186:363-71.

195. Pitman MB, Faquin WC. The fine-needle aspiration biopsy cytology of pancreatoblastoma. Diagn Cytopathol 2004;31:402-6.

196. Prinz RA, Dorsch TR, Lawrence AM. Clinical aspects of glucagon-producing islet cell tumors. Am J Gastroenterol 1981;76:125-31.

197. Rahier J, Guiot Y, Sempoux C. Persistent hyperinsulinaemic hypoglycaemia of infancy: a heterogeneous syndrome unrelated to nesidio-blastosis. Arch Dis Child Fetal Neonatal Ed 2000;82:F108-12.

198. Rahman A, Maitra A, Ashfaq R, Yeo CJ, Cameron JL, Hansel DE. Loss of p27 nuclear expression in a prognostically favorable subset of well-differentiated pancreatic endocrine neoplasms. Am J Clin Pathol 2003;120:685-90.

199. Reid JD, Yuh SL, Petrelli M, Jaffe R. Ductuloinsular tumors of the pancreas: a light, electron microscopic and immunohistochemical study. Cancer 1982;49:908-15.

200. Reyes CV, Wang T. Undifferentiated small cell carcinoma of the pancreas: a report of five cases. Cancer 1981;47:2500-2.

201. Rigaud G, Missiaglia E, Moore PS, et al. High resolution allelotype of nonfunctional pancreatic endocrine tumors: identification of two molecular subgroups with clinical implications. Cancer Res 2001;61:285-92.

202. Roggli VL, Judge DM, McGavran MH. Duodenal glucagonoma: a case report. Hum Pathol 1979;10:350-3.

203. Roth J, Kasper M, Stamm B, et al. Localization of proinsulin and insulin in human insulinoma: preliminary immunohistochemical results. Virchows Arch B Cell Pathol Incl Mol Pathol 1989;56:287-92.

204. Roth J, Klöppel G, Madsen OD, Storch MJ, Heitz PU. Distribution patterns of proinsulin and insulin in human insulinomas: an immunohistochemical analysis in 76 tumors. Virchows Arch B Cell Pathol Incl Mol Pathol 1992;63:51-61.

205. Ruttman E, Klöppel G, Bommer G, Kiehn M, Heitz PU. Pancreatic glucagonoma with and without syndrome. Immunocytochemical study of 5 tumour cases and review of the literature. Virchows Arch A Pathol Anat Histopathol 1980;388:51-67.

205a. Sakar A, Kara E, Aydede H, Ayhan S, Celik P, Yorgancioglu A. A case of small cell lung carcinoma presenting with jaundice due to pancreatic metastases. Tuberk Toraks 2005;53:181-4.

206. Saleh HA, Masood S, Khatib G. Percutaneous and intraoperative aspiration biopsy cytology of pancreatic neuroendocrine tumors: cytomorphologic study with an immunocytochemical contribution. Acta Cytol 1996;40:182-90.

207. Sanno N, Teramoto A, Osamura RY, et al. A growth hormone-releasing hormone-producing pancreatic islet cell tumor metastasized to the pituitary is associated with pituitary somatotroph hyperplasia and acromegaly. J Clin Endocrinol Metab 1997;82:2731-7.

208. Sempoux C, Guiot Y, Lefevre A, et al. Neonatal hyperinsulinemic hypoglycemia: heterogeneity of the syndrome and keys for differential diagnosis. J Clin Endocrinol Metab 1998;83:1455-61.

209. Serrano J, Goebel SU, Peghini PL, Lubensky IA, Gibril F, Jensen RT. Alterations in the p16INK4a/CDKN2A tumor suppressor gene in gastrinomas. J Clin Endocrinol Metab 2000;85: 4146-56.

210. Service FJ. Hypoglycemic disorders. N Engl J Med 1995;332:1144-52.

211. Service FJ, Dale AJ, Elveback LR, Jiang NS. Insulinoma: clinical and diagnostic features of 60 consecutive cases. Mayo Clin Proc 1976;51: 417-29.

212. Service FJ, McMahon MM, O'Brien PC, Ballard DJ. Functioning insulinoma—incidence, recurrence, and long-term survival of patients: a 60-year study. Mayo Clin Proc 1991;66:711-9.

213. Shames JM, Dhurandhar NR, Blackard WG. Insulin-secreting bronchial carcinoid tumor with widespread metastases. Am J Med 1968;44:632-7.

214. Shan L, Nakamura Y, Nakamura M, et al. Somatic mutations of multiple endocrine neoplasia type 1 gene in the sporadic endocrine tumors. Lab Invest 1998;78:471-5.

215. Shane E, Bilezikian JP. Parathyroid carcinoma: a review of 62 patients. Endocr Rev 1982;3:218-26.

216. Shaw JA, Vance RP, Geisinger KR, Marshall RB. Islet cell neoplasms. A fine-needle aspiration cytology study with immunocytochemical correlations. Am J Clin Pathol 1990;94:142-9.

217. Shetty MR, Boghossian HM, Duffell D, Freel R, Gonzales JC. Tumor-induced hypoglycemia: a result of ectopic insulin production. Cancer 1982;49:1920-3.

218. Shia J, Erlandson RA, Klimstra DS. Whorls of intermediate filaments with entrapped neurosecretory granules correspond to the "rhabdoid" inclusions seen in pancreatic endocrine neoplasms. Am J Surg Pathol 2004;28:271-3.

219. Shorter NA, Glick RD, Klimstra DS, Brennan MF, Laquaglia MP. Malignant pancreatic tumors in childhood and adolescence: the Memorial Sloan-Kettering experience, 1967 to present. J Pediatr Surg 2002;37:887-92.

219a. Singh R, Basturk O, Klimstra DS, et al. Lipid-rich variant of pancreatic endocrine neoplasms. Am J Surg Pathol 2006;30:194-200.

220. Smith AE, Levi AW, Nadasdy T, Campbell KA, Fishman EK, Hruban RH. The pigmented "black" neuroendocrine tumor of the pancreas: a question of origin. Cancer 2001;92:1984-91.

221. Sneige N, Ordonez NG, Veanattukalathil S, Samaan NA. Fine-needle aspiration cytology in pancreatic endocrine tumors. Diagn Cytopathol 1987;3:35-40.

221a. Soga J. Carcinoids of the pancreas: an analysis of 156 cases. Cancer 2005;104:1180-7.

222. Soga J, Yakuwa Y. Pancreatic polypeptide (PP)-producing tumors (PPomas): a review of the literature and statistical analysis of 58 cases. J Hepatobiliary Pancreat Surg 1994;1:556-63.

223. Soga J, Yakuwa Y. Somatostatinoma/inhibitory syndrome: a statistical evaluation of 173 reported cases as compared to other pancreatic endocrinomas. J Exp Clin Cancer Res 1999;18:13-22.

224. Soga J, Yakuwa Y. Vipoma/diarrheogenic syndrome: a statistical evaluation of 241 reported cases. J Exp Clin Cancer Res 1998;17:389-400.

225. Soga J, Yakuwa Y, Osaka M. Insulinoma/hypoglycemic syndrome: a statistical evaluation of 1085 reported cases of a Japanese series. J Exp Clin Cancer Res 1998;17:379-88.

226. Solcia E, Capella C, Klöppel G. Tumors of the pancreas. AFIP Atlas of Tumor Pathology, 3rd Series, Fascicle 20. Washington, DC: American Registry of Pathology; 1997.

227. Solcia E, Capella C, Riva C, Rindi G, Polak JM. The morphology and neuroendocrine profile of pancreatic epithelial VIPomas and extrapancreatic, VIP-producing, neurogenic tumors. Ann N Y Acad Sci 1988;527:508-17.

228. Speel EJ, Richter J, Moch H, et al. Genetic differences in endocrine pancreatic tumor subtypes detected by comparative genomic hybridization. Am J Pathol 1999;155:1787-94.

229. Speel EJ, Scheidweiler AF, Zhao J, et al. Genetic evidence for early divergence of small functioning and nonfunctioning endocrine pancreatic tumors: gain of 9Q34 is an early event in insulinomas. Cancer Res 2001;61:5186-92.

230. Stabile BE, Morrow DJ, Passaro E. The gastrinoma triangle: operative implications. Am J Surg 1984;147:25-31.

231. Stabile BE, Passaro E. Benign and malignant gastrinoma. Am J Surg 1985;149:144-50.

232. Stamm BH. Incidence and diagnostic significance of minor pathologic changes in the adult pancreas at autopsy: a systematic study of 112 autopsies in patients without known pancreatic disease. Hum Pathol 1984;15:677-83.

233. Stefanini P, Carboni M, Patrassi N, Basoli A. Beta-islet cell tumors of the pancreas: results of a study on 1,067 cases. Surgery 1974;75:597-609.

233a. Stelow EB, Bardales RH, Shami VM, et al. Cytology of pancreatic acinar cell carcinoma. Diagn Cytopathol 2006;34:367-72.

234. Stumpf E, Aalto Y, Hoog A, et al. Chromosomal alterations in human pancreatic endocrine tumors. Genes Chromosomes Cancer 2000;29:83-7.

235. Styne DM, Isaac R, Miller WL, et al. Endocrine, histological, and biochemical studies of adrenocorticotropin-producing islet cell carcinoma of the pancreas in childhood with characterization of proopiomelanocortin. J Clin Endocrinol Metab 1983;57:723-31.

The differential diagnosis in the pancreas is with other cellular neoplasms, most notably acinar cell carcinoma, pancreatic endocrine neoplasm, pancreatoblastoma, and solid-pseudopapillary neoplasm. Other small round blue cell neoplasms that can rarely involve the pancreas, such as PNET, must also be considered (see above). Most of these neoplasms can be excluded based on morphology alone but immunohistochemistry is helpful since these neoplasms have a characteristic immunohistochemical labeling profile.

Non-Hodgkin's Lymphoma

Lymphoma primary in the pancreas is much less common than secondary involvement by advanced stage lymphoma of other sites (see chapter 14). Most occur in the pancreatic head; thus, clinical presentation can mimic other more common primary pancreatic malignancies, especially ductal adenocarcinoma. Abdominal pain, nausea and vomiting, palpable abdominal mass, anorexia, weight loss, and obstructive jaundice are the most common presenting signs and symptoms. Reported neoplasms include *non-Hodgkin's lymphoma* of both B-cell and T-cell lineage, both low and high grade.

Of 72 patients reported with non-Hodgkin's lymphoma primarily involving the pancreas, there were 40 males and 32 females ranging in age from 37 to 86 years, with an average age of approximately 65 years (8,11,49,64,67,70). All patients were symptomatic, abdominal pain be-

ing the most common symptom. Jaundice was present in less than half of the patients, in contrast to the typical patient with an adenocarcinoma of the head of the pancreas where jaundice is almost universally present. The neoplastic masses ranged in size from 3 to 17 cm, with a mean of approximately 8 cm. Most (63 percent) were diffuse large B-cell lymphoma.

Similar to the gross appearance of lymphoma in lymph nodes, pancreatic lymphomas form a solid, homogenous, fleshy, tan mass (fig. 13-20). The histologic features of non-Hodgkin's lymphoma in the pancreas are similar to those described in lymph nodes and other parenchymal organs (14,75). Most lymphomas in the

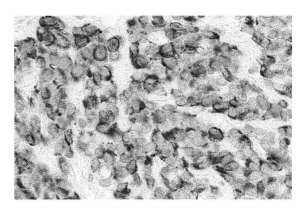

Figure 13-19

DESMOPLASTIC SMALL ROUND CELL TUMOR

A distinctive dot-like labeling pattern is seen with antibodies to desmin.

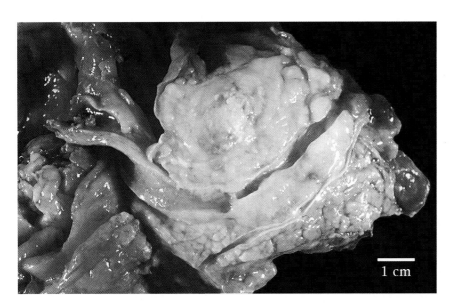

1 cm

Figure 13-20

NON-HODGKIN'S LYMPHOMA

The homogenous, fleshy tan mass in the pancreas is similar to the appearance of such lesions outside of the pancreas. This neoplasm compresses the bile duct.

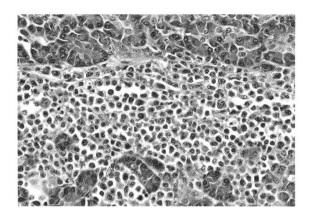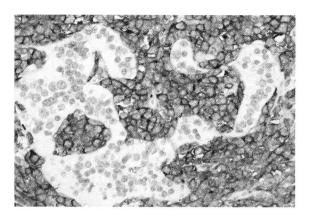

Figure 13-21

NON-HODGKIN'S LYMPHOMA: LARGE B-CELL LYMPHOMA

Left: A diffuse, nonorganoid proliferation of neoplastic cells infiltrates around and envelops normal pancreatic tissue.
Right: Immunolabeling of the cells for leukocyte common antigen (CD45) identifies the neoplasm as hematopoietic in origin. The entrapped acinar epithelial cells do not label and serve as an internal control.

pancreas are composed of large cells in a diffuse pattern without cohesion and organization. Cells permeate through the parenchyma, often entrapping normal structures (fig. 13-21, left). The neoplastic cells immunolabel for leukocyte common antigen (CD45) (fig. 13-21, right). Further subclassification of the lymphoma can be accomplished with a panel of other antibodies (described elsewhere in more detail [28]) on fixed or fresh tissue.

With adequate sampling and immunophenotypic analysis, fine needle aspiration biopsy can be used to diagnose and subclassify non-Hodgkin's lymphoma (11,24,59a,75). Proper specimen triage requires either a standard biopsy protocol for procuring fresh liquid-based tissue for immediate cytologic evaluation at the time of biopsy so that the lymphoid nature of the neoplasm can be recognized while additional tissue is still available for appropriate triage. Preoperative diagnosis is important for proper medical management, as lymphoma usually does not require surgical resection before therapy.

Cytologically, lymphoma is a noncohesive neoplasm, with the exception of an occasional "pseudocluster" which, regardless of subclassification, is a feature that helps in the distinction from carcinoma. The presence of stripped fragments of cytoplasm from the neoplastic lymphoid cells found in the background of aspirate smears, known as lymphoglandular

bodies (fig. 13-22), also supports a hematopoietic process but does not address malignancy.

The differential diagnosis depends on the type of lymphoma and is similar in histology and cytology. Cellular cohesion is absent in lymphoma and a feature of carcinomas and sarcomas. Large cell lymphomas are composed of cells with nuclei slightly larger than those of a histiocyte and small cell lymphomas are composed of cells slightly larger than mature lymphocytes. The nuclei are irregular in all cases, albeit subtly in small lymphocytic lymphoma. Although the nuclei of the more common large B-cell lymphomas are characteristically pleomorphic, they can range from relatively round and well differentiated, mimicking a pancreatic endocrine neoplasm, to anaplastic and bizarre, mimicking undifferentiated carcinoma or sarcoma. Distinguishing features include the chromatin pattern that is typically dispersed with peripheral clumping in lymphoma, coarse and speckled ("salt and pepper") in pancreatic endocrine tumors, and dense, irregular, and darkly staining in undifferentiated carcinoma and sarcoma. In addition, cytoplasmic features can help in the differential diagnosis. Large cell lymphomas often have relatively scant, eccentric cytoplasmic tags that can look like hand mirror handles on cytology smears, whereas pancreatic endocrine tumors have eccentric but more abundant, granular cytoplasm and undifferentiated

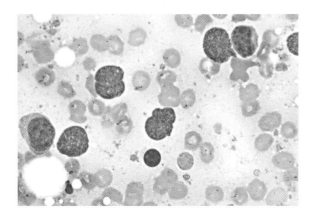

Figure 13-22

NON-HODGKIN'S LYMPHOMA:
LARGE B-CELL LYMPHOMA

A noncohesive population of large neoplastic cells, with peripherally clumped chromatin. The occasionally stripped cytoplasm forms globules in the background (lympho-glandular bodies) (direct smear; Romanowsky stain).

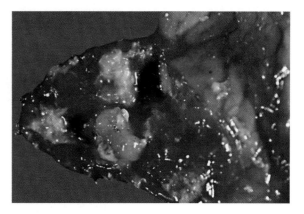

Figure 13-23

MATURE CYSTIC TERATOMA

The ectodermal, endodermal, and mesodermal compon-ents produce the variegated gross appearance of this neoplasm.

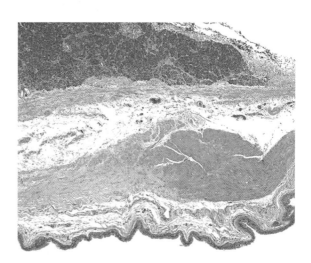

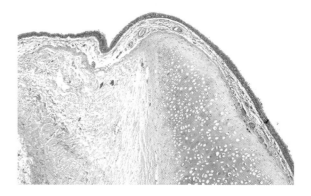

Figure 13-24

MATURE CYSTIC TERATOMA

Respiratory epithelium overlies mature cartilage on the bottom and smooth muscle at the top. Benign pancreatic parenchyma is on the very top.

carcinomas and sarcomas have more circumfer-ential and irregular cytoplasmic features.

The proposed treatment of patients with pri-mary pancreatic lymphoma varies from chemo-therapy alone (64,70) to combined chemo-therapy and radiation therapy (11). A more ag-gressive approach with surgical debulking prior to combined chemotherapy and radiotherapy has been proposed (8).

MISCELLANEOUS NEOPLASMS

Mature Cystic Teratoma

Mature cystic teratoma, a neoplasm with dif-ferentiation along lines of multiple germ cell layers, can arise in any organ, including the pan-creas (3,77). The radiologic appearance depends on the proportion of the ectodermal, endoder-mal, and mesodermal components. Similarly, the gross (fig. 13-23) and histologic appearances vary, but as in other sites, these neoplasms are recog-nized by the presence of mature tissue elements from the three germlines (fig. 13-24). Those re-ported in the pancreas have predominantly been monodermal teratomas with only ectodermal de-rivatives and are referred to as *dermoid cysts*. Ages reported range from 2 to 53 years, with a mean of 29 years (3). While children present with vom-iting, adults typically present with dyspepsia, malaise, epigastric discomfort, and weight loss. Most neoplasms are palpable and radiographic

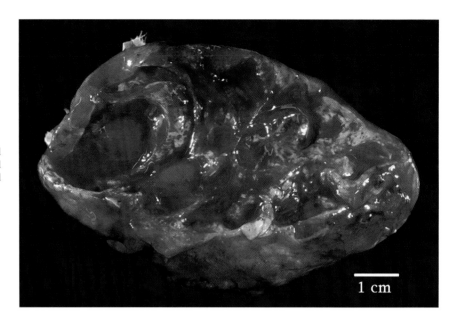

Figure 13-25

EXTRAADRENAL PARAGANGLIOMA

The cut surface is tan and fleshy but may be discolored red to brown from congestion and hemorrhage.

1 cm

evidence of a variegated solid and cystic mass with calcifications favors the diagnosis.

These neoplasms are invariably benign. Thorough gross and histologic examinations are warranted, however, to assess for any areas of firm, solid, fleshy, friable or necrotic tissue that may signify the presence of a carcinoma arising within the teratoma, a finding that portends a more aggressive biologic behavior, as in the ovary. Dermoid cysts are distinguished from lymphoepithelial cysts by the presence of dermal appendages or hair, features lacking in lymphoepithelial cysts, although sebaceous cells can be found in both dermoid and lymphoepithelial cysts.

Adenomatoid Tumor

Adenomatoid tumor, a benign neoplasm with mesothelial differentiation most common in the male and female genital tract, has been reported mimicking a pancreatic endocrine tumor clinically, radiologically, and cytologically (52). The neoplasm presented as a 1.5-cm, well-circumscribed, hypodense lesion in the pancreatic head of a 58-year-old woman. Endoscopic ultrasound-guided fine needle aspiration biopsy produced a bland, monotonous, predominantly non-cohesive epithelial cell proliferation with coarse chromatin and wispy cytoplasm, mimicking a pancreatic endocrine tumor. The characteristic histologic appearance of a spindled and epithelioid proliferation forming tubules, cords, and nests within a dense fibrous stroma and immuno-

histochemical analysis showing labeling with pancytokeratin, CK5/6, epithelial membrane antigen, calretinin, and CD99 led to the correct diagnosis of an adenomatoid tumor.

Extraadrenal Paraganglioma

Extraadrenal paraganglioma arises from the extraadrenal paraganglia, collections of neuroendocrine cells dispersed centripetally and symmetrically throughout the body. Paragangliomas also rarely arise in the ampulla of Vater and the retroperitoneum where they present in a peripancreatic location, mimicking a primary pancreatic neoplasm. Paragangliomas around the pancreas are associated with the sympathoadrenal neuroendocrine system.

Grossly, peripancreatic paraganglioma appears as a well-demarcated, firm, rubbery mass with pushing borders and a thin fibrous pseudocapsule. The cut surface of the neoplasm is tan and fleshy but may be discolored red to brown from congestion and hemorrhage (fig. 13-25). Cystic degeneration and necrosis occur. Needle puncture of paragangliomas is contraindicated due to the risk of hypertensive crisis (5).

Histologically and cytologically, the typical pattern is the "zellballen" arrangement of chief cells in varying sized organoid nests in an unpolarized, haphazard arrangement; true acini or rosettes as might be observed in pancreatic endocrine neoplasms are not observed (fig. 13-26). On histology and cytology, the chief cells have

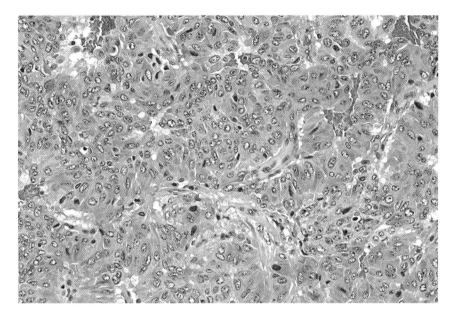

Figure 13-26

EXTRAADRENAL PARAGANGLIOMA

The neoplasm is characterized by the typical "zellballen" arrangement of unpolarized, haphazardly arranged neoplastic cells.

round, regular nuclei with basophilic cytoplasm than can sometimes appear granular. Large, bizarre cells with hyperchromatic nuclei and frequent intranuclear inclusions are common.

Peripancreatic paragangliomas are likely to be confused with pancreatic endocrine neoplasms, which can be histologically very similar and are much more common. Both neoplasms immunolabel for general endocrine markers, although chromogranin expression is usually more pronounced in paragangliomas. Expression of keratin and islet peptides favors a diagnosis of pancreatic endocrine neoplasm, whereas a well-formed sustentacular cell network that expresses S-100 protein is more common (though not exclusive) in paragangliomas. Most paragangliomas are peripancreatic rather than intrapancreatic, while well-differentiated pancreatic endocrine neoplasms are almost always intrapancreatic neoplasms.

REFERENCES

1. Abe H, Kubota K, Noie T, Bandai Y, Makuuchi M. Cystic lymphangioma of the pancreas: a case report with special reference to embryological development. Am J Gastroenterol 1997;92: 1566-7.
2. Adsay NV, Andea A, Basturk O, Kilinc N, Nassar H, Cheng JD. Secondary tumors of the pancreas: an analysis of a surgical and autopsy database and review of the literature. Virchows Arch 2004;444:527-35.
3. Adsay NV, Hasteh F, Cheng JD, Klimstra DS. Squamous-lined cysts of the pancreas: lymphoepithelial cysts, dermoid cysts (teratomas), and accessory-splenic epidermoid cysts. Semin Diagn Pathol 2000;17:56-65.
4. Adsay V, Cheng J, Athanasian E, Gerald W, Rosai J. Primary desmoplastic small cell tumor of soft tissues and bone of the hand. Am J Surg Pathol 1999;23:1408-13.
5. Akdamar MK, Eltoum I, Eloubeidi MA. Retroperitoneal paraganglioma: EUS appearance and risk associated with EUS-guided FNA. Gastrointest Endosc 2004;60:1018-21.
6. Argani P, Perez-Ordonez B, Xiao H, Caruana SM, Huvos AG, Ladanyi M. Olfactory neuroblastoma is not related to the Ewing family of tumors: absence of WES/FLI1 gene fusion and MIC2 expression. Am J Surg Pathol 1998;22:391-8.
7. Axelson J, Dawiskiba S, Akerman M, Ihse I. Connective tissue tumors. In: Howard JW, Idezuki Y, Ihes I, Prinz RA, eds. Surgical diseases of the pancreas, 3rd ed. Baltimore: Williams & Wilkins; 1998:633-6.

8. Behrns KE, Sarr MG, Strickler JG. Pancreatic lymphoma: is it a surgical disease? Pancreas 1994;9: 662-7.

9. Berman J, O'Leary TJ. Gastrointestinal stromal tumor workshop. Hum Pathol 2001;32:578-82.

10. Bigard MA, Boissel P, Regent D, Froment N. Intrapancreatic lipoma. First case in the literature. Gastroenterol Clin Biol 1989;13:505-7.

10a. Blackstein ME, Blay JY, Corless C, et al. Canadian Advisory Committee on GIST. Gastrointestinal stromal tumors: consensus statement on diagnosis and treatment. Can J Gastroenterol 2006;20:157-63.

11. Bouvet M, Staerkel GA, Spitz FR, et al. Primary pancreatic lymphoma. Surgery 1998;123:382-90.

12. Brown SZ, Owen DA, O'Connell JX, Scudamore CH. Schwannoma of the pancreas: a report of two cases and a review of the literature. Mod Pathol 1998;11:1178-82.

13. Bulchmann G, Schuster T, Haas RJ, Joppich I. Primitive neuroectodermal tumor of the pancreas. An extremely rare tumor. Case report and review of the literature. Klin Padiatr 2000;212: 185-8.

14. Cafferty LL, Katz RL, Ordonez NG, Carrasco CH, Cabanillas FR. Fine needle aspiration diagnosis of intra-abdominal and retroperitoneal lymphomas by a morphologic and immunocytochemical approach. Cancer 1990;65:72-7.

15. Casadei R, Minni F, Selva S, Marrano N, Marrano D. Cystic lymphangioma of the pancreas: anatomoclinical, diagnostic and therapeutic considerations regarding three personal observations and review of the literature. Hepatogastroenterology 2003;50:1681-6.

16. Chandrasoma P, Fitzgibbons P. Granular cell tumor of the intrapancreatic common bile duct. Cancer 1984;53:2178-82.

17. Chang WT, Lee KT, Yang SF. Cavernous hemangioma of the pancreas: report of a case. Pancreas 2003;26:310-2.

18. Coffin CM, Patel A, Perkins S, Elenitoba-Johnson KS, Perlman E, Griffin CA. ALK1 and p80 expression and chromosomal rearrangements involving 2p23 in inflammatory myofibroblastic tumor. Mod Pathol 2001;14:569-76.

19. Coffin CM, Watterson J, Priest JR, Dehner LP. Extrapulmonary inflammatory myofibroblastic tumor (inflammatory pseudotumor). A clinicopathologic and immunohistochemical study of 84 cases. Am J Surg Pathol 1995;19:859-72.

20. Danner DB, Hruban RH, Pitt HA, Hayashi R, Griffin CA, Perlman EJ. Primitive neuroectodermal tumor arising in the pancreas. Mod Pathol 1994;7:200-4.

21. de Alava E, Ladanyi M, Rosai J, Gerald WL. Detection of chimeric transcripts in desmoplastic small round cell tumor and related developmental tumors by reverse transcriptase polymerase chain reaction. A specific diagnostic assay. Am J Pathol 1995;147:1584-91.

22. Deb G, Jenkner A, De Sio L, et al. Spindle cell (kaposiform) hemangioendothelioma with Kasabach-Merritt syndrome in an infant: successful treatment with alpha-2A interferon. Med Pediatr Oncol 1997;28:358-61.

23. DiMaggio EM, Solcia M, Dore R, et al. Intrapancreatic lipoma: first case diagnosed with CT. AJR Am J Roentgenol 1996;167:56-7.

24. Dong HY, Harris NL, Preffer FI, Pitman MB. Fine-needle aspiration biopsy in the diagnosis and classification of primary and recurrent lymphoma: a retrospective analysis of the utility of cytomorphology and flow cytometry. Mod Pathol 2001;14:472-81.

25. Elliott GB, Kliman MR, Elliott KA. Persistence of lymphatico-venous shunts at the level of the microcirculation. Their relationship to "lymphangioma" of mesentery. Ann Surg 1970;172:131-6.

26. Elliott TE, Albertazzi VJ, Danto LA. Pancreatic liposarcoma: case report with review of retroperitoneal liposarcomas. Cancer 1980;45:1720-3.

27. Emerson L, Layfield LJ, Reiss R, Mulvihill S, Holden J. Malignant islet cell tumor with sarcomatous differentiation. Mod Pathol 2001;14:1187-91.

28. Ferry JA, Harris NL. Atlas of lymphoid hyperplasia and lymphoma. Philadelphia: W.B. Saunders; 1997:180-8.

29. Gerald WL, Rosai J. Case 2. Desmoplastic small cell tumor with divergent differentiation. Pediatr Pathol 1989;9:177-83.

30. Godart S. Embryological significance of lymphangioma. Arch Dis Child 1966;41:204-6.

31. Goldszmidt D, Pariente D, Yandza T, Dubousset AM, Valayer J. Kasabach-Merritt syndrome with pancreatic hemangioma in an infant. Arch Fr Pediatr 1993;50:593-7.

32. Griffin CA, Hawkins AL, Dvorak C, Henkle C, Ellingham T, Perlman EJ. Recurrent involvement of 2p23 inflammatory myofibroblastic tumors. Cancer Research 1999;59:2776-80.

33. Heywood G, Smyrk TC, Donohue JH. Primary angiomyolipoma of the pancreas. Pancreas 2004;28:443-5.

34. Hilliard RI, McKendry JB, Phillips MJ. Congenital abnormalities of the lymphatic system: a new clinical classification. Pediatrics 1990;86:988-94.

35. Hirose T, Maeda T, Furuya K, Kiyasu Y, Kawasaki H. Malignant peripheral nerve sheath tumor of the pancreas with perineurial cell differentiation. Ultrastruct Pathol 1998;22:227-31.

36. Ishikawa O, Matsui Y, Aoki Y, Iwanaga T, Terasawa T, Wada A. Leiomyosarcoma of the pancreas. Report of a case and review of the literature. Am J Surg Pathol 1981;5:597-602.

37. Katz DS, Hines J, Math KR, Nardi PM, Mindelzun RE, Lane MJ. Using CT to reveal fat-containing abnormalities of the pancreas. AJR Am J Roentgenol 1999;172:393-6.

38. Lae M, Roche PC, Jin L, Lloyd RV, Nascimento AG. Desmoplastic small round cell tumor: a clinicopathologic, immunohistochemical, and molecular study of 32 tumors. Am J Surg Pathol 2002;26:823-35.

39. Lazure T, Tebboune N, Ben Lagha N, Triller MF, Pariente D, Fabre M. [Pancreatic vascular tumours of childhood: a heterogeneous nosologic spectrum.] Ann Pathol 2002;22:226-9. [French.]

40. Lee JS, Kim HS, Jung JJ, et al. Ancient schwannoma of the pancreas mimicking a cystic tumor. Virchows Arch 2001;439:697-9.

41. Lüttges J, Mentzel T, Hubner G, et al. Solitary fibrous tumour of the pancreas: a new member of the small group of mesenchymal pancreatic tumours. Virchows Arch 1999;435:37-42.

42. Lüttges J, Pierre E, Zamboni G, et al. [Malignant non-epithelial tumors of the pancreas.] Pathologe 1997;18:233-7. [German.]

43. Lyons LL, North PE, Mac-Moune Lai F, Stoler MH, Folpe AL, Weiss SW. Kaposiform hemangioendothelioma: a study of 33 cases emphasizing its pathologic, immunophenotypic, and biologic uniqueness from juvenile hemangioma. Am J Surg Pathol 2004;28:559-68.

43a. Mizukami H, Yajima N, Wada R, et al. Pancreatic malignant fibrous histiocytoma, inflammatory myofibroblastic tumor, and inflammatory pseudotumor related to autoimmune pancreatitis: characterization and differential diagnosis. Virchows Arch 2006;448:552-60.

44. Monforte-Munoz H, Kapoor N, Albores-Saavedra J. Epstein-Barr virus-associated leiomyomatosis and posttransplant lymphoproliferative disorder in a child with severe combined immunodeficiency: case report and review of the literature. Pediatr Dev Pathol 2003;6:449-57.

45. Mori M, Miyazaki K, Motoyama K, Kitahara K. Benign nonepithelial fibroma in the pancreas. J Hepatobiliary Pancreat Surg 2002;9:646-9.

46. Movahedi-Lankarani S, Hruban RH, Westra WH, Klimstra DS. Primitive neuroectodermal tumors of the pancreas: a report of seven cases of rare neoplasm. Am J Surg Pathol 2002;26:1040-7.

47. Neibling HA. Primary sarcoma of the pancreas. Am Surg 1968;34:690-3.

48. Niedt GW, Greco MA, Wieczorek R, Blanc WA, Knowles DM 2nd. Hemangioma with Kaposi's sarcoma-like features: report of two cases. Pediatr Pathol 1989;5:567-75.

49. Nishimura R, Takakuwa T, Hoshida Y, Tsujimoto M, Aozasa K. Primary pancreatic lymphoma: clinicopathological analysis of 19 cases from Japan and review of the literature. Oncology 2001;60:322-9.

50. Nojiri T, Unemura Y, Hashimoto K, Yamazaki Y, Ikegami M. Pancreatic granular cell tumor combined with carcinoma in situ. Pathol Int 2001;51:879-82.

51. Ordonez NG. Desmoplastic small round cell tumor: II: an ultrastructural and immunohistochemical study with emphasis on new immunohistochemical markers. Am J Surg Pathol 1998;22:1314-27.

52. Overstreet K, Wixom C, Shabaik A, Bouvet M, Herndier B. Adenomatoid tumor of the pancreas: a case report with comparison of histology and aspiration cytology. Mod Pathol 2003;16:613-7.

53. Paal E, Thompson LD, Heffess CS. A clinicopathologic and immunohistochemical study of ten pancreatic lymphangiomas and a review of the literature. Cancer 1998;82:2150-8.

53a. Pascal RR, Sullivan L, Hauser L, Ferzli G. Primary malignant fibrohistiocytoma of the pancreas. Hum Pathol 1989;20:1215-7.

53b. Popescu LM, Hinescu ME, Ionescu N, Ciontea SM, Cretoiu D, Ardelean C. Interstitial cells of Cajal in the pancreas. J Cell Mol Med 2005;9:169-90.

54. Pungpapong S, Geiger XJ, Raimondo M. Inflammatory myofibroblastic tumor presenting as a pancreatic mass: a case report and review of the literature. JOP 2004;5:360-7.

55. Ramani P, Shah A. Lymphangiomatosis. Histologic and immunohistochemical analysis of four cases. Am J Surg Pathol 1993;17:329-35.

56. Ramuz O, Lelong B, Giovannini M, et al. "Sugar" tumor of the pancreas: a rare entity that is diagnosable on preoperative fine-needle biopsy. Virchows Arch 2005;446:555-9.

57. Raut CP, Fernandez-del Castillo C. Giant lipoma of the pancreas: case report and review of lipomatous lesions of the pancreas. Pancreas 2003;26:97-9.

58. Reith JD, Goldblum JR, Lyles RH, Weiss SW. Extragastrointestinal (soft tissue) stromal tumors: an analysis of 48 cases with emphasis on histologic predictors of outcome. Mod Pathol 2000;13:577-85.

59. Sabin FR. The lymphatic system in human embryos, with a consideration of the morphology of the system as a whole. Am J Anat 1909;9:43-91.

59a. Saif MW. Primary pancreatic lymphoma. JOP 2006;7:262-73.

60. Schulz AS, Urban J, Gessler P, Behnisch W, Kohne E, Heymer B. Anaemia, thrombocytopenia and coagulopathy due to occult diffuse infantile haemangiomatosis of spleen and pancreas. Eur J Pediatr 1999;158:379-83.

61. Shih SL, Chen BF, Chen SH, Chi T, Sheu CY. Spindle cell hemangioendothelioma of the pancreas treated with interferon-alpha2a. Pancreas 1998;16:215-6.

62. Tan G, Vitellas K, Morrison C, Frankel WL. Cystic schwannoma of the pancreas. Ann Diagn Pathol 2003;7:285-91.

63. Tebboune N, Lazure T, Fabre M, Pariente D. Pancreatic haemangioma in infancy: the place of radiology. Pediatr Radiol 2003;33:621-3.

64. Tuchek JM, De Jong SA, Pickleman J. Diagnosis, surgical intervention, and prognosis of primary pancreatic lymphoma. Am Surg 1993;59:513-8.

65. Urban BA, Fishman EK, Hruban RH, Cameron JL. CT findings in cystic schwannoma of the pancreas. J Comput Assist Tomogr 1992;16:492-3.

66. Villegas-Alvarez F, de Leon-Bojorge BY. [Hemangioendothelioma of the pancreas and choledochus, as a cause of cholestatic neonatal and Kasabach-Merrit syndromes.] Bol Med Hosp Infant Mex 1989;46:672-5. [Spanish.]

67. Volmar KE, Routbort MJ, Jones CK, Xie HB. Primary pancreatic lymphoma evaluated by fine-needle aspiration. Findings in 14 cases. Am J Clin Pathol 2004;121:898-903.

68. Wagliore MP, Stephens DH, Soule EH, McLeod RA. Lipomatous tumors of the abdominal cavity: CT appearance and pathologic correlation. AJR Am J Roentgenol 1981;137:539-45.

69. Walsh SV, Evangelista F, Khettry U. Inflammatory myofibroblastic tumor of the pancreaticobiliary region: morphologic and immunocytochemical study of three cases. Am J Surg Pathol 1998;22:412-8.

70. Webb TH, Lillemoe KD, Pitt HA, Jones RJ, Cameron JL. Pancreatic lymphoma. Is surgery mandatory for diagnosis or treatment? Ann Surg 1989;209:25-30.

71. Weidner N, Tjoe J. Immunohistochemical profile of monoclonal antibody 013: antibody that recognizes glycoprotein p30/32MIC2 and is useful in diagnosing Ewing's sarcoma and peripheral neuroepithelioma. Am J Surg Pathol 1994;18:486-94.

72. Wieczorek TJ, Faquin WC, Rubin BP, Cibas ES. Cytologic diagnosis of gastrointestinal stromal tumor with emphasis on the differential diagnosis with leiomyosarcoma. Cancer 2001;93:276-87.

73. Wreesmann V, van Eijck CH, Naus DC, van Velthuysen ML, Jeekel J, Mooi WI. Inflammatory pseudotumour (inflammatory myofibroblastic tumour) of the pancreas: a report of six cases associated with obliterative phlebitis. Histopathology 2001;38:105-10.

74. Yamaura K, Kato K, Miyazawa M, et al. Stromal tumor of the pancreas with expression of c-kit protein: report of a case. J Gastroenterol Hepatol 2004;19:467-70.

75. Young NA, Al-Saleem TI, Ehya H, Smith MR. Utilization of fine-needle aspiration cytology and flow cytometry in the diagnosis and subclassification of primary and recurrent lymphoma. Cancer 1998;84:252-61.

76. Yousem SA, Shaw H, Cieply K. Involvement of 2p23 in pulmonary inflammatory pseudotumors. Hum Pathol 2001;32:428-33.

77. Yu CW, Liu K, Lin WC, Li YW. Mature cystic teratoma of the pancreas in a child. Pediatr Radiol 2003;33:266-8.

78. Zalatnai A, Kovacs M, Flautner L, Sipos B, Sarkady E, Bocsi J. Pancreatic leiomyosarcoma. Case report with immunohistochemical and flow cytometric studies. Virchows Arch 1998;432:469-72.

79. Zamboni G, Pea M, Martignoni G, et al. Clear cell "sugar" tumour of the pancreas. A novel member of the family of lesions characterized by the presence of perivascular epithelioid cells. Am J Surg Pathol 1996;20:722-30.

80. Zukerberg LR, Nickoloff BJ, Weiss SW. Kaposiform hemangioendothelioma of infancy and childhood. An aggressive neoplasm associated with Kasabach-Merritt syndrome and lymphangiomatosis. Am J Surg Pathol 1993;17:321-8.

14 SECONDARY NEOPLASMS

Once only commonly diagnosed at autopsy, secondary neoplasms of the pancreas have been increasingly recognized in the antemortem period thanks to the improvements in imaging, the use of specific serum markers for the surveillance of patients with known malignancies, and the broader availability of fine needle aspiration biopsy. Although secondary neoplasms involving the pancreas can present significant clinical, radiologic, and diagnostic challenges, differentiating primary neoplasms from secondary pancreatic malignancies has important therapeutic implications. Most secondary neoplasms involving the pancreas are not treated surgically, although surgical resection is being increasingly performed for isolated metastases to the pancreas (22,25).

Secondary neoplasms involving the pancreas are less common than primary neoplasms, and pancreatic involvement as the sole site of metastatic disease is rare. The average age at presentation for patients with a secondary neoplasm involving the pancreas is 60 years, an age similar to that of patients with primary carcinomas of the pancreas (2,27). Most patients are asymptomatic, have vague, nonspecific symptoms, or have symptoms of disseminated malignancy (2,12). The most common symptoms include abdominal pain, jaundice, early satiety, and weight loss. Some patients present with pancreatitis. Gastrointestinal hemorrhage has been reported as a relatively unique presenting symptom of patients with metastatic renal cell carcinoma in some, but not all, series (2,12,38). Importantly, the majority of patients with secondary neoplasms involving the pancreas have a history of an extrapancreatic malignancy. A good clinical history is therefore extremely helpful when considering the diagnosis of a secondary neoplasm.

Neoplasms originating outside of the pancreas may secondarily involve the pancreas through direct extension, hematogenous or lymphatic metastases, or as a manifestation of systemic disease. In an autopsy series of 344 patients with secondary malignancies of the pancreas, 16 (5 percent) involved the pancreas by direct extension, 261 (75 percent) by hematogenous metastases, and 67 (19 percent) were systemic malignancies (lymphoma and leukemia) (10).

Carcinomas of the gastrointestinal tract are the neoplasms most likely to secondarily involve the pancreas by direct extension. These include carcinomas of the ampulla of Vater, extrahepatic bile ducts, duodenum, and stomach (27). Secondary neoplasms may also involve the pancreas by lymphatic or hematogenous metastases. The lymphatic system is the likely route of spread for carcinomas of the colon, given the pattern of lymphatic drainage along the mesocolon that overlies the pancreas (9). Similarly, renal cell carcinoma may metastasize to the pancreas from retrograde flow of lymph following lymphatic invasion within the kidney (36). Hematogenous spread, however, is much more common than lymphatic spread as evidenced by the lack of correlation between the intraparenchymal location of multiple metastatic deposits and the anatomic location of peripancreatic lymph nodes (12,33).

Carcinomas are by far the most common type of secondary neoplasm in the pancreas, but the prevalence and type of carcinoma are related to the population studied as well as the specimen types evaluated, e.g., autopsy versus surgical specimens (Tables 14-1, 14-2) (2). In autopsy series, the most common origin for metastases to the pancreas includes lung (25 percent), breast (13 percent), melanoma (11 percent), stomach (10 percent), colorectum (6 percent), kidney (4 percent), and ovary (4 percent) (Table 14-1). Since most such patients have widely disseminated disease, with the pancreas representing one of many involved organs, only a minority (8.5 percent) are clinically suspected of having primary pancreatic neoplasms prior to autopsy. The pancreas is diffusely involved in

Table 14-1

ORIGIN OF PANCREATIC METASTASES IN AUTOPSY SERIES[a]

Reference	Total Number	Lung	Breast	Melan-oma	Stomach	Colo-rectal	Kidney	Ovary	Other
Abrams (1)	116	16	23	0	28	6	2	10	31
Berge (5)	189	64	11	34	12	11	7	5	45
Cubilla (10)	261	49	51	23	19	25	7	13	74
Havig (17)	26	9	0	0	9	0	0	1	7
Willis (42)									
Personal series[b]	15	2	3	1	0	1	1	0	7
Literature[c]	127	34	12	31	0	0	12	0	38
Adsay (2)	81	34	3	2	10	6	4	1	21
Total	815	208(25%)	103(13%)	91(11%)	78(10%)	49(6%)	33(4%)	30(4%)	223(27%)[d]

[a]Table modified from reference 12.
[b]Personal review of cases by Willis.
[c]Literature review by Willis (42).
[d]Includes lymphoma/leukemia and metastatic neoplasms infrequently seen in any individual series including neoplasms of the soft tissues, esophagus, prostate gland, uterine cervix, liver, thyroid gland, biliary tract, small intestine, head and neck, salivary gland, urinary tract, adrenal gland, vulva, ovary, pleura, and skin.

Table 14-2

ORIGIN OF PANCREATIC METASTASES IN CLINICAL SERIES[a]

Reference	Total Number	Lung	Kidney	Breast	Colorectal	Melanoma	Liver	Other
Benning (4)	10	4	0	0	0	0	1	5
Biset (6)	7	2	3	0	0	0	0	2
Boudghene (7)	24	9	6	1	0	4	0	4
Carson (8)	11	4	1	1	1	0	1	3
Muranka (26)	30	10	1	5	2	2	3	7
Opacher (28)	13	1	6	1	0	0	2	3
Roland (31)	27	5	3	3	6	2	0	8
Rumancik (33)	7	0	2	2	0	1	0	2
Swenson (37)	12	3	0	0	3	0	1	5
Wernecke (40)	7	2	0	0	2	0	0	3
Whittington (41)	4	1	1	2	0	0	0	0
Adsay (2)	38	2	6	0	2	0	1	27[b]
Total	190	43(23%)	29(15%)	15(8%)	16(8%)	9(5%)	9(5%)	69(36%)[c]

[a]Table modified from reference 12.
[b]11 of the 27 other cases were non-Hodgkin's lymphoma.
[c]Includes leukemia and lymphoma, and metastases from primary sites infrequent in any individual series, such as primary neoplasms of the stomach, esophagus, uterus (fundus and cervix), ovary, prostate gland, skin, soft tissue sarcomas, lymphomas/leukemias, and neoplasms of unknown primary.

most cases (75 percent), but isolated metastatic deposits also develop, most often to the head of the pancreas. Most metastatic deposits are grossly evident, but 25 percent are only detected at the microscopic level.

In surgical series, the most common sites of origin for metastases to the pancreas are from the lung (23 percent), kidney (15 percent), breast (8 percent), colorectum (8 percent), and melanoma (5 percent) (Table 14-2). Compared to autopsy-

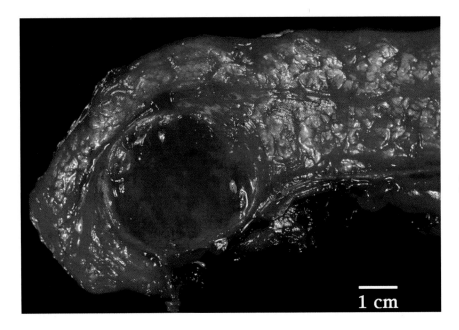

Figure 14-1

METASTATIC RENAL CELL CARCINOMA

Necrosis and hemorrhage in a well-circumscribed metastasis cause a red-brown discoloration.

1 cm

based series, many more (35 percent) of these surgically treated cases are clinically suspected of being primary pancreatic neoplasms, in many cases because the pancreas is the only site of metastatic involvement. Given that surgical exploration of pancreatic masses is biased toward those patients that present with pancreatic symptoms and/or are clinically suspected of having pancreatic primaries, autopsy analyses of secondary pancreatic neoplasms are more likely a better estimate of the relative frequency of the types of neoplasms that metastasize to the pancreas.

Only 2 to 4 percent of secondary neoplasms involving the pancreas are biopsied or resected (2,31). Secondary neoplasms that form solitary masses can clinically and radiologically mimic a primary pancreatic neoplasm. This is especially true of lymphoma and renal cell carcinoma (2,9). These solitary metastases to the pancreas can be diagnostically challenging, particularly if one is not aware of the patient's medical history (8,14).

Histologically, metastases often involve the pancreatic lobules, replacing normal acinar tissue and expanding the interlobular septa. The islets are usually spared and may be larger at the periphery of the metastatic deposit. This pattern of parenchymal involvement is not specific for metastases, however, the presence of one or more distinct, well-circumscribed nodules of neoplastic cells, not typical of the usual

ductal adenocarcinoma, should raise suspicion of a metastatic neoplasm.

METASTATIC RENAL CELL CARCINOMA

Renal cell carcinoma deserves special mention. Renal cell carcinoma has a propensity to metastasize as a solitary mass in the pancreas (30), it can metastasize years after the initial diagnosis of a renal primary (20), and patients with renal cell carcinoma can have a good long-term prognosis following surgical resection of the metastatic deposits (20,24,25,29). Any pancreatic mass in a patient with even a remote history of renal cell carcinoma should be clinically suspicious for a metastasis.

When it presents as a solitary metastasis, renal cell carcinoma can closely mimic a primary neoplasm. Radiologically, the lesion generally appears hypoechoic on ultrasound relative to the surrounding pancreatic parenchyma, whereas computerized tomography (CT) reveals an enhancing mass that may demonstrate hypervascularity on selective angiography (18). In a series of 21 cases of surgically resected metastatic renal cell carcinomas (38), the metastases ranged in size from 1.5 to 12.0 cm (mean, 4.0 cm) and involved the head alone (6 cases), the tail alone (4 cases), the body and tail (7 cases), or the entire pancreas (4 cases). Grossly, metastatic renal cell carcinoma forms well-circumscribed bright yellow-orange to red-brown to white-gray

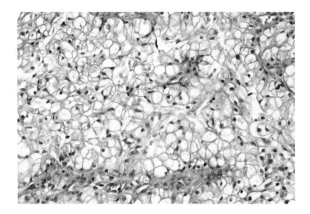

Figure 14-2

METASTATIC RENAL CELL CARCINOMA

Sheets, small nests, and cords of polygonal cells with abundant clear cytoplasm and bland, low-grade, slightly eccentric nuclei.

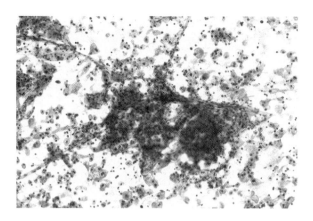

Figure 14-3

METASTATIC RENAL CELL CARCINOMA

A prominent vascular component is a common finding on aspirates of renal cell carcinoma (direct smear; Papanicolaou stain).

masses that occasionally show necrosis, hemorrhage, and cystic degeneration (fig. 14-1).

Conventional (clear cell) renal cell carcinoma is the most common histologic type to metastasize to the pancreas. As such, the predominant histologic pattern is one of sheets, small nests, and cords of polygonal cells with abundant clear cytoplasm and usually bland, low-grade, slightly eccentric nuclei with prominent nucleoli (fig. 14-2) (38). A rich sinusoidal vascular network separates the nests and cords of neoplastic cells, and hemorrhage is commonly present, including within neoplastic glandular lumens. This vascular network is recognized in aspirate smears as an arborizing proliferation of capillaries, and is a clue to the diagnosis (fig. 14-3) (39). A sarcomatoid component may be present, but this is also a rare finding and generally a minor component of an otherwise typical clear cell neoplasm.

Cytologically, cells of renal cell carcinoma appear as large polygonal clear cells arranged in cohesive clusters and as single cells. The nuclear features on fixed material show characteristic round, central nuclei and prominent, central nucleoli (fig. 14-4, left). Air-dried Romanowsky-stained smears enhance the microvesicular cytoplasm and show uniformly "punched out" cytoplasmic holes (fig. 14-4, right).

The differential diagnosis of a solid pancreatic clear cell neoplasm should include a primary ductal adenocarcinoma with clear cell or foamy gland change, a well-differentiated pan-

creatic endocrine neoplasm (PEN) with clear cell features, the extremely rare PEComa or "sugar tumor," solid serous adenoma, and other metastatic carcinomas with clear cells such as adenocarcinoma of the ovary.

Ductal adenocarcinoma of the pancreas with clear cell or foamy gland change enters the differential diagnosis primarily on fine needle aspiration biopsy (3). The cytology of aspirated single cells and nests of neoplastic cells of pure foamy gland adenocarcinoma can be difficult to distinguish from renal cell carcinoma. Both neoplasms are characterized by an abundance of clear cytoplasm with uniformly sized microvesicles and bland, slightly atypical nuclei. In difficult cases, the presence of a separate component of conventional ductal adenocarcinoma on cytology and cell block material can help establish the diagnosis of pancreatic carcinoma despite the presence of bland clear epithelial cells (35). Histochemical and immunohistochemical labeling of the cells can also distinguish the two neoplasms. Foamy gland adenocarcinoma contains mucin and stains with periodic acid–Schiff (PAS), resistant to diastase, as well as antibodies to carcinoembryonic antigen (CEA) and MUC1, albeit weakly. In contrast, renal cell carcinoma typically contains glycogen which is PAS positive but sensitive to diastase, labels with antibodies to renal cell carcinoma markers (RCCma) and CD10, but does not label with antibodies to CEA or MUC1 (3).

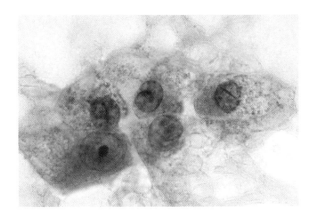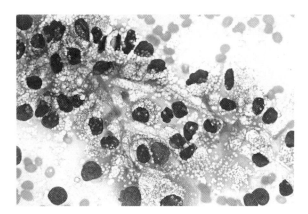

Figure 14-4

METASTATIC RENAL CELL CARCINOMA

Left: Round central nuclei and prominent central nucleoli are characteristic (direct smear; Papanicolaou stain).

Right: Air-dried Romanowsky-stained smears enhance the microvesicular cytoplasm with uniformly "punched out" cytoplasmic holes (direct smear; Romanowsky stain).

Well-differentiated PENs with clear cell change pose a diagnostic dilemma on both histology and cytology, especially in patients with von Hippel-Lindau (VHL) syndrome (19). Both renal cell carcinoma and PEN are common in patients with VHL syndrome, and the clear cell variant of PEN appears to be more common in these patients (23). Metastatic renal cell carcinoma to the pancreas, on the other hand, is unusual in patients with VHL (38), so the finding of a clear cell neoplasm in the pancreas of a patient with VHL favors a primary PEN over a metastatic neoplasm. Most clear cell PENs also have nonclear cells (19). The presence of a mixed clear cell and nonclear cell population of neoplastic cells on either cytology or histology favors a PEN. Immunohistochemical markers are helpful in difficult cases: in contrast to the clear cell PEN, metastatic renal cell carcinomas express CD10 and RCCma, but do not express endocrine markers.

PEComas are composed of a bland, glycogen-rich, clear epithelioid cell proliferation similar to renal cell carcinoma. Immunoreactivity of the neoplastic cells for HMB-45 and smooth muscle actin supports a diagnosis of a PEComa whereas the absence of such reactivity and immunolabeling of the cells for epithelial membrane antigen and vimentin support a diagnosis of metastatic renal cell carcinoma.

Solid serous adenoma has a similar architecture to renal cell carcinoma but lacks luminal hemorrhage and cytologic atypia, the nuclei usually being perfectly round and uniformly euchromatic. Both solid serous adenoma and renal cell carcinoma have cytoplasmic glycogen. Immunolabeling for RCCma, CD10, or vimentin suggests a diagnosis of renal cell carcinoma. Other clear cell carcinomas metastatic to the pancreas, such as from the ovary, should also be considered in the differential diagnosis.

Surgical resection of solitary metastases of renal cell carcinoma is the treatment of choice as patients have good long-term survival. Eleven of 23 patients with metastatic renal cell carcinoma underwent surgical resection in a series from the Mayo Clinic (7 distal and 3 total pancreatectomies, and 1 distal pancreatectomy followed by a total pancreatectomy 4 years later); 8 of the 11 were alive with a mean follow-up of 4 years, 6 of whom had no evidence of disease recurrence (15). A similarly good outcome was noted in a series of 16 patients by Stankard and Karl (34), with 12 patients alive 1 to 28 months postoperatively.

HEMATOPOIETIC MALIGNANCIES

Almost all hematopoietic malignancies, including leukemia (granulocytic sarcoma), non-Hodgkin's lymphoma, Hodgkin's disease, and extramedullary plasmacytoma, have been reported to involve the pancreas secondarily. *Non-Hodgkin's lymphoma (lymphoma)* is the most common. Although rare as a primary neoplasm

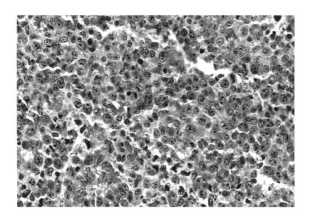 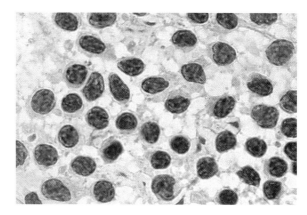

Figure 14-5

IMMUNOBLASTIC LYMPHOMA

Left: The more abundant cytoplasm and prominent nucleoli in immunoblastic lymphoma give the cells an epithelioid appearance.

Right: There is a diffuse, noncohesive population of small to medium-sized cells with little cytoplasm and peripherally clumped chromatin (direct smear; Papanicolaou stain).

in the pancreas, lymphoma commonly involves the pancreas secondarily: one third of the patients with lymphoma have pancreatic involvement (32). Like renal cell carcinoma, secondary involvement of the pancreas by lymphoma is prone to form solitary masses and therefore can mimic a primary neoplasm (2,4).

Histologic recognition of lymphoma is usually straightforward owing to the diffuse to nodular, nonorganoid proliferation of small blue cells that form an expansile mass lesion. Lymphomas composed of large cells, such as immunoblastic lymphoma (fig. 14-5, left), can be challenging because they have more abundant cytoplasm and prominent nucleoli, features that lend an epithelioid appearance to the cells. Entrapment of normal pancreatic structures can also be seen, and this is a helpful diagnostic feature.

The cytologic differential diagnosis is more challenging, as there are similarities in the aspirate smear pattern and cytomorphology between lymphoma and other cellular, solid neoplasms of the pancreas. Smears of lymphoma are highly cellular, often monotonous single cell proliferations of small to large cells with scant to no visible cytoplasm and round to angulated nuclei, peripheral chromatin, and occasionally prominent nucleoli (fig. 14-5, right). Acinar cell carcinoma, solid-pseudopapillary neoplasm, pancreatoblastoma, and PENs all produce cellu-

lar smears, but all usually demonstrate features of an epithelial neoplasm with cellular cohesion, polygonal cell shape, and relatively abundant cytoplasm compared to lymphoma. Aspirate smears and touch preparations suspicious for lymphoma should prompt additional sampling for flow cytometry immunophenotyping, thus allowing for subclassification and potentially precluding the need for additional sampling.

Plasmacytoma (multiple myeloma) may be confused with PENs on both histology (fig. 14-6) and cytology owing to the overlapping morphologic features of noncohesive single cells with eccentric cytoplasm that give a "plasmacytoid" appearance to the cells (13). Immunolabeling for cytokeratin, kappa and lambda light chains, chromogranin, and synaptophysin helps distinguish these two neoplasms.

METASTATIC MELANOMA

Surgical exploration of patients with abnormal *metastases from cutaneous melanoma* reveals pancreatic metastases in 16 percent (16). Metastatic deposits are usually solid black to brown masses, reflecting the presence of melanin pigment (fig. 14-7). Cystic degeneration is rare but can occur (11,21). Although most patients have a history of melanoma at the time of pancreatic biopsy, prompting complete immunophenotypic analysis of the neoplasm, it is estimated that 2 to 9 percent of patients with melanoma

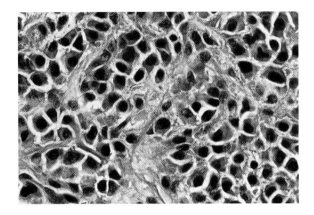

Figure 14-6

PLASMACYTOMA (MULTIPLE MYELOMA)

Epithelioid cells with eccentric cytoplasm mimic a pancreatic endocrine neoplasm.

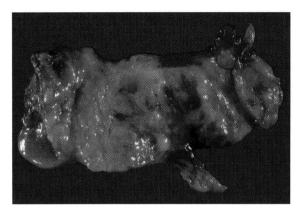

Figure 14-7

METASTATIC MALIGNANT MELANOMA

The black to brown discoloration reflects the presence of melanin pigment.

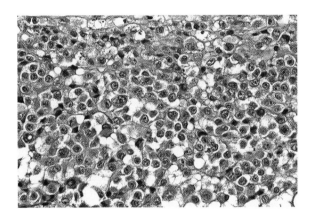

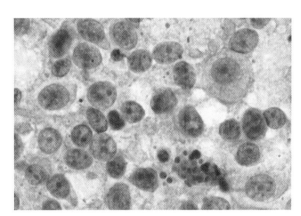

Figure 14-8

METASTATIC MALIGNANT MELANOMA

The classic histologic (left) and cytologic (right) appearance of melanoma is one of a diffuse, noncohesive and nonorganoid proliferation of an epithelioid neoplasm with large round nuclei, central macronucleoli, prominent nucleoli, and variably pigmented cytoplasm (direct smear; Papanicolaou stain).

metastatic to the pancreas have an occult primary and no known history (21), increasing the likelihood of a misdiagnosis of a primary pancreatic malignancy. The classic histologic (fig. 14-8, left) and cytologic (fig. 14-8, right) appearance of melanoma is a diffuse, noncohesive and nonorganoid proliferation of an epithelioid neoplasm, with large round nuclei, central macronucleoli, and moderate variably pigmented cytoplasm. Melanoma is known as "the great mimicker," because it can mimic all types of malignancies from lymphoma to carcinoma to sarcoma, as well as large cell, small cell, and spindle cell neoplasms. Intracytoplasmic and extracellular melanin pigment is not always present as a diagnostic clue, so immunolabeling for S-100 protein, HMB-45, Melan-A (MART-1), or other markers of melanocytic differentiation can aid the analysis of malignant epithelioid, spindle cell, and small cell neoplasms in the pancreas.

REFERENCES

1. Abrams HL, Spiro R, Goldstein N. Metastases in carcinoma; analysis of 1000 autopsied cases. Cancer 1950;3:74-85.
2. Adsay NV, Andea A, Basturk O, Kilinc N, Nassar H, Cheng JD. Secondary tumors of the pancreas: an analysis of a surgical and autopsy database and review of the literature. Virchows Arch 2004;444:527-35.
3. Adsay V, Logani S, Sarkar F, Crissman J, Vaitkevicius V. Foamy gland pattern of pancreatic ductal adenocarcinoma: a deceptively benign-appearing variant. Am J Surg Pathol 2000;24: 493-504.
4. Benning TL, Silverman JF, Berns LA, Geisinger KR. Fine needle aspiration of metastatic and hematologic malignancies clinically mimicking pancreatic carcinoma. Acta Cytol 1992;36:471-6.
5. Berge T, Lundberg S. Cancer in Malmo 1958-1969. An autopsy study. Acta Pathol Microbiol Scand Suppl 1977;260:1-235.
6. Biset JM, Laurent F, de Verbizier G, Houang B, Constantes G, Drouillard J. Ultrasound and computed tomographic findings in pancreatic metastases. Eur J Radiol 1991;12:41-4.
7. Boudghene FP, Deslandes PM, LeBlanche AF, Bigot JM. US and CT imaging features of intrapancreatic metastases. J Comput Assist Tomogr 1994;18:905-10.
8. Carson HJ, Green LK, Castelli MJ, Reyes CV, Prinz RA, Gattuso P. Utilization of fine-needle aspiration biopsy in the diagnosis of metastatic tumors to the pancreas. Diagn Cytopathol 1995;12:8-13.
9. Charnsangavej C, Whitley NO. Metastases to the pancreas and peripancreatic lymph nodes from carcinoma of the right side of the colon: CT findings in 12 patients. AJR Am J Roentgenol 1993;160:49-52.
10. Cubilla AL, Fitzgerald PF. Tumors of the exocrine pancreas. Atlas of Tumor Pathology, 2nd Series, Fascicle 19. Washington DC: Armed Forces Institute of Pathology; 1984:137.
11. DeWitt JM, Chappo J, Sherman S. Endoscopic ultrasound-guided fine-needle aspiration of melanoma metastatic to the pancreas; report of two cases and review. Endoscopy 2003;35:219-22.
12. Deziel DJ. Metastases to the pancreas. In: Howard JM, Idezuki Yk Ihse I, Prinz RA, eds. Surgical diseases of the pancreas, 3rd ed. Baltimore: Williams & Wilkins; 1998:643-648.
13. Dodd LG, Evans DB, Symmans F, Katz RL. Fine-needle aspiration of pancreatic extramedullary plasmacytoma: possible confusion with islet cell tumor. Diagn Cytopathol 1994;10:371-5.
14. Fritscher-Ravens A, Sriram PV, Krause C, et al. Detection of pancreatic metastases by EUS-guided fine-needle aspiration. Gastrointest Endosc 2001;53:65-70.
15. Ghavamian R, Klein KA, Stephens DH, et al. Renal cell carcinoma metastatic to the pancreas: clinical and radiological features. Mayo Clin Proc 2000;75:581-5.
16. Gutman H, Hess KR, Kokotsakis JA, Ross MI, Guinee VF, Balch CM. Surgery for abdominal metastases of cutaneous melanoma. World J Surg 2001;25:750-8.
17. Havig O. Some autopsy findings in malignant pancreatic lesions. Scand J Gastroenterol 1975; 10:23-4.
18. Hirota T, Tomida T, Iwasa M, Takahashi K, Kaneda M, Tamaki H. Solitary pancreatic metastasis occurring eight years after nephrectomy for renal cell carcinoma. A case report and surgical review. Int J Pancreatol 1996;19:145-53.
19. Hoang MP, Hruban RH, Albores-Saavedra J. Clear cell endocrine pancreatic tumor mimicking renal cell carcinoma: a distinctive neoplasm of von Hippel-Lindau disease. Am J Surg Pathol 2001;25:602-9.
20. Kassabian A, Stein J, Jabbour N, et al. Renal cell carcinoma metastatic to the pancreas: a single-institution series and review of the literature. Urology 2000;56:211-5.
21. Kitamura Y, Sakue M, Nishiyama K, et al. [A case of metastatic malignant melanoma mimicking pancreatic pseudocyst]. Gan No Rinsho 1987;33:748-52. [Japanese.]
22. Law CH, Wei AC, Hanna SS, et al. Pancreatic resection for metastatic renal cell carcinoma; presentation, treatment, and outcome. Ann Surg Oncol 2003;10:922-6.
23. Lubensky IA, Pack S, Ault D, et al. Multiple neuroendocrine tumors of the pancreas in von Hippel-Lindau disease patients: histopathological and molecular genetic analysis. Am J Pathol 1998;153:223-31.
24. McNichols DW, Segura JW, DeWeerd JH. Renal cell carcinoma: long-term survival and late recurrence. J Urol 1981;126:17-23.
25. Medina-Franco H, Helpern NB, Aldrete JS. Pancreaticoduodenectomy for metastatic tumors to the periampullary region. J Gastrointest Surg 1999;3:119-22.

26. Muranaka T, Teshima K, Honda H, Nanjo T, Hanada K, Oshiumi Y. Computed tomography and histologic appearance of pancreatic metastases from distant sources. Acta Radiol 1989;30:615-9.

27. Nakamura E, Shimizu M, Itoh T, Manabe T. Secondary tumors of the pancreas: clinicopathological study of 103 autopsy cases of Japanese patients. Pathol Int 2001;51:686-90.

28. Opocher E, Galeotti F, Spina GP, Battaglia G, Hernandez C. [Diagnosis of secondary tumors of the pancreas. Analysis of 13 cases.] Minerva Med 1982;73:577-81. [Italian.]

29. Ritchie AW, deKernion JB. The natural history and clinical features of renal carcinoma. Semin Nephrol 1987;7:131-9.

30. Robbins EG 2nd, Franceschi D, Barkin JS. Solitary metastatic tumors to the pancreas: a case report and review of the literature. Am J Gastroenterol 1996;91:2414-7.

31. Roland CF, van Heerden JA. Nonpancreatic primary tumors with metastasis to the pancreas. Surg Gynecol Obstet 1989;168:345-7.

32. Rosenberg SA, Diamond HD, Jaslowitz B, Craver LF. Lymphosarcoma: a review of 1269 cases. Medicine (Baltimore) 1961;61:31-84.

33. Rumancik WM, Megibow AJ, Bosniak MA, Hilton S. Metastatic disease to the pancreas: evaluation by computed tomography. J Comput Assist Tomogr 1984;8:829-34.

34. Stankard CE, Karl RC. The treatment of isolated pancreatic metastases from renal cell carcinoma: a surgical review. Am J Gastroenterol 1992;87:1658-60.

35. Stelow EB, Pambuccian SE, Bardales RH, et al. The cytology of pancreatic foamy gland adenocarcinoma. Am J Clin Pathol 2004;121:893-7.

36. Strijk SP. Pancreatic metastases of renal cell carcinoma: report of two cases. Gastrointest Radiol 1989;14:123-6.

37. Swensen T, Osnes M, Serck-Hanssen A. Endoscopic retrograde cholangio-pancreatography in primary and secondary tumours of the pancreas. Br J Radiol 1980;53:760-4.

38. Thompson LD, Heffess CS. Renal cell carcinoma to the pancreas in surgical pathology material. Cancer 2000;89:1076-88.

39. Weir M, Pitman MB. The vascular architecture of renal cell carcinoma in fine-needle aspiration biopsies. An aid in its distinction from hepatocellular carcinoma. Cancer 1997;81:45-50.

40. Wernecke K, Peters PE, Galanski M. Pancreatic metastases: US evaluation. Radiology 1986;160:399-402.

41. Whittington R, Moylan DJ, Dobelbower RR, Kramer S. Pancreatic tumours in patients with previous malignancy. Clin Radiol 1982;33:297-9.

42. Willis RA. Secondary tumors of the pancrea. In: Willis RA, ed. The spread of tumours in the human body, 3rd ed. London: Butterworths; 1973:216-7.

15 NON-NEOPLASTIC TUMORS AND TUMOR-LIKE LESIONS

A variety of solid and cystic lesions mimic pancreatic neoplasms at the clinical, radiographic, gross, and microscopic levels (Table 15-1). Recognition of their key diagnostic features is important for the proper clinical management of patients with pancreatic disease, and in some instances, histologic examination of the completely resected lesion may be required to exclude a neoplastic process. The sections that follow highlight the major diagnostic features

that can be used to distinguish each of these lesions from pancreatic neoplasms; more detailed information about the clinical manifestations, etiology, and pathogenesis of each entity is available elsewhere (106).

SOLID LESIONS OF THE EXOCRINE PANCREAS

Solid lesions most commonly mimic ductal adenocarcinomas since non-neoplastic solid

Table 15-1
NON-NEOPLASTIC TUMORS AND TUMOR-LIKE LESIONS

Lesion	Typical Configuration	Neoplasm Mimicked
Chronic pancreatitis	Solid	Ductal adenocarcinoma (C,G,M)[a]
Lymphoplasmacytic sclerosing pancreatitis	Solid	Ductal adenocarcinoma (C,G); lymphoma (M)
Reactive fibroinflammatory pseudotumor	Solid	Ductal adenocarcinoma (C,G); sarcoma (M)
Heterotopic pancreas	Solid	Extrapancreatic neoplasm (C,G)
Heterotopic spleen	Solid	Pancreatic endocrine neoplasm (C,G)
Hamartoma	Solid and cystic	Ductal adenocarcinoma (C,G); pancreatic endocrine neoplasm (C)
Sarcoidosis	Solid	Ductal adenocarcinoma (C,G)
Malakoplakia	Solid	Ductal adenocarcinoma (C,G)
Pseudocyst	Cystic	Mucinous cystic neoplasm (C,G,M); solid-pseudopapillary neoplasm (C,G,M)
Paraampullary duodenal wall cyst	Cystic and solid	Intraductal papillary mucinous neoplasm (C,G); ductal adenocarcinoma (C,G); sarcoma (M)
Ductal retention cyst	Cystic	Mucinous cystic neoplasm (C,G,M); macrocystic serous cystadenoma (C,G)
Congenital cyst	Cystic	Mucinous cystic neoplasm (C,G); macrocystic serous cystadenoma (C,G,M)
Lymphoepithelial cyst	Cystic	Mucinous cystic neoplasm (C,G)
Foregut cyst	Cystic	Mucinous cystic neoplasm (M); intraductal papillary mucinous neoplasm (C,G,M)
Islet hyperplasia	Microscopic	Pancreatic endocrine neoplasm (M)
Islet aggregation	Microscopic	Pancreatic endocrine neoplasm (M); ductal adenocarcinoma (M)
Nesidioblastosis	Solid or microscopic	Pancreatic endocrine neoplasm (C,G,M)
Islet dysplasia	Microscopic	Pancreatic endocrine neoplasm (M)

[a](C) = clinically; (G) = grossly; (M) = microscopically.

lesions are generally inflammatory in nature and therefore rather poorly circumscribed. In fact, chronic pancreatitis of alcoholic, obstructive, autoimmune, or other etiology is the primary entity in the histologic differential diagnosis of ductal adenocarcinoma. Not only are there radiographic and macroscopic similarities, but the microscopic appearance of non-neoplastic pancreatic ductules in regions of chronic pancreatitis may so closely simulate ductal adenocarcinoma that the distinction between the two entities represents one of the major challenges of diagnostic pathology. By some estimates, up to 5 percent of pancreatectomies performed for a preoperative diagnosis of a neoplasm will prove to contain a non-neoplastic lesion on pathologic examinaton (3a).

Chronic Pancreatitis

Definition. *Chronic pancreatitis* is inflammation of the pancreas with irreversible destruction of exocrine parenchyma along with fibrosis, and, in the late stages, destruction of endocrine parenchyma. Most cases in the United States are associated with long-term alcohol abuse (94,97,169). Other less common causes include longstanding obstruction of the pancreatic duct (from calculi, trauma, pancreas divisum) and inherited genetic disorders such as cystic fibrosis (31,38) and hereditary chronic pancreatitis due to a germline mutation in the cationic trypsinogen (*PRSS1*) or serine protease inhibitor, Kazal-type 1 *(SPINK1)* genes (62,184). *Tropical calcifying pancreatitis* is a particular type endemic in areas of Asia and Africa, related to chronic malnutrition and possibly germline *SPINK1* gene mutations, and associated with an increased risk of developing pancreatic carcinoma (112,147). An abnormal junction of the pancreatic and common bile ducts outside the duodenal wall ("abnormal pancreatobiliary duct junction") is a congenital condition most commonly reported in Asian patients that is associated with chronic pancreatitis (52,168). When the etiology of chronic pancreatitis is known, the condition is often designated more specifically, for example, *alcoholic chronic pancreatitis* or *obstructive chronic pancreatitis* (148).

Clinical Features. Clinically evident chronic pancreatitis affects approximately 3 to 4/100,000 people (185). Patients with alcoholic chronic pancreatitis have, by definition, a significant history of excessive alcoholic intake. Most patients have repeated episodes of acute pancreatitis accompanied by abdominal pain, nausea, malaise, and serum elevations in amylase and lipase; multiple attacks over periods of years are typical (10). Some patients, however, recount no specific bouts of acute pancreatitis but nonetheless have findings of chronic pancreatitis. The age of onset of patients with alcohol-related pancreatitis depends upon the severity of alcohol overuse, but significant chronic pancreatitis is present by the age of 40 years in some individuals.

In contrast to acute pancreatitis, the symptoms of chronic pancreatitis are more insidious. Since the initial result of chronic pancreatitis is loss of exocrine function due to loss of acinar elements, the clinical symptoms reflect a reduction in exocrine enzyme production. Intolerance of fatty foods is common, and chronic diarrhea, weight loss, and cachexia ultimately occur. The islets of Langerhans are relatively resistant to atrophy, so diabetes mellitus is usually a late complication. Biliary obstruction is uncommon but can occur (149).

Not all patients with pathologic evidence of chronic pancreatitis have a clinical history of pancreatic disease. Many older patients with normal exocrine and endocrine function have regions of chronic pancreatitis at autopsy, and it is common for some pancreatic lobules to show profound atrophy and fibrosis, whereas there remains normal parenchyma elsewhere in the gland. This sort of focal idiopathic chronic pancreatitis is not a major clinical problem, but localized chronic pancreatitis can produce a mass lesion on imaging studies. Furthermore, areas of chronic pancreatitis are commonly found adjacent to neoplasms. Biopsies from foci of chronic pancreatitis can be difficult to interpret, both because chronic pancreatitis can resemble ductal adenocarcinoma, resulting in an errant malignant diagnosis, and because sampling of a focus of chronic pancreatitis adjacent to a neoplasm may erroneously suggest a non-neoplastic process.

Since chronic pancreatitis may affect only a portion of the gland, radiographic studies may reveal a mass-like lesion resembling a pancreatic carcinoma. The areas of fibrosis often produce enlargement of the involved portion of the gland, and dilatation of the distal pancreatic duct is

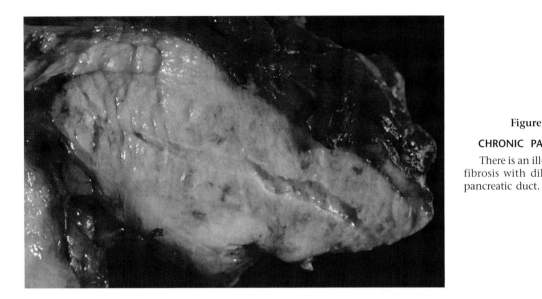

Figure 15-1

CHRONIC PANCREATITIS

There is an ill-defined area of fibrosis with dilatation of the pancreatic duct.

common. Features that suggest pancreatitis rather than carcinoma include calculi within the pancreatic ducts (139) and lack of involvement of the distal common bile duct (for lesions in the head of the gland). Pseudocyst formation in the peripancreatic tissue may also be seen radiographically. Diffuse involvement of the gland is more common in pancreatitis, although this appearance also may be produced by carcinomas of the head of the gland accompanied by obstructive pancreatitis in the tail. In the later stages of chronic pancreatitis, the atrophic, fibrotic parenchyma may be replaced by adipose tissue; in extreme cases, the substance of the pancreas is virtually indistinguishable from the surrounding retroperitoneal adipose tissue on imaging studies.

Gross Findings. Early in the course of chronic pancreatitis there is typically localized but irregular involvement of the pancreas. Localized chronic pancreatitis varies in extent from microscopic foci to large regions of fibrotic parenchyma simulating a neoplasm. Typically, localized chronic pancreatitis produces an ill-defined, firm white lesion, the borders of which may exhibit an infiltrative appearance at the interface with the normal parenchyma (fig. 15-1). Some cases are remarkably localized, reflecting involvement of the portions of the gland drained by a single major duct. These areas are firm but usually not gritty (in contrast to ductal adenocarcinoma). Calcifications may occur both within the ducts and in the peripancreatic tissues, and there may

be residual foci of fat necrosis from a recent episode of acute pancreatitis. The bile duct is usually not involved by the fibrotic process and is not constricted or proximally dilated.

Extensive involvement of the pancreas generally results in global atrophy of the gland. The normal soft, lobulated parenchyma is replaced with dense white fibrous tissue. The pancreatic ducts are generally dilated and distorted in alcoholic and obstructive chronic pancreatitis, and calculi may be found within them, especially in alcohol-related disease (fig. 15-2). Fatty replacement of the gland may also occur, and in extreme cases, there be such advanced atrophy and fatty infiltration that the pancreas is difficult to identify grossly. Chronic pancreatitis (especially from alcohol abuse) may be accompanied by pseudocyst formation (see below) (98).

Microscopic Findings. In typical cases, microscopic examination reveals variable degrees of involvement within the pancreas (40,94,97,154). Different lobules of the gland may exhibit different degrees of atrophy: some show only early loss of acinar cells and minimal fibrosis; others have near complete acinar atrophy but retention of ducts, ductules, and islets of Langerhans; while still other lobules show complete exocrine loss with only a few residual islets surrounded entirely by fat (fig. 15-3). In chronic pancreatitis due to ductal obstruction, the gland is more uniformly involved, with more pronounced fibrosis surrounding the dilated ducts than in the periphery (157).

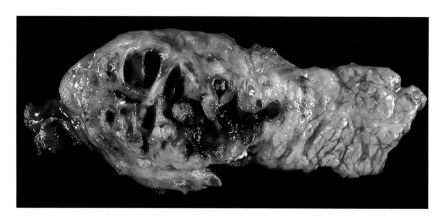

Figure 15-2

CHRONIC PANCREATITIS WITH LITHIASIS

Massively dilated, tortuous ducts contain irregular calculi.

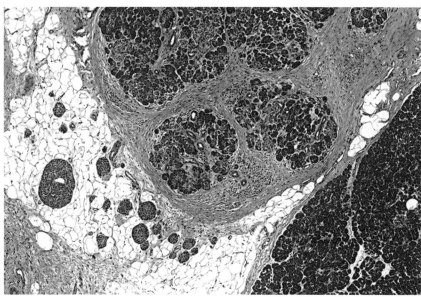

Figure 15-3

CHRONIC PANCREATITIS

There is variable involvement of lobules, some showing profound atrophy and consisting only of islets, some with moderate atrophy, and some minimally affected.

The key microscopic feature of chronic pancreatitis is that the underlying lobular architecture of the pancreas is retained (fig. 15-4). Inflammatory cells are usually sparse, consisting of scattered clusters of lymphocytes and histiocytes. The predominant finding is atrophy, with replacement of the normal parenchymal elements by fibrous tissue or fat. When the acini are lost, the residual ducts appear prominent, but there is no evidence that they are proliferating. Ductal dilatation is common, and luminal protein plugs may be found. Clusters of small ductules retain their inherent lobular organization, with larger ectatic ductules surrounded by clusters of small, round ductules (fig. 15-5). This lobular arrangement is the most helpful feature in establishing that this is a benign process. The stroma within the lobules is generally more loosely arranged than the interlobular stroma.

High-power microscopic examination reveals relatively uniform nuclei (fig. 15-5). If there is concurrent acute inflammation, there may be some reactive atypia, but the nuclei within each gland resemble each other in terms of size, shape, and location within the cell. Of course, foci of pancreatic intraepithelial neoplasia (PanIN) are common in areas of chronic pancreatitis, and these noninvasive lesions can show significant nuclear atypia. Other epithelial alterations may also occur in chronic pancreatitis, in particular, squamous metaplasia. Usually squamous metaplasia (fig. 15-6) is nonkeratinizing (also referred to as multilayered metaplasia), but sometimes keratinization does occur. In keeping with the maintenance of the lobular arrangement of the pancreas, individual glands are generally not found in abnormal locations such as adjacent to muscular vessels

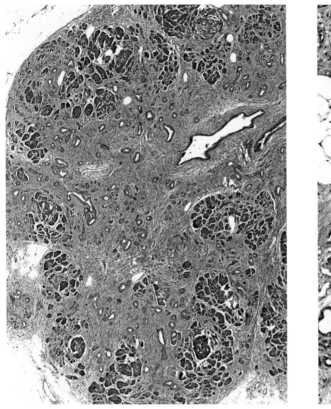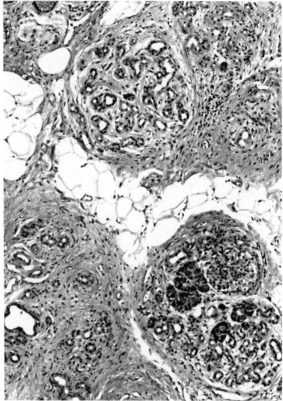

Figure 15-4

CHRONIC PANCREATITIS

Left: The underlying lobular architecture of the gland is preserved. Central ducts are surrounded by ductules and residual acini.

Right: With more pronounced atrophy, the lobules are widely separated.

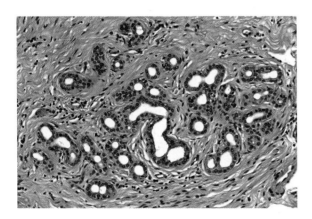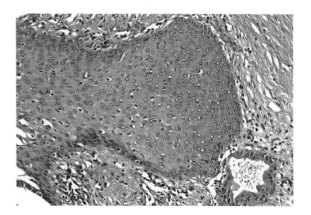

Figure 15-5

CHRONIC PANCREATITIS

At high-power microscopy, the remaining ductules retain a lobular arrangement, with smaller glands surrounding a larger, branched central gland. There is no significant nuclear atypia.

Figure 15-6

CHRONIC PANCREATITIS

Squamous metaplasia.

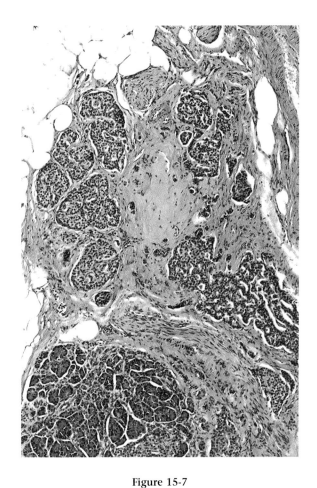

Figure 15-7

CHRONIC PANCREATITIS

Islet aggregation due to loss of exocrine parenchyma.

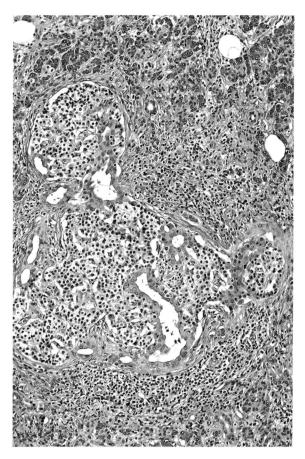

Figure 15-8

CHRONIC PANCREATITIS

Ductuloinsular complex.

(152), in the peripancreatic fat, within vessels, or wrapped around nerves.

A common finding in chronic pancreatitis is the aggregation of islets (fig. 15-7). Since islet cells are relatively resistant to atrophy, it is common to find some lobules in which the only remaining epithelial elements are the islet cells (17). With the loss of the exocrine parenchyma, the islets become concentrated together, resulting in an apparent increase in islet cell mass. Islet cells also may be admixed with small ductules, forming ductuloinsular complexes (fig. 15-8). Although this phenomenon has been labeled islet cell hyperplasia in the past, there is no evidence of true proliferation, and, in fact, many patients with chronic pancreatitis eventually develop diabetes mellitus; the

better term is islet aggregation. The histologic features of this process are discussed later.

It is common to find areas of pancreatitis adjacent to neoplasms, especially invasive ductal adenocarcinoma. This association has led to the suggestion that chronic pancreatitis may predispose to the development of pancreatic carcinoma, a complex and controversial topic (see chapter 7). On the other hand, chronic pancreatitis may result from local duct obstruction by the neoplasm. The histologic appearance of areas of chronic pancreatitis next to carcinomas is not sufficiently different from chronic pancreatitis of other etiologies to recognize it as peritumoral pancreatitis. Inflammatory cells may be more numerous than in alcoholic chronic pancreatitis, and luminal calcifications are less pronounced.

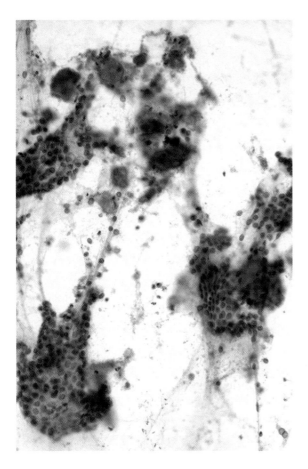

Figure 15-9

CHRONIC PANCREATITIS

Cytologic smear shows folded groups of bland ductal cells in a background of calcific debris (direct smear; Papanicolaou stain).

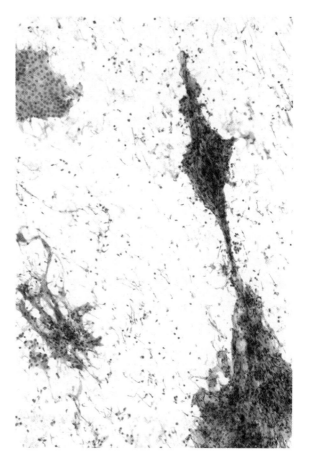

Figure 15-10

CHRONIC PANCREATITIS

Fibrotic and inflamed atrophic acinar tissue (lower right) associated with ductal cells (upper left) and background inflammation is characteristic of chronic pancreatitis on aspiration smears (direct smear; Papanicolaou stain).

Cytologic Findings. The cytologic diagnosis of chronic pancreatitis in patients with clinical and radiologic evidence of the disease is relatively straightforward (73,163). The most helpful cytologic findings include the presence of fibrotic parenchymal tissue, fragments of fibrous tissue, and chalky, granular calcified debris (fig. 15-9) (163). Although variable in quantity, mixed inflammation with histiocytes is also typically present. Ductal cells are almost always present, although they may be quite scanty and usually show minimal degrees of cytologic atypia, while maintaining the benign "honeycombed" pattern of nuclear spacing (fig. 15-10) (163). When ductal cells are scant, either fibrotic parenchyma or calcified debris predominates. The predominance of ductal cells without aci-

nar cells or calcified debris, a cytologic finding that suggests the diagnosis of adenocarcinoma, has not been described in patients with clinical and radiologic evidence of chronic pancreatitis. Attention should be paid to the presence of moderately atypical groups of ductal epithelium, and this finding should be commented upon in the cytology report as "atypical." Ductal cells that demonstrate a loss of the honeycombed nuclear spacing, with more crowding and nuclear irregularity, may indicate the presence of an associated adenocarcinoma (163), and further evaluation of the lesion is warranted.

Diagnostic difficulty arises most often when a mass lesion is radiographically apparent in the setting of chronic pancreatitis (53). The

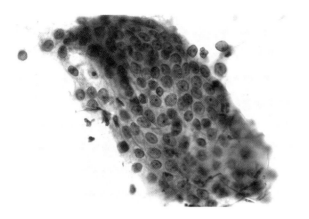
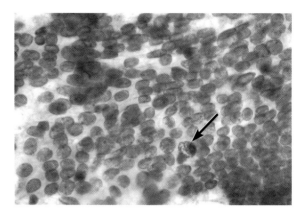

Figure 15-11

CHRONIC PANCREATITIS VERSUS WELL-DIFFERENTIATED ADENOCARCINOMA

Left: Cytology shows reactive ductal cells that are evenly arranged in sheets and groups. There is minimal nuclear crowding and overlapping, and the nuclear membranes are smooth.

Right: In contrast, well-differentiated carcinoma has nuclei that are more crowded and overlap, and nuclear membranes that are slightly grooved and indented. Note the mitotic figure in the carcinoma (arrow) (right and left: direct smears; Papanicolaou stain).

presence of an ill-defined lesion in the setting of chronic pancreatitis can lead to inaccurate biopsy needle placement and sampling error, causing false negative cytology results (53). Interpretation error is a minor reason for false negative results and occurs with well-differentiated adenocarcinoma (19,39a,113,146,187). False positive cytologic interpretations are extremely rare, since the specificity of fine needle aspiration for the diagnosis of pancreatic adenocarcinoma in most series is near 100 percent; however, chronic pancreatitis is often the culprit in false positive reports (181,183).

Differential Diagnosis. In the classic late stage of chronic pancreatitis, there is diffuse atrophy of the gland, ductal dilatation, and abundant calcification; this picture is not difficult to recognize. Many patients, however, have more localized involvement, with mass-like enlargement of a portion of the gland, and these cases of "tumoral pancreatitis" may closely mimic ductal adenocarcinoma. Features that favor a diagnosis of chronic pancreatitis include a retained lobular arrangement to the ducts and ductules; relative nuclear uniformity in terms of size, shape, and intracellular location; and the absence of glands in abnormal locations (perineurium, intravascular, extrapancreatic adipose tissue, or adjacent to muscular vessels). In contrast, ductal adenocarcinomas have haphazardly arranged glands with abnormal architectural features such as incomplete gland formation or solid cell clusters. Adenocarcinoma may show perineural or intravascular invasion, and the neoplastic glands may be adjacent to muscular vessels or in direct contact with adipocytes. Adenocarcinomas show marked (4 or more to 1) variation in nuclear area from cell to cell in a single gland, and the nuclei differ in shape and intracellular location. Also, stromal desmoplasia is frequent in ductal adenocarcinoma. Additional practical considerations regarding the distinction of chronic pancreatitis from ductal adenocarcinoma are presented in chapters 7 and 17.

Ductal adenocarcinoma is also in the differential diagnosis in cytologic material. In cytologic preparations of chronic pancreatitis, the overall cellularity of smears is relatively low (19, 146) and the smears contain a mixture of acinar epithelial cells and inflammatory cells, in contrast to a pure ductal cell population in adenocarcinoma. The cell groups in pancreatitis are flat, monolayered sheets of ductal cells with minimal crowding and nuclear overlap (fig. 15-11, left) compared to the subtle nuclear crowding in well-differentiated adenocarcinoma (fig. 15-11, right). Nuclear size is also more uniform in chronic pancreatitis, whereas nuclear enlargement and variation of nuclear size within a single group of cells favors adenocarcinoma (19,

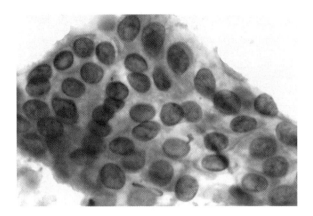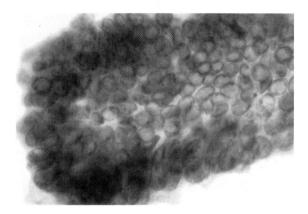

Figure 15-12

CHRONIC PANCREATITIS VERSUS WELL-DIFFERENTIATED ADENOCARCINOMA

Left: The chromatin pattern in reactive ductal cells is relatively euchromatic and evenly distributed.

Right: In well-differentiated carcinoma, the chromatin is unevenly distributed with peripheral clumping (parachromatin clearing). Note the difference in crowding, nuclear overlapping, and nuclear envelope contours.

37,113,146). Nuclear membrane abnormalities are also minimal in chronic pancreatitis (fig. 15-12, left), and there is evenly distributed granular chromatin, whereas the chromatin tends to dissipate in well-differentiated adenocarcinoma, yielding a clear-appearing nucleus (parachromatin clearing) (fig. 15-12, right) (113,146, 187). The cytoplasm of the ductal cells in chronic pancreatitis does not contain mucin visible by routine microscopy, but mucin may indeed be present and even abundant in well-differentiated adenocarcinoma. The cytologic distinction between benign ductal epithelium in chronic pancreatitis and malignant ductal epithelium in ductal adenocarcinoma is discussed further in chapter 7.

Other solid pancreatic neoplasms such as solid-pseudopapillary neoplasm, pancreatic endocrine neoplasm, and acinar cell carcinoma should be included in the cytologic differential diagnosis (105,181,183). Disrupted acinar cells forming irregular, papillary-like shapes and disorganized and noncohesive epithelium without the typical organoid grape-like clustering of benign acinar parenchyma can lead to misinterpretation as a neoplasm (see chapters 9 and 12) (42).

Lymphoplasmacytic Sclerosing Pancreatitis (Autoimmune Pancreatitis)

Definition. *Lymphoplasmacytic sclerosing pancreatitis* (LPSP) is a specific type of chronic pancreatitis that is characterized by a mixed inflammatory cell infiltrate centered around the pancreatic ducts along with venulitis. LPSP can produce a mass-like fibroinflammatory lesion and often simulates a carcinoma clinically and radiographically. LPSP is sometimes associated with other diseases of presumed autoimmune etiology. Synonyms include *sclerosing pancreatitis; nonalcoholic, duct-destructive chronic pancreatitis* (22,33, 46); and *autoimmune pancreatitis* (79,188).

Clinical Features. Most patients with LPSP are between the ages of 40 and 60 years. Men and women are equally affected. Most patients have no history of alcohol abuse or other predispositions to chronic pancreatitis (3). Presenting symptoms include abdominal pain, anorexia, and, for patients with involvement of the head of the gland, jaundice (92a,183,189). Many patients with LPSP have other associated disorders, including primary sclerosing cholangitis (48,90,127,130,155,175), lymphoplasmacytic cholecystitis (1), primary biliary cirrhosis (70), ulcerative colitis (15), and Sjögren's syndrome (55,92,127,130,155). Another family of disorders that has been encountered in these patients is the group of tumor-like lesions known as multifocal idiopathic fibrosclerosis (16,34,35, 39,70,86,110), including mediastinal and retroperitoneal fibrosis, Riedel's thyroiditis, and inflammatory pseudotumor of the orbit. All of these lesions have histologic features that overlap with those of LPSP. Several cases of LPSP associated with reactive fibroinflammatory

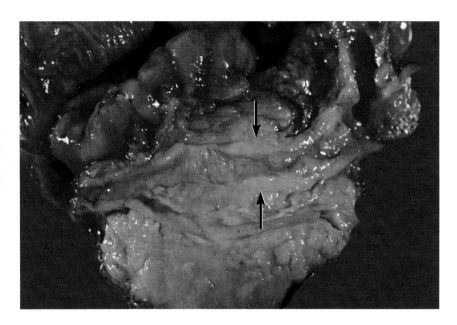

Figure 15-13

LYMPHOPLASMACYTIC SCLEROSING PANCREATITIS

An ill-defined firm mass fills the head of the pancreas and narrows the main pancreatic duct. There is associated thickening and stricture of the common bile duct (arrows).

pseudotumor formation (see below) have been described (93,133,137,172,180).

Based on these clinical associations, it is easy to see why LPSP is also designated autoimmune pancreatitis (79,96,188). Supporting this etiology, some patients have detectable autoantibodies, including antinuclear, antilactoferrin, antismooth muscle, and anticarbonic anhydrase II antibodies (79,131,172,177); elevations in rheumatoid factor and hypergammaglobulinemia have also been reported (79,177). Some patients have autoantibodies against pancreatic secretory trypsin inhibitor, a finding that may be related to the pathogenesis of the disease (12a). It has also been noted that elevations in serum immunoglobulin (Ig)G4 levels are common in LPSP patients, a finding that provides a potential diagnostic test for this disease. In one study, patients with LPSP had a mean serum IgG4 level of 663 mg/dL, compared with 51 mg/dL in normal individuals (66). Elevations in IgG4 have also been noted in patients with some of the other conditions associated with LPSP, such as sclerosing cholangitis, retroperitoneal fibrosis, and sialadenitis, suggesting that this constellation of disorders may represent a family of IgG4-related sclerosing diseases (86a). Associated autoimmune conditions are only found in 35 to 40 percent of patients with LPSP (46,183); thus, it may be premature to assume that all cases with the histologic appearance of LPSP are of autoimmune etiology.

Radiographic features (56,78,179) based on computerized tomography (CT) and magnetic resonance imaging (MRI) include a diffusely or segmentally enlarged pancreas with effacement of the normal lobular appearance and thickening of the common bile duct wall and gallbladder (89). The peripancreatic fat is not obscured. Ultrasound may show a diffusely swollen and hypoechoic pancreas that has been referred to as a "sausage-like" appearance.

Gross Findings. Most cases of LPSP involve the head of the pancreas, but disease restricted to the tail also occurs. The gross resemblance to carcinoma is striking. LPSP can produce an ill-defined, firm, tan-white mass; it can narrow the pancreatic and common bile ducts; and it can extend into the peripancreatic tissues (fig. 15-13).

Microscopic Findings. The histology of LPSP is distinctive (46,88,92a,97,150,183,189). A dense, mixed lymphoplasmacytic inflammatory infiltrate is centered on medium-sized to large pancreatic ducts (fig. 15-14). The ducts are sclerotic and stenotic (in contrast to the dilated ducts of alcoholic chronic pancreatitis), although obstructive dilatation of the ducts distal to the primary site of involvement may occur. Lymphocytes may be found within the epithelial layer of the pancreatic ducts, and there is evidence of destruction of the ductal epithelial cells. Cuff-like periductal fibrosis is characteristic. Although the inflammation is centered on the ducts, there is progressive atrophy of the

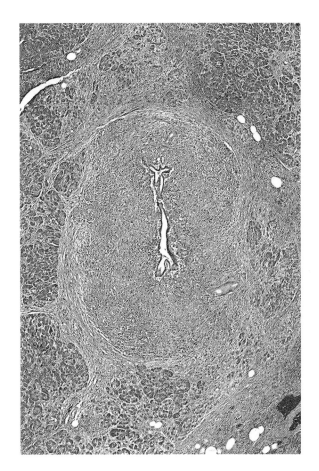 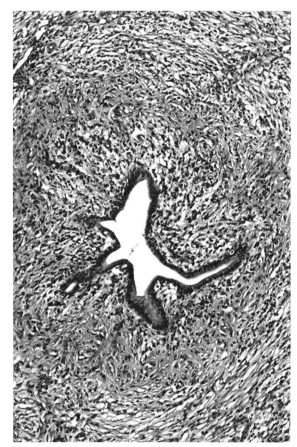

Figure 15-14

LYMPHOPLASMACYTIC SCLEROSING PANCREATITIS

Left: At low magnification, the inflammation is centered on the medium-sized ducts.
Right: Periductal fibrosis is present.

acinar elements and fibrosis. The inflammatory cells consist predominantly of lymphocytes and plasma cells, but it is common to find eosinophils (1) and occasional collections of neutrophils. Germinal centers may form. Aggregates of histiocytes may also be present, sometimes in vaguely granulomatous arrangements.

Another characteristic finding is the presence of inflammatory cells in the walls of small veins associated with luminal fibrosis (fig. 15-15). This "obliterative venulitis" is not a true necrotizing vasculitis, and the inflammatory cell composition is similar to that found around the ducts. Similar foci of venulitis are found in association with sclerosing cholangitis and lesions of the multifocal idiopathic fibrosclerosis family. Perineural aggregates of inflammatory cells have also been described in LPSP but are not specific.

The common bile duct and gallbladder in cases of LPSP may show inflammatory infiltrates that are similar to those surrounding the main pancreatic ducts (1,88). There may be a proliferation of periductal ductules, and the "onion skin" configuration of periductal fibrous tissue typically seen in sclerosing cholangitis may be found around the bile duct as well as within the pancreas. The stroma in areas of active involvement often has a storiform pattern of plump fibroblasts or myofibroblasts mixed with inflammatory cells (fig. 15-16) (183). The inflammation may extend into the peripancreatic adipose tissue.

In some cases of LPSP, there is pronounced expansion of the fibroinflammatory process, with complete replacement of the pancreatic parenchyma. This results in the formation of reactive

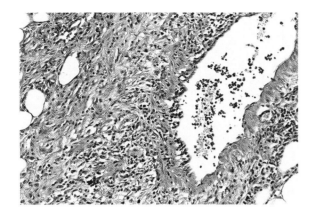
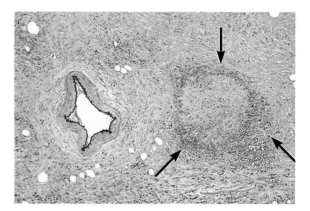

Figure 15-15

LYMPHOPLASMACYTIC SCLEROSING PANCREATITIS

Left: The inflammatory cells undermine and infiltrate the endothelium of a vein.
Right: Complete obliteration of a vein (arrows) is revealed by staining for elastin.

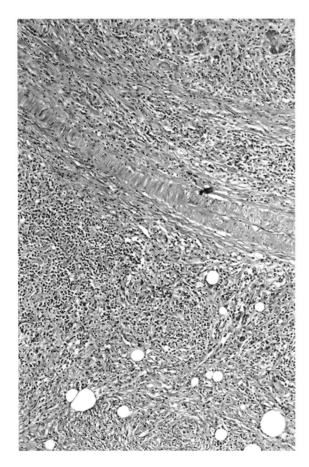

Figure 15-16

LYMPHOPLASMACYTIC SCLEROSING PANCREATITIS

Storiform pattern of inflammation and fibrosis.

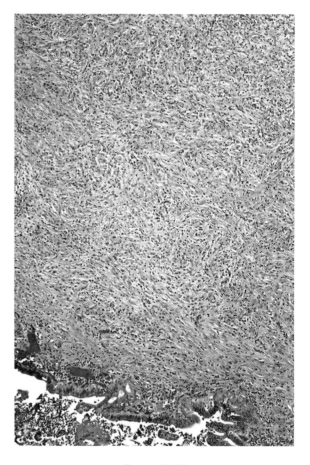

Figure 15-17

LYMPHOPLASMACYTIC SCLEROSING PANCREATITIS

Reactive fibroinflammatory pseudotumor formation. The deposition of collagen in this case formed a mass.

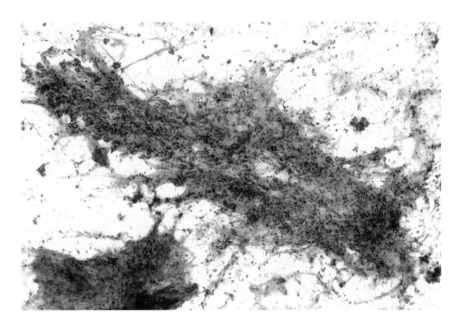

fibroinflammatory pseudotumors that measure 5 to 10 cm (fig. 15-17) (see below) (45,93,137).

Immunohistochemical labeling demonstrates a predominance of CD3-positive T lymphocytes in the periductal infiltrates, including a mixture of CD4 and CD8 cell types (86,189). Also present are CD20-positive B lymphocytes and macrophages that label for CD68. The plasma cells are polyclonal based on κ and λ immunolabeling. Antibodies to IgG4 label many plasma cells (86), and although this marker has not been shown to be entirely specific for LPSP, the finding of more than 50 IgG4-positive cells per high-power field is strongly suggestive of a diagnosis of LPSP and is not seen in the regions of pancreatitis accompanying pancreatic cancers (42a). Germinal centers (when present) consist mainly of B lymphocytes. The storiform fibroinflammatory stroma and the reactive fibroinflammatory pseudotumors are not positive for anaplastic lymphoma kinase (ALK), in contrast to many true inflammatory myofibroblastic tumors.

Cytologic Findings. The cytologic features of chronic pancreatitis and LPSP overlap, with both entities demonstrating mixed inflammation, fibrosis, atrophic pancreatic tissue, and disrupted acinar tissue; however, the constellation of background lymphocytes and cellular stromal fragments, with or without increased stromal lymphocytes, supports the interpretation of LPSP (fig. 15-18) (42). Although specific cytologic criteria for the diagnosis of LPSP have yet to be

established, correlation of these features with the clinical and radiologic features helps to suggest the diagnosis, allowing for serologic testing and other clinical investigations.

The presence of atrophic acinar parenchyma, lymphocytes, and cellular stromal fragments helps to distinguish LPSP from adenocarcinoma (42,189). In a patient with a clinical suspicion of pancreatic carcinoma, however, the findings on cytology may not be sufficiently specific to exclude a malignant neoplasm not sampled by the fine needle aspiration biopsy. In addition, reactive epithelial atypia in LPSP may mimic an adenocarcinoma.

Differential Diagnosis. Many of the studies of LPSP have emphasized the features distinguishing it from alcoholic pancreatitis (46,189). There are many histologic findings in LPSP that are absent in most cases of alcoholic pancreatitis, including dense lymphoplasmacytic inflammation, periductal inflammation, duct epithelial cell destruction, obliterative venulitis, and bile duct involvement. Furthermore, cases of LPSP lack pseudocyst formation, calculi, and irregular ductal dilatation, all common findings in alcoholic pancreatitis. The absence of a significant history of alcohol use in patients with LPSP is helpful.

The major entity in the clinical differential diagnosis of LPSP is not alcoholic pancreatitis, however, but infiltrating ductal adenocarcinoma (3,68,132,183). Both produce ill-defined masses, mostly in the head of the gland, and both can stricture the pancreatic and bile ducts. Patients with LPSP are usually younger than patients with ductal adenocarcinomas, and up to 40 percent have a prior history of another autoimmune-associated disease or fibroinflammatory lesion. If the possibility of LPSP is considered, an elevated serum IgG4 level may be particularly helpful. If the pancreas is resected, foci of LPSP may also resemble pancreatic carcinomas grossly, but the microscopic findings are usually not problematic. Dense periductal inflammation is not typical of ductal adenocarcinomas, and the pseudoinfiltrative appearance of ductules seen in alcoholic or idiopathic chronic pancreatitis is not prominent in LPSP. Areas of pancreatitis are commonly found adjacent to carcinomas, however, and areas of periductal inflammation, perineural inflammation, and even focal venulitis may accompany an invasive carcinoma. Thus, the ability to confirm a diagnosis of LPSP on the basis of a needle biopsy has been questioned.

Recently, the use of immunohistochemical labeling for IgG4 has been studied to distinguish LPSP from peritumoral pancreatitis adjacent to ductal adenocarcinomas. Although this technique is not completely sensitive, the finding of dense IgG4-positive plasma cells (more than 50 cells per high-power field) is highly specific for the diagnosis of LPSP and can be useful even in needle biopsy specimens that lack the characteristic histologic features of LPSP (42a).

Clearly, it is essential to interpret biopsy specimens in the light of the clinical information. It must always be recognized that a negative pancreatic biopsy does not exclude the possibility of a carcinoma, and many surgeons will be reluctant to treat a patient with a presumptive diagnosis of LPSP medically unless the clinical findings also strongly support that possibility. LPSP may also simulate lymphoma (76).

Treatment. Surgical resection is commonly performed for LPSP, especially since the disease often is not recognized preoperatively. Following surgery, strictures may recur in the biliary tree or mass lesions may develop elsewhere in the pancreas (68,183). In some of these patients, a favorable response to steroid therapy has been observed (75,91). In patients presenting with classic clinical findings, the diagnosis of LPSP may be strongly suggested preoperatively, allowing a trial of steroids as the primary therapy.

Reactive Fibroinflammatory Pseudotumor

Definition. *Reactive fibroinflammatory pseudotumor* is a mass lesion composed of a mixture of non-neoplastic inflammatory cells and fibroblasts. The term *inflammatory pseudotumor* has often been applied to these lesions when they occur in the pancreas. In other anatomic locations (e.g., the lung), the older term, inflammatory pseudotumor, has been largely replaced by the term *inflammatory myofibroblastic tumor*, since the neoplastic nature of these lesions in the lung and their principal cellular constituents have been clarified (165). Approximately 25 pancreatic lesions have been reported as inflammatory pseudotumors or inflammatory myofibroblastic tumors (142), but it is not clear that all such lesions are actually neoplastic inflammatory myofibroblastic tumors (44,84,103, 126a), and review of the reported cases actually suggests that many are non-neoplastic. The term reactive fibroinflammatory pseudotumor is proposed to specifically refer to non-neoplastic fibroinflammatory lesions; neoplastic inflammatory myofibroblastic tumors are discussed in chapter 13.

Clinical Features. Reactive fibroinflammatory pseudotumors usually occur in adults between the ages of 40 and 60 years; men and women are equally affected. Many reported pancreatic cases appear to have arisen in association with LPSP (45,137). These patients may have similar tumor-like lesions in other sites and probably have the syndrome of multifocal idiopathic fibrosclerosis. The head of the pancreas is preferentially involved. The presenting symptoms may be nonspecific, but jaundice has been reported when the pseudotumor involves the head of the gland. It is not clear whether the biliary obstruction is due to compression of the bile duct by the mass or strictures of the bile duct secondary to involvement by LPSP. In most cases, the finding on imaging studies of a mass of up to 5 cm suggests a pancreatic neoplasm, and resection is performed.

Pathologic Findings. Grossly, pancreatic reactive fibroinflammatory pseudotumors are relatively circumscribed, dense white masses adjacent to fibrotic pancreatic parenchyma. The histologic appearance somewhat resembles that of inflammatory myofibroblastic tumors, with variably collagenized fibrous tissue containing scattered lymphocytes, plasma cells, and histiocytes arranged in a vaguely storiform pattern (fig. 15-17) (93). Cytologically bland spindle cells, probably fibroblasts and myofibroblasts, are present between the bands of collagen. In contrast to neoplastic inflammatory myofibroblastic tumors, the cellularity is relatively low, there is more extensive collagenization, and the spindle cells have smaller, more regular nuclei. The process often extends into peripancreatic tissues, entrapping lobules of fat despite the grossly circumscribed appearance. Aggregates of lymphocytes, sometimes with follicle formation, are present, particularly at the periphery of the mass. Importantly, the adjacent pancreas often shows features of LPSP, including dense periductal lymphoplasmacytic inflammation and obliterative venulitis.

Differential Diagnosis. The differential diagnosis includes true neoplastic inflammatory myofibroblastic tumors, which usually occur in children and lack associated LPSP, as well as inflammatory fibrosarcoma (126a). The latter entity is also histologically similar to inflammatory myofibroblastic tumor but shows a denser spindle cellularity with cytologic atypia and abnormal mitoses. Inflammatory fibrosarcomas are probably part of the neoplastic spectrum of inflammatory myofibroblastic tumors but with overtly malignant features.

Prognosis. Although patients with reactive fibroinflammatory pseudotumors arising in the setting of LPSP are at risk for recurrence of fibroinflammatory processes elsewhere in the pancreatobiliary tree or in other anatomic locations, there is no evidence of malignant behavior.

Heterotopic Pancreas

Definition. *Heterotopic pancreas* consists of lobules of non-neoplastic pancreatic parenchyma located outside of the normal borders of the gland. Synonyms include *ectopic pancreas, adenomyoma* (in the ampulla or small bowel) (20), and *myoepithelial hamartoma.* This condition was first described by Schultz in 1727 by gross examination, and histologically by Klob in 1858. Heterotopic pancreas is found in up to 15 percent of autopsies (134). Common locations for heterotopic pancreas include the duodenum, stomach, liver (around bile ducts), gallbladder, ampulla of Vater, and small bowel, in particular, within Meckel diverticula (43,121). More distant

sites include the esophagus, lung, mediastinum, kidney, and thyroid gland (106). Heterotopic pancreas may originate from parenchyma displaced during embryonic migration of tissues.

The most commonly reported location of heterotopic pancreas is the second portion of the duodenum, although many apparent foci of pancreatic heterotopia in the proximal duodenum represent residual pancreatic elements associated with the minor papilla. In fact, when the histology of the minor papilla has been systematically investigated (21), most individuals have both gross and histologic evidence of residual ductal structures accompanied by variable amounts of acinar and endocrine tissue within the duodenal submucosa and wall. The high prevalence of these tissue elements in normal individuals suggests that pancreatic parenchyma in the region of the minor papilla is normal and therefore does not qualify as heterotopia.

Clinical Features. Foci of heterotopic pancreas range from microscopic clusters of acini to macroscopic nodules of parenchyma measuring several centimeters. Most microscopic foci are incidental findings and do not cause symptoms. Larger foci of heterotopic pancreas produce a range of symptoms depending upon their location. In the tubular gastrointestinal tract, bleeding, bowel obstruction, biliary obstruction (20), and intussusception may occur. Rare cases with superimposed pseudocyst formation are documented (28,47). Submucosal heterotopic pancreas can radiographically and endoscopically mimic a neoplasm such as a carcinoid tumor or gastrointestinal stromal tumor (49,140). Rarely, carcinomas arise in foci of heterotopic pancreas, producing symptoms generally similar to primary neoplasms arising in the same location.

Gross Findings. Most grossly evident foci of heterotopic pancreas occur in the tubular gastrointestinal tract. The nodules are firm, yellow to white, and submucosal. Larger foci cause umbilication of the overlying mucosa, sometimes with central ulceration. On cut section, normal parenchymal lobulations are often appreciable (fig. 15-19).

Microscopic Findings. All of the normal pancreatic epithelial elements may be found in heterotopic pancreas, but not every case demonstrates all three cell types (fig. 15-20). Most prevalent are ducts, and in some instances, these are

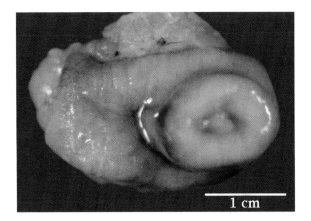
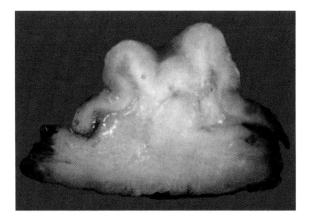

Figure 15-19

HETEROTOPIC PANCREAS INVOLVING STOMACH

Left: The lesion is umbilicated from the mucosal aspect.
Right: On cut section, there is a nodule of yellow tissue within the submucosa.

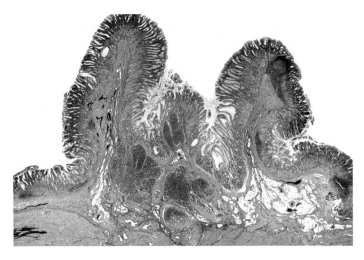

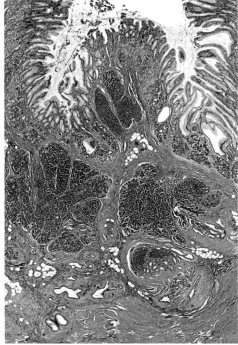

Figure 15-20

HETEROTOPIC PANCREAS

Above: Lobules of pancreatic tissue extend from the deep submucosa into the superficial muscularis propria.

Right: Some lobules contain abundant acini, others include only ducts.

the only epithelial structures identifiable. In the gastrointestinal tract, it is common to have smooth muscle surrounding these ducts, and examples lacking other pancreatic elements are commonly designated "adenomyoma" or "adenomyomatous hyperplasia." Acini are the second most frequent element, and it is their presence that clearly identifies the lesion as pancreatic. Up to 84 percent of heterotopic pancreas foci contain islets of Langerhans (134), and indi-

vidual endocrine cells may be identified in cases without discrete islets. Pseudocysts arising in heterotopic pancreas may obscure the pancreatic tissue, appearing as large, fibrous-walled cavities filled with purulent debris.

Some foci of heterotopic pancreas contain PanIN lesions; usually they are low grade. Also, a number of different neoplasms have been reported to arise in foci of heterotopic pancreas (118). Most are ductal adenocarcinomas, although acinar cell

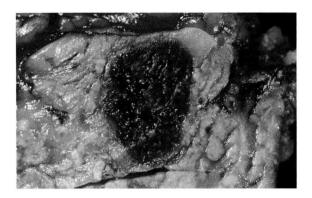
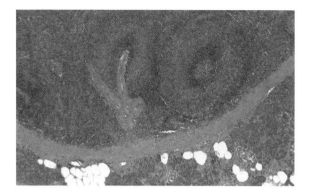

Figure 15-21

HETEROTOPIC SPLEEN IN PANCREATIC TAIL

Left: A sharply circumscribed nodule of red splenic tissue is surrounded by normal pancreas.
Right: Microscopically, normal red and white pulp is separated from the pancreatic tissue by a fibrous capsule.

carcinomas, solid-pseudopapillary neoplasms, and pancreatic endocrine neoplasms have also been described (13,72a). The histologic appearance of these neoplasms is similar to those arising in the pancreas proper. The possibility of origin of a carcinoma in heterotopic pancreatic tissue has been invoked to explain the occurrence of carcinomas with a pancreatic phenotype in extrapancreatic sites (such as an acinar cell neoplasm arising in the stomach [171]), even when residual elements of non-neoplastic pancreatic parenchyma cannot be identified.

Heterotopic Spleen

Nodules of *heterotopic splenic tissue* ("splenules" or "splenunculi") are found in the left upper quadrant of the abdomen in as many as 10 percent of autopsies (65). Although most occur in the soft tissues of the splenic hilum, heterotopic spleen may be found within the pancreatic parenchyma (65,108). Most intrapancreatic examples are found in the tail. They appear as soft, sharply circumscribed, reddish brown nodules surrounded by a thin fibrous capsule (fig. 15-21). They are usually small (less than 3 cm). Radiologic and gross examination reveal well-demarcated masses that may resemble small, solid pancreatic neoplasms, especially those with a rich vascularity such as pancreatic endocrine neoplasms, sugar tumors (PEComas), or small solid-pseudopapillary neoplasms. Microscopically, they consist of typical splenic parenchyma, including both red and white pulp, and are not diagnostically problematic. Rarely, epithelial cysts arise within nodules of intrapancreatic splenic tissue (see Cystic Lesions, below).

Hamartoma

A variety of different presumably non-neoplastic lesions in children and adults have been reported as *hamartomas of the pancreas* (29,51, 81,123,135a,136). Although in some cases it is difficult to discern the nature of these lesions based on the published details, two reports (51,136) have characterized a distinctive solid and cystic pancreatic hamartoma that meets the classic definition of a benign tumorous overgrowth of disorganized mature parenchymal elements native to the site of origin. All of the patients were female, aged 20 months, 36 years, and 55 years, who presented with abdominal pain. The 2.7-, 7.0-, and 9.0-cm lesions were well circumscribed and firm and contained scattered small cysts. Microscopically, variably cystic ductal structures were surrounded by disorganized acini and embedded in a fibroblastic, heavily collagenized stroma (fig. 15-22). One lesion also contained fat (51). There were no discrete islets, but scattered endocrine cells were identified by immunohistochemistry. These lesions were clearly benign and appeared non-neoplastic.

The microscopic differential diagnosis of pancreatic hamartoma includes localized chronic pancreatitis. Although pancreatitis can appear as a focal lesion, it is rarely as well circumscribed as a hamartoma. The absence of well-formed islets is another distinguishing feature, since

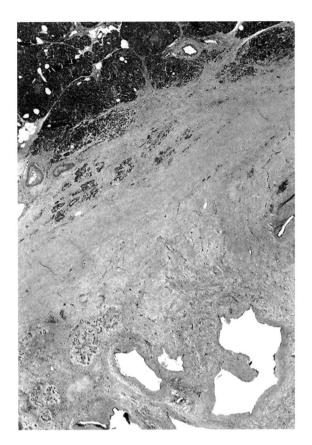 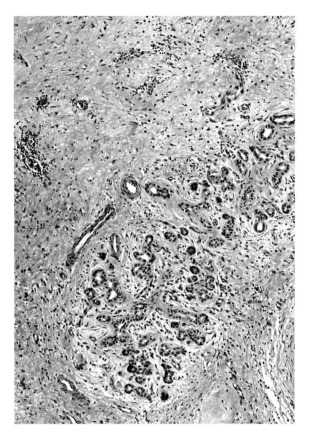

Figure 15-22

HAMARTOMA

Left: At low power the lesion is predominantly fibrotic and contains cystic ducts and lobules of atrophic parenchyma; the adjacent pancreas is normal.

Right: Higher power shows ducts and acini, but islets are not present.

even in the face of pronounced chronic pancreatitis the islets generally persist.

Another recently described pancreatic lesion (*cellular hamartoma resembling gastrointestinal stromal tumor*) consists of hypocellular fascicles of cytologically bland spindle cells with entrapped lobules of acinar cells (135a). Islets are not found. The spindle cells coexpress CD34, bcl-2, and c-kit (CD117) by immunohistochemistry, raising the possibility of a relationship to either solitary fibrous tumor or true gastrointestinal stromal tumor (see chapter 13).

Miscellaneous Solid Lesions

Lipomatous Pseudohypertrophy. Significant replacement of the exocrine elements by adipose tissue is referred to as lipomatous pseudohypertrophy. In most instances, lipomatous pseudohypertrophy is secondary to chronic pancreatitis (especially due to longstanding duct obstruction), cystic fibrosis, adult-onset diabetes mellitus, or Shwachman's syndrome (congenital lipomatosis) (16,151). Rare cases of primary lipomatous pseudohypertrophy have been described (157). In patients incidentally found to have lipomatous pseudohypertrophy without a known etiology, a neoplasm obstructing the proximal pancreatic duct should be ruled out. Patients may experience exocrine insufficiency (115).

Grossly, there is either diffuse enlargement of the gland or concentration of fat in the anterior head of the pancreas and in the uncinate process. The normal lobulation and overall configuration are maintained. Microscopically, mature adipose tissue and bands of fibrous tissue replace the acini and most of the ducts (fig. 15-23). The islets, however, are preserved and appear histologically normal.

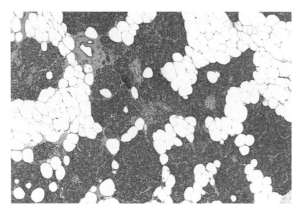

Figure 15-23

LIPOMATOUS PSEUDOHYPERTROPHY

The acinar tissue is replaced by mature adipose tissue.

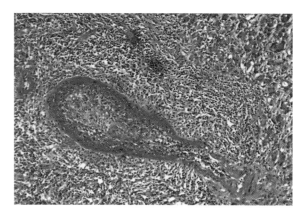

Figure 15-24

POLYARTERITIS NODOSA

A small muscular artery in the pancreas shows necrotizing vasculitis.

Nodular Lymphoid Hyperplasia. Aggregates of non-neoplastic lymphoid tissue may affect the pancreas. Some cases have been reported as *pseudolymphomas*, although this term is now discouraged. Nodular lymphoid hyperplasia may appear as a circumscribed soft yellow nodule or it may involve the gland more diffusely (72,129). The lymphoid tissue contains well-formed follicles and germinal centers surrounded by fibrotic stroma. Residual pancreatic parenchymal elements may be found among the lymphoid cells. As in other locations, nodular lymphoid hyperplasia of the pancreas must be distinguished from lymphoma (especially follicular lymphoma); both are equally rare in the pancreas.

Sarcoidosis. Sarcoidosis may involve the pancreas or peripancreatic lymph nodes, producing a mass (24,116,176). Most patients have a well-established diagnosis of sarcoidosis at the time the pancreatic involvement is detected. Histologically, the pancreas and lymph nodes contain numerous tightly formed, noncaseating granulomas with few multinucleated giant cells. In patients with a prior history of sarcoidosis, the presence of histologically typical granulomas is highly suggestive of pancreatic involvement, but stains for microorganisms as well as cultures are still recommended to exclude an infectious process. Granulomas of infectious etiology may also involve the pancreas and simulate a neoplasm (9).

Ectopic Adrenal Cortical Nodules. These nodules may rarely involve the pancreas where they can be confused with clear cell pancreatic endocrine neoplasm and metastatic renal cell carcinoma (8). Ectopic adrenal cortical nodules recapitulate the structure of the normal adrenal cortex and, in contrast to pancreatic endocrine neoplasms, are chromogranin negative.

Polyarteritis Nodosa. We have encountered a case of polyarteritis nodosa presenting as a mass lesion in the head of the pancreas, simulating a carcinoma. In addition to areas of fibrosis and atrophy, the pancreatic parenchyma displayed medium-sized arteries with necrotizing vasculitis (fig. 15-24).

Malakoplakia. This has rarely been reported as the cause of a pancreatic mass (104). The histologic features resemble those of malakoplakia occurring elsewhere, including the formation of Michaelis-Guttman bodies. In one patient this inflammatory mass was accompanied by a ductal adenocarcinoma (190).

Brunner Gland Hyperplasia. Rarely, when in the duodenal wall, this can be confused clinically for pancreatic carcinoma (156).

CYSTIC LESIONS OF THE EXOCRINE PANCREAS

Cystic lesions of the pancreas are detected more and more frequently with the increasing use of abdominal imaging. Although cystic neoplasms are relatively uncommon, they have their own host of non-neoplastic mimics. Since the majority of cystic lesions in the pancreas are pseudocysts that do not require surgical

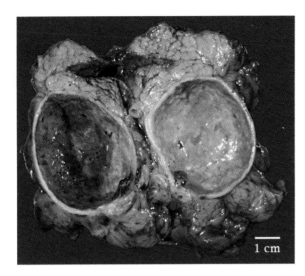

Figure 15-25

PSEUDOCYST

A unilocular cyst is adjacent to the pancreas. It is lined by hemorrhagic and necrotic tissue and surrounded by a thick fibrous pseudocapsule.

management, the preoperative distinction of benign cystic lesions from potentially malignant cystic neoplasms is of critical importance.

Pseudocyst

Definition. A *pseudocyst* is a grossly evident localized collection of necrotic-hemorrhagic material rich in pancreatic enzymes. Pseudocysts are surrounded by an inflamed fibrous capsule; no epithelial lining is present. Pseudocysts make up approximately 75 percent of the cystic lesions of the pancreas based on older studies (71), although with greater numbers of incidental retention cysts, small branch-duct type intraductal papillary mucinous neoplasms, and other cystic lesions detected by current imaging technologies, this percentage is likely decreasing (102).

Pseudocysts occur when acute injury to the pancreas results in the release and activation of pancreatic enzymes in peripancreatic tissues or in the pancreas itself. The digestive effects of these enzymes lead to tissue necrosis, particularly fat necrosis. The resulting liquefied material is surrounded by granulation tissue and ultimately enclosed within a fibrous capsule to form the lesion.

Clinical Features. Most patients with pseudocysts have a well-established history of acute pancreatitis, most commonly due to alcohol abuse but also possibly secondary to duct obstruction (e.g., by gallstones), trauma, and other causes (95). No cause is identifiable in the 13 percent of pseudocysts (122). Patients are usually middle-aged to older men, especially when the etiology is alcohol related. Those resulting from trauma or biliary disease occur in younger patients and have an equal gender predilection (95).

Pseudocysts develop in about 10 percent of patients with acute pancreatitis, more frequently in those with severe bouts or repeated episodes. Infection of a pseudocyst leads to a peripancreatic abscess and is a dire complication. Erosion into adjacent structures or rupture may occur. Pseudocyst formation has been reported rarely in foci of heterotopic pancreas (see above).

Gross Findings. Most pseudocysts appear as unilocular, well-demarcated cysts in the peripancreatic tissues, densely adherent to the pancreas itself (fig. 15-25). About 65 percent affect the tail (122). They range from a few to 20 cm and occasionally are multiple. The cyst contents are viscous, oily, and hemorrhagic. The fibrous wall is lined by shaggy necrotic debris and measures several millimeters to several centimeters in thickness. Erosion into the pancreatic ducts may result in continuity of the cyst lumen with the ductal system.

Microscopic Findings. The wall of a pseudocyst is composed of granulation tissue and variably organized fibroinflammatory tissue (fig. 15-26). The wall varies from actively inflamed, with a plump myofibroblastic cell component, to densely hyalinized, with only scattered spindled fibroblasts embedded in bands of collagen. Fresh and organizing hemorrhage is common. The luminal aspect has no epithelial lining; there is only fibrin, necrotic debris, remnants of fat necrosis, and aggregates of foamy histiocytes. Pseudocysts are usually surrounded by additional fibrous tissue that blends imperceptibly into the adjacent fibrotic pancreatic parenchyma.

Pseudocysts also occur as a complication of eosinophilic pancreatitis, a condition characterized by massive infiltration of the pancreas by eosinophils, with associated fibrosis and atrophy (2). Peripheral eosinophilia is characteristically present.

Cytologic Findings. Pancreatic pseudocysts are typically aspirated when the radiologic diagnosis is uncertain. Access to the cyst is via fine needle aspiration biopsy, increasingly performed under EUS guidance. The cyst fluid aspirated from an uncomplicated pseudocyst is generally thin, cloudy, and nonmucinous. A complicated pseudocyst, however, may contain thick fluid owing to the presence of hemorrhage or marked inflammation (25). The characteristic cytologic appearance of pseudocyst fluid is one of degenerative cyst debris containing inflammatory cells, histiocytes, hemosiderin (free and in histiocytes), and often bile (fig. 15-27). By definition, pseudocysts should not have epithelial cells on cytologic examination; however, histiocytes can be mistaken for epithelial cells, particularly mucinous epithelial cells (fig. 15-27). Foamy histiocytes in pseudocysts are mucin negative with special stains for mucin; this is important since mucin-positive histiocytes may be the only cytologic evidence of a mucin-producing neoplastic cyst.

Differential Diagnosis. In patients with a well-established history of acute or chronic pancreatitis, the suspicion that a peripancreatic cystic lesion likely represents a pseudocyst is high, and biopsies of such lesions are seldom performed. However, pseudocyst-like changes are often found focally in several pancreatic neoplasms (mucinous cystic neoplasms, solid-pseudopapillary neoplasms, and microcystic serous

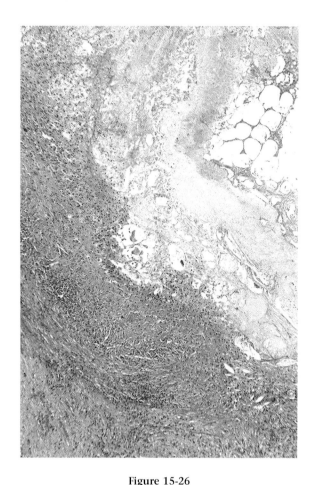

Figure 15-26

PSEUDOCYST

An inflamed fibrotic pseudocapsule surrounds necrotic adipocytes.

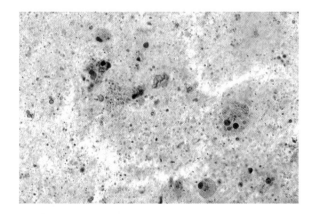
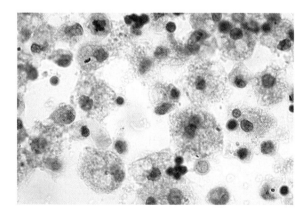

Figure 15-27

PSEUDOCYST

Left: The characteristic cytologic features include amorphous cyst debris with inflammatory cells, histiocytes, hemosiderin, and bile, but no epithelial cells (cytospin preparation; Papanicolaou stain).

Right: Histiocytes, especially foamy histiocytes, can mimic epithelial cells (ThinPrep®; Papanicolaou stain).

cystadenomas), and the distinction of these neoplasms from a pseudocyst may be problematic, including on cytology, where nonmucinous cyst fluid lacking epithelial cells may be found (182). The possibility of a neoplasm with pseudocyst-like degenerative changes should be considered when the patient lacks a history of pancreatitis or when the adjacent pancreatic parenchyma is histologically normal. In these instances the specimen should be extensively sampled. Any epithelial elements within the cyst suggest an alternative diagnosis to pseudocyst.

Mucinous cystic neoplasms generally have a tall columnar, mucinous epithelial lining that is at least focally preserved; in the event of extensive denudation, the presence of cellular ovarian-like stroma in the cyst wall is helpful. This specialized stroma can be distinguished from the reactive myofibroblastic cells of a pseudocyst by immunohistochemical labeling for estrogen or progesterone receptors and inhibin, all of which may be expressed by the stroma of mucinous cystic neoplasms. The residual epithelial elements of solid-pseudopapillary neoplasms generally are found within the lumen of the cyst. Serous cystadenomas are recognized by small cysts lined by cuboidal cells with clear cytoplasm.

Levels of cyst fluid amylase and carcinoembryonic antigen (CEA) distinguish pseudocysts from neoplastic cysts (26,32,54,67,111,138,158). Amylase is consistently elevated (thousands of U/L) in pseudocysts. Other than intraductal papillary mucinous neoplasms that connect to the pancreatic ducts, amylase levels are rarely as elevated in neoplastic cysts. Elevated amylase levels can sometimes be seen in serous and mucinous cystic neoplasms, but cyst fluid with a very low amylase level is highly unlikely to be a pseudocyst. Elevated cyst fluid CEA levels suggest a mucinous epithelium-lined cyst. A CEA level over 200 ng/mL is the most specific marker for identifying mucinous cysts (26) and is not usually encountered in pseudocysts. Contamination of a cytologic specimen with epithelial or mesothelial cells may falsely suggest an epithelium-lined cyst.

Paraampullary Duodenal Wall Cyst (Groove Pancreatitis)

Definition. *Paraampullary duodenal wall cysts are non-neoplastic inflammatory cystic lesions* that arise in a specific location adjacent to the minor papilla. They most likely develop in submucosal pancreatic tissue associated with remnants of the minor papilla. They are associated with pancreatitis in the region of the pancreas between the superior aspect of the pancreatic head, the common bile duct, and the duodenum (the "groove" region). Paraampullary duodenal wall cysts are dilated, partially de-epithelialized ductal structures. Alternative names include *cystic dystrophy of the duodenal wall* (59,141), *groove pancreatitis* (18,51,153,164), and *paraduodenal pancreatitis* (5a).

Clinical Features. Most patients are men in their forties. Alcohol use and cigarette smoking are commonly reported. Symptoms include abdominal pain, weight loss, vomiting, and, less commonly, jaundice. Upper endoscopy may reveal an intramural mass or duodenal stenosis in the region proximal to the major papilla. On CT scans there is thickening of the duodenum, in many cases associated with cyst formation in the duodenal wall or in the subjacent head of the pancreas (80,141). Strictures in the distal common bile duct or main pancreatic duct may be present. In the two thirds of cases with prominent cyst formation, the radiographic appearance resembles that of a pseudocyst, duodenal duplication cyst, or cystic pancreatic neoplasm, although familiarity with the entity may suggest the correct diagnosis (21). The cases without radiographically evident cystic change more commonly simulate pancreatic or periampullary neoplasms. In many of the reported cases, pancreatoduodenectomy has been performed for both diagnostic and therapeutic reasons.

Gross Findings. Grossly, paraampullary duodenal wall cysts are divided into cystic and solid types (21). In both types the duodenal wall and underlying pancreatic parenchyma are thickened and fibrotic, often in the region of the minor papilla. The more common cystic variant consists of one to several cysts in the duodenal wall and pancreatic head; each cyst measures 1 to 10 cm (fig. 15-28). Fibrous thickening of the duodenal wall is the predominant finding of the solid variant, although smaller (less than 1 cm) cystic structures may be found on close inspection. The pancreatic parenchyma in the groove region is fibrotic and expanded, and

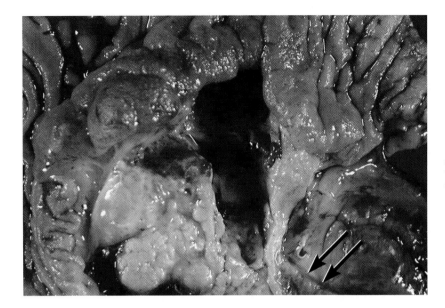

Figure 15-28

PARAAMPULLARY DUODENAL WALL CYST

The cysts in the duodenal wall and subjacent pancreas are unilocular. The arrows indicate the pancreatic duct.

there may be fibrotic strictures of the common bile duct and main pancreatic duct.

Microscopic Findings. Grossly identifiable cysts consist of massively dilated ducts, some of which are still partially lined by ductal epithelium (fig. 15-29) (21,168). Smaller dilated ducts are also seen microscopically. The lining epithelium may be mucinous or may have reactive cytologic atypia. Characteristically, the cysts contain large, eosinophilic, amorphous inspissated enzymatic secretions, some with a vaguely crystalline structure. The walls of the cysts are composed of markedly inflamed fibrous tissue, including lymphocytes, plasma cells, and neutrophils. Luminal and mural calcifications are common. A striking reactive spindle cell proliferation is usually present, including smooth muscle cells and myofibroblasts associated with inflammatory cells. The smooth muscle cells immunolabel for actin as well as desmin. Pancreatic elements including both acini and islets may be found in the duodenal submucosa and muscularis (59). In the groove region the underlying pancreatic parenchyma demonstrates atrophy, fat necrosis, and dense fibrosis. If the process significantly compresses the main pancreatic duct, obstructive chronic pancreatitis may extend into the remainder of the gland.

Differential Diagnosis. It is important to appreciate the anatomic distribution of the process to recognize this entity, especially in cases without prominent cyst formation. The pancre-

atitis can resemble pancreatitis of alcoholic or other nonspecific etiology, and cysts lacking an epithelial lining can mimic pseudocysts. The inspissated enzymatic secretions are highly characteristic, although similar secretions can accumulate in ducts obstructed by other processes. Microscopically, the reactive fibroinflammatory proliferation is often extremely exuberant, resembling an inflammatory myofibroblastic tumor or even a sarcoma. The participation of desmin-positive true smooth muscle cells may lead to the erroneous impression of a leiomyosarcoma if the other associated findings (i.e., the cysts) are not considered.

Discussion. Recent studies have clarified both the histologic features as well as the possible pathogenesis of this condition. The location of the cysts and the association with pancreatic parenchyma in the duodenal wall suggest that the cysts arise from dilated ducts associated with the minor papilla (fig. 15-30) (21, 153,170). It has been speculated that pancreatic secretions from this submucosal parenchyma normally pass into the duodenum through a patent minor papilla, and that obstruction of the small duct leading into the minor papilla and the consequent inflammatory process result in paraampullary duodenal wall cysts (52). In fact, serial sectioning of paraampullary duodenal wall cysts has failed to demonstrate a connection of the cysts to the duct of Santorini and the duodenal lumen, in

357

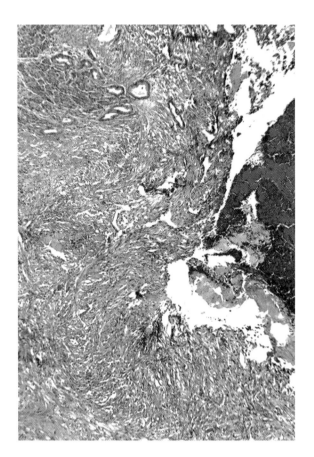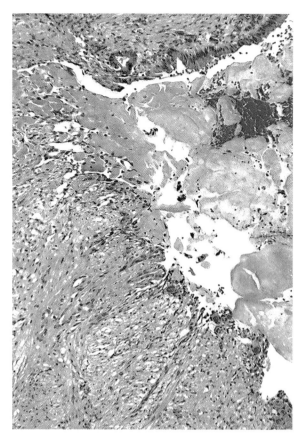

Figure 15-29

PARAAMPULLARY DUODENAL WALL CYST

Left: An irregular cystic cavity is filled with blood and amorphous proteinaceous secretions. The wall is lined by spindle cells and inflammation.

Right: At higher power, residual ductal epithelium (top) focally lines the cyst.

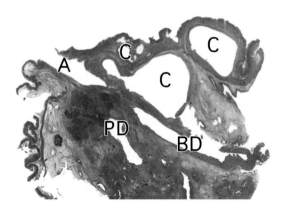

Figure 15-30

PARAAMPULLARY DUODENAL WALL CYST

Whole mount section shows the relationship of the cysts to the minor papilla and duodenal wall. (A = ampulla; BD = bile duct; PD = pancreatic duct; C = cysts). (Courtesy of Dr. Giuseppe Zamboni, Verona, Italy.)

contrast to the situation in the minor papilla of normal individuals (21). It is still not clear whether the primary pathology is alcoholic chronic pancreatitis that affects both the duodenal submucosal parenchyma as well as the pancreas itself, or whether the initiating event is the obstruction of the minor papilla, with pancreatitis in the gland proper only occurring as a secondary event. Cases with involvement limited to the duodenal wall would support the latter hypothesis.

Ductal Retention Cyst and Mucinous Non-neoplastic Cyst

Definition. A *ductal retention cyst* is a non-neoplastic unilocular cyst formed by the dilatation of an obstructed pancreatic duct and lined by a simple epithelial layer. An alternative term is

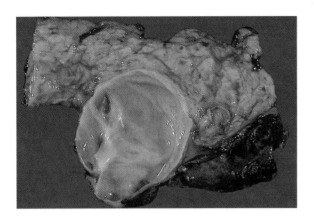

Figure 15-31

RETENTION CYST

The cyst is unilocular and has a smooth lining lacking papillae.

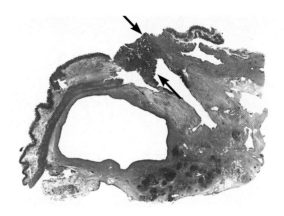

Figure 15-32

RETENTION CYST

Whole mount section shows a large retention cyst secondary to a small obstructing carcinoma in the ampulla of Vater (arrows).

simple cyst. Some authors restrict the term "retention cyst" to those examples lined by normal ductal epithelium composed of cuboidal cells lacking significant apical mucin (95). Simple cysts with a tall columnar mucinous lining are then designated as *mucinous non-neoplastic cysts* (27), although they can alternatively be regarded as *retention cysts involved by low-grade PanIN* (77).

Most patients are adults. There may be chronic pancreatitis or a neoplasm elsewhere within the pancreas. Patients with cystic fibrosis develop multiple retention cysts filled with viscous secretions (95). Since retention cysts result from ductal obstruction, it is important to ensure that they are not caused by a small obstructing carcinoma located proximal to the cyst. Most patients are asymptomatic and the cysts are detected incidentally on imaging studies or grossly. Retention cysts are increasingly identified with the greater use of abdominal CT scanning, and their preoperative distinction from cystic neoplasms is an area of difficulty. Cyst loculations, cyst complexity, or mural nodules should raise concerns that a pancreatic cyst is not simply a retention cyst.

Pathologic Findings. Ductal retention cysts may occur anywhere in the pancreas and vary from small (3- to 5-mm) thin-walled cysts surrounded by normal parenchyma to sizeable (over 5-cm) cysts with a fibrotic wall in regions of atrophic pancreatitis (figs. 15-31, 15-32). They are usually single and unilocular, but sometimes may appear more complex, with haustrations of the wall, or they may be multiple. The lining is usually smooth and glistening. Careful examination may reveal stenosis or obstruction of the pancreatic duct system.

Microscopically, retention cysts have a simple epithelial lining. In strictly defined cases, the cells are cuboidal without obvious accumulation of apical mucin and resemble normal or attenuated ductal epithelium (fig. 15-33). PanIN may involve retention cysts, and a simple columnar mucinous lining may be present (fig. 15-34). These cysts are also designated mucinous non-neoplastic cysts. The nuclei are uniform, round, and basally located. Papillae are not encountered in retention cysts, and their presence suggests a diagnosis of branch duct intraductal papillary mucinous neoplasm (see below). Inflammation is present in the wall of some cysts, with pericystic fibrosis. The lining may be partially denuded, simulating a pseudocyst.

The cytologic features are not clearly defined and aspiration biopsy is essentially nondiagnostic. The procurement of mucoid fluid, however, can lead to an erroneous cytologic diagnosis of a mucin-producing neoplastic cyst. In retention cysts secondary to obstructing carcinomas, the adenocarcinoma may colonize the cyst.

Differential Diagnosis. Retention cysts may resemble mucinous cystic neoplasms, macrocystic serous cystadenomas, branch duct intraductal papillary mucinous neoplasms, and

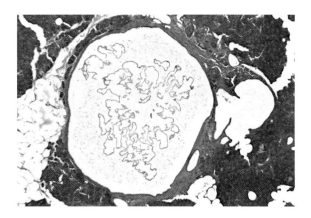
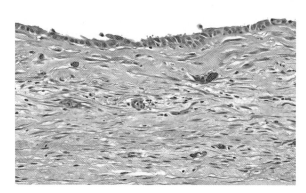

Figure 15-33

RETENTION CYST

Dilated duct without papillae (left) is lined by normal-appearing ductal epithelium (right).

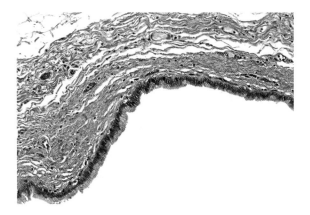

Figure 15-34

RETENTION CYST

Involvement of the cyst by pancreatic intraepithelial neoplasia (PanIN-1A).

pseudocysts. Other than pseudocysts, all of these entities are usually multilocular or multicystic. Pseudocysts usually affect patients with a history of acute pancreatitis and completely lack an epithelial lining, so if careful examination of a fibrous-walled cyst with mural inflammation fails to identify epithelium, the diagnosis of pseudocyst should be favored. Mucinous cystic neoplasms have the characteristic hypercellular ovarian-like stroma underlying the epithelium; in addition, the epithelium is often papillary and may show significant nuclear atypia. Macrocystic serous cystadenomas, like retention cysts, have a simple layer of cuboidal epithelium but the cytoplasm is clear due to glycogen accumu-

lation. Branch duct intraductal papillary mucinous neoplasms may be extremely hard to distinguish from retention cysts when the latter are involved by low-grade PanIN (77). If there are multiple dilated ducts and papillae, a diagnosis of intraductal papillary mucinous neoplasm is suggested. It has been recognized, however, that large foci of PanIN may be nearly impossible to distinguish from small intraductal papillary mucinous neoplasms, and it is difficult to exclude the possibility that a cystic duct lined by flat mucinous epithelium and surrounded by ducts with more exuberant papillae may be a retention cyst in a region extensively involved by PanIN. International guidelines have recently been developed to distinguish retention cysts from intraductal papillary mucinous neoplasms and PanIN (77), but cysts exist that defy rigid classification.

Congenital Cyst

A *congenital cyst* is an uncommon unilocular cyst that does not communicate with the ductal system and is lined by a single layer of nonmucinous epithelium. Also known as *dysgenetic cysts*, congenital cysts are presumably present at birth and are not associated with ductal obstruction or other specific abnormalities in the pancreas. Small solitary congenital cysts are asymptomatic and many are undetected. Some are multiple, as in cases associated with cysts of the kidney and liver (135). The multiple cysts of von Hippel-Lindau syndrome may be congenital cysts (157), although their glycogen-rich clear cell lining more resembles that of serous cystadenoma (notably, macrocystic serous cystadenoma). Congenital cysts may be found at any age but are most often reported in children (82, 120,125). They are usually 1 to 2 cm in diameter and lined by cuboidal epithelium resembling that of normal ducts. In adults, congenital cysts may be microscopically indistinguishable from retention cysts, the diagnosis that is favored in the presence of pancreatitis or mass lesions elsewhere in the gland.

Lymphoepithelial Cyst

Definition. *Pancreatic lymphoepithelial cysts* are unilocular or multilocular cystic lesions lined predominantly by mature squamous epithelium and surrounded by non-neoplastic lymphoid elements. Nearly 50 cases have been reported (4,5). Lymphoepithelial cysts are the most common pancreatic cyst lined by squamous epithelium, the other entities being epidermoid cyst in intrapancreatic heterotopic spleen and mature cystic teratoma (dermoid cyst). Malignant transformation has not been described in pancreatic lymphoepithelial cysts.

Clinical Features. Although initially reported exclusively in men, lymphoepithelial cysts are now known to occur in women as well, but with a 4 to 1 male predominance. Most patients are older adults (mean age, 56 years). The symptoms are nonspecific and include pain, nausea, anorexia, and fever. There are no reported associations with conditions related to lymphoepithelial cysts of the parotid gland or head and neck region, such as Sjögren's syndrome, human immunodeficiency virus, or autoimmune diseases. Pancreatic lymphoepithelial cysts are evenly distributed throughout the gland and may project into the peripancreatic tissues; their sharp delineation from the pancreatic parenchyma may help suggest the diagnosis radiographically.

Gross Findings. Lymphoepithelial cysts range from 1.2 to 17.0 cm (mean, 4.7 cm), and are either unilocular (40 percent) or multilocular (60 percent). They are well circumscribed and sharply separate from the adjacent pancreas (fig. 15-35), sometimes appearing to be peripancreatic. The cyst wall is usually 1 to 3 mm thick. The cysts are filled with cheesy keratinaceous debris. If the cyst contents are removed, the lining of the cysts can be seen to be smooth to granular.

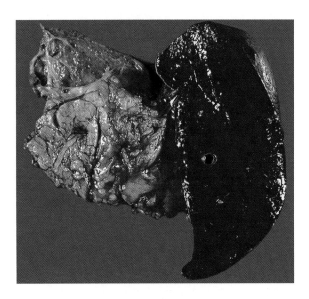

Figure 15-35

LYMPHOEPITHELIAL CYST

The peripancreatic unilocular cyst superior to the pancreas contains keratin debris, which is adherent to the otherwise smooth lining.

Lymphoepithelial cysts with abundant lymphoid tissue may have a band of tan soft tissue surrounding the wall of the cyst. Multilocular cysts have thin septa between the locules.

Microscopic Findings. The cysts are lined by mature, stratified squamous epithelium, usually with keratinization (fig. 15-36). In some cases, there may be a superimposed acute inflammatory infiltrate and reactive epithelial atypia, but dysplasia is not encountered. Other types of epithelia may be found, including non-keratinizing squamous epithelium, flat cuboidal epithelium, and transitional epithelium. Rarely, there are scattered sebaceous and mucinous cells; no skin adnexal structures should be found. The lymphoid tissue is immediately beneath the epithelium, and lymphocytes rarely extend into the squamous layer. Germinal center formation is common. The solid lymphoepithelial islands that are commonly found in salivary lymphoepithelial cysts are rare in the pancreatic counterpart but have been described (5). Small microcystic structures may be found in the lymphoid layer. Epithelioid granulomas, cholesterol clefts, and areas of stromal hyalinization may be present. The adjacent pancreas is usually unremarkable.

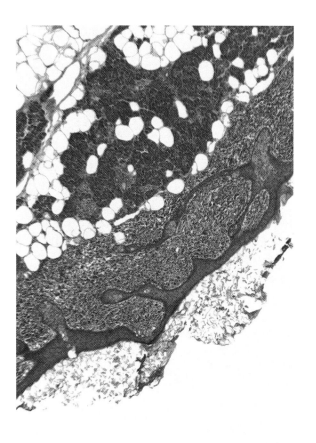
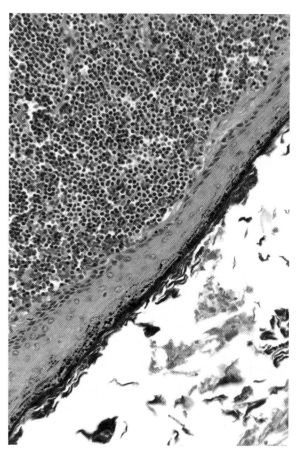

Figure 15-36

LYMPHOEPITHELIAL CYST

Left: The squamous epithelial lining of the cyst is surrounded by a dense band of lymphocytes.
Right: The epithelium is keratinizing and exhibits a granular cell layer.

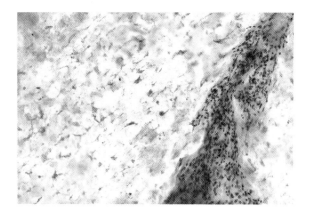

Figure 15-37

LYMPHOEPITHELIAL CYST

A fibrous tissue fragment of cyst wall with embedded lymphocytes (right) is associated with a background of keratinaceous debris (direct smear; Papanicolaou stain).

Cytologic Findings. The cytologic examination of a lymphoepithelial cyst may be diagnostic provided an adequate sample is obtained (23, 30,32,50,114,126). The characteristic appearance on cytology reflects the histologic appearance: cyst debris containing nucleated and anucleated squamous cells, keratinaceous and cholesterol debris, and scattered histiocytes and rare lymphocytes in the background. Fibrous tissue fragments with embedded lymphocytes and squamous cells may be noted (fig. 15-37).

Differential Diagnosis. Most cystic neoplasms of the pancreas are lined exclusively by glandular (serous or mucinous) epithelium, so their distinction from lymphoepithelial cysts is not problematic. Grossly, lymphoepithelial cysts may resemble pseudocysts since the keratinaceous debris of lymphoepithelial cysts is

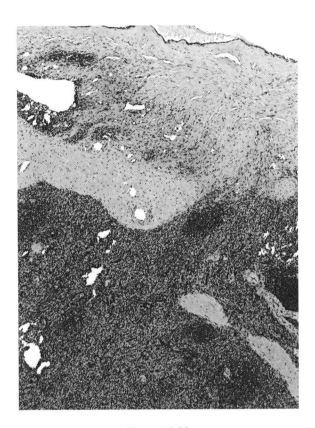

Figure 15-38

**EPIDERMOID CYST IN
INTRAPANCREATIC HETEROTOPIC SPLEEN**

The cyst (top) has a thin epithelial lining surrounded by splenic red and white pulp. (Courtesy of Dr. N. Volkan Adsay, Detroit, MI.)

similar to the necrotic material of pseudocysts and both are often peripancreatic. Microscopically, however, the principal differential diagnostic entity is mature cystic teratoma and epidermoid cyst in intrapancreatic heterotopic spleen. In contrast with these entities, lymphoepithelial cysts have a male predominance and occur in an older age group (5). Since lymphoepithelial cysts may have small foci of sebaceous or mucinous differentiation, there is histologic overlap with mature cystic teratomas. If adnexal structures, hair, or other types of epithelium (intestinal, respiratory) are present, the lesion is a teratoma. Extensive sebaceous or mucinous elements are also more suggestive of a teratoma. A dense band of lymphoid tissue surrounding a squamous-lined cyst generally signifies a lymphoepithelial cyst, especially when germinal centers are present. If splenic red pulp is found adjacent to the cyst, the diagnosis is epidermoid cyst in intrapancreatic heterotopic spleen.

On cytology, the presence of squamous cells and keratinaceous debris excludes pseudocyst as well as serous and mucinous cysts. Analysis of cyst fluid may be misleading, however, with markedly elevated CEA levels incorrectly suggesting a malignant mucin-producing cystic neoplasm (32,85).

Discussion. The origin of pancreatic lymphoepithelial cysts is uncertain. Speculations have included origin from epithelial inclusions in peripancreatic lymph nodes (although such inclusions have only exceptionally been demonstrated, and the lymphoid elements of most lymphoepithelial cysts do not have the features of a residual lymph node), squamous metaplasia of the pancreatic ductal epithelium, derivation as a form of monodermal teratoma, and displacement of a branchial cleft cyst. Another intriguing suggestion is that there is an interaction between a subset of lymphocytes and the pancreatic ductal epithelium that results in squamous differentiation and proliferation, with cyst formation initially due to secretory activity of the lining cells (5). Whatever the mechanism of formation, pancreatic lymphoepithelial cysts are benign lesions that are cured by conservative resection.

Epidermoid Cyst in
Intrapancreatic Heterotopic Spleen

Heterotopic splenic tissue is rarely found in the tail of the pancreas. Even more exceptional is the occurrence of *epidermoid cysts within intrapancreatic heterotopic spleen* (5,128). Since 10 percent of nonparasitic splenic cysts are epidermoid, the occasional appearance of an epidermoid cyst in intrapancreatic splenic tissue is not unexpected. All of the reported cases have occurred in the tail of the pancreas. They usually are diagnosed in adults (mean age, 37 years), and occur in both men and women equally. Symptoms include epigastric pain and nausea. The lesions are well-demarcated and average 4.5 cm. Both unilocular and multilocular cases have been reported.

The cysts contain serous fluid or keratinaceous debris and are lined by stratified keratinizing squamous epithelium (fig. 15-38). The surrounding splenic tissue is usually unremarkable other than its ectopic location, although white pulp elements may be sparse. Malignancy has not been described in epidermoid cysts in intrapancreatic heterotopic spleen.

The differential diagnosis includes lymphoepithelial cyst (see above) and dermoid cyst (mature cystic teratoma). Recognition of the splenic elements allows a correct diagnosis.

Miscellaneous Cystic Lesions

Foregut (Enteric) Cyst. Very rare foregut cysts, or gastrointestinal duplication cysts, are usually found adjacent to the pancreas rather than within it and originate from the wall of the stomach or duodenum (100). Some communicate with the pancreatic ducts. Foregut cysts are congenital. They may cause pancreatitis and often present in childhood (41,74,82,109,117). Most are found in the head of the gland, although some also affect the tail (101). Foregut cysts are simple cysts lined by a variety of epithelia including gastric, small intestinal, squamous, and ciliated columnar (11,100). The wall of the cyst contains bundles of smooth muscle. The muscle layer is relatively well-oriented and skin adnexal structures are lacking, allowing distinction from mature cystic teratomas.

Duodenal Diverticula. These appear as unilocular intrapancreatic or peripancreatic cysts when they occur on the pancreatic side of the duodenum. Thus, they may simulate primary pancreatic cystic lesions such as retention cysts, pseudocysts, or cystic neoplasms (69). Duodenal diverticula are outpouchings of the duodenum, and the lumen of the cyst (as well as the mucosa) is contiguous with the duodenal lumen. Small diverticula are not uncommon close to the ampulla of Vater (124). Duodenal diverticula should be distinguished from foregut cysts, which do not communicate with the duodenal lumen.

Endometriotic Cyst. These are extremely rare in the pancreas (119). As in other locations, they occur in reproductive-aged women and are lined by endometrial epithelium with endometrial-type stroma and hemorrhage in the wall. Endometriotic cysts can be confused with mucinous cystic neoplasms, since the later also have a cellular stromal component. Mucinous cystic neoplasms, however, usually have an abundantly mucinous lining and lack significant stromal hemorrhage.

Parasitic Cyst. Rarely, hydatid cysts occur in the pancreas and mimic primary cystic neoplasms (87,102a). In one study, 4 of 280 patients (1.4 percent) with hydatid disease had pancreatic involvement (102a), all in the head of the gland. The diagnosis should be considered in regions in which echinococcal disease is endemic.

LESIONS OF THE ENDOCRINE PANCREAS

Islet Hyperplasia

Islet hyperplasia is an absolute increase in islet mass resulting from an increase in islet cell number. It is important to recognize that there are age-related differences in islet cell mass (143), so a volume of islets that may represent hyperplasia in an adult could be normal in an infant. Islet hyperplasia results from an increase either in all cell types or in β cells alone. Islet cell hyperplasia can be observed in infants of diabetic mothers and in patients with Beckwith-Wiedemann syndrome, erythroblastosis fetalis, hereditary tyrosinemia, Zellweger's syndrome, and leprechaunism (49,60,61,157,162). The aggregation of islets that occurs secondary to chronic pancreatitis (see below) should not be confused with true islet hyperplasia.

Hyperplastic islets of Langerhans are usually more than 250 μm in diameter (157). In infants of diabetic mothers, the islets are larger and more numerous than in the normal pancreas. In addition, they show β-cell hypertrophy. In patients with Beckwith-Wiedemann syndrome, the pancreas is often increased in size and shows massive diffuse islet hyperplasia with abnormally large and confluent islets of Langerhans. They may be clustered in the center of the lobules and surrounded by a rim of acinar cells (162). In all other conditions mentioned above, the islet hyperplasia is similar to that seen in infants of diabetic mothers. The normal distribution of the different islet cell types is maintained in islet hyperplasia, allowing the distinction of a hyperplastic islet from an endocrine microadenoma. The presence of pancreatitis in the adjacent parenchyma suggests that the islet clustering is due to islet aggregation rather than hyperplasia.

Islet Aggregation

Definition. *Islet aggregation* is a clustering of architecturally normal or distorted, non-neoplastic

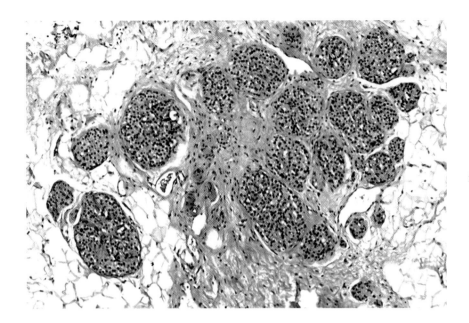

Figure 15-39

ISLET AGGREGATION

Aggregation of compact islets with nesting architecture.

islets, usually encountered in the setting of chronic pancreatitis. The term islet cell hyperplasia has been misapplied to these lesions.

General Features. Islet aggregation is a commonly encountered phenomenon. Since the endocrine elements of the pancreas are relatively resistant to the atrophy that affects the acini and, subsequently, the ducts during the evolution of chronic pancreatitis, islets of Langerhans often remain after loss of the exocrine components. Due to the loss of substantial parenchymal volume, the remaining islets appear more densely clustered than in the normal pancreas. The inflammation and fibrosis that occur in chronic pancreatitis may cause architectural abnormalities in these islets, resulting in pseudoinfiltrative patterns. Thus, islet aggregation may simulate both exocrine and endocrine neoplastic processes (see Differential Diagnosis, below) (17,157). There are no data demonstrating that the total endocrine cell mass is increased relative to the normal pancreas (in fact, endocrine function is usually decreased), and proliferation studies fail to demonstrate increased mitotic activity or DNA synthesis in areas of islet aggregation.

Pathologic Findings. Islet aggregation is not apparent grossly, other than generally involving regions of fibrotic parenchyma. Thus, a pancreas grossly harboring foci of chronic pancreatitis is likely to display some degree of islet aggregation microscopically.

To some extent, the histologic appearance of islet aggregation depends upon the region of the pancreas that is involved. In most of the pancreas (superior head, body, and tail), the majority of islets of Langerhans are of the compact type (see chapter 1). When the parenchyma from these regions undergoes atrophy, the well-circumscribed nests of endocrine cells that constitute the residual compact islets cluster together and are surrounded by variably dense bands of collagenized stroma (fig. 15-39). Often, the islet morphology is preserved, and although the individual islets of Langerhans may vary in size (as they normally do), they are readily recognizable as islets. In the inferior portion of the pancreatic head, however, most of the islets of Langerhans are of the diffuse type, consisting mainly of pancreatic polypeptide (PP) cells, and when atrophy affects this region, the interlacing strands of endocrine cells assume an exaggerated trabecular arrangement, often having a pseudoinfiltrative appearance within the surrounding fibrotic stroma. In both types of islet aggregation, the nuclear features are those of normal islet cells, including the presence of occasional enlarged nuclei; no true pleomorphism is found. Close association between islets and small ducts is common, resulting in ductulo-insular complexes resembling those of nesidioblastosis (see Differential Diagnosis, below).

Additional diagnostic difficulties arise when there has been more active stromal remodeling

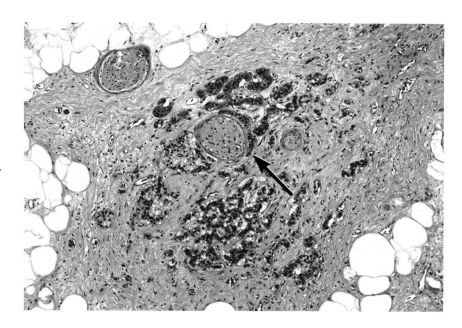

Figure 15-40

ISLET AGGREGATION

Perineural "invasion" (arrow).

in regions of parenchymal atrophy. The normal shape of the islet may then be distorted, accentuating the pseudoinfiltrative appearance. Extension of non-neoplastic islets into peripancreatic fat also occurs, especially when there is a concomitant fatty infiltration of the pancreas. Finally, islet cells may extend into perineural spaces (fig. 15-40). It is not clear how the islet cells become draped around nerves without having true invasive capabilities; normal islets are not supplied with nerves of the size commonly surrounded by islet cells in islet aggregation. Presumably the juxtaposition results from tissue remodeling during scarring from chronic pancreatitis, but the possibility of actual perineural invasion by non-neoplastic islet cells cannot be excluded.

The normal number and distribution of the peptide cell types can be demonstrated immunohistochemically in islet aggregation (including a significant population of PP cells in the diffuse islets).

Differential Diagnosis. The differential diagnosis includes endocrine microadenoma, islet hyperplasia or nesidioblastosis, and invasive carcinoma. Since endocrine neoplasms, including microadenomas, have an altered peptide cell composition (microadenomas are commonly α-cell or PP-cell predominant), they can be distinguished from islet aggregation by labeling for the four normal islet cell peptides: insulin, glucagon, somatostatin, and pancreatic polypeptide. The

terms islet hyperplasia and nesidioblastosis are often mistakenly used for islet aggregation. Both of these much rarer conditions are strictly defined and associated with characteristic clinical syndromes. In the absence of hyperinsulinemic hypoglycemia, a diagnosis of nesidioblastosis should not be made, and most cases occur in neonates. There is no evidence of chronic pancreatitis, endocrine cells are seen abutting small ducts as well as in irregular clusters, and marked nuclear enlargement is commonly present. Islet hyperplasia may consist simply of enlarged (greater than 250 μm) islets, but again the surrounding exocrine pancreas is usually normal.

Some foci of islet aggregation have a sufficiently pseudoinfiltrative pattern to suggest a diagnosis of an invasive neoplasm. This is particularly problematic in needle biopsy or frozen section specimens, where the strands of endocrine cells can resemble a poorly differentiated ductal adenocarcinoma. Perineural invasion by islet cells may complete the false picture of carcinoma. If the possibility of islet aggregation is considered, immunohistochemical labeling for chromogranin or synaptophysin will readily distinguish the process from carcinoma. Histologic features suggesting aggregation of diffuse islets include relative nuclear uniformity, a coarsely clumped chromatin pattern, perineural invasion by only solid nests or strands of cells without lumen formation, and absence of stromal desmoplasia.

Nesidioblastosis

Nesidioblastosis is a descriptor of the morphologic findings accompanying functional disorders of β cells associated with hyperinsulinemic hypoglycemia in the absence of an insulinoma. The histologic changes vary depending upon the clinical setting (neonates and infants versus adults) and the underlying genetic abnormalities. These morphologic abnormalities include hypertrophic β cells within the islets and, particularly in neonates, close association of islet cells with small pancreatic ducts (ductulo-insular complexes) and abnormal aggregation of islets. Patients with nesidioblastosis are usually neonates and infants with hyperinsulinism (persistent neonatal hyperinsulinemic hypoglycemia [PNHH]) (40,64,157,166,167). Rarely, adults with hypoglycemia have similar histologic findings (persistent adult hyperinsulinemic hypoglycemia [PAHH]) (7,12,63,178), but insulinomas are much more common in the pediatric patient population.

The term nesidioblastosis has been incorrectly used to refer to a variety of abnormal endocrine lesions in other contexts, in particular to islet aggregation associated with chronic pancreatitis. Histologically similar ductuloinsular complexes can be found in both circumstances. The use of the term nesidioblastosis, however, should be restricted to cases with clear functional abnormalities in β cells. In fact, some authors (83,143,166) advocate using the term only as a purely morphologic descriptor of the presence of endocrine cells associated with small ducts, as originally described (107,186), and instead propose using "hyperinsulinism" to refer to the clinicopathologic process described herein (58).

Nesidioblastosis in Neonates and Infants. *Clinical Features and Genetics.* PNHH is usually seen in neonates and presents within the first year of life in 70 percent of cases (157). The symptoms of hypoglycemia include pallor, sweating, seizures, motor abnormalities, and macrosomia (14). There is inadequate suppression of insulin at low plasma concentrations of glucose, so the serum insulin levels may not be absolutely elevated but are abnormally high for the level of glucose (161).

Study of the genetics of PNHH has revealed a number of different mutations in genes encoding the adenosine triphosphate (ATP)-sensitive potassium channel (K_{ATP}) in the cell membrane of β cells (such as *ABCC8* and *KCNJ11*) (173,174) or in the glutamate dehydrogenase, glucokinase, or short-chain L-3-hydroxyacyl-CoA dehydrogenase genes (36,57,160), demonstrating that this disorder clearly has a functional basis and does not simply reflect an increase in the β-cell mass. The severity of symptoms reflects the specific mutation from which the patient suffers (166). Most cases are sporadic, although familial cases have been recorded.

Gross Findings. In most instances, the gross appearance of the pancreas is normal. In the 25 to 50 percent of patients with the focal form of the disease (see below), a localized nodule resembling a small pancreatic endocrine neoplasm is found (60). Even the focal form is usually grossly inapparent, leading to difficulties in localization and treatment (6).

Microscopic Findings. Many reports have been published over the last 30 years regarding the histologic features and classification of the resected pancreata from patients with PNHH. Despite some discrepancies among the reports, most agree that nesidioblastosis can be divided into two general types, diffuse and focal (60,83, 143,145,151a,166,167).

The diffuse form of nesidioblastosis shows islet abnormalities throughout the gland but no discrete localized aggregation. The key finding is the presence of enlarged and hyperchromatic β-cell nuclei (fig. 15-41). Per islet, there are usually one or two β cells with a prominent giant nucleus. The size of the nuclei in β cells varies somewhat in normal neonates, but in nesidioblastosis there is a 40 percent increase in nuclear volume compared with age-matched controls. As a general rule, a three-fold increase relative to the nuclei of adjacent islet cells is found (167). Other changes include abnormal islet shapes, enlarged islets, and ductuloinsular complexes, but these findings may not be abnormal compared to age-matched controls (64,166).

In focal nesidioblastosis there is a localized nodular lesion that may be similar histologically to an insulinoma (adenoma-like), but more commonly there is simply an aggregate of ill-formed islet-like clusters associated with ductuloinsular complexes (fig. 15-42). Some of the nuclei within the lesion are enlarged

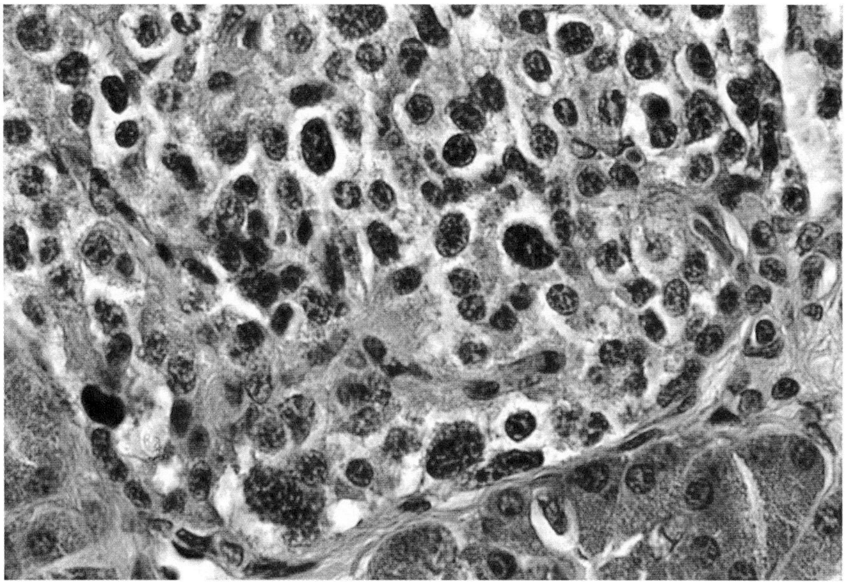

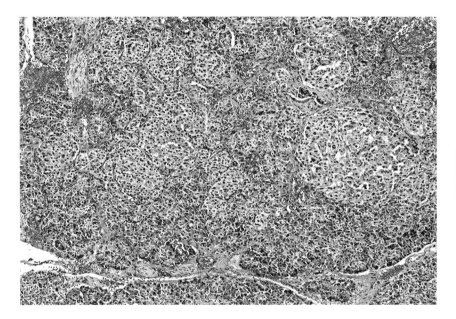

Figure 15-41

DIFFUSE NESIDIOBLASTOSIS

Some islet cells show marked nuclear enlargement.

Figure 15-42

FOCAL NESIDIOBLASTOSIS

Clusters of islet cells with nuclear enlargement are separated by thin bands of acinar cells. This is also known as adenomatous hyperplasia.

(thought to be polyploid). Thin rims of acini separate the cell clusters, and the endocrine cell clusters do not disrupt the original boundaries of the pancreatic lobules. These foci are designated adenomatous hyperplasia, and the endocrine elements should occupy at least 40 percent of the involved area (167). In the focal form of the disease, the islets of Langerhans in the surrounding pancreas are normal. Some patients have multifocal disease, for instance, one focus in the head and one in the tail (61,145). The foci of adenomatous hyperplasia are usually smaller than 1 cm (159).

Immunohistochemical labeling of the adenoma-like lesions as well as the foci of adenomatosis demonstrates a normal spatial distribution of the different islet cell types, suggesting a hyperplastic lesion, in contrast to insulinomas.

Differential Diagnosis. In neonates with the characteristic clinical findings, the chief differential diagnosis is not between nesidioblastosis and other lesions but between the focal and diffuse forms of nesidioblastosis. Since focal nesidioblastosis can be successfully treated by localized pancreatectomy (6), the distinction is important (144,167). Identification of an adenoma-like lesion or adenomatous hyperplasia suggests the focal form. Examination of the islets away from the lesion is suggested to confirm normal nuclear morphology. The presence of markedly enlarged nuclei in β cells from different regions of the pancreas strongly suggests the diffuse form of the disease, requiring a near-total (95 percent) pancreatectomy in cases refractory to medical management (166).

From a histologic standpoint, other endocrine lesions in chronic pancreatitis resemble the changes of nesidioblastosis, including islet cell clusters (islet aggregation) and ductuloinsular complexes. Usually there are other obvious features of chronic pancreatitis in the surrounding pancreas. In the absence of clinical evidence of hyperinsulinism, these lesions should be designated descriptively and the term nesidioblastosis should be avoided.

Nesidioblastosis in Adults. A diagnosis of nesidioblastosis in an adult with hyperinsulinemic hypoglycemia should be made with great caution, since most such patients have insulinomas, which can be small and difficult to locate. Rare cases of adult nesidioblastosis do occur, however, in which the only histologic finding may be β-cell nuclear hypertrophy, although the nuclei do not show as much enlargement as in the neonatal form. Occasionally, there is an increase in the number of islets and significant variability in their size and shape (7,12,63,176a,178). Rare cases of hyperinsulinism without a solitary insulinoma have also been attributed to microadenomatosis, in which multiple endocrine microadenomas produce insulin (11a). Thus, a diagnosis of nesidioblastosis in an adult requires systematic examination of the resected pancreas, with serial sections to exclude an insulinoma.

Islet Dysplasia

Islet dysplasia refers to cytologic and architectural alterations in islets, mostly in patients with multiple endocrine neoplasia, type 1 (MEN1). Dysplastic islets are enlarged and have a trabecular architecture as well as nuclear enlargement and mild atypia (99,157). They measure less than 0.5 mm. The normal peptide cell types are present but their proportions and topography are abnormal.

The term islet dysplasia is specifically intended to refer to the abnormal islets encountered in pancreata from MEN1 patients that are not large enough to be regarded as microadenomas. Enlarged or abnormal islets encountered in other settings should not be regarded as dysplastic, since there is no evidence of neoplastic potential in most of these cases.

REFERENCES

1. Abraham SC, Cruz-Correa M, Argani P, Furth EE, Hruban RH, Boitnott JK. Lymphoplasmacytic chronic cholecystitis and biliary tract disease in patients with lymphoplasmacytic sclerosing pancreatitis. Am J Surg Pathol 2003;27:441-51.
2. Abraham SC, Leach S, Yeo CJ, et al. Eosinophilic pancreatitis and increased eosinophils in the pancreas. Am J Surg Pathol 2003;27:334-42.
3. Abraham SC, Wilentz RE, Yeo CJ, et al. Pancreaticoduodenectomy (Whipple resections) in patients without malignancy: are they all 'chronic pancreatitis'? Am J Surg Pathol 2003;27:110-20.
3a. Adsay NV, Basturk O, Klimstra DS, Klöppel G. Pancreatic pseudotumors: non-neoplastic solid lesions of the pancreas that clinically mimic pancreas cancer. Semin Diagn Pathol 2004;21:260-7.
4. Adsay NV, Hasteh F, Cheng JD, et al. Lymphoepithelial cysts of the pancreas: a report of 12 cases and a review of the literature. Mod Pathol 2002;15:492-501.
5. Adsay NV, Hasteh F, Cheng JD, Klimstra DS. Squamous-lined cysts of the pancreas: lymphoepithelial cysts, dermoid cysts (teratomas), and accessory-splenic epidermoid cysts. Semin Diagn Pathol 2000;17:56-65.
5a. Adsay NV, Zamboni G. Paraduodenal pancreatitis: a clinico-pathologically distinct entity unifying "cystic dystrophy of heterotopic pancreas," "para-duodenal wall cyst," and "groove pancreatitis." Semin Diagn Pathol 2004;21:247-54.

6. Adzick NS, Thornton PS, Stanley CA, Kaye RD, Ruchelli E. A multidisciplinary approach to the focal form of congenital hyperinsulinism leads to successful treatment by partial pancreatectomy. J Pediatr Surg 2004;39:270-5.

7. Albers N, Lohr M, Bogner U, Loy V, Klöppel G. Nesidioblastosis of the pancreas in an adult with persistent hyperinsulinemic hypoglycemia. Am J Clin Pathol 1989;91:336-40.

8. Albores-Saavedra J. The pseudometastasis. Patologia 1994;32:63-71.

9. Alvarez M, Rodriguez A, Zabaleta S, Basterra G, Galdos J, Campos F. [Pseudotumor pancreatic tuberculosis]. Rev Esp Enferm Dig 1994;86:625-6. {Spanish.]

10. Ammann RW, Akovbiantz A, Largiader F, Schueler G. Course and outcome of chronic pancreatitis. Longitudinal study of a mixed medical-surgical series of 245 patients. Gastroenterology 1984;86:820-8.

11. Andersson R, Lindell G, Cwikiel W, Dawiskiba S. Retroperitoneal bronchogenic cyst as a differential diagnosis of pancreatic mucinous cystic tumor. Dig Surg 2003;20:55-7.

11a. Anlauf M, Schlenger R, Bauersfeld J, et al. Microadenomatosis of the endocrine pancreas in patients with and without the multiple endocrine neoplasia type 1 syndrome. Am J Surg Pathol 2006;30:560-74.

12. Anlauf M, Wieben D, Perren A, et al. Persistent hyperinsulinemic hypoglycemia in 15 adults with diffuse nesidioblastosis: diagnostic criteria, incidence, and characterization of beta-cell changes. Am J Surg Pathol 2005;29:524-33.

12a. Asada M, Nishio A, Uchida K, et al. Identification of a novel autoantibody against pancreatic secretory trypsin inhibitor in patients with autoimmune pancreatitis. Pancreas 2006;33:20-6.

13. Ashida K, Egashira Y, Tutumi A, et al. Endocrine neoplasm arising from duodenal heterotopic pancreas: a case report. Gastrointest Endosc 1997;46:172-6.

14. Aynsley-Green A, Hussain K, Hall J, et al. Practical management of hyperinsulinism in infancy. Arch Dis Child Fetal Neonatal Ed 2000;82:F98-F107.

15. Barthet M, Hastier P, Bernard JP, et al. Chronic pancreatitis and inflammatory bowel disease: true or coincidental association? Am J Gastroenterol 1999;94:2141-8.

16. Bartholomew LG, Cain JC, Woolner LB, Utz DC, Ferris DO. Sclerosing cholangitis: its possible association with Riedel's struma and fibrous retroperitonitis. Report of two cases. N Engl J Med 1963;269:8-12.

17. Bartow SA, Mukai K, Rosai J. Pseudoneoplastic proliferation of endocrine cells in pancreatic fibrosis. Cancer 1981;47:2627-33.

18. Becker V, Mischke U. Groove pancreatitis. Int J Pancreatol 1991;10:173-82.

19. Bentz JS, Kochman ML, Faigel DO, Ginsberg GG, Smith DB, Gupta PK. Endoscopic ultrasound-guided real-time fine-needle aspiration: clinicopathologic features of 60 patients. Diagn Cytopathol 1998;18:98-109.

20. Bill K, Belber JP, Carson JW. Adenomyoma (pancreatic heterotopia) of the duodenum producing common bile duct obstruction. Gastrointest Endosc 1982;28:182-4.

21. Bogina G, Scarpa A, Mombello A, et al. Cystic dystrophy of the duodenal wall is a pancreatitis of the intraduodenal pancreas caused by the obstruction of papilla minor. Am J Surg Pathol. [In press.]

22. Bogomoletz WV. Duct destructive chronic pancreatitis. A new insight into the pathology of idiopathic non-alcoholic chronic pancreatitis. Gut 1997;41:272-3.

23. Bolis GB, Farabi R, Liberati F, Maccio T. Lymphoepithelial cyst of the pancreas. Report of a case diagnosed by fine needle aspiration biopsy. Acta Cytol 1998;42:384-6.

24. Brady MS, Garfein CF, Klimstra DS, Brenann MF. Sarcoidosis of the pancreas. J Surg Oncol 1993;54:132-7.

25. Brugge WR, Lauwers GY, Sahani D, Fernandez-del Castillo C, Warshaw AL. Cystic neoplasms of the pancreas. N Engl J Med 2004;351:1218-26.

26. Brugge WR, Lewandrowski KB, Lee-Lewandrowski E, et al. Diagnosis of pancreatic cystic neoplasms: a report of the cooperative pancreatic cyst study. Gastroenterology 2004;126:1330-6.

27. Brunner A, Ladurner R, Kosmahl M, Mikuz G, Tzankov A. Mucinous non-neoplastic cyst of the pancreas accompanied by non-parasitic asymptomatic liver cysts. Virchows Arch 2004;444:482-4.

28. Burke GW, Binder SC, Barron AM, Dratch PL, Umlas J. Heterotopic pancreas: gastric outlet obstruction secondary to pancreatitis and pancreatic pseudocyst. Am J Gastroenterol 1989;84:52-5.

29. Burt TB, Condon VR, Matlak ME. Fetal pancreatic hamartoma. Pediatr Radiol 1983;13:287-9.

30. Cappellari JO. Fine-needle aspiration cytology of a pancreatic lymphoepithelial cyst. Diagn Cytopathol 1993;9:77-81.

31. Castellani C, Bonizzato A, Rolfini R, Frulloni L, Cavallini GC, Mastella G. Increased prevalence of mutations of the cystic fibrosis gene in idiopathic chronic and recurrent pancreatitis. Am J Gastroenterol 1999;94:1993-5.

32. Centeno BA, Stockwell JW, Lewandrowski KB. Cyst fluid cytology and chemical features in a case of lymphoepithelial cyst of the pancreas: a rare and difficult preoperative diagnosis. Diagn Cytopathol 1999;21:328-30.

33. Chung JP, Na SK, Park YN, et al. Non-alcoholic duct-destructive chronic pancreatitis: recognition before definitive treatment. Yonsei Med J 1999;40:518-22.

34. Chutaputti A, Burrell MI, Boyer JL. Pseudotumor of the pancreas associated with retroperitoneal fibrosis: a dramatic response to corticosteroid therapy. Am J Gastroenterol 1995;90:1155-8.

35. Clark A, Zeman RK, Choyke PL, et al. Pancreatic pseudotumors associated with multifocal idiopathic fibrosclerosis. Gastrointest Radiol 1988;13:30-2.

36. Clayton PT, Eaton S, Aynsley-Green A, et al. Hyperinsulinism in short-chain L-3-hydroxyacyl-CoA dehydrogenase deficiency reveals the importance of beta-oxidation in insulin secretion. J Clin Invest 2001;108:457-65.

37. Cohen MB, Egerter DP, Holly EA, Ahn DK, Miller TR. Pancreatic adenocarcinoma: regression analysis to identify improved cytologic criteria. Diagn Cytopathol 1991;7:341-5.

38. Cohn JA, Friedman KJ, Noone PG, Knowles MR, Silverman LM, Jowell PS. Relation between mutations of the cystic fibrosis gene and idiopathic pancreatitis. N Engl J Med 1998;339:653-8.

39. Comings DE, Skubi KB, Van Eyes J, Motulsky AG. Familial multifocal fibrosclerosis. Findings suggesting that retroperitoneal fibrosis, mediastinal fibrosis, sclerosing cholangitis, Riedel's thyroiditis, and pseudotumor of the orbit may be different manifestations of a single disease. Ann Intern Med 1967;66:884-92.

39a. David O, Green L, Reddy V, et al. Pancreatic masses: a multi-institutional study of 364 fine-needle aspiration biopsies with histopathologic correlation. Diagn Cytopathol 1998;19:423-7.

40. De Angelis C, Valente G, Spaccapietra M, et al. Histological study of alcoholic, nonalcoholic, and obstructive chronic pancreatitis. Pancreas 1992;7:193-6.

41. Demetriadis D, Ververidis M, Papathanasiou D, Bania D, Giannoulopoulos G. Pancreatitis due to cystic duodenal duplication in a 12-year-old child. Eur J Pediatr Surg 1997;7:109-11.

42. Deshpande V, Mino-Kenudson M, Brugge WR, et al. Endoscopic ultrasound guided fine needle aspiration biopsy of autoimmune pancreatitis: diagnostic criteria pitfalls. Am J Surg Pathol 2005;29:1464-71.

42a. Dhall D, Suriawinata A, Shia J, Tang L, Klimstra D. Immunohistochemical detection of IgG4-positive plasma cells helps distinguish lympho-plasmacytic sclerosing pancreatitis (LPSP) from pancreatitis associated with carcinoma or other conditions. Mod Pathol 2006;29:272a.

43. Dolan RV, ReMine WH, Dockerty MB. The fate of heterotopic pancreatic tissue. A study of 212 cases. Arch Surg 1974;109:762-5.

44. Dudiak KM. Abdominal case of the day. Inflammatory pseudotumor of the pancreas. AJR Am J Roentgenol 1993;160:1324-5.

45. Eckstein RP, Hollings RM, Martin PA, Katelaris CH. Pancreatic pseudotumor arising in association with Sjögren's syndrome. Pathology 1995;27:284-8.

46. Ectors N, Maillet B, Aerts R, et al. Non-alcoholic duct destructive chronic pancreatitis. Gut 1997;41:263-8.

47. Eisenberger CF, Kropp A, Langwieler TE, Gocht A, Izbicki JR, Knoefel WT. Heterotopic pancreatitis: gastric outlet obstruction due to an intramural pseudocyst and hamartoma. Z Gastroenterol 2002;40:259-62.

48. Epstein O, Chapman RW, Lake-Bakaar G, Foo AY, Rosalki SB, Sherlock S. The pancreas in primary biliary cirrhosis and primary sclerosing cholangitis. Gastroenterology 1982;83:1177-82.

49. Fekete F, Noun R, Sauvanet A, Flejou JF, Bernades P, Belghiti J. Pseudotumor developing in heterotopic pancreas. World J Surg 1996;20:295-8.

50. Fitko R, Kampmeier PA, Batti FH, Benjoya RA, Rao SM. Lymphoepithelial cyst of the pancreas with sebaceous differentiation. Int J Pancreatol 1994;15:145-7.

51. Flaherty MJ, Benjamin DR. Multicystic pancreatic hamartoma: a distinctive lesion with immunohistochemical and ultrastructural study. Hum Pathol 1992;23:1309-12.

52. Flejou JF, Potet F, Molas G, Bernades P, Amouyal P, Fekete F. Cystic dystrophy of the gastric and duodenal wall developing in heterotopic pancreas: an unrecognised entity. Gut 1993;34:343-7.

53. Fritscher-Ravens A, Brand L, Knofel WT, et al. Comparison of endoscopic ultrasound-guided fine needle aspiration for focal pancreatic lesions in patients with normal parenchyma and chronic pancreatitis. Am J Gastroenterol 2002;97:2768-75.

54. Frossard JL, Amouyal P, Amouyal G, et al. Performance of endosonography-guided fine needle aspiration and biopsy in the diagnosis of pancreatic cystic lesions. Am J Gastroenterol 2003;98:1516-24.

55. Frulloni L, Morana G, Bovo P, et al. Salivary gland involvement in patients with chronic pancreatitis. Pancreas 1999;19:33-8.

56. Furukawa N, Muranaka T, Yasumori K, Matsubayashi R, Hayashida K, Arita Y. Autoimmune pancreatitis: radiologic findings in three histologically proven cases. J Comput Assist Tomogr 1998;22:880-3.

57. Glaser B, Kesavan P, Heyman M, et al. Familial hyperinsulinism caused by an activating glucokinase mutation. N Engl J Med 1998;338:226-30.

58. Glaser B, Thornton P, Otonkoski T, Junien C. Genetics of neonatal hyperinsulinism. Arch Dis Child Fetal Neonatal Ed 2000;82:F79-F86.

59. Glaser M, Roskar Z, Skalicky M, Krajnc I. Cystic dystrophy of the duodenal wall in a heterotopic pancreas. Wien Klin Wochenschr 2002;114:1013-6.

60. Goossens A, Gepts W, Saudubray JM, et al. Diffuse and focal nesidioblastosis. A clinicopathological study of 24 patients with persistent neonatal hyperinsulinemic hypoglycemia. Am J Surg Pathol 1989;13:766-75.

61. Goossens A, Heitz PU, Klöppel G. Pancreatic endocrine cells and their non-neoplastic proliferations. In: Dayal Y, ed. Endocrine pathology of gut and pancreas. Boca Raton, Fla.: CRC Press; 1991:69-104.

62. Gorry MC, Gabbaizedeh D, Furey W, et al. Mutations in the cationic trypsinogen gene are associated with recurrent acute and chronic pancreatitis. Gastroenterology 1997;113:1063-8.

63. Gould VE, Chejfec G, Shah K, Paloyan E, Lawrence AM. Adult nesidiodysplasia. Semin Diagn Pathol 1984;1:43-53.

64. Gould VE, Memoli VA, Dardi LE, Gould NS. Nesidiodysplasia and nesidioblastosis of infancy: structural and functional correlations with the syndrome of hyperinsulinemic hypoglycemia. Pediatr Pathol 1983;1:7-31.

65. Halpert B, Gyorkey F. Lesions observed in accessory spleens of 311 patients. Am J Clin Pathol 1959;32:165-8.

66. Hamano H, Kawa S, Horiuchi A, et al. High serum IgG4 concentrations in patients with sclerosing pancreatitis. N Engl J Med 2001;344:732-8.

67. Hammel P, Levy P, Voitot H, et al. Preoperative cyst fluid analysis is useful for the differential diagnosis of cystic lesions of the pancreas. Gastroenterology 1995;108:1230-5.

68. Hardacre JM, Iacobuzio-Donahue CA, Sohn TA, et al. Results of pancreaticoduodenectomy for lymphoplasmacytic sclerosing pancreatitis. Ann Surg 2003;237:853-9.

69. Hariri A, Siegelman SS, Hruban RH. Duodenal diverticulum mimicking a cystic pancreatic neoplasm. Br J Radiol 2005;78:562-4.

70. Hastier P, Buckley MJ, Le Gall P, Bellon S, Dumas R, Delmont J. First report of association of chronic pancreatitis, primary biliary cirrhosis, and systemic sclerosis. Dig Dis Sci 1998;43:2426-8.

71. Hastings PR, Nance FC, Becker WF. Changing patterns in the management of pancreatic pseudocysts. Ann Surg 1975;181:546-51.

72. Hatzitheoklitos E, Buchler MW, Friess H, et al. Pseudolymphoma of the pancreas mimicking cancer. Pancreas 1994;9:668-70.

72a. Hennings J, Garske U, Botling J, Hellman P. Malignant insulinoma in ectopic pancreatic tissue. Dig Surg 2005;22:377-9.

73. Hollerbach S, Klamann A, Topalidis T, Schmiegel WH. Endoscopic ultrasonography (EUS) and fine-needle aspiration (FNA) cytology for diagnosis of chronic pancreatitis. Endoscopy 2001;33:824-31.

74. Holstege A, Barner S, Brambs HJ, Wenz W, Gerok W, Farthmann EH. Relapsing pancreatitis associated with duodenal wall cysts. Diagnostic approach and treatment. Gastroenterology 1985;88:814-9.

75. Hong SP, Park SW, Chung JP, et al. Autoimmune pancreatitis with effective steroid therapy. Yonsei Med J 2003;44:534-8.

76. Horiuchi A, Kaneko T, Yamamura N, et al. Autoimmune chronic pancreatitis simulating pancreatic lymphoma. Am J Gastroenterol 1996;91:2607-9.

77. Hruban RH, Takaori K, Klimstra DS, et al. An illustrated consensus on the classification of pancreatic intraepithelial neoplasia and intraductal papillary mucinous neoplasms. Am J Surg Pathol 2004;28:977-87.

78. Irie H, Honda H, Baba S, et al. Autoimmune pancreatitis: CT and MR characteristics. AJR Am J Roentgenol 1998;170:1323-7.

79. Ito T, Nakano I, Koyanagi S, et al. Autoimmune pancreatitis as a new clinical entity. Three cases of autoimmune pancreatitis with effective steroid therapy. Dig Dis Sci 1997;42:1458-68.

80. Itoh S, Yamakawa K, Shimamoto K, Endo T, Ishigaki T. CT findings in groove pancreatitis: correlation with histopathological findings. J Comput Assist Tomogr 1994;18:911-5.

81. Izbicki JR, Knoefel WT, Muller-Hocker J, Mandelkow HK. Pancreatic hamartoma: a benign tumor of the pancreas. Am J Gastroenterol 1994;89:1261-2.

82. Jaffe R. The pancreas. In: Wigglewsorth JS, Singer DB, eds. Textbook of fetal and perinatal pathology, 2nd ed. Malden, Mass: Blackwell Scientific; 1980:1021-55.

83. Jaffe R, Hashida Y, Yunis EJ. The endocrine pancreas of the neonate and infant. Perspect Pediatr Pathol. 1982;7:137-65.

84. Johnson RL, Page DL, Dean RH. Pseudotumor of the pancreas. South Med J 1983;76:647-9.

85. Kaiserling E, Seitz KH, Rettenmaier G, et al. Lymphoepithelial cyst of the pancreas. Clinical, morphological, and immunohistochemical findings. Zentralbl Pathol 1991;137:431-8.

86. Kamisawa T, Funata N, Hayashi Y, et al. Close relationship between autoimmune pancreatitis and multifocal fibrosclerosis. Gut 2003;52:683-7.

86a. Kamisawa T, Nakajima H, Egawa N, Funata N, Tsuruta K, Okamoto A. IgG4-related sclerosing disease incorporating sclerosing pancreatitis, cholangitis, sialadenitis and retroperitoneal fibrosis with lymphadenopathy. Pancreatology 2006;6:132-7.

87. Kattan YB. Hydatid cysts in pancreas. Br Med J 1975;4:729-30.

88. Kawaguchi K, Koike M, Tsuruta K, Okamoto A, Tabata I, Fujita N. Lymphoplasmacytic sclerosing pancreatitis with cholangitis: a variant of primary sclerosing cholangitis extensively involving pancreas. Hum Pathol 1991;22:387-95.

89. Kawamoto S, Siegelman SS, Hruban RH, Fishman EK. Lymphoplasmacytic sclerosing pancreatitis with obstructive jaundice: CT and pathology features. AJR Am J Roentgenol 2004;183:915-21.

90. Kazumori H, Ashizawa N, Moriyama N, et al. Primary sclerosing pancreatitis and cholangitis. Int J Pancreatol 1998;24:123-7.

91. Kim KP, Kim MH, Song MH, Lee SS, Seo DW, Lee SK. Autoimmune chronic pancreatitis. Am J Gastroenterol 2004;99:1605-16.

92. Kino-Ohsaki J, Nishimori I, Morita M, et al. Serum antibodies to carbonic anhydrase I and II in patients with idiopathic chronic pancreatitis and Sjogren's syndrome. Gastroenterology 1996;110:1579-86.

92a. Klimstra DS, Adsay NV. Lymphoplasmacytic sclerosing (autoimmune) pancreatitis. Semin Diagn Pathol 2004;21:237-46.

93. Klimstra DS, Conlon KC, Adsay NV. Lymphoplasmacytic sclerosing pancreatitis with pseudotumor formation. Pathol Case Rev 2001;6:94-9.

94. Klöppel G. Pathology of chronic pancreatitis and pancreatic pain. Acta Chir Scand 1990;156:261-5.

95. Klöppel G. Pseudocysts and other non-neoplastic cysts of the pancreas. Semin Diagn Pathol 2000;17:7-15.

96. Klöppel G, Lüttges J, Lohr M, Zamboni G, Longnecker D. Autoimmune pancreatitis: pathological, clinical, and immunological features. Pancreas 2003;27:14-9.

97. Klöppel G, Maillet B. Pseudocysts in chronic pancreatitis: a morphological analysis of 57 resection specimens and 9 autopsy pancreata. Pancreas 1991;6:266-74.

98. Klöppel G, Maillet B. Pathology of acute and chronic pancreatitis. Pancreas 1993;8:659-70.

99. Klöppel G, Willemer S, Stamm B, Hacki WH, Heitz PU. Pancreatic lesions and hormonal profile of pancreatic tumors in multiple endocrine neoplasia type I. An immunocytochemical study of nine patients. Cancer 1986;57:1824-32.

100. Kohzaki S, Fukuda T, Fujimoto T, et al. Case report: ciliated foregut cyst of the pancreas mimicking teratomatous tumour. Br J Radiol 1994;67:601-4.

101. Komminoth P, Seelentag WK, Saremaslani P, Heitz PU, Roth J. CD44 isoform expression in the diffuse neuroendocrine system. II. Benign and malignant tumors. Histochem Cell Biol 1996;106:551-62.

102. Kosmahl M, Pauser U, Peters K, et al. Cystic neoplasms of the pancreas and tumor-like lesions with cystic features: a review of 418 cases and a classification proposal. Virchows Arch 2004;445:168-78.

102a. Krige JE, Mirza K, Bornman PC, Beningfield SJ. Primary hydatid cysts of the pancreas. S Afr J Surg 2005;43:37-40.

103. Kroft SH, Stryker SJ, Winter JN, Ergun G, Rao MS. Inflammatory pseudotumor of the pancreas. Int J Pancreatol 1995;18:277-83.

104. Kulatunga A, Kyllonen AP, Dammert K. Malakoplakia of the pancreas. A case report. Acta Pathol Microbiol Immunol Scand [A] 1987;95:127-9.

105. Labate AM, Klimstra DS, Zakowski MF. Comparative cytologic features of pancreatic acinar cell carcinoma and islet cell tumor. Diagn Cytopathol 1997;16:112-6.

106. Lack EE. Pathology of the pancreas, gallbladder, extrahepatic biliary tract, and ampullary region. Oxford: Oxford University Press; 2003.

107. Laidlaw GF. Nesidioblastoma, the islet tumor of the pancreas. Am J Pathol 1938;14:125-34.

108. Landry ML, Sarma DP. Accessory spleen in the head of the pancreas. Hum Pathol 1989;20:497.

109. Lavine JE, Harrison M, Heyman MB. Gastrointestinal duplications causing relapsing pancreatitis in children. Gastroenterology 1989;97:1556-8.

110. Levey JM, Mathai J. Diffuse pancreatic fibrosis: an uncommon feature of multifocal idiopathic fibrosclerosis. Am J Gastroenterol 1998;93:640-2.

111. Lewandrowski KB, Lee J, Southern J, Centeno BA, Warshaw A. Cyst fluid analysis in the differential diagnosis of pancreatic cysts: a new approach to the preoperative assessment of pancreatic cystic lesions. AJR Am J Roentgenol 1995;164:815-9.

112. Lin CC, Wang HP, Chen MF, et al. Chronic calcifying pancreatitis in Taiwan: a multicentric study and comparison with western countries. Hepatogastroenterology 1997;44:842-8.

113. Lin F, Staerkel G. Cytologic criteria for well differentiated adenocarcinoma of the pancreas in fine-needle aspiration biopsy specimens. Cancer 2003;99:44-50.

114. Liu J, Shin HJ, Rubenchik I, Lang E, Lahoti S, Staerkel GA. Cytologic features of lymphoepithelial cyst of the pancreas: two preoperatively diagnosed cases based on fine-needle aspiration. Diagn Cytopathol 1999;21:346-50.

115. Lozano M, Navarro S, Perez-Ayuso R, et al. Lipomatosis of the pancreas: an unusual cause of massive steatorrhea. Pancreas 1988;3:580-2.

116. Maher L, Choi H, Dodds WJ. Noncaseating granulomas of the pancreas. Probable sarcoidosis. Am J Gastroenterol 1981;75:222-5.

117. Mahmood K, Butt MM, Haleem A. Duplication of the duodenum exhibiting heterotropia in the pancreas: report of a case. Ann Saudi Med 1989; 9:602-4.

118. Makhlouf HR, Almeida JL, Sobin LH. Carcinoma in jejunal pancreatic heterotopia. Arch Pathol Lab Med 1999;123:707-11.

119. Marchevsky AM, Zimmerman MJ, Aufses AH Jr, Weiss H. Endometrial cyst of the pancreas. Gastroenterology 1984;86:1589-91.

120. Mares AJ, Hirsch M. Congenital cysts of the head of the pancreas. J Pediatr Surg 1977;12: 547-52.

121. Martinez NS, Morlock CG, Dockerty MB, Waugh JM, Weber HM. Heterotopic pancreatic tissue involving the stomach. Ann Surg 1958; 147:1-12.

122. Maule WF, Reber HA. Diagnosis and management of pancreatic pseudocysts, pancreatic ascites, and pancreatic fistulas. In: Go VL, Gardner JD, Brooks FP, Lebenthal E, DiMagno EP, Scheele GA, eds. The exdocrine pancreas: biology, pathobiology and diseases. New York: Raven Press; 1986:601-10.

123. McFaul CD, Vitone LJ, Campbell F, et al. Pancreatic hamartoma. Pancreatology 2004;4:533-7.

124. Mester Z, Csanaky G, Mocsay L, Epstein O. Anatomy of duodenal papilla and genesis of pancreatic reflux. Arch Surg 1963;87:775-87.

125. Miles RM. Pancreatic cyst in the newborn; a case report. Ann Surg 1959;149:576-81.

126. Mitchell ML. Fine needle aspiration biopsy of peripancreatic lymphoepithelial cysts. Acta Cytol 1990;34:462-3.

126a. Mizukami H, Yajima N, Wada R, et al. Pancreatic malignant fibrous histiocytoma, inflammatory myofibroblastic tumor, and inflammatory pseudotumor related to autoimmune pancreatitis: characterization and differential diagnosis. Virchows Arch 2006;448:552-60.

127. Montefusco PP, Geiss AC, Bronzo RL, Randall S, Kahn E, McKinley MJ. Sclerosing cholangitis, chronic pancreatitis, and Sjogren's syndrome: a syndrome complex. Am J Surg 1984; 147:822-6.

128. Morohoshi T, Hamamoto T, Kunimura T, et al. Epidermoid cyst derived from an accessory spleen in the pancreas. A case report with literature survey. Acta Pathol Jpn 1991;41:916-21.

129. Nakashiro H, Tokunaga O, Watanabe T, Ishibashi K, Kuwaki T. Localized lymphoid hyperplasia (pseudolymphoma) of the pancreas presenting with obstructive jaundice. Hum Pathol 1991;22:724-6.

130. Nieminen U, Koivisto T, Kahri A, Farkkila M. Sjögren's syndrome with chronic pancreatitis, sclerosing cholangitis, and pulmonary infiltrations. Am J Gastroenterol 1997;92:139-42.

131. Nishimori I, Yamamoto Y, Okazaki K, et al. Identification of autoantibodies to a pancreatic antigen in patients with idiopathic chronic pancreatitis and Sjögren's syndrome. Pancreas 1994;9:374-81.

132. Notohara K, Burgart LJ, Yadav D, Chari S, Smyrk TC. Idiopathic chronic pancreatitis with periductal lymphoplasmacytic infiltration: clinicopathologic features of 35 cases. Am J Surg Pathol 2003;27:1119-27.

133. Ohana M, Okazaki K, Hajiro K, Kobashi Y. Multiple pancreatic masses associated with autoimmunity. Am J Gastroenterol 1998;93:99-102.

134. Pang LC. Pancreatic heterotopia: a reappraisal and clinicopathologic analysis of 32 cases. South Med J 1988;81:1264-75.

135. Pasternack A, Hjelt L. Cystic disease of the kidneys, liver, and pancreas. Ann Paediatr Fenn 1961;7:138-45.

135a. Pauser U, da Silva MT, Placke J, Klimstra DS, Klöppel G. Cellular hamartoma resembling gastrointestinal stromal tumor: a solid tumor of the pancreas expressing c-kit (CD117). Mod Pathol 2005;18:1211-6.

136. Pauser U, Kosmahl M, Kruslin B, Klimstra DS, Klöppel G. Pancreatic solid and cystic hamartoma in adults: characterization of a new tumorous lesion. Am J Surg Pathol 2005;29:797-800.

137. Petter LM, Martin JK Jr, Menke DM. Localized lymphoplasmacellular pancreatitis forming a pancreatic inflammatory pseudotumor. Mayo Clin Proc 1998;73:447-50.

138. Pinto MM, Meriano FV. Diagnosis of cystic pancreatic lesions by cytologic examination and carcinoembryonic antigen and amylase assays of cyst contents. Acta Cytol 1991;35:456-63.

139. Pitchumoni CS, Mohan AT. Pancreatic stones. Gastroenterol Clin North Am 1990;19:873-93.

140. Pitt HA. Pseudotumor developing in heterotopic pancreas. World J Surg 1997;21:123.

141. Procacci C, Graziani R, Zamboni G, et al. Cystic dystrophy of the duodenal wall: radiologic findings. Radiology 1997;205:741-7.

142. Pungpapong S, Geiger XJ, Raimondo M. Inflammatory myofibroblastic tumor presenting as a pancreatic mass: a case report and review of the literature. JOP 2004;5:360-7.

143. Rahier J, Guiot Y, Sempoux C. Persistent hyperinsulinaemic hypoglycaemia of infancy: a heterogeneous syndrome unrelated to nesidioblastosis. Arch Dis Child Fetal Neonatal Ed 2000;82:F108-12.

144. Rahier J, Sempoux C, Fournet JC, et al. Partial or near-total pancreatectomy for persistent neonatal hyperinsulinaemic hypoglycaemia: the pathologist's role. Histopathology 1998;32:15-9.

145. Reinecke-Luthge A, Koschoreck F, Klöppel G. The molecular basis of persistent hyperinsulinemic hypoglycemia of infancy and its pathologic substrates. Virchows Arch 2000;436:1-5.

146. Robins DB, Katz RL, Evans DB, Atkinson EN, Green L. Fine needle aspiration of the pancreas. In quest of accuracy. Acta Cytol 1995;39:1-10.

147. Rossi L, Whitcomb DC, Ehrlich GD, et al. Lack of R117H mutation in the cationic trypsinogen gene in patients with tropical pancreatitis from Bangladesh. Pancreas 1998;17:278-80.

148. Sarles H. Definitions and classifications of pancreatitis. Pancreas 1991;6:470-4.

149. Scott J, Summerfield JA, Elias E, Dick R, Sherlock S. Chronic pancreatitis: a cause of cholestasis. Gut 1977;18:196-201.

150. Scully KA, Li SC, Hebert JC, Trainer TD. The characteristic appearance of non-alcoholic duct destructive chronic pancreatitis: a report of 2 cases. Arch Pathol Lab Med 2000;124:1535-8.

151. Seifert G. Lipomatous atrophy and other forms. In: Klöppel G, Heitz PH, eds. Pancreatic pathology. Edinburgh: Churchill Livingston; 1984:27-31.

151a. Sempoux C, Guiot Y, Lefevre A, et al. Neonatal hyperinsulinemic hypoglycemia: heterogeneity of the syndrome and keys for differential diagnosis. J Clin Endocrinol Metab 1998;83:1455-61.

152. Sharma S, Green KB. The pancreatic duct and its arteriovenous relationship: an underutilized aid in the diagnosis and distinction of pancreatic adenocarcinoma from pancreatic intraepithelial neoplasia. A study of 126 pancreatectomy specimens. Am J Surg Pathol 2004;28: 613-20.

153. Shudo R, Yazaki Y, Sakurai S, et al. Groove pancreatitis: report of a case and review of the clinical and radiologic features of groove pancreatitis reported in Japan. Intern Med 2002;41: 537-42.

154. Singh SM, Reber HA. The pathology of chronic pancreatitis. World J Surg 1990;14:2-10.

155. Sjögren I, Wengle B, Korsgren M. Primary sclerosing cholangitis associated with fibrosis of the submandibular glands and the pancreas. Acta Med Scand 1979;205:139-41.

156. Skellenger ME, Kinner BM, Jordan PH Jr. Brunner's gland hamartomas can mimic carcinoma of the head of the pancreas. Surg Gynecol Obstet 1983;156:774-6.

157. Solcia E, Capella C, Klöppel G. Tumors of the pancreas. AFIP Atlas of Tumor Pathology, 3rd Series, Fascicle 20. Washington, DC: American Registry of Pathology; 1997.

158. Sperti C, Pasquali C, Pedrazzoli S, Guolo P, Liessi G. Expression of mucin-like carcinoma-associated antigen in the cyst fluid differentiates mucinous from nonmucinous pancreatic cysts. Am J Gastroenterol 1997;92:672-5.

159. Stanley CA. Advances in diagnosis and treatment of hyperinsulinism in infants and children. J Clin Endocrinol Metab 2002;87:4857-9.

160. Stanley CA, Lieu YK, Hsu BY, et al. Hyperinsulinism and hyperammonemia in infants with regulatory mutations of the glutamate dehydrogenase gene. N Engl J Med 1998;338:1352-7.

161. Stanley CA, Thornton PS, Ganguly A, et al. Preoperative evaluation of infants with focal or diffuse congenital hyperinsulinism by intravenous acute insulin response tests and selective pancreatic arterial calcium stimulation. J Clin Endocrinol Metab 2004;89:288-96.

162. Stefan Y, Bordi C, Grasso S, Orci L. Beckwith-Wiedemann syndrome: a quantitative, immunohistochemical study of pancreatic islet cell populations. Diabetologia 1985;28:914-9.

163. Stelow EB, Bardales RH, Lai R, et al. The cytological spectrum of chronic pancreatitis. Diagn Cytopathol 2005;32:65-9.

164. Stolte M, Weiss W, Volkholz H, Rosch W. A special form of segmental pancreatitis: "groove pancreatitis." Hepatogastroenterology 1982;29: 198-208.

165. Su LD, Atayde-Perez A, Sheldon S, Fletcher JA, Weiss SW. Inflammatory myofibroblastic tumor: cytogenetic evidence supporting clonal origin. Mod Pathol 1998;11:364-8.

166. Suchi M, MacMullen C, Thornton PS, Ganguly A, Stanley CA, Ruchelli ED. Histopathology of congenital hyperinsulinism: retrospective study with genotype correlations. Pediatr Dev Pathol 2003;6:322-33.

375

167. Suchi M, Thornton PS, Adzick NS, et al. Congenital hyperinsulinism: intraoperative biopsy interpretation can direct the extent of pancreatectomy. Am J Surg Pathol 2004;28:1326-35.

168. Suda K, Miyano T, Suzuki F, et al. Clinicopathologic and experimental studies on cases of abnormal pancreatico-choledocho-ductal junction. Acta Pathol Jpn 1987;37:1549-62.

169. Suda K, Mogaki M, Oyama T, Matsumoto Y. Histopathologic and immunohistochemical studies on alcoholic pancreatitis and chronic obstructive pancreatitis: a special emphasis on ductal obstruction and genesis of pancreatitis. Am J Gastroenterol 1990;85:271-6.

170. Suda K, Takase M, Shiono S, et al. Duodenal wall cysts may be derived from a ductal component of ectopic pancreatic tissue. Histopathology 2002;41:351-6.

171. Sun Y, Wasserman PG. Acinar cell carcinoma arising in the stomach: a case report with literature review. Hum Pathol 2004;35:263-5.

172. Taniguchi T, Seko S, Azuma K, et al. Autoimmune pancreatitis detected as a mass in the tail of the pancreas. J Gastroenterol Hepatol 2000; 15:461-4.

173. Thomas P, Ye Y, Lightner E. Mutation of the pancreatic islet inward rectifier Kir6.2 also leads to familial persistent hyperinsulinemic hypoglycemia of infancy. Hum Mol Genet 1996;5: 1809-12.

174. Thomas PM, Cote GJ, Wohllk N, et al. Mutations in the sulfonylurea receptor gene in familial persistent hyperinsulinemic hypoglycemia of infancy. Science 1995;268:426-9.

175. Thompson JN, Collier NA, Blumgart LH. Pancreatitis in primary sclerosing cholangitis. Dig Surg 1985;2:98-103.

176. Tsou E, Romano MC, Kerwin DM, Soteropoulos GC, Katz S. Sarcoidosis of anterior mediastinal nodes, pancreas, and uterine cervix: three unusual sites in the same patient. Am Rev Respir Dis 1980;122:333-8.

176a. Tsujino M, Sugiyama T, Nishida K, et al. Non-insulinoma pancreatogenous hypoglycemia syndrome: a rare case of adult-onset nesidioblastosis. Intern Med 2005;44:843-7.

177. Uchida K, Okazaki K, Konishi Y, et al. Clinical analysis of autoimmune-related pancreatitis. Am J Gastroenterol 2000;95:2788-94.

178. van der Wal BC, de Krijger RR, de Herder WW, et al. Adult hyperinsulinemic hypoglycemia not caused by an insulinoma: a report of two cases. Virchows Arch 2000;436:481-6.

179. Van Hoe L, Gryspeerdt S, Ectors N, et al. Non-alcoholic duct-destructive chronic pancreatitis: imaging findings. AJR Am J Roentgenol 1998; 170:643-7.

180. Venu RP, Radke JS, Brown RD, et al. Autoimmune pancreatitis, pancreatic mass, and lower gastrointestinal bleed. J Clin Gastroenterol 1999;28:364-7.

181. Voss M, Hammel P, Molas G, et al. Value of endoscopic ultrasound guided fine needle aspiration biopsy in the diagnosis of solid pancreatic masses. Gut 2000;46:244-9.

182. Warshaw AL, Compton CC, Lewandrowski KB, Cardenosa G, Mueller PR. Cystic tumors of the pancreas. New clinical, radiologic, and pathologic observations in 67 patients. Ann Surg 1990;212:432-45.

183. Weber SM, Cubukcu-Dimopulo O, Palesty JA, et al. Lymphoplasmacytic sclerosing pancreatitis: inflammatory mimic of pancreatic carcinoma. J Gastrointest Surg 2003;7:129-37.

184. Whitcomb DC, Gorry MC, Preston RA, et al. Hereditary pancreatitis is caused by a mutation in the cationic trypsinogen gene. Nat Genet 1996;14:141-5.

185. Worning H. Incidence and prevalence of chronic pancreatitis. In: Beger HG, Büchler M, Ditschuneit H, Malfertheiner P, eds. Chronic pancreatitis: research and clinical management. Berlin: Springer-Verlag; 1990:8-14.

186. Yakovac WC, Baker L, Hummeler K. Beta cell nesidioblastosis in idiopathic hypoglycemia of infancy. J Pediatr 1971;79:226-31.

187. Ylagan LR, Edmundowicz S, Kasal K, Walsh D, Lu DW. Endoscopic ultrasound guided fine-needle aspiration cytology of pancreatic carcinoma: a 3-year experience and review of the literature. Cancer 2002;96:362-9.

188. Yoshida K, Toki F, Takeuchi T, Watanabe S, Shiratori K, Hayashi N. Chronic pancreatitis caused by an autoimmune abnormality. Proposal of the concept of autoimmune pancreatitis. Dig Dis Sci 1995;40:1561-8.

189. Zamboni G, Lüttges J, Capelli P, et al. Histopathological features of diagnostic and clinical relevance in autoimmune pancreatitis: a study on 53 resection specimens and 9 biopsy specimens. Virchows Arch 2004;445:552-63.

190. Zuk RJ, Neal JW, Baithun SI. Malakoplakia of the pancreas. Virchows Arch A Pathol Anat Histopathol 1990;417:181-4.

16 DISSECTION AND REPORTING OF PANCREATIC RESECTION SPECIMENS

Recommended protocols for the gross examination and reporting of pancreatic specimens containing malignant neoplasms have been published by the College of American Pathologists (2) and the Association of Directors of Anatomical and Surgical Pathology (1,4,5). We present here our collective experience and preference for the gross dissection, sectioning, and reporting of pancreatic specimens (6).

DISSECTION

Pancreatoduodenectomy (Whipple) Specimen

Since Alan Oldfather Whipple popularized the surgical resection of carcinoma of the head of the pancreas in the 1930s (7), the standard pancreaticoduodenectomy specimen has been known as the Whipple specimen. The Whipple procedure can be used to resect neoplasms of the pancreatic head, duodenum, ampulla of Vater, and distal common bile duct. The standard pancreaticoduodenectomy specimen consists of the distal stomach; the proximal duodenum from the pylorus to the ligament of Treitz, including the ampulla of Vater; the head and neck of the pancreas; and the distal common bile duct. The gallbladder is also typically removed during the procedure and may be attached to the specimen but is often submitted separately. The distal stomach is not resected in pylorus-preserving pancreatoduodenectomies. This modified procedure leaves the entire stomach and pyloric sphincter intact and provides a better functional outcome.

Gross Description. The specimen should be identified by the labeled information on the specimen container, including the patient's name, medical record number, and specimen type (e.g., standard versus pylorus-preserving pancreatoduodenectomy; partial versus total pancreatectomy). Document whether the specimen was received fresh or fixed. If the specimen was partially dissected for frozen section diagnosis, this fact, too, should be noted.

The initial orientation of the specimen is crucial prior to measurement and dissection. Gross photographs at this point are generally uninformative. Initial orientation starts with identifying the proximal and distal ends of the duodenum. If the pylorus is present, the orientation is obvious; if the pylorus is not present, the shorter segment of duodenum is almost always proximal and the longer segment is distal. Placing the duodenum in its in situ "C-shape" should position the pancreatic head properly. The uncinate is a hook-shaped process that extends caudally and dorsally from the pancreas. Cupping the fingers and thumb simulates the anatomy of the pancreas with the superior mesenteric artery and vein situated between the pancreatic neck and body (the fingers) and the uncinate process (the thumb) (fig. 16-1). A groove, or indentation into the pancreatic parenchyma, created by the superior mesenteric artery and vein is often appreciated. The head of the pancreas sits in the "C" created by the duodenum. Measure the size of each organ (the pancreas, the duodenum, the stomach, and, if present, the gallbladder) in three dimensions.

After the specimen has been oriented and the external examination completed the duodenum can be opened along the aspect opposite the pancreas so as to avoid the ampulla. If staples are present at one or both of the duodenal margins, simply cut the margins off in a strip as close to the staples as possible. Gently rinse any contents and evaluate the duodenal mucosa for any lesions, especially the ampulla. A photograph of any visible duodenal lesions may be appropriate at this point, making sure that the lesion fills the view finder of the camera. A low-power photograph of the entire Whipple specimen with a small periampullary mass is useless. If an ampullary mass is present, take measurements, document if it is endophytic or exophytic, describe the features of the lesion (color, consistency, presence or absence

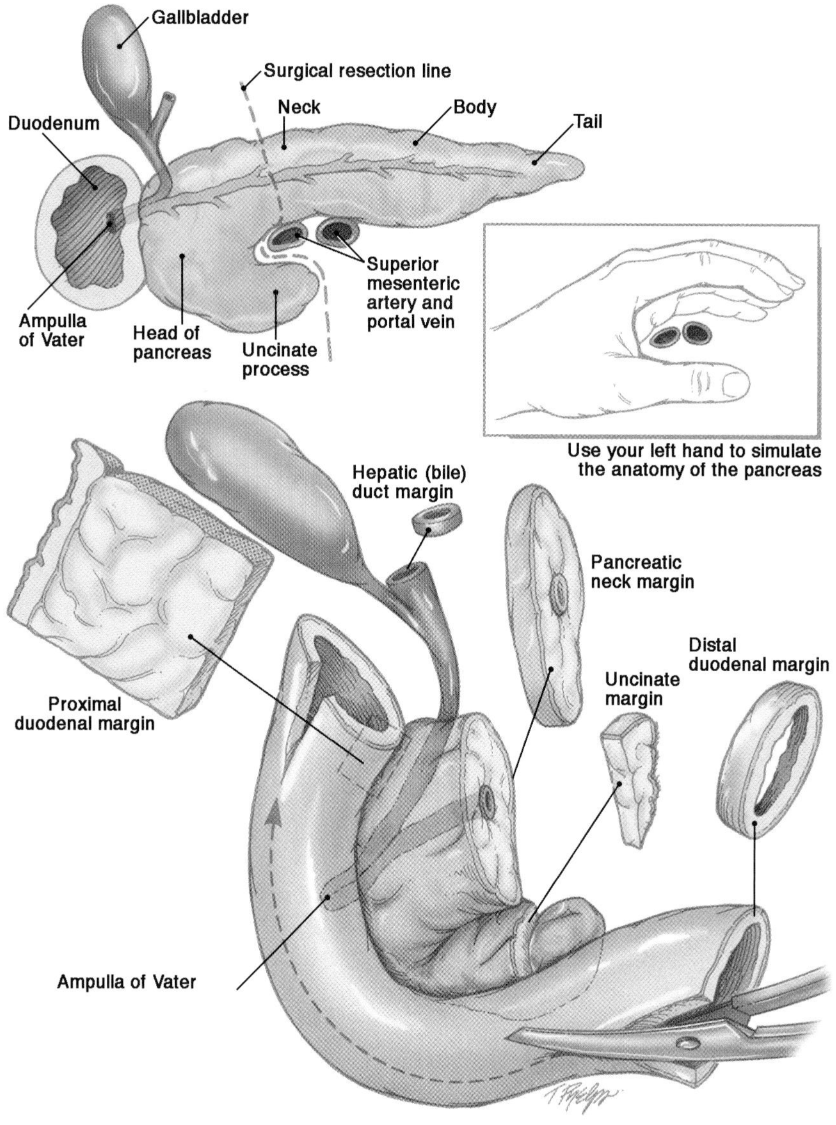

Figure 16-1

**PANCREATIC ANATOMY
AND THE
WHIPPLE SPECIMEN**

The orientation and important margins of a pancreatic-oduodenectomy (Whipple) specimen. (Artwork adapted by Jennifer Parsons Brumbaugh from a figure in Westra WH, Hruban RH, Phelps TH, Isacson C. Surgical pathology dissection, an illustrated guide, 2nd ed. New York: Springer; 2002:90.)

of ulceration), and carefully document the relationship of the lesion to the ampulla of Vater.

Next, find the common bile duct. The common bile duct is recognized by its tubular shape and typically green-tinged mucosa. If the gallbladder is present, use the insertion of the cystic duct to find the common bile duct and follow the common bile duct to the bile duct resection margin. Alternatively, the bile duct and margin can be found by probing the duct from the ampulla of Vater if there is no obstruction.

The distal pancreatic neck margin will appear as an oval of cut parenchyma with cautery artifact and a central duct. At this point, if pancreatic divisum is in the differential diag-

nosis, pass a probe through the transected pancreatic duct visible at the pancreatic neck margin and determine if the probe exists from the major or minor papilla.

Once the landmarks have been identified, proper inking of the soft tissue margins is in order. Blot the ink dry. This takes just a few minutes. The ink can obliterate anatomic landmarks and cause disorientation, so some prefer to ink the various margins with different colors. Document the designations of the inks used in the gross description.

Dissection. With the specimen oriented and inked, some of the margins should be taken for histologic evaluation before the specimen is further dissected. The standard margins include the proximal enteric margin (either the stomach or duodenum), the distal duodenal margin, the pancreatic neck resection margin with pancreatic duct, the common bile duct margin, the posterior or retroperitoneal soft tissue margin(s), the uncinate margin(s), and the anterior pancreatic soft tissue margin (fig. 16-1). We like to obtain shave sections of the bile duct, pancreatic neck, and enteric margins prior to further dissection, and perpendicular sections of the uncinate and soft tissue margins after the neoplasm has been dissected. Although the benefit of histologic sampling of grossly negative enteric margins is debatable, these sections not only document a negative margin, but they also serve as a representative sample of the duodenum and stomach, reducing the need for additional sampling of those organs. For neoplasms not externally visible, palpation of the pancreatic parenchyma will help to identify the location of the neoplasm and determine the best area for the closest possible margins. En face margins should be placed in the cassette with the true margin facing down so that the true margin is in the block facing the microtome blade for sectioning. Additional radial sections of soft tissue margins may be taken after further dissection.

The bile duct and pancreatic duct should now be probed for patency and to establish their relationship with any lesion, especially cystic neoplasms. If the pancreatic duct connects with a neoplastic cyst with mucin, the neoplasm is classified as an intraductal pancreatic mucinous neoplasm; the vast majority of mucinous cystic neoplasms do not connect to the pancreatic duct. At this point the bile duct can be opened along the posterior surface of the gland using scissors. Bile duct strictures should be documented, and, when present, strictures can help identify subtle neoplasms. The pancreatic parenchyma is then sectioned at 2-mm intervals in a bread loaf fashion using a sharp knife or long blade (fig. 16-2). Alternatively, the specimen can be bivalved along the plane created by the pancreatic and bile ducts. If the later approach is chosen, a very sharp long knife can be used to bivalve the head of the pancreas along probes placed through the pancreatic and common bile ducts. This approach clarifies the relationship of the lesion

to the surrounding parenchyma, pancreatic duct, bile duct, and duodenal wall. If there is a stricture present, this process can still be performed up to the stricture from both directions.

This is an ideal time to take pertinent photographs. Remember to fill the camera view finder as much as possible with the lesion and related adjacent tissue! The cut surface of the pancreas and lesion should be examined unfixed for color, texture, consistency, interfaces between normal and abnormal tissue, and relationships between the lesion and surrounding tissues, including the pancreatic parenchyma, the larger pancreatic ducts, the duodenum, the bile duct, the ampulla, and other organs. The exact location of the neoplasm should be described, for example, in the uncinate process. For adenocarcinomas that involve both the pancreatic duct and intrapancreatic common bile duct, it can be very difficult to determine the site of origin on histology. The best way to assess the site of origin is often from gross inspection. The bulk of the neoplasm is typically centered on the duct of origin, and this should be documented in the gross description.

For cystic masses, the cyst contents should be described: bloody, serous, mucoid, necrotic. Observe whether the cysts are unilocular or multilocular and note their size range. Describe the features of any septa (thick or thin), and the cyst lining (smooth or papillary), and always remember to determine whether the cysts communicate with the larger pancreatic ducts. Finally, and most importantly, examine the cysts for mural nodules. Photograph any identifiable mural masses. Table 16-1 lists the important gross features to document.

If lymphoma is suspected, an appropriate section of tumor should be submitted fresh for flow cytometry. As molecular tests are becoming increasingly important in the characterization of pancreatic neoplasms, it is prudent to freeze a section of tumor, if in excess, in liquid nitrogen and store at -80°C to preserve the DNA, mRNA, and protein. The specimen should now be fixed in 10 percent buffered formalin overnight for best results with further dissection and sectioning for histology.

Tissue Sections. The purpose of histologic evaluation of any specimen is for diagnosis and to guide patient therapy and management. This

Table 16-1

CHECKLIST OF GROSS CHARACTERISTICS OF PANCREAS SPECIMENS

Gross Feature	Description
Specimen identification	Received fresh or fixed, postfrozen section; labeled with patient's name, unit number, written description on label
Type of specimen	Pancreatoduodenectomy (standard vs. pylorus-sparing), distal pancreatectomy, total pancreatectomy, enucleation of mass
Organs present	Identify all organs submitted
Measurements	Individual organs and mass lesion in three dimensions
Location of mass	Exact location, e.g., pancreatic head centered around pancreatic or bile duct
Relationship of mass to surrounding structures	Relative to margins, pancreatic and bile duct, duodenal wall, ampulla, spleen, major vessels, etc.
Characteristics of the mass:	
Overall	Solid: diffuse, nodular, lobulated, hemorrhage, necrosis
	Cystic: unilocular or multilocular, size of cysts, septa (thick, thin, nodules), cyst lining (smooth, papillary), cyst contents (thick or thin mucoid, serous, bloody), hemorrhage, necrosis
Interface	Encapsulated, circumscribed; do the cysts communicate with the pancreatic ducts?; is there a mass in the wall of the cyst?
Color	Tan, white, brown, red, yellow, variegated
Texture and consistency	Soft, fleshy, firm, scirrous, friable, spongy

can readily be accomplished with efficient sampling of the specimen. Care should be taken to ensure that every section has a purpose and provides useful information. For example, it is not necessary to have three sections of normal duodenum, 10 sections of a serous cystadenoma, or to submit an entire ductal adenocarcinoma for histologic evaluation. Conversely, it is important to remember that benign-appearing mucinous cystic neoplasms and intraductal papillary mucinous neoplasms can harbor an invasive carcinoma even when a mural nodule is not visible on gross inspection. As such, neoplastic mucinous cysts should be either entirely submitted for histologic examination, or sections should at least be submitted until an invasive carcinoma is identified.

Understanding the important aspects of tumor staging and the information desired in the final histologic report will assist in taking appropriate sections. For example, the pathologic staging (pT) of ductal adenocarcinoma depends on the size of the neoplasm (a gross evaluation) and invasion of the neoplasm outside of the pancreas. A pT3 neoplasm directly invades the duodenum, extrapancreatic bile duct, or peripancreatic soft tissues. Such invasion is visible on gross examination and need only be

documented with one or two sections. The distinction between fibrosis and invasive tumor can be impossible by gross examination, so radial sections of pancreatic tissue effaced by firm white tissue is warranted to properly evaluate the size of the neoplasm and the margins, especially the retroperitoneal or posterior margin that often harbors microscopic tumor.

The relationship of the tumor to the ampulla of Vater, the duodenum, the pancreas, and the bile duct is illustrated by a section taken parallel to the pancreatic and biliary ducts. This should include the neoplasm, the duodenal mucosa, the profiles of the pancreatic and biliary ducts, and the parenchyma of the pancreatic head (figs. 16-2, 16-3).

Lymph nodes are easier to find in the fixed specimen as formalin tends to harden the nodes, making them easier to distinguish from fat. Knowing where to look for nodes is helpful (see chapter 1). A useful hint is that lymph nodes often sit in the groove created by the junction of the pancreas and the bowel wall. It is not necessary to report the nodal groups separately. The TNM staging system simply documents the absence (pN0) or presence of one (pN1A) or multiple (pN1B) positive nodes. All nodes should be submitted entirely, with accurate

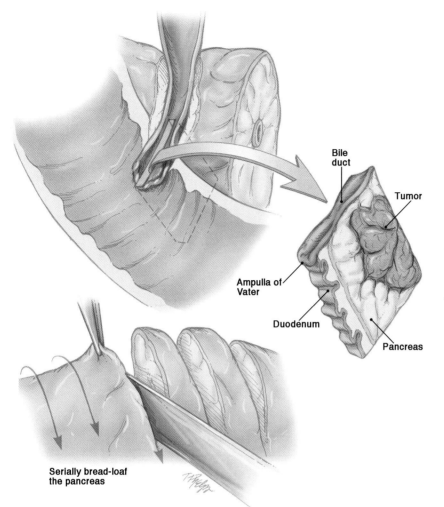

Figure 16-2

DISSECTION OF A PANCREATICODUODENECTOMY (WHIPPLE) SPECIMEN WITH OPTIMAL SECTIONING OF A NEOPLASM IN THE PANCREATIC HEAD

A section through the ampulla of Vater can be used to demonstrate the relationship of the tumor to the ampulla, to the bile duct, to the duodenum, and to the pancreas (see fig. 16-3 for examples). (Artwork adapted by Jennifer Parsons Brumbaugh from a figure in Westra WH, Hruban RH, Phelps TH, Isacson C. Surgical pathology dissection, an illustrated guide, 2nd ed. New York: Springer; 2002:91.)

documentation as to whether the nodes are bisected or trisected in a block or if more than one block represents a single large node.

Table 16-2 lists section codes from a typical Whipple specimen.

Distal Pancreatectomy

A distal pancreatectomy can be used to resect neoplasms of the body and tail of the pancreas. The resection typically includes the pancreatic tail with varying portions of the pancreatic body, peripancreatic soft tissue with nodes, spleen, and splenic vessels.

Gross Description and Dissection. The specimen should be identified by the labeled information on the specimen container, including the patient's name, medical record number, and specimen type including all organs re-

ceived (e.g., distal pancreatectomy with attached spleen). Document whether the specimen was received fresh or fixed, and if the specimen was partially dissected for frozen section.

Measure the overall specimen and each organ individually. Document the exact location, extent, and size of any externally visible masses. Take special note of the peripancreatic and proximal pancreatic margins for gross involvement by the neoplasm. Keep in mind that a neoplasm that invades the spleen is staged as pT4. Do not photograph at this point unless there is an external finding worth noting. A photograph of an undissected specimen is usually useless.

Ink and blot dry the proximal and peripancreatic margins. A shave, or depending on local preferences, a series of perpendicular sections of the proximal pancreatic margin can be taken

381

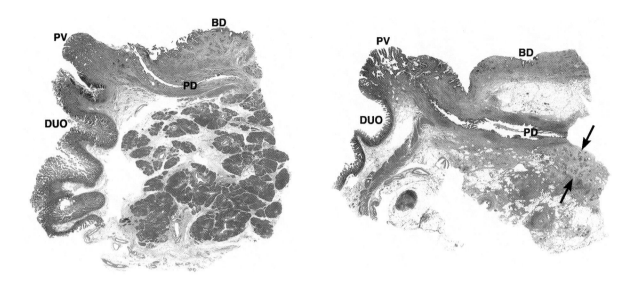

Figure 16-3

WHOLE MOUNT SECTIONS OF THE AMPULLA OF VATER AS ILLUSTRATED IN FIGURE 16-2

Histologic sections taken through the ampulla of Vater demonstrate the relationships among the bile duct (BD), the papilla of Vater (PV), the pancreatic duct (PD), and the duodenum (DUO). Note the invasive carcinoma of the bile duct in the left figure and the in situ carcinoma in the pancreatic duct and the infiltrating carcinoma (arrows) in the pancreatic parenchyma in the right figure.

Table 16-2

RECOMMENDED TISSUE SECTIONS FOR STANDARD PANCREATIC SPECIMENS

Cassette Number	Pancreatoduodenectomy	Distal Pancreatectomy
1	Proximal enteric margin (en face)	Proximal pancreatic margin with duct
2	Distal enteric margin (en face)	Anterior peripancreatic soft tissue margin
3	Distal pancreatic margin with pancreatic duct (en face)	Posterior peripancreatic soft tissue margin
4	Common bile duct margin (en face)	Closest soft tissue margin radially
5	Posterior (retroperitoneal) margin (radial)	Representative splenic vessels if negative; interface with mass if positive
6	Uncinate margin (radial)	Mass-pancreatic duct interface
7	Anterior margin (radial)	Mass-spleen interface (if present)
8	Section through the ampulla of Vater	Mass-normal pancreas interface (if present)
9	Mass-duodenum interface	Mass-other organ interface (if present)
10	Mass-bile duct interface	Additional representative mass (1 per cm)
11	Mass-normal pancreatic tissue interface	Additional representative mass (1 per cm)
12	Additional representative mass (if large)	Representative spleen-normal or metastatic deposit
13	Non-neoplastic pancreas	Non-neoplastic pancreas
14-x	Remainder of any cystic mass	Remainder of any cystic mass
y-z	Peripancreatic lymph nodes	Peripancreatic nodes

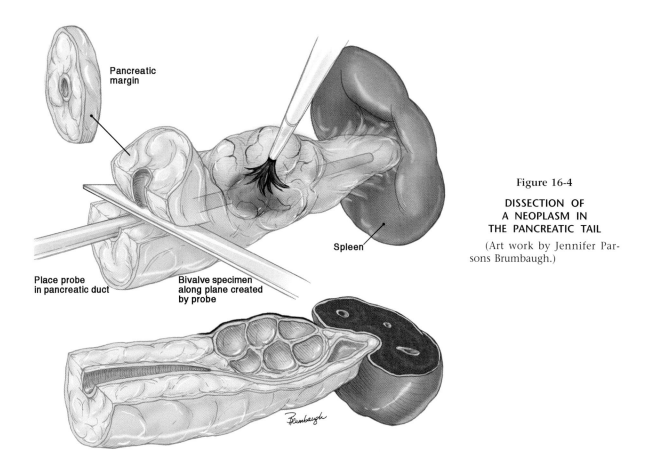

Pancreatic margin

Spleen

Place probe in pancreatic duct

Bivalve specimen along plane created by probe

Figure 16-4

DISSECTION OF A NEOPLASM IN THE PANCREATIC TAIL

(Art work by Jennifer Parsons Brumbaugh.)

at this time. Next, place a probe into the pancreatic duct and longitudinally bivalve the pancreas along the probe with a long sharp knife (fig. 16-4). Note the relationship of any lesions to the spleen, to peripancreatic soft tissue margins, and to the pancreatic duct. If the lesion is cystic, document the cyst contents and whether or not the cysts connect to the larger pancreatic ducts. Measure the lesion and describe the characteristics of the mass as detailed above for a Whipple specimen (Table 16-1). Now is a good time for a close photograph. If the spleen is uninvolved by the neoplasm, it can be serially sectioned at 1-cm intervals and assessed for disease. The entire specimen can then be fixed in 10 percent buffered formalin overnight prior to further dissection.

Tissue Sections. Tissue sections should be taken with the purpose of documenting the type and extent of the disease process. Peripancreatic soft tissue margins can be taken either as perpendicular margins or as en face margins depending on local preferences. Remember to place en face sections so that the true margin is sectioned for histology. A section of the splenic vessels is appropriate if grossly negative and is necessary if grossly positive. In addition to sections that demonstrate the tumor, sections should be obtained which show the relationship of the tumor to the larger pancreatic ducts, to the extrapancreatic soft tissues, and to the spleen. All lymph nodes should be submitted entirely with accurate documentation of the number of blocks for each node and whether a single block contains a bisected or trisected node. Grossly evident direct extension of the disease process into the spleen or separate metastatic deposits require only a single section for documentation. A grossly negative spleen requires only a single representative section. See Table 16-2 for a list of sections appropriate for a typical distal pancreatectomy specimen.

Table 16-3

SAMPLE REPORT TEMPLATE FOR DUCTAL ADENOCARCINOMA

Patient Name: _____   Pathology Number: _____

Pancreas, Resection

        Type of resection: pancreaticoduodenectomy, distal pancreatectomy, other _____

        Tumor type according to AFIP[a] Classification _____

        Specific site of origin, i.e., head, body, tail

        Size _____ cm (in greatest dimension)

Tumor Stage Summary: pT___ N____ M____   (See Note For Synoptic Report).

NOTE:

Histologic Grade:
- ☐ GX (cannot be assessed)
- ☐ G1 (well differentiated)
- ☐ G2 (moderately differentiated)
- ☐ G3 (poorly Undifferentiated)
- ☐ G4 (undifferentiated)

Extent of Invasion:
- ☐ pT1 (intrapancreatic ≤cm)
- ☐ pT2 (intrapancreatic >2cm)
- ☐ pT3 (extrapancreatic; not involving celiac axis or SMA)[b] local extension: _____ (duodenum, extrapancreatic bile duct, peripancreatic soft tissues [specify margin])
- ☐ pT4 (extrapancreatic involving celiac axis or SMA)

Lymphatic Invasion: ☐ absent   ☐ present

Vascular Invasion: ☐ absent   ☐ present

Perineural Invasion: ☐ absent   ☐ present

Major Vessel Invasion: ☐ absent   ☐ present—(specify: celiac axis, SMA[b])

Margins:

   Distal Pancreatic:
- ☐ uninvolved (clearance: ___ mm)
- ☐ involved
- ☐ involved by PanIN[b] (3)
- ☐ involved by IPMN[b] (adenoma, borderline or carcinoma)

   Uncinate:
- ☐ uninvolved (clearance: ___ mm)
- ☐ involved

   Posterior (Retroperitoneal):
- ☐ uninvolved (clearance: ___ mm)
- ☐ involved

   Anterior Pancreatic:
- ☐ uninvolved (clearance: ___ mm)
- ☐ involved

   Common Bile Duct:
- ☐ uninvolved (clearance: ___ mm)
- ☐ involved

   Enteric Margins:
- ☐ uninvolved (stomach and duodenum)
- ☐ involved (specify: _____)

Lymph Nodes:
- ☐ pNX (none assessed)
- ☐ pN0 (all negative)
- Total nodes examined (=____)
- ☐ pN1a (positive)
- ☐ pN1b (positive)
- Total nodes positive (=_____)

Metastases:
- ☐ pMX (cannot be assessed)
- ☐ pM0 (none)
- ☐ pM1 (present)
- (specify sites: _____)

Non-neoplastic Pancreas:

Comment:

---

[a]AFIP = Armed Forces Institute of Pathology.

[b]SMA = Superior mesenteric artery; PanIN = pancreatic intraepithelial neoplasia; IPMN = intraductal papillary mucinous neoplasm.

THE PATHOLOGY REPORT

Pathology reports document important information for the treatment and management of the patient. For resection specimens intended for cure, standard information such as tumor type, tumor size, tumor grade, resection margins, and nodal status are crucial. For endocrine neoplasms, the presence or absence of small versus large vessel invasion, direct invasion into adjacent organs, metastases, necrosis, and mitotic index are important. Pathology reports have become increasingly complex and detailed, and the need to be able to accurately compare data internationally has led to the acceptance of the TNM staging system (chapter 3) (3). In addition, complete reports are often required for patient eligibility in clinical trials. As such, the standardized report has gained wide spread acceptance. The standardized report not only ensures that a complete report is generated, it serves as a useful teaching tool for residency training programs. Table 16-3 outlines a sample template for ductal adenocarcinoma.

REFERENCES

1. Albores-Saavedra J, Heffess C, Hruban RH, Klimstra D, Longnecker D. Recommendations for the reporting of pancreatic specimens containing malignant tumors. The Association of Directors of Anatomic and Surgical Pathology. Am J Clin Pathol 1999;111:304-7.
2. Compton CC, Henson DE. Protocol for the examination of specimens removed from patients with carcinoma of the exocrine pancreas: a basis for checklists. Cancer Committee, College of American Pathologists. Arch Pathol Lab Med 1997;121:1129-36.
3. Hermanek P, Hutter RV, Sobin LH, Wagner G, Wittekind CH. TNM atlas: illustrated guide to the TNM/pTNM classification of malignant tumours, 4th ed. Berlin: Springer-Verlag; 1997: 144-52.
4. Recommendations for the reporting of pancreatic specimens containing malignant tumors. Association of Directors of Anatomic and Surgical Pathology. Hum Pathol 1998;29:893-5.
5. Recommendations for reporting resected pancreatic neoplasms. The Association of Directors of Anatomic and Surgical Pathology. Mod Pathol 1998;11:500-4.
6. Westra WH, Hruban RH, Phelps TH, Isacson C, eds. Surgical pathology dissection: an illustrated guide, 2nd ed. New York: Springer-Verlag; 2003:88-92.
7. Whipple AO, Parsons WW, Mullin CR. Treatment of carcinoma of the ampulla of Vater. Ann Surg 1935;102:763-9.

17

DIAGNOSTIC EVALUATION OF PANCREATIC NEOPLASMS

Pancreatic neoplasms are best diagnosed through an integration of the gross, microscopic, clinical, and radiographic findings. Simply knowing the age and gender of the patient, whether a neoplasm is solid or cystic, its location within the pancreas, and the patient's presenting symptoms can establish the most likely diagnoses prior to microscopic evaluation. Tables 17-1 and 17-2 and figure 17-1 present the gender ratios, age distribution, presenting symptoms, and usual location within the pancreas for the more common pancreatic neoplasms. A simplified algorithmic approach to the diagnosis of pancreatic neoplasms is presented in figure 17-2. The sections that follow provide a practical approach to the common diagnostic situations that arise in the pathologic evaluation of pancreatic neoplasms. Although we recognize that some of the material presented here repeats information found elsewhere in this Fascicle, we believe it is useful to provide a single chapter dedicated to the practical evaluation of pancreatic neoplasms.

DIAGNOSIS OF DUCTAL ADENOCARCINOMA

Biopsy Interpretation

Given the high proportion of pancreatic neoplasms that are invasive ductal adenocarcinomas and their highly aggressive clinical course,

the proper identification of this neoplasm is the most important pathologic diagnosis related to the pancreas. Most often, ductal adenocarcinomas present at an advanced clinical stage, so a diagnosis must be based on biopsy or cytology material from the primary neoplasm or its metastases, often in the intraoperative setting. Non-neoplastic lesions can simulate ductal adenocarcinoma in both the primary location and in several common sites of metastatic disease, and the diagnostic issues encountered during the evaluation of these specimens vary according to the type of specimen and its source.

Frozen sections are best evaluated with an understanding of the impact the diagnosis will have on intraoperative decision making. Although treatment algorithms vary somewhat by institution and by surgeon, there are several common themes, such as the use of intraoperative frozen sections to evaluate margins and to establish the presence of metastases. Well-defined diagnostic criteria need to be rigorously applied whenever adenocarcinoma of the pancreas is considered.

Patients explored operatively with a presumptive diagnosis of pancreatic cancer may or may not have a definitive preoperative diagnosis of malignancy. If the mass appears resectable, many surgeons will perform a pancreatectomy without a preoperative or intraoperative

Table 17-1

SEX RATIOS AND LOCATIONS OF PANCREATIC NEOPLASMS

Neoplasm	M:F	Location	Gross Configuration
Ductal adenocarcinoma	1.3:1	Head > Tail	Solid
Intraductal papillary mucinous neoplasm	1.5:1	Head > Tail	Cystic/Intraductal
Mucinous cystic neoplasm	1:20	Tail	Cystic
Serous cystadenoma	1:2.3	Head = Tail	Cystic
Acinar cell carcinoma	3.6:1	Head = Tail	Solid
Pancreatoblastoma	1.3–2.0:1	Head = Tail	Solid
Pancreatic endocrine neoplasm	1:1	Head = Tail	Solid
Solid-pseudopapillary tumor	1:9	Head = Tail	Solid/Cystic

diagnosis of malignancy (6). This practice has achieved wide acceptance due to the difficulty of establishing a definitive diagnosis using pre-

operative cytology or needle biopsy, or even intraoperative direct biopsy analysis. The false negative rate for such biopsy procedures ranges from 10 to 30 percent (17,30), usually because the desmoplastic reaction associated with most neoplasms results in low neoplastic cellularity, and the diagnostically challenging nature of the specimens themselves means that even biopsies taken from the center of a clinically obvious cancer may fail to yield diagnostic tissue.

In the event that a resection is planned without a pathologic diagnosis, intraoperative frozen sections are often submitted from possible metastases identified during laparotomy or laparoscopy (12). If an intraoperative biopsy from a distant site reveals metastatic pancreatic carcinoma, the planned resection of the primary neoplasm is usually aborted. Therefore, if a metastasis is misinterpreted on frozen section as a benign lesion, an unnecessary radical operation may ensue. It is particularly important to correctly diagnose small foci of metastatic carcinoma in biopsies from the liver or peritoneum, and multiple frozen section levels should be obtained if necessary (e.g., in the event of a

Table 17-2
PRESENTING MANIFESTATIONS OF PANCREATIC NEOPLASMS

Ductal adenocarcinoma	Jaundice, pain, weight loss, cachexia
Intraductal papillary mucinous neoplasm	Exocrine insufficiency, pain
Mucinous cystic neoplasm	Nonspecific[a]
Serous cystadenoma	Nonspecific
Acinar cell carcinoma	Nonspecific; lipase hypersecretion (fat necrosis, polyarthralgia)
Pancreatoblastoma	Nonspecific
Pancreatic endocrine neoplasm	Nonspecific; endocrine paraneoplastic syndromes (hyperinsulinism, Zollinger-Ellison, Verner-Morrison, etc)
Solid-pseudopapillary neoplasm	Nonspecific

[a]Abdominal pain, gastrointestinal symptoms, enlarging mass.

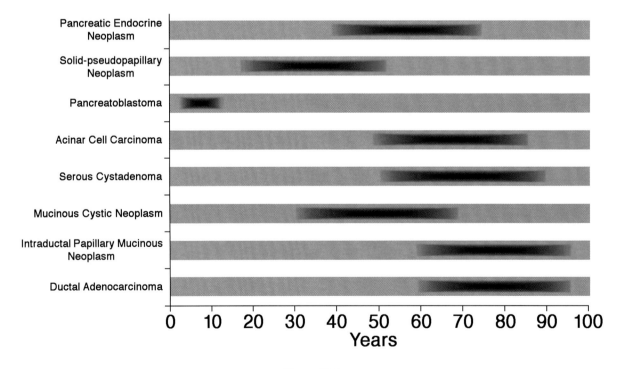

Figure 17-1

AGE DISTRIBUTION OF PATIENTS WITH MAJOR TYPES OF PANCREATIC NEOPLASIA

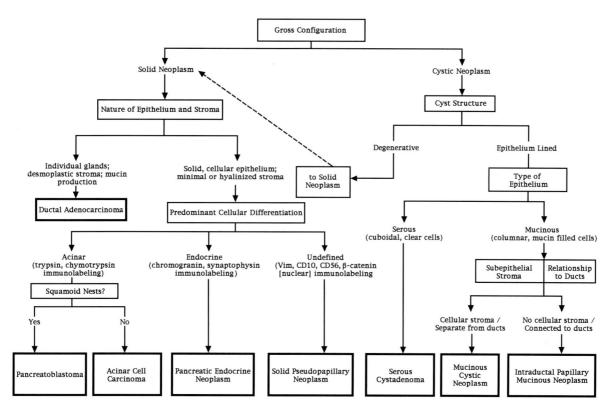

Figure 17-2

SIMPLE DIAGNOSTIC ALGORITHM FOR THE EVALUATION OF PANCREATIC NEOPLASMS

liver biopsy with a lesion identified by the surgeon that shows only normal liver parenchyma on the initial frozen section level).

Biopsy interpretation of a primary pancreatic lesion can be even more challenging, particularly the distinction between ductal adenocarcinoma and chronic pancreatitis. We have found eight features helpful in this distinction (Table 17-3, fig. 17-3). 1) The loss of a lobular arrangement (which is usually preserved in areas of atrophic chronic pancreatitis), resulting in a haphazard arrangement of the glands, is the single most helpful feature in separating ductal adenocarcinoma from benign processes. If the glands are too sparse to evaluate the architecture (or the biopsy is distorted), careful examination of the nuclear features may help establish the diagnosis. 2) Variation in nuclear area greater than 4 to 1 from cell to cell in a single gland is very specific for adenocarcinoma. 3) Prominent and multiple nucleoli support a diagnosis of carcinoma. If two cytologically different populations of glands are present

Table 17-3		
FEATURES HELPFUL IN DISTINGUISHING DUCTAL ADENOCARCINOMA FROM CHRONIC PANCREATITIS		
Feature	**Carcinoma**	**Pancreatitis**
Glandular architecture	Haphazard	Lobular
Variation in nuclear size	Variable (4:1 or more)	Uniform
Nucleoli	Huge irregular nucleoli	Single, regular
Incomplete glands	May be present	Absent
Luminal necrosis	May be present	Absent
Glands immediately adjacent to muscular artery	May be present	Absent
Perineural invasion	May be present	Absent
Vascular invasion	May be present	Absent

in a biopsy, it can be helpful to contrast the nuclear features of a clearly benign population with those of subtly atypical malignant glands. 4) The neoplastic glands of invasive

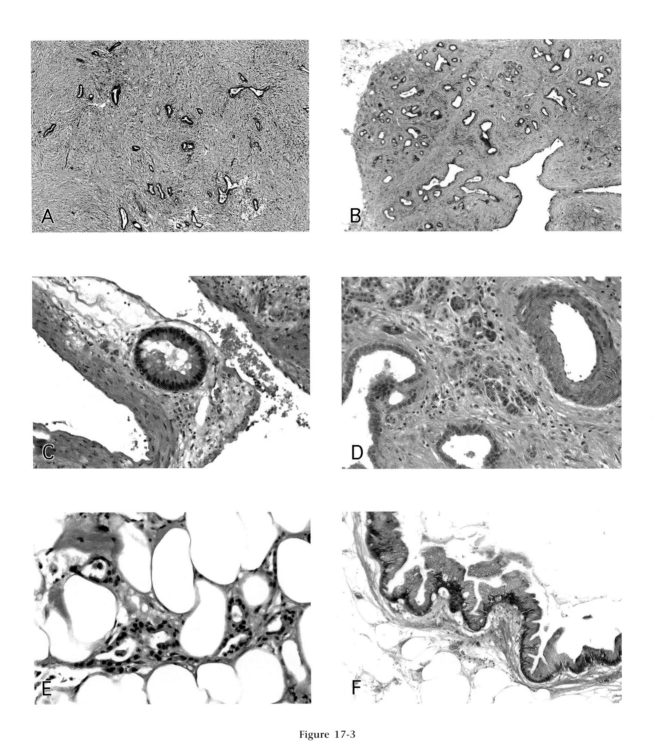

Figure 17-3

COMPARATIVE HISTOLOGIC FEATURES OF DUCTAL
ADENOCARCINOMA (LEFT) AND CHRONIC PANCREATITIS (RIGHT)

Haphazard glands of carcinoma (A) versus lobular architecture of chronic pancreatitis (B). Malignant gland adjacent to a muscular artery (C) versus ducts separated from the vessels in atrophic pancreatitis (D). Malignant glands immediately apposed to adipocytes (E) versus fatty infiltration of the pancreas, with a layer of collagen separating the benign gland from the fat (F). Perineural invasion by carcinoma with an evident glandular lumen (G) versus non-neoplastic perineural islet cells (H). Nuclear features of adenocarcinoma with marked variation in size and shape (I) versus the uniform nuclear morphology of ductules in chronic pancreatitis (J).

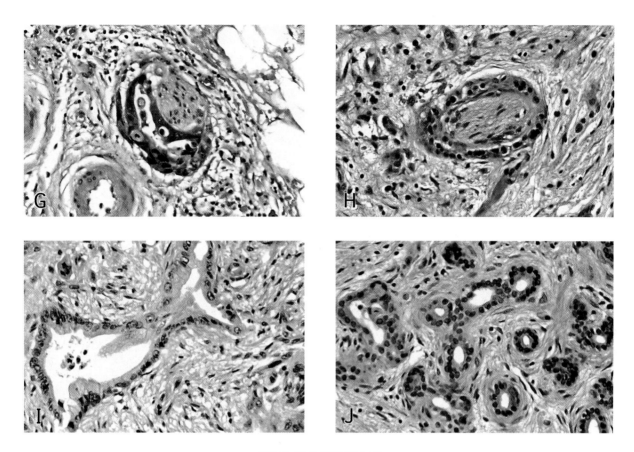

Figure 17-3 (Continued)

adenocarcinoma are often incomplete; i.e., tubular structures are only partially lined by epithelium, with naked stroma forming part of the lining of the lumen. 5) Intraluminal necrosis supports the diagnosis of carcinoma, as does 6) the presence of a gland adjacent to a muscular vessel (41). 7) Perineural invasion by glands (solid nests of cells may be perineural non-neoplastic islet cells) and 8) vascular invasion support the diagnosis. If invasion into nerves, vessels, or lymphatics is found, the diagnosis of carcinoma is almost certain, but this is an uncommon finding in biopsy specimens.

Mitoses may be found in adenocarcinoma, and atypical mitoses are highly suggestive of that diagnosis, although uncommonly found in biopsies. The location of glands adjacent to adipocytes can also help distinguish invasive carcinoma from reactive glands, since even in profound atrophy with fatty infiltration into the parenchyma of the pancreas, there is usually a layer of fibrous stroma maintained around each

ductule. Stromal hypercellularity may suggest the desmoplasia of ductal adenocarcinoma; this finding alone will not allow a definitive diagnosis but suggests that additional levels of the lesion should be evaluated or additional biopsies procured. The quantity of inflammation is usually not helpful, since chronic pancreatitis often has minimal inflammation, and some ductal adenocarcinomas may have inflammatory cells associated with the desmoplastic stroma. Dense periductal chronic inflammation raises the possibility of lymphoplasmacytic sclerosing (autoimmune) pancreatitis (46,47); foci of the characteristic obliterative venulitis should be sought to further support this diagnosis in suspicious cases.

When infiltrating adenocarcinoma of the pancreas grows into preexisting epithelium such as the duodenal mucosa, the cancer can grow along the epithelial surface and mimic a noninvasive adenoma (fig. 17-4). In these cases, an examination of deeper tissues will usually reveal the underlying invasive carcinoma.

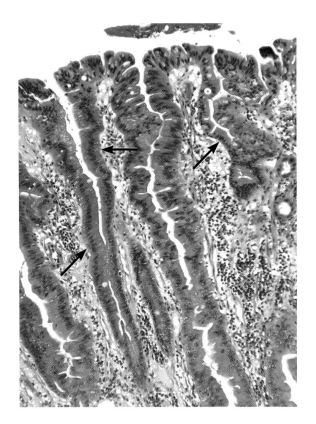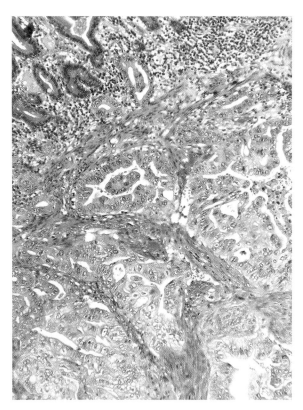

Figure 17-4

INFILTRATING DUCTAL ADENOCARCINOMA REPLACING THE DUODENAL MUCOSA

Left: As the malignant glands colonize the mucosal basement membrane, they become better differentiated and resemble a primary duodenal adenoma. The interposed normal epithelium (arrows) is a clue to the correct diagnosis.

Right: The tissues deep to the mucosa contain the contiguous, moderately differentiated ductal adenocarcinoma from the pancreas.

Table 17-4

IMMUNOHISTOCHEMICAL LABELING IN THE DIAGNOSIS OF DUCTAL ADENOCARCINOMA

	Benign Glands (Chronic Pancreatitis, Benign Bile Duct Lesions) (% Abnormal	Ductal Adenocarcinoma Expression)
CEA (monoclonal)[a]	10	90
B72.3	5	92
CA125[b]	0	45
p53[c]	0	60
Smad4 (Dpc4)[d]	0	55
Mesothelin	5	95

[a]CEA = carcinoembryonic antigen; abnormal expression is cytoplasmic reactivity.
[b]CA = carbohydrate antigen.
[c]Abnormal expression is reactivity in >20% of nuclei.
[d]Abnormal expression is loss of cytoplasmic and nuclear labeling.

In difficult cases, immunohistochemistry may be used to support the diagnosis of ductal adenocarcinoma (Table 17-4). Aberrant expression of tumor-associated glycoproteins, such as B72.3, carbohydrate antigen (CA)125, or carcinoembryonic antigen (CEA) (using monoclonal antibodies) is much more frequent in invasive carcinomas or foci of high-grade pancreatic intraepithelial neoplasia (PanIN) than in non-neoplastic ducts (20). Loss of expression of Smad4 (Dpc4) is essentially diagnostic of carcinoma, provided there is labeling of the non-neoplastic tissues to serve as an internal control (44). Strong expression of p53, mesothelin, or prostate stem cell antigen also supports a malignant diagnosis.

Biopsies of regions of chronic pancreatitis may mimic invasive carcinoma particularly if they yield ducts involved by PanIN. An individual glandular profile containing PanIN may be very difficult to distinguish from invasive carcinoma (Table 17-5, fig. 17-5), since the overall lobular architecture of the glands may not be apparent and the cells have all the features of a neoplasm (indeed, they *are* neoplastic, just not invasive). Features that favor a focus of PanIN rather than a well-differentiated invasive carcinoma include round, regular glandular profiles; a distinct separation of the gland from muscular arteries; lack of a thick, apical eosinophilic cytoplasmic layer (characteristic of well-differentiated ductal adenocarcinoma with a foamy gland pattern [3]); lack of small solid clusters of cells in the adjacent stroma; bland hypocellular stroma; and absence of intraluminal necrosis and incomplete glands. Most foci of PanIN are low to intermediate grade (PanIN-1 and -2), so significant cytoarchitectural atypia is much more common in invasive carcinoma. Of course, finding atypical glands in an abnormal location (see above) is strong evidence that the neoplastic proliferation is indeed invasive.

Other pancreatic neoplasms can be mistaken for ductal adenocarcinoma based on biopsy evaluation. Pancreatic endocrine neoplasms may mimic ductal adenocarcinoma, especially on a biopsy or frozen section, where the typical organoid architecture of a pancreatic endocrine

Table 17-5

FEATURES HELPFUL IN DISTINGUISHING WELL-DIFFERENTIATED DUCTAL ADENOCARCINOMA FROM PANCREATIC INTRAEPITHELIAL NEOPLASIA (PanIN)

	Invasive Carcinoma	PanIN
Gland location	May be abnormal[a]	Normal
Glandular architecture	Haphazard	Lobular
Apical eosinophilic layer	May be present	Usually absent
Incomplete glands	May be present	Usually absent
Solid cell clusters	May be present	Usually absent
Stroma	Desmoplastic	Hyalinized
Cytologic atypia	Marked	Mild to moderate
Glandular profiles	Irregular	Lobular

[a]Such as adjacent to muscular vessels, within duodenal muscularis, perineural, intravascular, and adjacent to adipocytes.

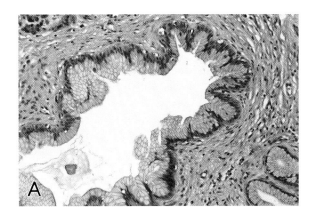

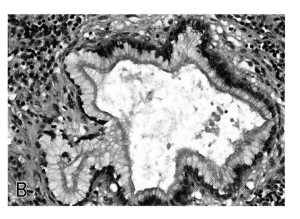

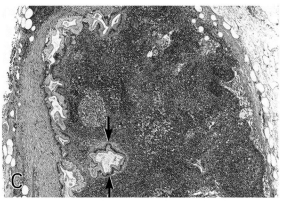

Figure 17-5

COMPARATIVE HISTOLOGIC FEATURES OF PANCREATIC INTRAEPITHELIAL NEOPLASIA AND WELL-DIFFERENTIATED INFILTRATING DUCTAL ADENOCARCINOMA

A: Low-grade pancreatic intraepithelial neoplasia (PanIN) consists of tall columnar mucinous cells with uniform, basally oriented nuclei.

B: The invasive ductal adenocarcinoma has similar cytologic features, but the gland is more irregular and there is a thick apical eosinophilic border.

C: The malignant gland in B actually represents a lymph node metastasis (arrows).

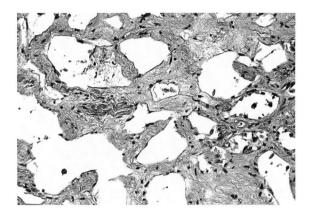 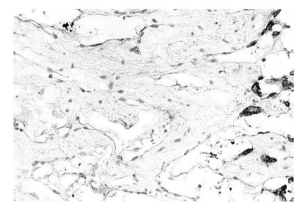

Figure 17-6

PANCREATIC ENDOCRINE NEOPLASM

Left: Loss of the epithelial cells leaves the stromal framework, resembling a hemangioma.
Right: Immunolabeling for chromogranin reveals a few remaining neoplastic cells.

neoplasm may be difficult to appreciate. The finding of solid nests in a fibrotic stroma or gland formation in an endocrine neoplasm may incorrectly suggest the diagnosis of ductal adenocarcinoma. Touch preparations can be particularly helpful in distinguishing ductal adenocarcinomas from endocrine neoplasms. In addition, recognition of the wide array of morphologic patterns encountered in pancreatic endocrine neoplasms helps avoid confusion. Immunohistochemical labeling for chromogranin and synaptophysin establishes the diagnosis in most cases.

An interesting phenomenon may occur in pancreatic endocrine neoplasms and other well-differentiated endocrine neoplasms when subjected to needle biopsy (particularly their hepatic metastases). The more fragile nests of neoplastic cells may become disrupted, leaving behind only the more rigid stromal framework. The resulting fragments often resemble cavernous hemangiomas (fig. 17-6, left) or, if a few neoplastic cells remain adherent to the stroma, irregular gland-forming neoplasms such as adenocarcinomas. In almost all cases, there are sufficient cells attached to the stroma for immunohistochemical identification (fig. 17-6, right).

Liver and Peritoneal Biopsies

The liver is often biopsied when searching for metastatic pancreatic cancer since this is the most commonly involved organ. Small, radio-graphically occult liver metastases are often subcapsular, appearing as firm white nodules or plaques on the liver surface. Several benign primary liver lesions have a similar gross appearance, including bile duct hamartomas (9), bile duct adenomas (8,14), and focal subcapsular scars, which may contain reactive bile ductular proliferations. Histologically, these lesions may resemble a metastatic well-differentiated ductal adenocarcinoma (Table 17-6).

Bile duct hamartomas (von Meyenburg complexes) are commonly multiple and are composed of ectatic bile ductules containing bile and surrounded by bland fibrous stroma (fig. 17-7). The epithelial cells are usually cuboidal to flattened, and they lack atypia and mucinous cytoplasm. The finding of bile within a glandular proliferation in the liver almost always indicates a bile duct hamartoma, although colonization of the bile ducts by metastatic carcinoma may, rarely, result in the presence of bile within the lumens of malignant glands.

Bile duct adenomas are usually solitary benign biliary neoplasms that consist of unencapsulated nodular collections of small bile ductules of relatively uniform size and even distribution (fig. 17-8). Again, the cells are cuboidal rather than columnar, but cytoplasmic mucin may be found. Areas of stromal hyalinization may occur in the center of bile duct adenomas, and some have an associated lymphocytic infiltrate. Since they are neoplastic, there may be enlargement and mild

Table 17-6

FEATURES HELPFUL IN DISTINGUISHING BENIGN BILE
DUCTULAR LESIONS FROM METASTATIC DUCTAL ADENOCARCINOMA

	Bile Duct Hamartoma	Bile Duct Adenoma	Reactive Bile Ductular Proliferation	Ductal Adenocarcinoma
Size	1-3 mm	1-20 mm	Variable	Variable
Number	May be multiple	Usually solitary	Variable	Multiple
Gland spacing	Regular	Regular	Variable; may be lobular	Irregular
Gland shape	Ectatic	Tubular/acinar	Tubular/acinar	Irregular
Luminal bile	Present	Absent	Absent	Absent
Nuclear morphology	Bland	Mildly atypical	Reactive features	Moderately to markedly atypical
Stroma	Hyalinized	Hyalinized/inflamed	Variable	Desmoplastic
Cytoplasmic mucin	Absent	May be present	Absent	Often present

irregularities in the nuclei, although frank pleomorphism is rare. The atypia may be noticeable in comparison with adjacent non-neoplastic bile ducts, sometimes leading to the false impression of malignancy.

The nonspecific reactive bile ductular proliferations that often accompany scars and other localized lesions in the liver have no reproducible histologic features. Sometimes the biliary ductules retain a lobular arrangement; however, a patternless arrangement of small ductules also occurs, usually trailing through the fibrotic liver tissue without the formation of nodules. Acute inflammation can cause a troubling degree of reactive nuclear atypia.

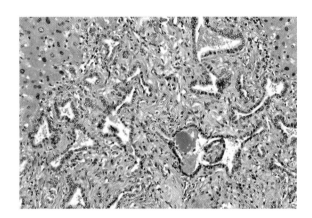

Figure 17-7

BILE DUCT HAMARTOMA

Ectatic bile ductules with luminal bile.

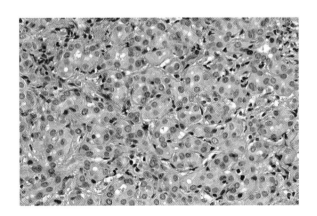

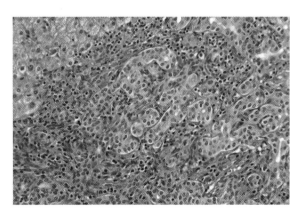

Figure 17-8

BILE DUCT ADENOMA

Left: Back-to-back tubular glands with relatively uniform nuclear features.
Right: An inflammatory stroma is present here.

The features that help distinguish metastatic ductal adenocarcinoma from these benign biliary lesions are similar to those used to distinguish carcinoma from chronic pancreatitis. The neoplastic glands of metastatic ductal adenocarcinoma are arranged haphazardly and vary in size and shape. The nuclei usually show significant enlargement and vary in shape, location, and size between adjacent cells within the individual glands. Cytoplasmic mucin is usually more evident in metastatic ductal adenocarcinoma than in any of the benign biliary lesions. If desmoplastic stroma is present, it is a helpful feature as well. Metastases to the liver are usually multiple; if an individual biopsy is problematic at the time of frozen section, it may be prudent for the surgeon to sample another lesion.

In some cases, the distinction of benign biliary lesions from metastatic carcinoma may be problematic even on permanent sections. Immunohistochemistry has proven useful in these instances, and it is best to prepare additional unstained slides at the time of frozen section to ensure that the diagnostic tissue is not lost during reprocessing of the paraffin sections. Immunohistochemical stains useful for distinguishing benign biliary lesions from metastatic pancreatic carcinoma include the same antigens used in the separation of carcinoma from benign ductules of chronic pancreatitis (CEA, B72.3 [TAG-72], CA125, p53, Dpc4, and mesothelin) (16). Studies have shown that nearly all of the benign biliary lesions exhibit normal expression of these markers, so abnormal expression in an atypical glandular lesion strongly supports the diagnosis of a metastasis, especially when several markers are abnormally expressed (16,43).

When peritoneal metastases are suspected, the differential diagnosis is less problematic. Well-formed glands directly opposed to adipocytes are almost always malignant. Reactive mesothelial hyperplasia may be found in peritoneal biopsies, but the proliferating epithelioid cells are usually located on the surface of the peritoneum, and there are no glandular formations deep in the fat. In females, endosalpingiosis or endometriosis can result in benign glands within the peritoneum. The uniformity of the nuclei and the association with endometrial stroma or hemorrhage (in the case of endometriosis) allow a correct diagnosis.

DIAGNOSIS OF THE SOLID CELLULAR PANCREATIC NEOPLASM

Whereas the most common pancreatic neoplasm, ductal adenocarcinoma, usually appears as a relatively hypocellular solid tumor due to its prominent stromal component, a number of other histologically similar entities consist of solid masses with a densely cellular low-power microscopic appearance. In this group of "solid cellular" pancreatic neoplasms are pancreatic endocrine neoplasms, acinar cell carcinomas, pancreatoblastomas, and solid-pseudopapillary neoplasms (fig. 17-9) (18,19). In addition to their characteristic clinical and histologic features, each of these neoplasms has a reproducible immunohistochemical phenotype that may be essential for proper diagnosis.

Age at presentation, and to some extent gender, may help narrow the diagnostic choices (see Table 17-1). Although both acinar cell carcinomas and pancreatoblastomas occur at any age, pancreatoblastomas are much more common in children, specifically in the first decade of life (mean age, 9.8 years), and acinar cell carcinomas generally affect older adults (mean age, 58.3 years). Solid-pseudopapillary neoplasms are more common in females than males and usually occur between the ages of 20 and 30 years. Pancreatic endocrine neoplasms occur at any age but are uncommon in children.

The presence of a paraneoplastic syndrome also provides an important diagnostic clue. The many different endocrine syndromes that accompany pancreatic endocrine neoplasms are well known, and some patients with acinar cell carcinomas have the lipase hypersecretion syndrome manifested by subcutaneous fat necrosis, polyarthralgia, and peripheral eosinophilia. Most patients with pancreatic endocrine neoplasms and acinar cell carcinomas, however, as with solid-pseudopapillary neoplasms and pancreatoblastomas, present without specific tumor-associated syndromes, with symptoms related only to the local affects of the enlarging mass.

Histologically, all of these entities share a cellular low-power appearance and usually have a relatively circumscribed periphery and a pushing growth pattern (fig. 17-9). Features that help distinguish these neoplasms are listed in Table 17-7. Whereas all four may have areas with a solid nesting pattern, specific architectural

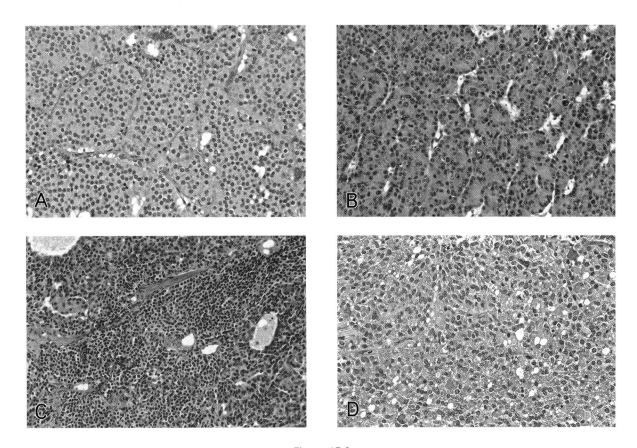

Figure 17-9

SOLID CELLULAR PANCREATIC NEOPLASMS

A relatively similar low-power pattern is found in pancreatic endocrine neoplasm (A), acinar cell carcinoma (B), pancreatoblastoma (C), and solid-pseudopapillary neoplasm (D).

Table 17-7

DISTINGUISHING FEATURES OF SOLID CELLULAR NEOPLASMS

	Acinar Cell Carcinoma	Pancreatic Endocrine Neoplasm	Pancreato-blastoma	Solid-Pseudopapillary Neoplasm
Solid nesting pattern	++[a]	++	++	++
Glands or acini	++	+	++	–
Pseudopapillae	–	–	–	++
Squamoid nests	–	–	++	–
Trabecular pattern	–	+	–	–
Abundant stroma	–	+	+[b]	+
Granular eosinophilic cytoplasm	++	+	++	+
Hyaline globules	–	–	–	++
Nuclear grooves	–	–	–	++
Nucleoli	++	+	++	–

[a]++ = usually present; + = may be present; – = usually absent.
[b]Often hypercellular.

arrangements are generally present as well. Pseudopapillae formed by degenerative changes of noncohesive epithelial cells are highly characteristic, if not pathognomonic, of solid-pseudopapillary neoplasm. Aggregates of foam cells, hyaline globules, and cholesterol crystals are also typical of this neoplasm. Squamoid nests are largely restricted to pancreatoblastomas, and a variety of different organoid patterns (trabecular, gyriform, nested) typify pancreatic endocrine neoplasms. Acinar spaces are found in 75 percent of acinar cell carcinomas, but identical structures are also found in pancreatoblastomas (a neoplasm that also has predominantly acinar differentiation), and similar small glandular spaces occur in pancreatic endocrine neoplasms as well. Solid-pseudopapillary neoplasms, however, completely lack gland formation, so the presence of true lumens in a solid cellular pancreatic neoplasm excludes this diagnosis.

The amount and character of the stroma may be helpful diagnostically. Of these four neoplasms, acinar cell carcinomas usually contain the least stroma. Both solid-pseudopapillary neoplasms and pancreatic endocrine neoplasms often have more abundant fibrotic stroma, and in pancreatic endocrine neoplasms there may be extracellular amyloid deposition. The stroma of pancreatoblastomas is cellular, especially in neoplasms occurring in children.

Nuclear features are also useful. Single prominent nucleoli are characteristic of acinar cell carcinomas, while solid-pseudopapillary neoplasms have oval nuclei with longitudinal grooves. Pancreatic endocrine neoplasms often exhibit the classic stippled ("salt and pepper") chromatin pattern of well-differentiated endocrine neoplasms, but they may also have a wide array of alternate cytologic appearances (including prominent nucleoli on occasion). Pancreatoblastomas lack distinctive cytologic features but may contain a more primitive-appearing, small cell component, and the nuclei in the squamoid nests are larger and have a more open chromatin pattern than those in the surrounding elements. A high mitotic rate is unusual in pancreatoblastomas, pancreatic endocrine neoplasms, and solid-pseudopapillary neoplasms and thus should suggest acinar cell carcinoma.

The cytoplasm of acinar cell carcinomas and some pancreatoblastomas is finely granular and eosinophilic. In solid-pseudopapillary neoplasms, clusters of cells contain large cytoplasmic hyaline globules. The cytoplasmic appearance of pancreatic endocrine neoplasms varies widely, from faintly basophilic to oncocytic to clear.

There is sufficient overlap among these solid cellular neoplasms to justify the use of immunohistochemistry in all but the most histologically classic examples. Special stains such as mucicarmine and periodic acid-Schiff with diastase (dPAS) may provide some clues but are often not fully diagnostic. The widely recognized positivity of acinar cell carcinomas for dPAS, which stains the zymogen granules, is also widely overstated. Only the most highly granulated acinar cell carcinomas display sufficient dPAS positivity for this stain to be useful. Focal mucin positivity may be found in pancreatic endocrine neoplasms, acinar cell carcinomas, and pancreatoblastomas; only solid-pseudopapillary neoplasms are totally negative. Immunohistochemistry is therefore needed to define the direction of differentiation of the neoplasm (18).

Antibodies are available to recognize endocrine differentiation (e.g., chromogranin and synaptophysin), acinar differentiation (e.g., trypsin and chymotrypsin), and ductal differentiation (e.g., CK19, CA19.9, and CEA). Bearing in mind that minor components with divergent differentiation may be found in almost all pancreatic neoplasms, the labeling profile with these antibodies is usually adequate to establish a diagnosis (Table 17-8). Thus, pancreatic endocrine neoplasms label with antibodies to chromogranin and synaptophysin, acinar cell carcinomas label with antibodies to trypsin and chymotrypsin, and pancreatoblastomas express both acinar and endocrine differentiation and sometimes ductal differentiation as well (but are predominantly acinar). Solid-pseudopapillary neoplasms generally express no specific cell lineage markers (except that some express synaptophysin and all immunolabel with CD56); however, they do express CD10 (36) and show abnormal nuclear labeling with antibodies to beta-catenin (1). The combined use of this panel of stains also helps define the rare mixed carcinomas of the pancreas, many of which exhibit acinar differentiation in addition to either endocrine or ductal differentiation (or both). Mixed carcinomas

Table 17-8

IMMUNOHISTOCHEMICAL STAINING OF SOLID CELLULAR NEOPLASMS

	Acinar Cell Carcinoma	Pancreatic Endocrine Neoplasm	Pancreato-blastoma	Solid-Pseudopapil-lary Neoplasm
CAM5.2	++[a]	++	++	F
Vimentin	–	–	–	++
Trypsin/chymotrypsin	++	–	++	–
Chromogranin	F	++	+	–
Synaptophysin	F	++	+	+
CD56	F	++	+	++
CK19	–	+	+	–
CA19.9	–	+	+	–
Alpha-1-antitrypsin	++	+	++	++
CD10	–	–	–	++
Beta-catenin[b]	+	–	+	++

[a]++ = usually positive; + = may be positive; F = may be focally positive; – = usually negative.
[b]Nuclear staining.

Table 17-9

CYSTIC LESIONS OF THE PANCREAS

	Type of Cyst	No. of Locules	Size of Cysts
Non-neoplastic Cysts			
Pseudocyst	Degenerative	Unilocular	Macrocystic
Ductal retention cyst	True cyst	Unilocular	Macrocystic
Lymphoepithelial cyst	True cyst	Oligolocular	Macrocystic
Squamous cyst in heterotopic spleen	True cyst	Oligolocular	Macrocystic
Paraduodenal wall cyst	Degenerative	Uni/oligolocular	Macrocystic
Benign Cystic Neoplasms			
Microcystic serous cystadenoma	True cyst	Multilocular	Microcystic
Macrocystic serous cystadenoma	True cyst	Oligolocular	Macrocystic
Acinar cell cystadenoma	True cyst	Oligo/multilocular	Microcystic
Dermoid cyst	True cyst	Oligolocular	Macrocystic
Malignant or Premalignant Cystic Neoplasms			
Mucinous cystic neoplasm	True cyst	Oligolocular	Macrocystic
Intraductal papillary mucinous neoplasm	Ductal dilation	Oligolocular	Macrocystic
Intraductal oncocytic papillary neoplasm	Ductal dilation	Oligolocular	Macrocystic
Acinar cell cystadenocarcinoma	True cyst	Multilocular	Microcystic
Primary Solid Neoplasms with Secondary Cystic Changes			
Solid-pseudopapillary neoplasm	Degenerative	Uni/oligolocular	Varies
Ductal adenocarcinoma	Various[a]	Uni/oligolocular	Microcystic
Pancreatic endocrine neoplasm	Degenerative	Oligolocular	Macrocystic

[a]Ductal adenocarcinoma may have unilocular degenerative cysts (macrocystic) or cystic dilatation of invasive glands that are true multiple microcysts.

are defined as having at least 25 percent of each cellular component (21).

DIAGNOSIS OF THE CYSTIC PANCREATIC NEOPLASM

A wide array of benign and malignant pancreatic neoplasms and other lesions appear cystic, and the differential diagnosis of the cystic pancreatic mass is a common clinical problem (2,7,24). The preoperative diagnosis of cystic lesions is particularly important since some (pseudocysts, some serous cystic neoplasms) may be managed nonsurgically, while others are fully malignant neoplasms requiring resection.

Table 17-9 lists cystic lesions that are encountered in the pancreas.

Cystic neoplasms can be divided into microcystic and macrocystic types. In microcystic neoplasms, the individual locules range from less than 1 mm to approximately 1 cm in diameter, and the cut section of the tumor may even appear solid in some regions. Macrocystic neoplasms usually have fewer locules that are one to several centimeters in diameter.

Cystic changes occur in pancreatic neoplasms via three different mechanisms. Some neoplasms are fundamentally cystic, in the sense that the cysts are lined by neoplastic epithelium and presumably result from the accumulation of fluid secreted by the neoplastic cells into glandular lumens. Serous cystic neoplasms, mucinous cystic neoplasms, and acinar cystic neoplasms are examples. In other instances, the cystic change results from cellular degeneration or necrosis within a fundamentally solid neoplasm. In these cases, the cysts may be lined by neoplastic cells, but there is no continuous well-oriented epithelial cell layer, and often the cyst is lined by fibrin or necrotic debris. Degenerative cystic change is typical of the solid-pseudo-papillary neoplasm but may also occur in ductal adenocarcinomas, pancreatic endocrine neoplasms, and other usually solid neoplasms of the pancreas. Other than in solid-pseudopapillary neoplasm, these degenerative cysts are generally unilocular. Finally, some radiographically cystic neoplasms are in fact dilated preexisting ducts (e.g., intraductal papillary mucinous neoplasms and intraductal oncocytic papillary neoplasms). Some intraductal neoplasms are very localized, producing a solitary unilocular cyst (as in branch duct intraductal papillary mucinous neoplasms [45]). In more extensive examples, the cystic change diffusely affects the branching ductal system, resulting in the appearance of multiple separate cysts on cross sectional imaging studies.

The differential diagnosis of a cystic pancreatic neoplasm begins with the patient demographics (see Table 17-1) and radiologic findings. Several of the most common cystic neoplasms are highly characteristic in their age of onset, gender predilection, or location within the pancreas. For instance, mucinous cystic neoplasms almost always occur in the tail of

Table 17-10

FEATURES HELPFUL IN DISTINGUISHING MUCINOUS CYSTIC NEOPLASMS (MCN) FROM INTRADUCTAL PAPILLARY MUCINOUS NEOPLASMS (IPMN)

	MCN	IPMN
Relationship to larger pancreatic ducts	None	Arise within larger ducts
Cellular stroma	Present	Absent
Cystic configuration	Single multilocular	Multiple separate
Sex ratio (M:F)	1:20	1.5:1
Mean age	45	63
Location	Tail	Head > Tail
Papilla formation	Focal	Extensive
Papilla type	Gastric foveolar, pancreatobiliary	Gastric foveolar, intestinal, pancreatobiliary
Peripheral capsule	Present	Absent

the pancreas of a middle-aged female. Solid-pseudopapillary neoplasms are also more common in females but usually occur between the ages of 20 and 30 years. Intraductal papillary mucinous neoplasms, by contrast, typically arise in the head of the gland.

The macrocystic versus microcystic nature of the lesion can often be determined radiographically. Some radiographic studies (endoscopic retrograde cholangiopancreatography [ERCP] or magnetic resonance cholangiopancreatography [MRCP]) can be used to establish the intraductal location of intraductal papillary mucinous neoplasms and intraductal oncocytic papillary neoplasms.

Once the neoplasm has been resected, the histologic differential diagnosis is usually not problematic. Serous cystic neoplasms are lined by cuboidal cells with clear PAS-positive cytoplasm. Solid-pseudopapillary neoplasms, cystic endocrine neoplasms, and ductal adenocarcinomas demonstrate characteristic histologic findings in their noncystic regions.

Two neoplasms that can be difficult to distinguish histologically are mucinous cystic neoplasms and intraductal papillary mucinous neoplasms (Table 17-10). Generally, mucinous cystic neoplasms appear as a single mass containing multiple cysts, while intraductal papillary mucinous neoplasms appear as multiple separate cysts (fig. 17-

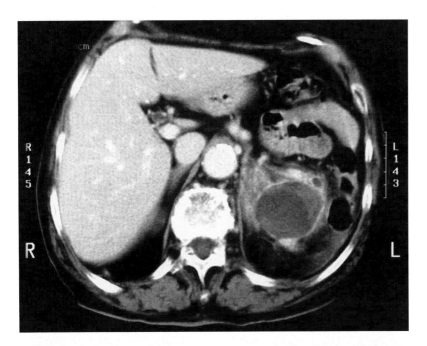

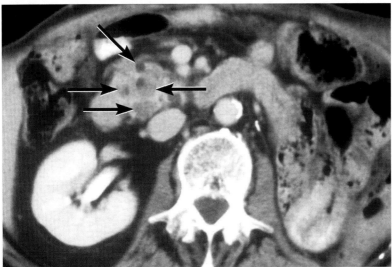

Figure 17-10

MUCINOUS CYSTIC NEOPLASM AND INTRADUCTAL PAPILLARY MUCINOUS NEOPLASM

Top: Radiologically, mucinous cystic neoplasms usually have a single multi-locular cyst.

Bottom: Intraductal papillary mucinous neoplasms often have multiple separate cysts (arrows).

10). Two features distinguish these neoplasms. First, intraductal papillary mucinous neoplasms involve the larger pancreatic ducts, while the vast majority of mucinous cystic neoplasms do not. Documenting the relationship of the cysts to the pancreatic duct can be accomplished easily by passing a probe into the pancreatic duct at the time of gross dissection (see chapter 16). In some intraductal papillary mucinous neoplasms, particularly the branch duct variety, it may be difficult to demonstrate continuity between the pancreatic ducts and the cysts. In these cases, the presence or absence of ovarian-type stroma establishes the diagnosis: mucinous cystic neoplasms, by definition, have this distinctive stroma. In difficult cases, this stroma can be highlighted with immunolabeling for progesterone receptors and inhibin.

Macrocystic serous cystadenomas may be radiographically confused with branch duct intraductal papillary mucinous neoplasms, pseudocysts, and mucinous cystic neoplasms. If there are foci of PanIN adjacent to a macrocystic serous cystadenoma, it may be mistaken microscopically for a branch duct intraductal papillary mucinous neoplasm unless the clear

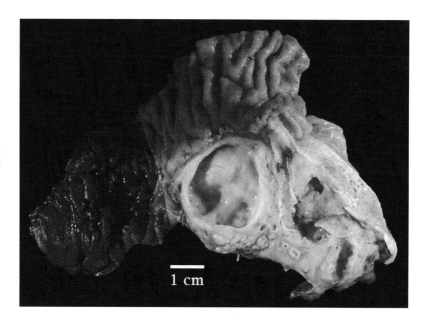

Figure 17-11

INFILTRATING DUCTAL ADENOCARCINOMA WITH RETENTION CYST

The gross appearance is dominated by a large unilocular cyst secondary to an adjacent invasive carcinoma.

1 cm

cuboidal lining of some of the cystic spaces is noted. In all of these instances, the distinctive glycogen-rich cuboidal lining establishes the diagnosis of a macrocystic serous cystadenoma.

Cystic change also occurs in 8 percent of ductal adenocarcinoma by several mechanisms (23a). Degenerative cystic change due to necrosis (mentioned above) is probably the most common (28). Also, obstruction of the pancreatic ducts by the invasive carcinoma may result in distal ductal dilatation that produces a ductal retention cyst (22). These cysts may be mistaken grossly as the principal lesion in the gland, with the more significant invasive carcinoma blending into apparent areas of chronic pancreatitis (fig. 17-11). Also, individual neoplastic glands in a ductal adenocarcinoma may be massively dilated, to the extent that they are seen grossly as microcystic structures; this phenomenon is often marked in the glands infiltrating the duodenal muscularis propria. Finally, there may be pseudocyst formation due to carcinoma-associated pancreatitis (23a).

It should be remembered, however, that the majority of cystic lesions represent pseudocysts. A history of alcohol abuse, bouts of acute pancreatitis, and symptoms of chronic pancreatitis are helpful in the diagnosis of a pseudocyst, and biopsy of the lesion is seldom necessary. Several cystic neoplasms of the pancreas may simulate a pseudocyst histologically, however. It is well known that the epithelium of mucinous cystic neoplasms can be focally denuded, with inflammation and reactive changes in the thick outer capsule of the neoplasm. Biopsy of such an area may lead to the false impression of a pseudocyst. Clinical and radiographic clues to the correct diagnosis include occurrence in a relatively young female, a multilocular nature to the cyst, and a normal appearance to the uninvolved pancreas. Histologically, pseudocyst-like areas of mucinous cystic neoplasms may be indistinguishable from true pseudocysts, however, if elements of the hypercellular ovarian-type stroma of mucinous cystic neoplasms are found, the correct diagnosis can be made. Immunohistochemical labeling (see above) distinguishes the characteristic cellular stroma of mucinous cystic neoplasms from the reactive myofibroblastic proliferation that can occur in the wall of a pseudocyst.

Other cystic pancreatic neoplasms that can develop degenerative changes that histologically simulate pseudocysts are serous cystadenomas, which may have subtotal infarction following fine needle aspiration, or solid-pseudopapillary neoplasms, which typically exhibit widespread degenerative changes and may have a fibrotic capsule like the wall of a pseudocyst. Again, the lack of clinical findings predisposing to pseudocyst formation is helpful in suggesting an alternative diagnosis, but regions with intact neoplastic elements must be present to allow a definite diagnosis.

CYTOLOGIC EVALUATION OF PANCREATIC NEOPLASMS

Cytologic specimens, generally in the form of brushings of the bile duct or ampulla or fine needle aspiration biopsies of solid or cystic masses, are commonly used in the evaluation of pancreatic lesions. The specific cytologic features of each tumor type are discussed with each entity; however, there are some general considerations when evaluating these specimens that parallel those of the histologic evaluation discussed above.

Specimen Preparation

The cells aspirated from either a solid or cystic mass in the pancreas can be prepared in a number of ways: direct smears, cytospins (Thermo-Shandon Instruments), liquid-based preparations (Thinprep® [Cytyc Corporation, Marlborough, MA] or SurePath™ prep [TriPath Inc, Burlington, NC]), and cell blocks. Direct smears are the most common and cell block preparations are optimal, since the formalin-fixed, paraffin-embedded tissue can be used readily for ancillary studies. A centrifuged cell button of needle rinsings and visible tissue fragments can be prepared and processed as a cell block. Aspirates rinsed in saline can be used for flow cytometry analysis in cases suspicious of lymphoma. Liquid-based preparations eliminate obscuring blood and inflammation and provide excellent cellular preservation; however, familiarity with the differences in cellular and extracellular material, such as mucin, should be attained prior to the interpretation of this preparation type (13,32,33).

Bile Duct Brushing Cytology

Pancreatic neoplasms involving the bile duct can be detected with direct bile duct sampling, brushing cytology being the favored technique. Brush cytology has virtually replaced direct bile sampling and bile duct washing due to its increased sensitivity and specificity (4,25,26,39). The use of brushing cytology, however, results in a higher false positive and negative rate than does fine needle aspiration biopsy (15).

False negative results are mostly due to sampling error attributable either to the lack of invasion into the bile duct lumen or the charac-teristic abundant desmoplastic stroma of ductal adenocarcinomas with low neoplastic cellularity. Cell loss during the retrieval of the brush also contributes to a low cell yield. Cells obscured by preparation artifact also preclude optimal evaluation. Solutions to these problems include repeated brushings (three or more per case) (38), disrupting the lining epithelium with a stent or stiff brush (37), protecting the cell-laden brush with a sheath during removal and salvage cytology of the brush sheath (5,27), and rinsing stents after they are removed (42).

False positive cytology interpretations occur with biliary epithelial dysplasia and marked reactive atypia from instrumentation and indwelling stents, changes that are nearly indistinguishable from carcinoma (23,26,27). Many patients with a bile duct stricture will have a stent in place, and a very high threshold for a malignant diagnosis should be established in such cases. The diagnosis of malignancy appears most accurate when using the "overall features of malignancy" as assessed by an experienced cytopathologist (39). High cellularity, background necrosis, and individual atypical cells establish a low-power suspicion of malignancy. Nuclear molding, chromatin clumping, and increased nuclear to cytoplasmic ratio are the most helpful features on high-power microscopy (11). Any doubt of a malignant diagnosis after the first few seconds of review should prompt an indeterminate (atypical or suspicious) interpretation when dealing with bile duct brushing specimens.

Fine Needle Aspiration Biopsy

The interpretation of aspiration cytology smears is influenced by the technique used to obtain the specimen. Computerized tomography (CT)-guided percutaneous fine needle aspiration biopsy is most commonly used, however, endoscopic ultrasound (EUS)-guided biopsy is becoming increasingly utilized due to the higher resolution of the latter (0.5 cm versus 1.0 cm) and the ability with EUS to perform biopsies of multiple sites and thus stage the neoplasm during the same procedure. In contrast to percutaneous biopsies, EUS-guided biopsies traverse the stomach or duodenal wall and can introduce epithelial and mucin contamination from these sites. The challenge of identifying gastrointestinal epithelial contamination is generally not

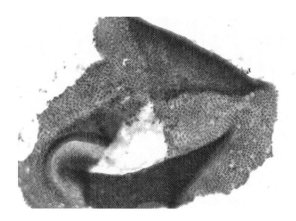

Figure 17-12

DUODENAL EPITHELIUM

Duodenal epithelium is recognized by the presence of large, often folded sheets of glandular epithelium with evenly spaced nuclei, a luminal edge with brush border, and scattered goblet cells. The cytoplasm is dense and non-mucinous (direct smear; Papanicolaou stain).

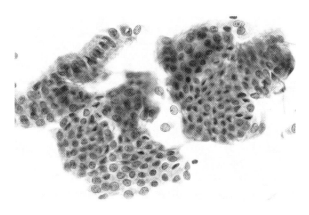

Figure 17-13

GASTRIC EPITHELIUM

Gastric epithelium frequently presents as smaller, monolayered sheets of glandular epithelial cells without a luminal edge or brush border and generally no goblet cells. The cytoplasm is usually nonmucinous (direct smear; Papanicolaou stain).

an issue with poorly differentiated neoplasms where two populations of cells (one benign and one malignant) are readily recognized, but it can be a significant issue with well-differentiated adenocarcinomas and pancreatic cysts.

The initial approach to all aspiration cytology smears should include a low-power evaluation of the overall cellularity, cellular composition, architectural arrangement of cell groups, cohesiveness of the cells, and background elements such as inflammation, mucin, and necrosis. High-power evaluation of the cytomorphologic features of the individual cells then follows where nuclear size, nuclear shape, chromatin pattern, nucleoli, and cytoplasmic features aid in determining the degree of atypia and cell type. Combining all of these elements of the smear with the clinical and radiologic information establishes the cytologic diagnosis.

Gastrointestinal Contamination

The recognition of gastric and duodenal epithelial contamination is critical for the accurate interpretation of EUS-guided biopsies. Gastritis and duodenitis with injury and repair of the epithelium can lead to a false positive interpretation of carcinoma, and neoplastic groups of well-differentiated adenocarcinoma can be mistakenly disregarded as gastrointestinal contamination. It is especially difficult to distin-

guish the glandular epithelium and mucin of the duodenum and stomach from the cyst lining of a mucin-producing cystic neoplasm.

Duodenal epithelium is recognized by the large, folded, sheet-like arrangement of evenly spaced cells studded with goblet cells (fig. 17-12). A luminal edge of contiguous nonmucinous cytoplasm with a brush border is often present (35). Difficulty arises when folds in sheets appear "papillary," nuclear chromatin appears somewhat cleared, or the epithelium fragments into smaller groups. Duodenal nuclei, however, are generally uniformly small, round, and regularly spaced in a group or sheet, and the cytoplasm does not appear clear or vacuolated (except for the occasional goblet cell).

Gastric epithelial contamination may also occur as large sheets, but more commonly occurs as smaller, flat monolayered groups (fig. 17-13). Luminal edges are not as common as with duodenal epithelium and a brush border is absent. The epithelium of the stomach is predominantly nonmucinous, however, foveolar cells may display apical cytoplasmic mucin in groups (fig. 17-14) and singly, thus causing difficulty in the interpretation of cyst aspirates (34,35).

Background mucin can be a contaminant from the gastrointestinal tract. The quality of the mucin is important. Mucin that is thick and viscous, a feature often first appreciated at the

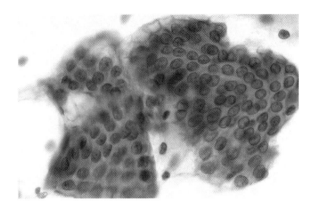

Figure 17-14

GASTRIC EPITHELIUM

Gastric foveolar cells may display apical cytoplasmic mucin, a diagnostic pitfall particularly when compared with mucin-producing cysts with low-grade dysplasia (direct smear; Papanicolaou stain).

time of aspiration of a cyst, forms a film over the slide and appears "colloid-like." This type of mucin is virtually diagnostic of a mucin-producing neoplasm and should not be dismissed as gastrointestinal contamination. Entrapped inflammatory cells, histiocytes, and degenerated cells within the mucin also support an origin from a neoplastic cyst. Mucin from the gastrointestinal tract may be focally thick or thin and is often associated with the contaminating epithelium. Other lesions that can produce thick mucin include pancreatic duct obstruction in chronic pancreatitis and extrapancreatic cysts such as enteric duplication cysts. Attention to the radiologic and clinical features of the pancreatic lesion are helpful; for example, duct obstruction does not typically produce a large unilocular or multilocular cyst.

Solid Masses

Usually the fine needle aspiration biopsy of a solid pancreatic mass is performed for the diagnosis of ductal adenocarcinoma. In contrast to benign and reactive processes such as pancreatitis, the primary entities in the differential diagnosis, percutaneous aspiration biopsy of carcinoma generally produces cellular smears in which glandular epithelial cells predominate. The characteristic desmoplastic reaction associated with many invasive carcinomas may lead to a paucicellular specimen, so it is difficult to establish the absolute number of ductal groups

required for a malignant interpretation. In addition, gastrointestinal contamination can contribute to what appears to be a highly cellular specimen on EUS-guided biopsy and care must be taken to carefully distinguish epithelium from the stomach and duodenum from pancreatic ductal epithelium (see above). High cellularity is not as important a criterion for poorly differentiated adenocarcinoma as it is for well-differentiated adenocarcinoma, and there is no established minimum number of malignant cells or groups of cells for the diagnosis of poorly differentiated adenocarcinoma (10,31,40). Greater than 90 percent accuracy with at least six groups of cells in well-differentiated carcinoma has been reported (40). Other neoplasms in the differential diagnosis of a solid mass, including acinar cell carcinoma, pancreatic endocrine neoplasm, pancreatoblastoma, and solid-pseudopapillary neoplasm, almost always produce richly cellular smears, and high cellularity should be a requirement for the diagnosis of these neoplasms (Table 17-11).

The composition of the cellular elements on the slide is important in distinguishing benign from malignant processes. Smears of carcinoma should be relatively pure, with only ductal groups for adenocarcinoma, only acinar cells for acinar cell carcinoma, and only endocrine cells for a pancreatic endocrine neoplasm. Aspirates of pancreatoblastoma are dominated by acinar cells. Smears containing acinar, ductal, and endocrine cells should be interpreted with caution as they may represent non-neoplastic pancreas. Similarly, granulation tissue and fibrous tissue fragments with inflammation are features associated with pancreatitis, and the cytologic diagnosis of carcinoma in this setting should be made with extreme caution. Background necrosis and intact single atypical cells are features that suggest malignancy.

The architectural arrangement of carcinoma cells ranges from large crowded sheets, to small three-dimensional clusters and balls of cells, to single cells. Poorly differentiated ductal adenocarcinoma typically produces smaller, less cohesive groups of cells and single cells with overt cytologic features of malignancy (fig. 17-15, lower right). The arrangement of the cells in groups and sheets is important in distinguishing benign ductal groups from well-differentiated ductal

Table 17-11

CYTOLOGIC FEATURES OF PANCREATIC NEOPLASMS

Neoplasm	Typical Cytologic Features	Variant Cytologic Features
Ductal adeno- carcinoma	Glandular epithelium with slightly (well-differentiated) to markedly (poorly differentiated) atypical, unevenly spaced nuclei with irregular nuclear membranes Scant to voluminous and obviously mucinous cytoplasm Single malignant cells, mitoses, and coagulative necrosis	Squamous differentiation Signet ring cells Pleomorphic mononuclear and multinucleated giant cells Malignant mononuclear cells with benign osteoclast-like giant cells
Pancreatic endo- crine neoplasm	Monotonous, small polygonal, often plasmacytoid cells, mostly singly Stippled "salt and pepper" chromatin Cytoplasm either wispy and ill-defined or intact and well defined Fibrovascular stroma	Small cell carcinoma Poorly differentiated large cell endocrine carcinoma
Acinar cell carcinoma	Loosely cohesive, large to small cellular groups, single cells, and many stripped nuclei Prominent macronucleoli Granular cytoplasm Fibrovascular stroma	Nucleoli may not be prominent Cytoplasm may not appear granular Plasmacytoid cells may mimic endocrine neoplasms
Pancreato- blastoma	Predominantly acinar cell differentiation with similar cytologic features to acinar cell carcinoma Squamoid corpuscles (on cell blocks)	Primitive cells without well-developed acinar differentiation No discernible squamoid corpuscles
Solid-pseudo- papillary neoplasm	Papillary structures with a central fibrovascular core occasionally surrounded by myxoid stroma Uniform small cells with oval nuclei Even chromatin Frequent nuclear grooves	No apparent papillary architecture Single cell pattern can mimic endocrine neoplasms
Intraductal papil- lary mucinous neoplasm	Thick, "colloid-type" background mucin Papillary fragments of mucinous epithelium Variable atypia	Scant mucin No mucinous epithelium Absent papillary epithelial fragments
Mucinous cystic neoplasm	Thick, "colloid-type" background mucin Groups and single mucinous epithelial cells Variable atypia	Scant mucin No mucinous epithelium
Serous cyst- adenoma	Scantily cellular smears Nonmucinous background Few groups of cuboidal cells Round, uniform nuclei Scant, finely vacuolated cytoplasm	Acellular aspirates Cells may resemble histiocytes

carcinoma. Nuclei that are crowded, that over-lap, that have lost nuclear polarity, or that display an uneven distribution in a sheet are associated with malignancy. In contrast, benign nuclei maintain order, polarity, and a uniform distribution within the sheet or group (fig. 17-15, upper left). Single intact cells are common in poorly differentiated carcinoma. Single malignant cells may be scattered in the smear background but may also be seen at the edge of more cohesive groups. The presence of intact individual atypical epithelial cells in well-differentiated carcinoma is significant and supports a malignant interpretation.

The smear pattern and architectural arrangement of cells are also important features of acinar cell carcinoma, pancreatic endocrine neoplasm, and solid-pseudopapillary neoplasm. In contrast to the cohesive, grape-like clustering of benign acinar cells, acinar cell carcinoma produces solid sheets and many single cells, especially stripped, naked nuclei. Endocrine neoplasms classically present in a noncohesive, single cell fashion with few cohesive groups of cells. Solid-pseudopapillary neoplasms yield papillary tissue fragments as well as single cells and small clusters. Due to the predominance of acinar cells in pancreatoblastoma, clinical

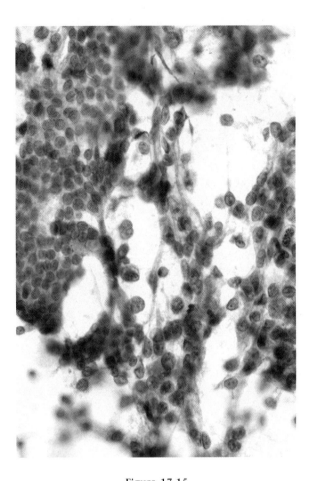

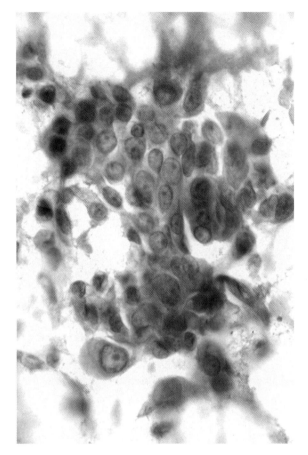

Figure 17-15

POORLY DIFFERENTIATED ADENOCARCINOMA

Overt features of malignancy signify poorly differentiated adenocarcinoma and clearly distinguish the malignant groups of cells (lower right) from benign ductal groups (upper left) and gastrointestinal contamination (direct smear; Papanicolaou stain).

Figure 17-16

WELL-DIFFERENTIATED ADENOCARCINOMA

Slight nuclear crowding and overlapping, parachromatin clearing, and subtly irregular nuclear membranes signify a well-differentiated adenocarcinoma (direct smear; Papanicolaou stain).

correlation is important to distinguish this neoplasm from acinar cell carcinoma.

Although smear pattern is helpful, no pattern is specific to any one entity. The individual cellular features are most important in the cytologic diagnosis. Poorly differentiated ductal carcinoma cells display large, pleomorphic, often angulated nuclei with hyperchromatic chromatin and generally prominent nucleoli. The very high nuclear to cytoplasmic ratio results in scant cytoplasm. Well-differentiated ductal carcinoma cells are often characterized by pale nuclei with parachromatin clearing and subtly irregular nuclear membranes (fig. 17-16). Endocrine cells display round nuclei with coarse, stippled "salt and pepper" chromatin (fig. 17-17) while the nuclei of solid-pseudopapillary neoplasm are bland and uniform with evenly disbursed chromatin, no nucleoli, and occasional nuclear grooves and/or perinuclear vacuoles (fig. 17-18). The presence of cytoplasmic mucin signifies an adenocarcinoma, in contrast to the dense, granular cytoplasm that can be seen in acinar cell carcinoma or endocrine neoplasms. Metastases to the pancreas, although relatively rare, must always be kept in mind. All ancillary tests applicable to the histologic specimen can also be applied to cytology material to help in the differential diagnosis (see above).

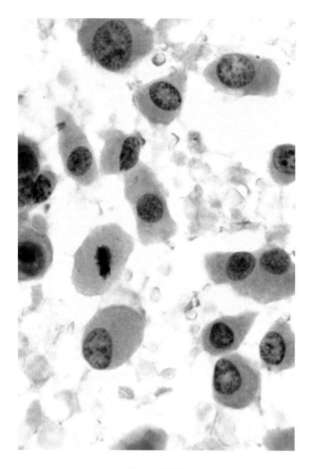

Figure 17-17

PANCREATIC ENDOCRINE NEOPLASM

Mostly single cells with round nuclei and coarse, stippled chromatin on a cellular smear are consistent features of most neuroendocrine neoplasms (direct smear; Papanicolaou stain).

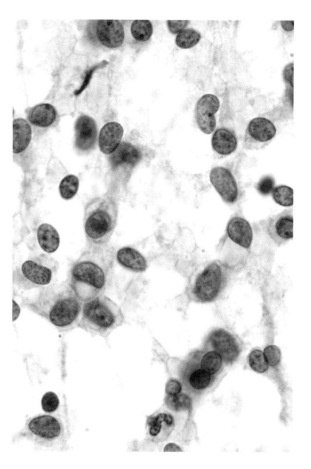

Figure 17-18

SOLID-PSEUDOPAPILLARY NEOPLASM

The nuclei are round or oval, with evenly disbursed chromatin, smooth nuclear membranes, and occasional perinuclear vacuoles in contrast to pancreatic endocrine neoplasm (direct smear; Papanicolaou stain).

Cystic Lesions

The first clue to the cytologic diagnosis is often gleaned from the gross characteristics of the cyst fluid at the time of aspiration. Thin, bloody or brown fluid is commonly obtained from pseudocysts whereas very little fluid is aspirated from most serous cystic neoplasms. Thick viscous mucoid fluid obtained from a true cyst is virtually diagnostic of a mucin-producing cystic neoplasm, either mucinous cystic neoplasm or intraductal papillary mucinous neoplasm. Thin, clear, not apparently mucoid fluid ~ific, and may in fact represent gas-~ntamination.

~ cyst fluid, if sufficient in prepare cytospin slides

for mucin stains (mucicarmine and Alcian blue at pH 2.5) to assess for both extracellular and intracellular mucin. Although no study has assessed the diagnostic utility of these mucin stains, in our experience they aid in the identification of background mucin and intracytoplasmic mucin in cases where these features are difficult to appreciate on the routinely prepared specimen. Gastrointestinal contamination can be a pitfall and must be kept in mind. It is important to remember, however, that the absence of mucin by these special stains does not exclude the diagnosis of a mucin-producing cystic neoplasm.

By definition, pseudocysts do not contain an epithelial lining, so epithelial cells should be absent from the cytologic preparation. The recognition of gastrointestinal epithelial contamination becomes especially important in these cases. Bland-appearing glandular epithelium with nonmucinous cytoplasm in a background of histiocytes, inflammation, and cyst debris, especially bile and hemosiderin-laden debris, should raise the possibility of gastrointestinal contamination. Normal tissue from the pancreas and surrounding structures can also contaminate the specimen obtained by CT- and EUS-guided biopsies. Serous cystic neoplasms produce scantily cellular specimens containing few small groups of cuboidal cells with round, regular nuclei and scant, nonmucinous cytoplasm. The specific diagnosis of a mucin-producing cystic neoplasm is unlikely on cytology alone unless large papillary fragments, consistent with an intraductal papillary neoplasm, are identified. The aspirates from most mucinous cystic neoplasms without invasion are typically scantily cellular and the epithelial cells are nonspecific in architecture: they are arranged in flat sheets, small groups, and singly. Cytoplasmic mucin vacuoles may or may not be apparent (Table 17-11) (34).

Solid neoplasms with cystic degeneration (especially cystic endocrine neoplasms) should always be kept in the differential diagnosis of all cyst aspirates. Very cellular cyst fluid with round cells, coarse speckled chromatin, and no overt features of malignancy, is suspicious for a cystic pancreatic endocrine neoplasm.

Cyst fluid analysis has been studied as a means of distinguishing benign cysts from those requiring surgical resection (2,7,29). Elevations in cyst fluid amylase accompanied by a low viscosity (less than that of serum) and a low CEA level suggests a pseudocyst. Intraductal papillary mucinous neoplasms, because they involve the pancreatic ducts, also usually contain fluid rich in amylase. Since most of the potentially malignant cystic lesions have a mucinous epithelial lining, detection of elevated levels of glycoproteins such as CEA in the cyst fluid suggests that the cyst must be removed. Intraductal papillary mucinous neoplasms and mucinous cystic neoplasms typically have an elevated CEA level (above 200 ng/mL), with very high levels (thousands ng/mL) associated with malignancy (29).

REFERENCES

1. Abraham SC, Klimstra DS, Wilentz RE, et al. Solid-pseudopapillary tumors of the pancreas are genetically distinct from pancreatic ductal adenocarcinomas and almost always harbor beta-catenin mutations. Am J Pathol 2002;160:1361-9.
2. Adsay NV, Klimstra DS, Compton CC. Cystic lesions of the pancreas. Introduction. Semin Diagn Pathol 2000;17:1-6.
3. Adsay NV, Logani S, Sarkar F, Crissman J, Vaitkevicius V. Foamy gland pattern of pancreatic ductal adenocarcinoma: a deceptively benign-appearing variant. Am J Surg Pathol 2000;24:493-504.
4. Bardales RH, Stanley MW, Simpson DD, et al. Diagnostic value of brush cytology in the diagnosis of duodenal, biliary, and ampullary neoplasms. Am J Clin Pathol 1998;109:540-8.
5. Baron TH, Lee JG, Wax TD, Schmitt CM, Cotton PB, Leung JW. An in vitro, randomized, prospective study to maximize cellular yield during bile duct brush cytology. Gastrointest Endosc 1994;40:146-9.
6. Bottger TC, Junginger T. Treatment of tumors of the pancreatic head with suspected but unproved malignancy: is a nihilistic approach justified? World J Surg 1999;23:158-62.
7. Brugge WR, Lauwers GY, Sahani D, Fernandez-del Castillo C, Warshaw AL. Cystic neoplasms of the pancreas. N Engl J Med 2004;351:1218-26.
8. Cho C, Rullis I, Rogers LS. Bile duct adenomas as liver nodules. Arch Surg 1978;113:272-4.
9. Chung EB. Multiple bile-duct hamartomas. Cancer 1970;26:287-96.
10. Cohen MB, Egerter DP, Holly EA, Ahn DK, Miller TR. Pancreatic adenocarcinoma: regression analysis to identify improved cytologic criteria. Diagn Cytopathol 1991;7:341-5.
11. Cohen MB, Wittchow RJ, Johlin FC, Bottles K, Raab SS. Brush cytology of the extrahepatic biliary tract: comparison of cytologic features of adenocarcinoma and benign biliary strictures. Mod Pathol 1995;8:498-502.

12. Conlon KC, Dougherty E, Klimstra DS, Coit DG, Turnbull AD, Brennan MF. The value of minimal access surgery in the staging of patients with potentially resectable peripancreatic malignancy. Ann Surg 1996;223:134-40.

13. de Luna R, Eloubeidi MA, Sheffield MV, et al. Comparison of ThinPrep and conventional preparations in pancreatic fine-needle aspiration biopsy. Diagn Cytopathol 2004;30:71-6.

14. Govindarajan S, Peters RL. The bile duct adenoma. A lesion distinct from Meyenburg complex. Arch Pathol Lab Med 1984;108:922-4.

15. Henke AC, Jensen CS, Cohen MB. Cytologic diagnosis of adenocarcinoma in biliary and pancreatic duct brushings. Adv Anat Pathol 2002;9:301-8.

16. Hornick JL, Lauwers GY, Odze RD. Immunohistochemistry can help distinguish metastatic pancreatic adenocarcinomas from bile duct adenomas and hamartomas of the liver. Am J Surg Pathol 2005;29:381-9.

17. Isaacson R, Weiland LH, McIlrath DC. Biopsy of the pancreas. Arch Surg 1974;109:227-30.

18. Klimstra DS. Cell lineage in pancreatic neoplasms. In: Sarkar FH, Dugan MC, eds. Pancreatic cancer: advances in molecular pathology, diagnosis and clinical management. Natick: BioTechniques Books; 1998:21-47.

19. Klimstra DS, Adsay NV. Pancreas cancer: pathology. In: Kelsen DP, Daly JM, Kern SE, Levin B, Tepper JE, eds. Gastrointestinal oncology: principles and practices. Philadelphia: Lippincott, Williams & Wilkins; 2002:459-76.

20. Klimstra DS, Hameed MR, Marrero AM, Conlon KC, Brennan MF. Ductal proliferative lesions associated with infiltrating ductal adenocarcinoma of the pancreas. Int J Pancreatol 1994;16:224-5.

21. Klimstra DS, Rosai J, Heffess CS. Mixed acinar-endocrine carcinomas of the pancreas. Am J Surg Pathol 1994;18:765-78.

22. Klöppel G. Pseudocysts and other non-neoplastic cysts of the pancreas. Semin Diagn Pathol 2000;17:7-15.

23. Kocjan G, Smith AN. Bile duct brushings cytology: potential pitfalls in diagnosis. Diagn Cytopathol 1997;16:358-63.

23a. Kosmahl M, Pauser U, Anlauf M, Klöppel G. Pancreatic adenocarcinoma with cystic features: neither rare nor uniform. Mod Pathol 2005;18: 1157-64.

24. Kosmahl M, Pauser U, Peters K, et al. Cystic neoplasms of the pancreas and tumor-like lesions with cystic features: a review of 418 cases and a classification proposal. Virchows Arch 2004;445:168-78.

25. Kurzawinski T, Deery A, Davidson BR. Diagnostic value of cytology for biliary stricture. Br J Surg 1993;80:414-21.

26. Layfield LJ, Wax TD, Lee JG, Cotton PB. Accuracy and morphologic aspects of pancreatic and biliary duct brushings. Acta Cytol 1995;39:11-8.

27. Lee JG, Leung JW, Baillie J, Layfield LJ, Cotton PB. Benign dysplastic or malignant—making sense of endoscopic bile duct brush cytology: results in 149 consecutive patients. Am J Gastroenterol 1995;90:722-6.

28. Lee LY, Hsu HL, Chen HM, Hsueh C. Ductal adenocarcinoma of the pancreas with huge cystic degeneration: a lesion to be distinguished from pseudocyst and mucinous cystadenocarcinoma. Int J Surg Pathol 2003;11:235-9.

29. Lewandrowski KB, Southern JF, Pins MR, Compton CC, Warshaw AL. Cyst fluid analysis in the differential diagnosis of pancreatic cysts. A comparison of pseudocysts, serous cystadenomas, mucinous cystic neoplasms, and mucinous cystadenocarcinoma. Ann Surg 1993;217:41-7.

30. Lightwood R, Reber HA, Way LW. The risk and accuracy of pancreatic biopsy. Am J Surg 1976; 132:189-94.

31. Lin F, Staerkel G. Cytologic criteria for well differentiated adenocarcinoma of the pancreas in fine-needle aspiration biopsy specimens. Cancer 2003;99:44-50.

32. Michael CW, Hunter B. Interpretation of fine-needle aspirates processed by the ThinPrep technique: cytologic artifacts and diagnostic pitfalls. Diagn Cytopathol 2000;23:6-13.

33. Michael CW, McConnel J, Pecott J, Afify AM, Al Khafaji B. Comparison of ThinPrep and TriPath PREP liquid-based preparations in nongynecologic specimens: a pilot study. Diagn Cytopathol 2001;25:177-84.

34. Michaels PJ, Brachtel EF, Bounds BC, Brugge WR, Bishop PM. Intraductal papillary mucinous neoplasm of the pancreas: cytologic features predict histologic grade. Cancer 2006;108:163-73.

35. Nagle JA, Wilbur DC, Pitman MB. Cytomorphology of gastric and duodenal epithelium and reactivity to B72.3: a baseline for comparison to pancreatic neoplasms aspirated by EUS-FNAB. Diagn Cytopathol 2005;33:381-6.

36. Notohara K, Hamazaki S, Tsukayama C, et al. Solid-pseudopapillary tumor of the pancreas: immunohistochemical localization of neuroendocrine markers and CD10. Am J Surg Pathol 2000;24:1361-71.

37. Parasher VK, Huibregtse K. Endoscopic retrograde wire-guided cytology of malignant biliary strictures using a novel scraping brush. Gastrointest Endosc 1998;48:288-90.

38. Rabinovitz M, Zajko AB, Hassanein T, et al. Diagnostic value of brush cytology in the diagnosis of bile duct carcinoma: a study in 65 patients with bile duct strictures. Hepatology 1990;12:747-52.

39. Renshaw AA, Madge R, Jiroutek M, Granter SR. Bile duct brushing cytology: statistical analysis of proposed diagnostic criteria. Am J Clin Pathol 1998;110:635-40.

40. Robins DB, Katz RL, Evans DB, Atkinson EN, Green L. Fine needle aspiration of the pancreas. In quest of accuracy. Acta Cytol 1995;39:1-10.

41. Sharma S, Green KB. The pancreatic duct and its arteriovenous relationship: an underutilized aid in the diagnosis and distinction of pancreatic adenocarcinoma from pancreatic intraepithelial neoplasia. A study of 126 pancreatectomy specimens. Am J Surg Pathol 2004;28:613-20.

42. Simsir A, Greenebaum E, Stevens PD, Abedi M. Biliary stent replacement cytology. Diagn Cytopathol 1997;16:233-7.

43. Suriawinata A, Klimstra DS. Distinguishing bile duct adenoma, hamartoma and ductular proliferation from metastatic pancreatic adenocarcinoma in the liver by immunohistochemistry. Mod Pathol 2002;15:294A.

44. Tascilar M, Offerhaus GJ, Altink R, et al. Immunohistochemical labeling for the Dpc4 gene product is a specific marker for adenocarcinoma in biopsy specimens of the pancreas and bile duct. Am J Clin Pathol 2001;116:831-7.

45. Terris B, Ponsot P, Paye F, et al. Intraductal papillary mucinous tumors of the pancreas confined to secondary ducts show less aggressive pathologic features as compared with those involving the main pancreatic duct. Am J Surg Pathol 2000;24:1372-7.

46. Weber SM, Cubukcu-Dimopulo O, Palesty JA, et al. Lymphoplasmacytic sclerosing pancreatitis: inflammatory mimic of pancreatic carcinoma. J Gastrointest Surg 2003;7:129-37.

47. Zamboni G, Lüttges J, Capelli P, et al. Histopathological features of diagnostic and clinical relevance in autoimmune pancreatitis: a study on 53 resection specimens and 9 biopsy specimens. Virchows Arch 2004;445:552-63.

Index*

---

*Numbers in boldface indicate table and figure pages.

W

Z